Practical Guide
to the Care of the
Psychiatric Patient

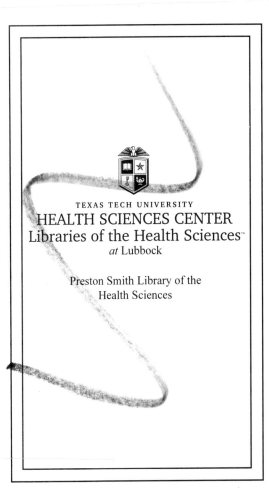

Series Editor

Fred F. Ferri, MD, FACP

Clinical Professor
Brown Medical School
Providence, Rhode Island

OTHER VOLUMES IN THE "PRACTICAL GUIDE SERIES"

Wachtel, et al: *Practical Guide to the Care of the Geriatric Patient*

Danakas: *Practical Guide to the Care of the Gynecologic/Obstetric Patient*

Alario, et al: *Practical Guide to the Care of the Pediatric Patient*

Ferri: *Practical Guide to the Care of the Medical Patient*

Practical Guide to the Care of the Psychiatric Patient

3rd Edition

Richard J. Goldberg, MD, MS

Professor
Department of Psychiatry and Human Behavior
Brown University
Psychiatrist-in-Chief, Department of Psychiatry
Rhode Island Hospital, The Miriam Hospital
Providence, Rhode Island

MOSBY

ELSEVIER

1600 John F. Kennedy Blvd.
Ste 1800
Philadelphia, PA 19103-2899

PRACTICAL GUIDE TO THE CARE   ISBN: 978-0-323-03683-2
OF THE PSYCHIATRIC PATIENT

Notice

Knowledge and best practice in this field are constantly changing. As new research
and experience broaden our knowledge, changes in practice, treatment and drug
therapy may become necessary or appropriate. Readers are advised to check
the most current information provided (i) on procedures featured or (ii) by the
manufacturer of each product to be administered, to verify the recommended dose
or formula, the method and duration of administration, and contraindications. It is
the responsibility of the practitioner, relying on their own experience and knowledge
of the patient, to make diagnoses, to determine dosages and the best treatment for
each individual patient, and to take all appropriate safety precautions. To the fullest
extent of the law, neither the Publisher nor the Editors assumes any liability for any
injury and/or damage to persons or property arising out of or related to any use of the
material contained in this book.

The Publisher

Library of Congress Cataloging-in-Publication Data
Practical guide to the care of the psychiatric patient / [edited by]
Richard J. Goldberg. — 3rd ed.
  p. ; cm. – (Practical guide series)
  Rev. ed. of: Practical guide to the care of the psychiatric patient /
Richard J. Goldberg. 2nd ed. c1998.
  Includes bibliographical references and index.
  ISBN 978-0-323-03683-2
  1. Psychotherapy patients–Care–Handbooks, manuals, etc. I.
Goldberg, Richard J., II. Goldberg, Richard J., Practical guide to the
care of the psychiatric patient. III. Series: Practical guide series (Philadelphia, Pa.)
  [DNLM: 1. Mental Disorders–diagnosis–Handbooks. 2. Mental Disorders–therapy–
Handbooks. WM 34 P8943 2007]
RC454.G5885 2007
616.89–dc22   2006037788

  Acquisitions Editor: James Merritt
  Developmental Editor: Andrea Deis
  Publishing Services Manager: Linda Van Pelt
  Project Manager: Joan Nikelsky
  Design Direction: Ellen Zanolle

Working together to grow
libraries in developing countries
www.elsevier.com | www.bookaid.org | www.sabre.org

ELSEVIER   BOOK AID International   Sabre Foundation

Printed in the United States of America

Last digit is the print number: 9 8 7 6 5 4 3 2 1

To the staff of the Departments of Psychiatry at Rhode Island and The Miriam Hospitals for their support and for their excellence as scholars and clinicians

Contributors

Daniela A. Boerescu, MD
Attending Psychiatrist, Department of Psychiatry
Rhode Island Hospital
Providence, Rhode Island
Personality Disorders

Mark B. Elliot, MD
Assistant Clinical Professor, Department of Psychiatry
    and Human Behavior
Brown University
Attending Psychiatrist, Partial Hospitalization Program
Department of Psychiatry
Rhode Island Hospital
Providence, Rhode Island
Eating Disorders, Obesity, and Nicotine Dependence

Richard J. Goldberg, MD, MS
Professor, Department of Psychiatry
    and Human Behavior
Brown University
Psychiatrist-in-Chief, Department of Psychiatry
Rhode Island Hospital and The Miriam Hospital
Providence, Rhode Island
*Psychiatric Interview and Database; Medical Evaluation
    of Psychiatric Symptoms; Alzheimer's Disease:
    Diagnosis and Treatment; Anxiety Disorders:
    Diagnosis and Management; Treatment of Anxiety:
    Medications and Therapies; The P450 System:
    Drug Interactions*

Colin J. Harrington, MD
Associate Professor, Clinician Educator
Department of Psychiatry and Human Behavior
Brown University
Director, Division of Consultation Psychiatry
Rhode Island Hospital
Providence, Rhode Island
Somatoform Disorders

Sandra A. Jacobson, MD
Assistant Professor, Department of Psychiatry
    and Human Behavior
Brown University
Director, Division of Consultation Liaison Psychiatry
The Miriam Hospital
Providence, Rhode Island
Delirium, Dementia, and Other Cognitive Disorders

Ali Kazim, MD
Clinical Assistant Professor, Department of Psychiatry
    and Human Behavior
Brown University
Director, Division of Emergency Psychiatry
Rhode Island Hospital
Providence, Rhode Island
Behavioral Emergencies and Forensic Issues

Roger Lowell McRoberts III, MD
Clinical Assistant Professor, Department of Psychiatry
    and Human Behavior
Brown University
Attending Psychiatrist, Department of Psychiatry
Rhode Island Hospital
Providence, Rhode Island
Role of Psychiatric Factors in Medical Practice

Richard P. Millman, MD
Professor, Department of Medicine
Brown University
Director, Sleep Disorders Center of Lifespan Hospitals
Rhode Island Hospital
Providence, Rhode Island
Sleep Problems and the Use of Hypnotics

Joseph V. Penn, MD, CCHP
Clinical Assistant Professor, Department of Psychiatry
    and Human Behavior
Brown University
Director, Child and Adolescent Forensic Psychiatry
Department of Psychiatry
Rhode Island Hospital
Providence, Rhode Island
Child and Adolescent Psychiatry

Donn Posner, PhD
Clinical Assistant Professor, Department of Psychiatry
  and Human Behavior
Brown University
Assistant Director, Division of Outpatient Psychiatry, and
  Director of Adult Psychology
Department of Psychiatry
Rhode Island Hospital
Providence, Rhode Island
*Anxiety Disorders: Diagnosis and Management; Treatment of Anxiety:
  Medications and Therapies*

Michael A. Posternak, MD
Clinical Assistant Professor, Department of Psychiatry
  and Human Behavior
Brown University
Research Psychiatrist, Department of Psychiatry
Rhode Island Hospital
Providence, Rhode Island
Depression: Identification and Diagnosis; Antidepressants

Moataz M. Ragheb, MD, PhD
Assistant Clinical Professor, Department of Psychiatry
  and Human Behavior
Brown University; Providence, Rhode Island
Assistant Clinical Professor, Ain Shams University Faculty of Medicine
Department of Neuropsychiatry; Cairo, Egypt
Attending Psychiatrist, Department of Psychiatry
Rhode Island Hospital; Providence, Rhode Island
Psychotic Symptoms, Schizophrenia, and Antipsychotic Agents

David A. Solomon, MD
Clinical Associate Professor
Department of Psychiatry and Human Behavior
Brown University
Associate Director, Inpatient Psychiatry
Assistant Director, Mood Disorders Program
Department of Psychiatry
Rhode Island Hospital
Providence, Rhode Island
Electroconvulsive Therapy

Michael D. Stein, MD
Professor of Medicine and Community Health, Department of Medicine
Brown University
Director, Substance Abuse Research Unit
Division of General Internal Medicine
Rhode Island Hospital
Providence, Rhode Island
Alcohol and Substance Abuse

Christine J. Truman, MD
Psychiatrist, Finney Psychotherapy Associates
Norfolk, Virginia
Bipolar Disorder and Mood-Stabilizing Drugs

John P. Wincze, PhD
Adjunct Professor, Department of Psychiatry and Human Behavior
Adjunct Professor, Department of Psychology
Brown University
Providence, Rhode Island
Sexual Disorders

Mark Zimmerman, MD
Associate Professor, Department of Psychiatry and Human Behavior
Brown University
Director, Division of Outpatient Psychiatry
Rhode Island Hospital
Providence, Rhode Island
*Depression: Identification and Diagnosis; Antidepressants; Treatment of
  Anxiety: Medications and Therapies*

Preface

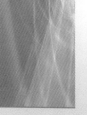

This book is intended to provide practical guidance for diagnosing and treating psychiatric problems. The overall goals of the book include the following:

Clarifying diagnostic categories and terminology
Improving recognition of psychiatric problems
Demystifying the mental status examination
Detailing the proper use of psychiatric medications

The text is presented in outline form for clarity, with sequential diagnostic and management strategies. However, it is *not* intended to be superficial in approach, and the content is, whenever possible, based on documented and referenced sources.

The use of the *Diagnostic and Statistical Manual of Mental Disorders*, edition 4-TR (*DSM-IV-TR*), is generally followed. However, some of the categories are simplified for purposes of clarity. This text (unlike the *DSM*) is not intended primarily for research purposes, but is meant to be clinically useful. Readers are urged to obtain a copy of the *DSM-IV-TR* for reference. References at the end of each chapter direct the reader to worthwhile supplementary information.

The "essentials" approach of this book emerges from more than 25 years of teaching psychiatry to practicing physicians, medical students, and residents in both psychiatry and primary care medicine. The intent is to provide clear and practical approaches and guidelines. This core information will serve as a solid foundation and organization to which more detailed readings can be added.

This book is intended to be useful for the following individuals:

Medical students looking for a basic guide to psychiatry for their clerkship.

Primary care residents looking for practical information that can be applied to the psychiatric problems of their patients.

Primary care physicians and providers wanting to organize psychiatric knowledge already gathered through experience and to obtain updates on new terms and treatments.

Medical specialists who realize that many patient problems are complicated by psychiatric issues—for example, that gastrointestinal symptoms are often a somatic manifestation of depression, and atypical chest pain is frequently a result of an underlying anxiety disorder.

Mental health clinicians (nurse clinician specialists, social workers, psychologists, etc.) who look for a concise summary of psychiatric issues that present in their practices.

Richard J. Goldberg

Acknowledgments

I wish to acknowledge the contributions of William "Curt" LaFrance, Jr., MD, whose neuropsychiatric knowledge was valuable in reviewing Chapter 3 on the Medical Evaluation of Psychiatric Symptoms. Dr. LaFrance is an Assistant Professor, Departments of Psychiatry and Neurology (Research), Brown University, and the Director of Neuropsychiatry, Rhode Island Hospital.

I would like to thank Dawn T. Orsini for her assistance in the project management for this book.

Contents

1   Role of Psychiatric Factors in Medical Practice, 1
Roger Lowell McRoberts III

1.1   Prevalence of Mental Health and Substance Abuse Disorders, 1
1.2   Use of Psychiatric Services, 1
1.3   Functional and Economic Impact of Mental Health and Substance Abuse Disorders, 1
1.4   Prevalence of Mental Health and Substance Abuse Disorders in Medical Practice, 2
1.5   Psychiatric Problems in Primary Care, 5
1.6   Impact of Mental Health and Substance Abuse Problems on Medical Costs, 8
1.7   Cost–Benefit Issues Involving Mental Health and Substance Abuse Services, 9
1.8   Strategic Questions for Assessing Integration of Medical and Psychiatric Services, 9

2   Psychiatric Interview and Database, 12
Richard J. Goldberg

2.1   Psychiatric Interview, 12
2.2   Psychiatric Database, 13
2.3   Mental Status Examination, 30

3   Medical Evaluation of Psychiatric Symptoms, 33
Richard J. Goldberg

3.1   Medical Causes of Symptoms, 33
3.2   Diagnostic Testing, 41

4   Delirium, Dementia, and Other Cognitive Disorders, 50
Sandra A. Jacobson

4.1   Delirium, 50
4.2   Dementia, 54

4.3   Amnestic Disorders, 60

4.4   Cognitive Mental Status Examination, 61

5   Alzheimer's Disease: Diagnosis and Treatment, 64
Richard J. Goldberg

5.1   Overview, 64

5.2   Behavioral Symptoms, 65

5.3   Medications to Treat Agitation and Psychosis, 68

5.4   Cognitive Symptoms, 76

5.5   Anxiety, 78

5.6   Depression, 79

5.7   Some Common Medical Issues, 80

5.8   Omnibus Budget Reconciliation Act Regulations, 83

6   Depression: Identification and Diagnosis, 86
Michael A. Posternak and Mark Zimmerman

6.1   General Issues of Identification, 86

6.2   Strategy for Evaluating Depression, 86

6.3   Mood Disorder Resulting from a General Medical Condition, 89

6.4   Major Depressive Disorder (Major Depression), 90

6.5   Adjustment Disorder with Depressed Mood, 101

6.6   Dysthymic Disorder, 102

6.7   Mixed Anxiety and Depression, 103

6.8   Premenstrual Dysphoric Disorder, 105

6.9   Minor Depression (Subthreshold Depression), 106

7   Antidepressants, 108
Michael A. Posternak and Mark Zimmerman

7.1   Overview, 108

7.2   Specific Issues in Using Antidepressants, 110

7.3   Tricyclic Antidepressants, 120

7.4   Second-Generation Antidepressants, 121

7.5   Uncommon (But Important) Medical Complications of the SSRIs and SNRIs, 127

7.6   Stimulants as Antidepressants, 131

7.7   Monoamine Oxidase Inhibitors, 132

8   Bipolar Disorder and Mood-Stabilizing
         Drugs, 137
         Christine J. Truman
         8.1   Bipolar Disorder, 137
         8.2   Manic, Hypomanic, Mixed, Cyclothymic, and Rapid
                Cycling Episodes, 138
         8.3   Lithium, 144
         8.4   Valproic Acid, 147
         8.5   Carbamazepine, 150
         8.6   Oxcarbazepine, 153
         8.7   Lamotrigine, 154
         8.8   Atypical Antipsychotics, 155
         8.9   Benzodiazepines, 155
         8.10   Nonmedication Dimensions of Treatment, 156
         8.11   Electroconvulsive Therapy, 156

9   Anxiety Disorders: Diagnosis and
         Management, 158
         Richard J. Goldberg and Donn Posner
         9.1   Overview and Background, 158
         9.2   Diagnostic Approach to Anxiety Symptoms, 158
         9.3   Panic Disorder, 159
         9.4   Obsessive-Compulsive Disorder, 166
         9.5   Generalized Anxiety Disorder, 168
         9.6   Phobias, 170
         9.7   Adjustment Disorder with Anxiety, 172
         9.8   Acute Stress Disorder, 173
         9.9   Posttraumatic Stress Disorder, 175

10   Treatment of Anxiety: Medications and
         Therapies, 178
         Richard J. Goldberg, Donn Posner, and Mark Zimmerman
         10.1   Benzodiazepines, 178
         10.2   Azapirones, 185
         10.3   Comparison of Benzodiazepines and Azapirones, 186
         10.4   Antidepressants for Anxiety, 187
         10.5   Other Sedative–Hypnotics, 188
         10.6   Cognitive Behavior Therapy, 189

11 Sleep Problems and the Use of
Hypnotics, 195
Richard P. Millman
11.1   Overview, 195
11.2   Evaluation of Sleep Problems, 195
11.3   Hypersomnia, 197
11.4   Insomnia, 200
11.5   Sleep Disorders Related to Another
Mental Disorder, 203
11.6   Sleep Disorders Associated with
Medications, 203
11.7   Parasomnias, 204
11.8   Hypnotic Drugs, 205

12 Psychotic Symptoms, Schizophrenia, and
Antipsychotic Agents, 210
Moataz M. Ragheb
12.1   Identification of Psychotic Symptoms, 210
12.2   Differential Diagnosis of Psychotic Symptoms, 212
12.3   Schizophrenia, 214
12.4   Antipsychotic Agents Used to Treat Schizophrenia
and Other Psychotic Disorders, 219
12.5   Alternatives to Antipsychotics for Psychotic Symptoms
of Schizophrenia, 251
12.6   Nonpharmacological Aspects of Treating
Schizophrenia, 251

13 Somatoform Disorders, 253
Colin J. Harrington
13.1   Overview, 253
13.2   Somatization Disorder, 254
13.3   Acute Somatized Symptoms, 257
13.4   Conversion Disorder, 258
13.5   Pain Disorder, 262
13.6   Hypochondriasis, 263
13.7   Body Dysmorphic Disorder, 265
13.8   Factitious Disorder, 266
13.9   Malingering, 268
13.10 Somatoform Disorders Not Otherwise
Specified, 268

14   Behavioral Emergencies and Forensic
         Issues, 271
         Ali Kazim
         14.1   Behavioral Emergencies, 271
         14.2   Suicide Evaluation, 277
         14.3   Evaluation of the Violent or Homicidal Patient, 281
         14.4   Use of Physical Restraints, 283
         14.5   Commitment Under Mental Health Statutes, 284
         14.6   Competence Evaluations, 285

15   Alcohol and Substance Abuse, 287
         Michael D. Stein
         15.1   Alcohol Abuse, 287
         15.2   Alcohol Dependence, 288
         15.3   Alcohol Intoxication, 290
         15.4   Alcoholic Paranoia, 290
         15.5   Pathologic Intoxication, 291
         15.6   Wernicke-Korsakoff Syndrome (Alcohol Amnestic
                 Syndrome), 291
         15.7   Alcoholic Hallucinosis, 291
         15.8   Alcoholic Dementia, 292
         15.9   Hepatic Encephalopathy, 292
         15.10   Fetal Alcohol Syndrome, 292
         15.11   Alcohol Comorbidities, 292
         15.12   Alcohol and Sedative Withdrawal, 293
         15.13   Blood Alcohol Level, 300
         15.14   Abuse of Cocaine and Other Stimulants, 301
         15.15   Hallucinogens, 305
         15.16   Issues in Narcotic Use, 305
         15.17   Psychotropics as Analgesic Augmentors, 314
         15.18   Marijuana Abuse, 315

16   Electroconvulsive Therapy, 317
         David A. Solomon
         16.1   Overview, 317
         16.2   Indications, 317
         16.3   Contraindications, 318
         16.4   Adverse Effects, 318
         16.5   Drug Interactions, 321
         16.6   Procedure, 321
         16.7   Considerations with Specific Medical Diseases, 324

17   Personality Disorders, 328
Daniela A. Boerescu
  17.1   Overview, 328
  17.2   Paranoid Personality Disorder, 330
  17.3   Schizoid and Schizotypal Personality Disorder, 332
  17.4   Antisocial Personality Disorder, 333
  17.5   Borderline Personality Disorder, 334
  17.6   Histrionic Personality Disorder, 335
  17.7   Narcissistic Personality Disorder, 336
  17.8   Avoidant Personality Disorder, 337
  17.9   Dependent Personality Disorder, 338
  17.10 Obsessive–Compulsive Personality Disorder, 339
  17.11 Depressive Personality Disorder, 340
  17.12 Passive–Aggressive (Negativistic)
          Personality Disorder, 340

**18   Eating Disorders, Obesity, and Nicotine
        Dependence, 343**
Mark B. Elliot
  18.1   Anorexia Nervosa, 343
  18.2   Bulimia Nervosa, 348
  18.3   Obesity, 351
  18.4   Nicotine Dependence, 355

19   Sexual Disorders, 363
John P. Wincze
  19.1   Phases of Sexual Function, 363
  19.2   Sexual History, 363
  19.3   Sexual Dysfunction, 364
  19.4   Paraphilias, 375
  19.5   Gender Identity Disorder, 376

20   The P450 System: Drug Interactions, 378
Richard J. Goldberg
  20.1   Definition, 378
  20.2   P450 System Terminology, 378
  20.3   Genetic Polymorphism, 382
  20.4   Age Effects, 383
  20.5   P450 Inhibitors, 383
  20.6   P450 Substrates, 384
  20.7   P450 Inducers, 386
  20.8   Therapeutic Implications, 386

21 Child and Adolescent Psychiatry, 389
Joseph V. Penn
21.1   General Principles, 389
21.2   Anxiety Disorders, 390
21.3   Attention-Deficit/Hyperactivity Disorder, 409
21.4   Disruptive Behavior Disorders, 414
21.5   Depressive Disorders, 418
21.6   Learning Disorders, 433
21.7   Mental Retardation and Developmental Disabilities, 435

22 Formulary, 442

Index, 505

Role of Psychiatric Factors in Medical Practice

Roger Lowell McRoberts III

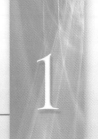

1.1 Prevalence of Mental Health and Substance Abuse Disorders

The National Comorbidity Survey presents data from the first survey to administer a structured psychiatric interview to a national probability sample in the United States. In this project, trained research assistants conducted door-to-door structured interviews of a national sample of more than 8000 people.

1. Data from this survey provide estimates of the lifetime and 12-month prevalence of psychiatric disorders in adults (ages 18 to 55 years) in the United States (Table 1-1).
2. About 28% of Americans older than 18 years (a group of more than 52 million) suffer from a mental or addictive disorder in a 1-year period.

1.2 Use of Psychiatric Services

1. Each year more than 20 million people older than 18 years make out-patient visits to mental health professionals or volunteer resources for mental health or substance abuse reasons, for an annual total of more than 325 million visits.
2. About 1.5 million Americans have at least one inpatient mental health or addiction admission during a 1-year period.

1.3 Functional and Economic Impact of Mental Health and Substance Abuse Disorders

Mental health disorders have a documented severe impact on people's lives and ability to function.

1. Functional impact of depression. Patients with depression tend to show impaired functioning comparable to or worse than that associated with eight chronic medical conditions (hypertension, diabetes, advanced coronary artery disease, angina, arthritis, back problems, lung problems, and gastrointestinal disorders).
2. Depression and disability.
   a. Depression is a major diagnosis associated with disability.
   b. Depression accounts for more than half the disability days associated with mental disorders.

Table 1-1 **Prevalence of Psychiatric Disorders in the United States**		
	Prevalence (%)	
Disorder	**Lifetime**	**12-Month**
Any psychiatric disorder	*48.0*	*29.5*
Any affective disorder	*19.3*	*11.3*
Major depression, all	16.2	6.6
Major depression, male	12.7	7.7
Major depression, female	21.3	12.9
Any anxiety disorder	*24.9*	*17.2*
Social phobia	13.3	7.9
Panic disorder	3.5	2.3
Any substance abuse	*26.6*	*11.3*
Alcohol dependence	14.1	7.2

Data from Kessler RC, Berglund P, Demler O, et al: *JAMA* 289(23):3095-3105, 2003; Kessler RC, McGonagle KA, Zhao S, et al: *Arch Gen Psychiatry* 51:8-19, 1994.

    c. Depression accounts for more disability days and recidivism than heart disease, diabetes, high blood pressure, or low back pain.

    d. In patients who are disabled for 40 days or more, depression is the single most common diagnosis.

ECONOMIC COSTS OF MENTAL HEALTH AND SUBSTANCE ABUSE DISORDERS

Overall, mental health and substance abuse (MHSA) services account for between 4% and 13% of the health care dollars in various managed care plans across the United States (Table 1-2). The cost of mental illness in the United States exceeds $160 billion annually.

1. The continued pressure to reduce the amount allocated for MHSA services has created the feeling in many locations that services have been reduced beyond a reasonable minimum level.

2. Below an adequate level, shifting of problems into the general medical sector begins increasing use of services in that area.

TREATMENT SUCCESS RATES FOR MENTAL HEALTH AND SUBSTANCE ABUSE DISORDERS

A common misconception is that mental health treatment is not successful. However, the success rates for the treatment of many common mental disorders equal or exceed the success rates for many other medical disorders (Table 1-3).

1.4 Prevalence of Mental Health and Substance Abuse Disorders in Medical Practice

1. Most treatment for psychiatric problems takes place in the general medical care setting, not in specialty psychiatry or mental health programs (Table 1-4). Nearly half (48%) of respondents to a National Mental Health survey stated that their primary care or family physician

Table 1-2 Costs of Mental Health and Substance Abuse Disorders (in billions of dollars, 1990)

Category	Mental Disorders	Alcohol Abuse	Drug Abuse	Total
Direct treatment	66.8	14.3	4.0	85.1
Productivity losses	73.2	75.2	14.0	162.4
Non–health-related costs	8.0	9.5	49.0	66.5
TOTALS	148.0	99.0	67.0	314.0

Data from Substance Abuse and Mental Health Services Administration: Report No. 1995-PHDG 78. Washington, DC, US Public Health Service, 1995.

Table 1-3 Success Rates for the Treatment of Common Medical Disorders

Disorder	Treatment Success Rate (%)
Mental Health	
Panic	80
Bipolar	80
Major depression	65-80
Schizophrenia	60
OCD	60
Cardiovascular	
Arthrectomy	52
Angioplasty	41

OCD, obsessive–compulsive disorder.

Table 1-4 Where Patients with Mental Disorders Receive Treatment: First Source of Help

Source of Care	Public Seeking Treatment
Primary care physician	31%
Family or friends	32%
Psychiatrist, psychologist, other mental health worker	14%
Clergy	5%
Health organization	2%
Advocacy organization	3%

Note: 10.5% of the U.S. population seeks mental health treatment each year: Data from the Substance Abuse and Mental Health Services Administration, Office of Applied Studies: National Household Survey on Drug Abuse, 2000 and 2001. Available at www.samhsa.gov.

Table 1-5 **Prevalence of Mental Health Disorders in Primary Care Practice***	
Mental Disorder	**Percent**
None	61.4
Somatoform	14.6
Major depression	11.5
Dysthymia	7.8
Minor depression	6.4
Major depression in partial remission	6.3
Generalized anxiety	7.0
Panic	3.6
Other anxiety	9.0
Alcohol	5.1
Binge eating	3.0

*Evaluation of 1000 patients.
Data from Spitzer RL, Williams JBW, Kroenke K, et al: *JAMA* 272:1749-1756, 1994.

was the first to diagnose their mental health disorder. Therefore, physicians need increased training in the recognition and management of psychiatric disorders.

2. Patients with mental disorders constitute 5% to 20% of general medical patients and are 1.5 to 2 times as likely to visit the medical setting as patients without those disorders.

3. More than 50% of patients with a diagnosable mental disorder have had an outpatient general health visit within a 6-month period, compared with about 12% who visited a mental health specialist.
   a. Approximately 15% of primary care patients have current anxiety or depression.
   b. One thousand patients at four primary care sites were evaluated using a two-stage screening and interviewing process that addressed 18 specific mental disorders (Table 1-5).

4. There is a significant lack of recognition of mental disorders in general practice.
   a. One study found that although 26.7% of patients in a large primary practice had a mental disorder, less than 10% were recognized by the primary care physicians.
   b. Other studies have shown that only one third to one half of mental disorders are recognized in primary care. Only half of the cases of anxiety and depression in medical settings are recognized, and most cases are undertreated. In one study, 84% of patients with anxiety or depressive disorders sought treatment from a primary care clinician, and only 19% received care that met criteria for adequacy as defined by treatment guidelines.

MEDICAL ILLNESS AND DRUG EFFECTS MASQUERADING AS PSYCHIATRIC PROBLEMS

See Chapter 3.

1.5 Psychiatric Problems in Primary Care

Psychiatric comorbidity in medical practice affects the course, outcome, and cost of medical care.

1. Psychiatric problems increase medical length of stay and use of medical services, decrease functional level, and have a negative impact on overall prognosis and outcome. Studies have documented a direct correlation between the prevalence of mood and anxiety disorders and the number of a patient's physical complaints.
2. Disorders related to smoking, drinking, and drug use account for a significant portion of the health care dollar.
3. The elderly medical population has a high prevalence of psychiatric comorbidity, which often goes unrecognized.
   a. Approximately 15% to 20% suffer from depressive symptoms.
   b. Forty percent of patients with Parkinson's disease and 20% to 30% of those with stroke have depression.
   c. Approximately 20% of the elderly have substance abuse disorders. In fact, the rates of hospitalization in the elderly for alcohol-related problems are similar to those for myocardial infarction.
   d. Between 10% and 20% suffer from anxiety disorders, including phobias. In fact, phobia is the most common psychiatric disorder in women older than 65 years.
   e. Between 6% and 10% have progressive dementias. Among those with Alzheimer's disease, 30% to 40% have delusions or hallucinations.
4. A significant prevalence of psychiatric comorbidity has been repeatedly documented in medical inpatients. Psychiatric consultation for medical inpatients with psychiatric complications has been demonstrated to reduce the costs and improve the effectiveness of treatment.

EXAMPLES OF PSYCHIATRIC PROBLEMS IN PRIMARY CARE

Table 1-6 lists psychiatric problems in primary medical practice.

1. Fatigue.
   a. Fatigue is one of the most common presenting complaints in primary care.
   b. Between 20% and 40% of these patients have underlying depressive disorders, which are generally not recognized or treated.
   c. These patients are often high users of medical services and suffer from significant impairment.
2. Insomnia.
   a. Insomnia is a common presenting complaint in primary care.
   b. Insomnia is a common presenting complaint for patients with depression.
   c. Between one third and two thirds of patients with chronic insomnia have a psychiatric disorder.
3. Chronic medical conditions. Patients with chronic medical conditions have a significantly increased prevalence of psychiatric disorders.

Table 1-6 **Psychiatric Problems in Medical Care**	
Problem	**Issue**
Fatigue	Between 20% and 40% caused by underlying depression
Insomnia	One third to two thirds of patients have a psychiatric disorder
Chronic medical conditions	Increased prevalence of psychiatric disorder
Myocardial infarction	Twenty percent fail to recover fully because of depression
Generalized anxiety	Manifests as repeated physical symptoms
Elderly	Significant rates of overlooked psychiatric diagnoses
Depression	Adversely affects medical outcomes
Panic disorder	Accounts for many misdiagnosed cardiac and pulmonary symptoms
Somatization disorder	High users of medical resources
Substance abuse	Major contributor to use of medical services and to multiple diseases
Psychosocial problems	The underlying driving force for many patients to seek medical care

4. Myocardial infarction (MI).
   a. Twenty percent of patients who have medically recovered from MI fail to return to their previous level of function.
      (1) The most likely reason for this failure of recovery involves psychiatric problems, especially depression.
      (2) Patients who remain depressed 3 months after a heart attack tend to remain depressed for the next 12 to 18 months without some intervention.
   b. The mortality rate for depressed survivors of MI appears to be five times higher than for nondepressed survivors, and depression is as strong a predictor of mortality as left ventricular function.
5. Chronic somatic symptoms.
   a. Generalized anxiety disorder (GAD) often presents as somatization. The estimated prevalence of GAD in primary care practice is about 15%.
   b. Patients with GAD usually have such symptoms as breathing problems, nonspecific complaints, sexual dysfunction, and irritable bowel symptoms.
   c. Depression is another common cause of somatization.
   d. Somatization disorder, especially a subsyndromal variant, is another common cause (see Chapter 13).
6. Depression.
   a. Depression has been shown to adversely affect the course of patients with a variety of medical disorders, including chronic renal failure, congestive heart failure, and irritable bowel syndrome.

  b. The medical outcomes of depressed patients may be adversely affected by noncompliance or other self-destructive behavior (see Chapter 6).
7. Panic disorder (see Chapter 9).
  a. Panic disorder accounts for 9% of ambulatory patients referred for cardiac disease (usually consisting of atypical chest pain).
  b. It accounts for 17% of patients referred for pulmonary function testing.
  c. Symptoms of panic disorder often confound medical diagnosis and lead to needless expenditures, such as unnecessary angiograms.
  d. A study of 334 consecutive patients with acute chest pain seen in an urban hospital emergency department (ED) found panic disorder in 17.5% and depression in 23.1%. It is likely that these psychiatric symptoms significantly affect use of medical resources and outcome.
  e. The direct and indirect cost of inadequately treated panic disorder is about $18,000 per year, compared with about $1000 per year for successful treatment.
8. Somatization (see Chapter 13).
  a. The per capita expenditures for these patients are six times greater than the average for hospital costs, 14 times greater for physician charges, and nine times greater for personnel health.
  b. These patients often receive unnecessary surgery and diagnostic procedures, leading to iatrogenic disorders.
  c. Although somatization is difficult to manage, there is evidence that management guidelines can reduce the use of medical services by these patients.
9. Tobacco, drug, and alcohol use.
  a. These behavioral problems are associated with more than $170 billion per year in health care costs.
  b. Together, they account for 60% of all preventable deaths.
  c. More than one third of admissions to the adult intensive care unit (ICU) at Johns Hopkins Hospital have been reported to be directly related to alcohol, tobacco, or other drug use. Drug-abusing patients stayed in the ICU longer and had higher medical bills than other patients.
  d. Physicians' failure to recognize alcohol abuse continues to be a problem.
  e. Evidence suggests that costs can be positively affected by treating alcoholism.
10. Psychosocial difficulties.
  a. Psychosocial difficulties are important determinants of why patients visit their doctor and affect both physical and mental health. For example:
    (1) Repeated emergency visits for chest pain might actually represent emotional reactions to ongoing family discord.
    (2) Domestic violence and sexual abuse can produce a variety of otherwise puzzling medical presentations.
    (3) Bereavement can produce facsimiles of medical symptoms.

b. Although about 50% of primary care patients have some significant psychosocial distress, it has been estimated that only about one third of this is detected by physicians.

11. Trauma patients. A study of a sample of trauma patients seen in a New Jersey hospital found that 58% had abused substances in the 3 months before the trauma, 40% had an anxiety disorder, 37% an affective disorder, and 30% had posttraumatic stress disorder.

1.6 Impact of Mental Health and Substance Abuse Problems on Medical Costs

1. Depression and anxiety add costs in primary care.
   a. In one study, primary care patients with one of these psychiatric problems had markedly higher yearly costs (about $2300 per year versus about $1200 per year) than patients without one of these problems, after adjusting for medical morbidity.
   b. Additional studies noted that among patients who used more medical care, systematic identification and treatment of depression produced significant and sustained improvements in clinical outcomes as well as significant decreases in health services costs. Cost differential reflected greater use of general medical services, not increased mental health care costs.
   c. In a study conducted by a major provider, primary care physicians with a higher percentage of recorded mental health diagnoses generated significantly lower panel member costs, with fewer avoidable hospitalizations.

2. A large fraction of adult ICU admissions are related to substance abuse, particularly among uninsured patients.
   a. Twenty-eight percent of ICU admissions, generating 39% of costs, were related to substance abuse. These admissions were significantly longer and more expensive than admissions not related to substance abuse.
   b. Forty-four percent of admissions in the uninsured group were related to substance abuse, generating 61% of all ICU costs in this group.

3. Unrecognized panic disorder and depression account for significant costs in the ED.
   a. There is a high comorbidity of panic disorder and depression in patients with acute chest pain in the ED.
   b. Panic disorder often manifests as acute chest pain (also as neurologic, gastrointestinal, and pulmonary problems).
   c. The health care system probably spends millions of dollars unnecessarily on patients with undiagnosed panic disorder who come to the ED with repeated physical complaints.
   d. Depression is also known to be associated with high use of medical resources.
   e. ED use could probably be reduced by providing adequate screening for some high-risk populations, such as patients with acute chest pain, although no definitive study has been done to prove the positive cost benefit of providing such screening and treatment.

4. Psychiatric comorbidity is associated with prolonged medical length of stay (LOS). Significant association has been consistently found between increased LOS and delirium, dementia, depression, and some personality variables, even when the data are controlled for degree of physical impairment, emergency versus elective admission status, and medical versus surgical service status.

1.7 Cost–Benefit Issues Involving Mental Health and Substance Abuse Services

1. Psychiatric intervention reduces medical LOS in elderly patients with hip fracture. In a study of 452 patients 65 years of age or older, admitted to two general hospitals for surgical repair of fractured hip, LOS was compared between a "control" year and a year when psychiatric consultation and screening were provided to every patient. As a result of screening, psychiatric interventions were provided as indicated clinically. These interventions resulted in an average reduction in LOS of about 2 days.
2. Treatment for behavioral health problems reduces overall health costs (data from Substance Abuse and Mental Health Services Administration [SAMHSA]). This report presented conclusions drawn from a review of a number of studies done between 1988 and 1994.
   a. Total health care costs of treated alcoholics declined 23% to 55% from pretreatment levels.
   b. Untreated alcoholics spend twice as much on health care as patients without alcohol problems.
   c. Treatment of mental disorders is associated with about a 20% reduction in overall costs of health care services.
3. Behavioral interventions can reduce use of medical services by patients with somatization.
   a. A significant number of medical visits are by the "worried well," people with no diagnosable medical disorder. People with problems of psychosocial origin account for many of these visits.
   b. A study done in a large health maintenance organization (HMO) in Boston looked at high users of primary care who experienced physical symptoms associated with significant psychosocial components. After 6 months, the patients who had received a group therapy intervention had reduced their medical visits, and their medical costs were $4000 lower for the study period.
4. Psychotherapy can have a cost benefit by reducing use of medical services. A classic paper reported the effectiveness of brief psychotherapy in decreasing use of medical services. The costs of the mental health treatment were more than offset by the savings in medical care use.

1.8 Strategic Questions for Assessing Integration of Medical and Psychiatric Services

1. Accessibility. Is there a single number access for MHSA services?

2. Integration.
   a. Are MHSA staff located within primary care settings?
   b. Are there any joint management-planning teams?
   c. Are any MHSA issues used as quality indicators in tracking primary medical care?
3. Screening.
   a. Are MHSA screening instruments used in primary care?
   b. Are high-risk populations (such as patients with trauma, chest pain, or cancer) being screened?
4. Treatment quality.
   a. What is being done to ensure adequate treatment of depression and anxiety?
   b. What is being done to ensure that panic disorder and substance abuse are being recognized in the ED?
5. Interface between primary care and mental health care. Are primary care physicians being trained adequately to perform the role of gatekeeper for mental health problems?
6. Outcomes. Are outcome measures being used to assess efficacy of programs and progress in mental health in the community?

SUGGESTED READINGS

Campbell TL, Franks P, Fiscella K, et al: Do physicians who diagnose more mental health disorders generate lower health care costs? *J Fam Pract* 49(4):305-310, 2000.

Druss BG, Rosenheck RA, Sledge WH: Health and disability costs of depressive illness in a major U.S. corporation. *Am J Psychiatry* 157(8):1274-1278, 2000.

Frank RG, McGuire TG, Normand SL, Goldman HH: The value of mental health care at the system level: The case of treating depression. *Health Aff (Millwood)* 18(5):71-88, 1999.

Hendrie HC: Epidemiology of dementia and Alzheimer's disease. *Am J Geriatr Psychiatry* 6(2 Suppl 1):S3-S18, 1998.

Katon WJ, Lin E, Russo J, Unutzer J: Increased medical costs of a population-based sample of depressed elderly patients. *Arch Gen Psychiatry* 60(9):897-903, 2003.

Kessler RC, Berglund P, Demler O, et al: The epidemiology of major depressive disorder: Results from the National Comorbidity Survey Replication (NCS-R). *JAMA* 289(23):3095-3105, 2003.

Kessler RC, Frank RG: The impact of psychiatric disorders on work loss days. *Psychol Med* 27:861-873, 1997.

Kessler RC, McGonagle KA, Zhao S, et al: Lifetime and 12-month prevalence of DSM-III-R psychiatric disorders in the United States. Results from the National Comorbidity Survey. *Arch Gen Psychiatry* 51:8-19, 1994.

Lerner D, Adler DA, Chang H, et al: Unemployment, job retention, and productivity loss among employees with depression. *Psychiatr Serv* 55(12):1371-1378, 2004.

Lyness JM, Caine ED, King DA, et al: Psychiatric disorders in older primary care patients. *J Gen Intern Med* 14:249-254, 1999.

Murray CJL, Lopez AD (eds): The Global Burden of Disease: A Comprehensive Assessment of Mortality and Disability from Diseases, Injuries, and Risk Factors in 1990 and Projected to 2020. Cambridge, Mass, Harvard University Press, 1998.

Sartorius N, Ustun TB, Lecrubier Y, Wittchen HU: Depression comorbid with anxiety: Results from the WHO study on psychological disorders in primary health care. *Br J Psychiatry Suppl* (30):38-43, 1996.

Simon G, Ormel J, VonKorff M, Barlow W: Health care costs associated with depressive and anxiety disorders in primary care. *Am J Psychiatry* 152(3):352-357, 1995.

Simon GE, Barber C, Birnbaum HG, et al: Depression and work productivity: The comparative costs of treatment versus nontreatment. *J Occup Environ Med* 43(1):2-9, 2001.

Simon GE, Manning WG, Katzelnick DJ, et al: Cost-effectiveness of systematic depression treatment for high utilizers of general medical care. *Arch Gen Psychiatry* 58(2):181-187, 2001.

Stewart WF, Ricci JA, Chee E, et al: Cost of lost productive work time among US workers with depression. *JAMA* 289(23):3135-3144. Erratum in JAMA 290(16):2218, 2003.

Wang PS, Beck AL, Berglund P, et al: Effects of major depression on moment-in-time work performance. *Am J Psychiatry* 161(10):1885-1891, 2004.

World Health Organization: *The World Health Report 2001—Mental Health: New Understanding, New Hope.* Geneva, World Health Organization, 2001.

Young AS, Klap R, Sherbourne CD, Wells KB: The quality of care for depressive and anxiety disorders in the United States. *Arch Gen Psychiatry* 58:55-61, 2001.

Psychiatric Interview and Database

2

Richard J. Goldberg

2.1 Psychiatric Interview

1. Establish privacy.
   a. Establish conditions in which the patient can speak confidentially.
   b. When consulting on medical inpatients, try to leave a two- or four-bed room for a more private area.
2. Ensure safety.
   a. If there is any question about potential danger, conduct the interview in a safe place with other staff or security available.
   b. Avoid settings without access to a door, especially when interviewing a paranoid or potentially agitated patient.
3. Establish a time frame. Let patients know in advance about the length of the interview. This allows patients to adjust their level of detail. Also it removes patients' fantasies that the interview is being ended prematurely because they are boring or difficult or that it is being extended because they are special.
4. Give the reason for the interview.
   a. As with any medical interview, establish the chief complaint by asking the patient, "What do you hope to accomplish by meeting with me today?"
   b. If the interview has been set up as a result of a consultation request, some patients may be unclear about the purpose of the meeting.
5. Identify yourself by name, position, and profession.
6. Address the patient with respect. Patients should be addressed by courtesy title and last name.
7. Avoid obvious barriers.
   a. Try not to take detailed notes in front of the patient.
   b. Create a reasonable physical distance between you and the patient—not too far or too close.
   c. Be sure the patient, especially if elderly, can hear you.
   d. Do not sit in the blind spot of a patient who has had a stroke.
8. Inform the patient about what will happen after the interview.
   a. For example, "After we finish today, I will give you my assessment of the problem and discuss what to do next. This may involve some diagnostic studies, an additional interview, or a referral to some other person if I feel that is necessary."

b. Some patients assume that the interviewer will automatically become their therapist or provider. If this is not the case, let the patient know that your role is limited to evaluation and that a referral, if appropriate, will be made afterward.

9. Basic issues of confidentiality.

a. Do not communicate with anyone about the patient without permission.

b. Obtaining or providing records usually requires signed written consent, except in emergency situations.

c. If the interview will result in a report to someone else (such as a judge, worker's compensation board, or supervisor), make sure the patient understands and is willing to be interviewed under such circumstances.

d. Remember that medical records are public documents. Most states do not have laws that protect the privacy of psychiatric records. Although important information should be recorded, use some discretion recording sensitive material.

2.2 Psychiatric Database

OVERVIEW

1. The psychiatric database (example as in Fig. 2-1) is a means to an end, not an end in itself.

2. A database ensures that necessary data for a differential diagnosis are recorded systematically.

3. A database serves quality assurance and teaching functions.

4. The database should not be a barrier. Extensive note taking should be avoided.

5. The time required to complete a database depends on the setting and the goal. In an emergency evaluation, the relevant database can be covered in about 30 minutes. More extended outpatient evaluations can take several hours.

6. Not every item of the database must be obtained on every patient. For example, when assessing delirium, a developmental history is unnecessary. Conversely, some sections of this database are not extensive enough for some specialized problems.

7. The database is not the final evaluation. Greater detail in specific areas is obtained in ongoing treatment. For example, it may be enough in an initial interview to identify some significant family problems. A more thorough family assessment may be needed to define the problem fully.

8. Sometimes the database cannot be completed in an initial interview. In that case, indicate that the interview has not been sufficient to define the problem and that another meeting is necessary.

9. The database should allow the clinician to formulate a multiaxial DSM-IV (*Diagnostic and Statistical Manual of Mental Disorders, 4th edition*) diagnosis (Box 2-1). DSM-IV axes are listed in Box 2-2.

SECTION I: SOCIODEMOGRAPHICS

1. When presenting a case, present demographics first, because these define risk factors and influence clinical thinking. For example,

INITIAL EVALUATION

Date of Evaluation: _____

First   Last

NAME: _____

mo - day - yr

DOB: _____   M_____   F_____

CHIEF COMPLAINT

_____
_____
_____
_____

HISTORY OF PRESENT ILLNESS AND CURRENT PSYCHIATRIC TREATMENT

_____
_____
_____
_____

PAST PSYCHIATRIC HISTORY   Not Applicable

_____
_____
_____

Figure 2-1   Psychiatric interview and database.

diagnostic possibilities for an elderly widow in a nursing home are different from those for a postpartum mother living alone and receiving welfare.

2. Specific items.
   a. Some items have obvious administrative value: name, record number, address, phone number, date of birth, and sex.
   b. Marital status. Separation or divorce is one of the most stressful life events. Divorced and separated persons have poorer mental and physical health than their single, married, or even widowed counterparts.
   c. Education. If the patient has not completed high school, you may want to inquire about the reason. Were there some major life events, a history of learning disability, or a behavior problem? Can the patient read? Note any disparity between the level of education and work level.
   d. Religion. A patient's religion has potential significance if there is a strong religious affiliation and can influence ways of understanding and dealing with medical problems.
   e. Insurance status. Unfortunately, insurance status is a major determinant of access to care. There are also complicated rules in many

SUICIDE HISTORY   Not Applicable

| If yes, How many: _____ Last Attempted _____ |
| Consequences_____ |
| _____ |
| _____ |
| _____ |
| **Behaviors:** (cutting, burning, head banging, etc.) |
| _____ |
| _____ |
| _____ |

ASSAULT / LEGAL HISTORY (Other pertinent past history)

| _____ |
| _____ |
| _____ |
| _____ |

SUBSTANCE ABUSE   Denied

| SUBSTANCE   AMOUNT / FREQUENCY / ROUTE   LAST USE   SXS OF WITHDRWAL |
| HX OF DETOX   (When/Where/Last) |
| |
| |
| |

| Consequence of substance abuse: Neurological   Physical   Legal   School   Social   Family |
| Describe:_____ |
| _____ |
| _____ |

ALLERGIES:

| _____ |
| _____ |
| _____ |

Figure 2-1, Cont'd.

plans for authorization of treatment, copayments, deductibles, and total limits of coverage.

f. Responsible person. The billing office is interested in who is responsible for the patient's bill. The clinician is interested in identifying the significant other, such as spouse, parent, or roommate. The absence of such a person indicates serious isolation. Consider when this person should be part of the evaluation (if the patient consents).

2—Psychiatric Interview and Database

MEDICAL HISTORY   Not Applicable   **PRIMARY CARE PHYSICIAN:**

NEUROLOGICAL HISTORY AND PAST INVESTIGATIONS (CT, MRI, EEG, NEUROPSYCH TESTING, ETC.):

CURRENT MEDICATION (PSYCHIATRIC AND OTHER):   Not Applicable

FAMILY PSYCHIATRIC HISTORY   Not Applicable

DEVELOPMENTAL AND CHILDHOOD HISTORY *(Please clarify all 'yes' answers)*   Not Applicable

Problems with
pregnancy/delivery:_____

Early medical problems:

Problems with language/motor development:

ABUSE HISTORY   Not Applicable

History of:	Sexual abuse	Physical abuse	Emotional abuse	Verbal abuse

Figure 2-1, Cont'd.

g. Referrer. The referring professional should send pertinent background information and should receive a letter summarizing the findings. No information can be obtained or sent without patient permission. If a patient does not want information shared, it is important to understand why.

h. Reason. The "reason" refers to the reason given by the referring person (or the patient's reason if self-referred). Often there is

SOCIAL HISTORY (marital status, employment, education, children, social support, current living situation, etc.):

```
_____
_____
_____
_____
_____
```

REVIEW OF SYSTEMS (If applicable)

PULSE_____BLOOD PRESSURE_____

TEMPERATURE_____

Constitutional		Skin		Eyes		Endocrine	ENT	Heme
CV	Resp		GI		GU	Neuro		MS

MEDICAL CLEARANCE THROUGH E.D: Reviewed   Not Reviewed

MENTAL STATUS   (DESCRIBE ALL POSITIVE FINDINGS)
GENERAL APPEARANCE & BEHAVIOR   Unremarkable

withdrawn	poor eye contact	crying	distinguishing features (scars, tattoos, tobacco-stained fingers, etc.)
Other:_____			

MANNER (check at least one)   (DESCRIBE ALL POSITIVE FINDINGS)

cooperative	guarded	angry	hostile	inappropriately friendly
Other:				

MOTOR

Unremarkable	restless agitated	retarded	abnormal movements:

SPEECH/LANGUAGE   **Not Applicable**   (DESCRIBE ALL POSITIVE FINDINGS)

Abnormal rate:	rapid	pressured	slowed
Abnormal volume:	loud	soft	whisper
Abnormal amount:	monosyllable	mute	hypertalkative
Articulation difficulty:	mumbled	slurred	
Language comprehension:	poor		
Language expression:	poor		
Nonverbal communication:	inappropriate		

Figure 2-1, Cont'd.

significant discrepancy between the stated reason for the referral and the real reason. The referring physician may state that the reason is "to evaluate depression" but really means, "I am frustrated with this patient's noncompliance."

MOOD AND AFFECT   Not Applicable   (DESCRIBE ALL POSITIVE FINDINGS)

Patient quote _____

Abnormal: depressed/sad   angry   euphoric   anxious   irritable

    flat   blunted

Inappropriate   Labile

History of Mania / Hypomania (document symptoms) _____

ANXIETY SYMPTOMS (Panic, agoraphobia, OCD, GAD, PTSD, phobias, etc.):

THOUGHT PROCESS   Not Applicable   (DESCRIBE ALL POSITIVE FINDINGS)

no	yes	Abnormal:	circumstantial	tangential	loose	flight of ideas
no	yes	Incoherent				
no	yes	Illogical				
no	yes	Blocking				
no	yes	Distractible				

THOUGHT CONTENT   Not Applicable   (DESCRIBE ALL POSITIVE FINDINGS)

no	yes	Suicidal			
no	yes	Passive death wishes			
no	yes	Homicidal/Violence			
no	yes	Guilt/Worthlessness			
no	yes	Obsessions			
no	yes	Overvalued ideas			
no	yes	Hypochondriacal			
no	yes	Delusions:	thought broadcasting	thought withdrawal	thought insertion
	control	reference	grandiose	paranoid	somatic

PERCEPTION   Not Applicable   (DESCRIBE ALL POSITIVE FINDINGS)

no	yes	Hallucinations: auditory	visual	olfactory	tactile
no	yes	Illusions			
no	yes	Flashbacks			

COGNITIVE FUNCTIONING   Not Applicable   (DESCRIBE ALL POSITIVE FINDINGS)

no	yes	Altered level of consciousness:		drowsy	stupor
no	yes	Disoriented:	time	place	person
no	yes	Memory loss:	recent	remote	
no	yes	Difficulty concentrating/attending			
no	yes	Mental retardation			

VEGETATIVE SYMPTOMS   Not Applicable   (DESCRIBE ALL POSITIVE FINDINGS)

Appetite	Weight	Sleep	Energy	Interest
	Concentration	Libido		

Figure 2-1, Cont'd.

INTELLECT:	above average	average	below average
INSIGHT:	poor	fair	good
JUDGMENT:	poor	fair	good

_____

_____

PATIENT/FAMILY STRENGTHS & RESOURCES   *(Please list specific examples in checked categories)*

Hobbies: _____

Extensive support system: _____

Sports/Recreation: _____

Extracurricular activities: _____

Community service: _____

Academics: _____

Previous successful therapies: _____

Employment: _____

Supportive/Cooperative family: _____
Other: _____

INITIAL DIAGNOSES

Axis I:

(Principal) _____

(Secondary)_____

(Secondary)_____

Axis II:

Axis III:

Axis IV: Problems with:	Primary support group	Economics	Occupation
Social environment	Access to health care services	Housing	
Education	Legal system		
Other social/environmental factors			

Axis V: GAF (1-100)   current_____highest past year

_____

ADDITIONAL COMMENTS:

_____

_____

_____

Figure 2-1, Cont'd.

SECTION II: CHIEF COMPLAINT

1. As with any medical interview, establish the chief complaint, which forms the basis for the subsequent history.
2. In patients with multiple complaints, try to establish a hierarchical list. Ask the patient to define what seems to be the most important

INITIAL TREATMENT PLAN   **Describe if applicable**

Inpatient _____

Outpatient _____

Partial Hospital _____

Individual Therapy _____

Couples / Marital Therapy _____

Laboratory Investigations _____

Medication_____

_____

OTHER INTERVENTIONS:

_____

_____

_____

_____

SIDE EFFECTS / DRUG INTERACTIONS, ETC.:

Risks / Benefits /Side effects / drug interactions reviewed	Yes	No
Patient understands	Yes	No
Patient agrees	Yes	No
Patient refuses	Yes	No
Clinical condition precludes patient education	Yes	No

_____

_____

Signature: MD   RN   SW   Student   Date

ATTENDING NOTE (If applicable):

_____

_____

_____

_____

_____

_____

_____

_____

Signature_____   Date_____

Figure 2-1, Cont'd.

of the problems mentioned. The chief complaint may be elicited by the question, "What is it you hope to accomplish by meeting with me today?"

3. The patient might have no chief complaint if the referral was made for a consultation. In such cases, the patient should be told the reason for

BOX 2-1   Multiaxial Evaluation Report Form

Axis I: Clinical Disorders

Other conditions that may be a focus of clinical attention

Diagnostic code					DSM-IV name

Axis II: Personality Disorders

Mental retardation

Diagnostic code					DSM-IV name

Axis III: Medical Conditions

ICD-9-CM code					ICD-9-CM name

Axis IV: Psychosocial and Environmental Problems

Problems with primary support group. Specify:

Problems related to social environment. Specify:

Educational problems. Specify:

Occupational problems. Specify:

Housing problems. Specify:

Economic problems. Specify:

Problems with access to health care services. Specify:

Problems related to interaction with the legal system or crime. Specify:

Other psychosocial or environmental problems. Specify:

Axis V: Global Assessment of Functioning

See Box 2-4 to determine score.

Global assessment of functioning scale score:

> ### BOX 2-2   Psychiatric Axes
>
> Axis I: Psychiatric clinical disorders
> Axis II: Personality disorders
> Axis III: General medical conditions
> Axis IV: Psychosocial and environmental problems
> Axis V: A rating number derived from the Global Assessment of
>   Functioning Scale (see Box 2-4)

the referral. For example, if the consultation is to evaluate depression, you might say, "Dr. X has asked me to meet with you because of some difficulties managing stress." In patients uncomfortable with psychiatry, such an opening may be more facilitative than saying, "I'm here to evaluate your depression."

SECTION III: HISTORY OF PRESENT ILLNESS

1. The history of present illness (HPI) in psychiatry does not differ from that in other areas of medical practice. Identify the time and setting of the onset of the symptoms and trace their development to the present.
2. Do not assume you know what a patient means by words such as "depression," "confusion," "upset," "anxiety," or "nervous breakdown." Always ask patients to define what they mean.
3. Always find out, "Why now?" What were the precipitating factors? Include a question such as, "Are there any other stresses, changes, or losses that have been an issue for you?"
4. If the patient does not speak English, find a competent interpreter. Using family members can be a problem because of confidentiality and distortions.
5. Time segments of the interview.
   a. Try to reserve the first portion of the interview for the patient to talk freely without too much structured questioning, which prematurely closes off potential problems. Inquiries should start with open-ended questions and become more specific.
   b. The second portion of the initial interview should cover remaining aspects of the database, including the mental status.
6. Process of the interview.
   a. Summarize your understanding of the problem, allowing the patient a chance to correct it.
   b. Ask "Is there anything else you want to tell me?"
   c. Determine patient's expectations, fears, and interpretation of symptoms, with questions such as:
      (1) "What worries or fears do you have about your health, condition, or situation?"
      (2) "What do you think is the cause of your symptoms?"

SECTION IV: PAST PSYCHIATRIC HISTORY

1. Psychiatric hospitalizations. Inquire about any psychiatric (or substance abuse) admissions.
   a. Record the number of admissions, dates, and locations.
   b. Obtain a release of information to request records.
2. Outpatient treatment. Inquire about outpatient psychiatric or substance abuse treatment.
   a. Record the names of providers and dates of treatment.
   b. Obtain a signed release to request summaries.
   c. Ask what was helpful or problematic about previous treatment in order to continue what worked or avoid repeating mistakes.
3. Significant symptoms without treatment. Ask, "Are there times you had some nervous difficulties but did not see anyone for help?" Many patients have histories of significant psychiatric symptoms without formal psychiatric treatment.

SECTION V: DEVELOPMENTAL HISTORY

1. A developmental history is not necessary for every patient. For example, an elderly patient evaluated for a change in mental status would not require a developmental history.
2. Many adults have behavioral problems with developmental determinants. The reasons for obtaining developmental data include the following.
   a. Perinatal or childhood insults to the central nervous system may be associated with delayed maturation, increased risk of seizures, and behavioral and cognitive problems.
   b. Some adult behavior problems are strongly influenced by childhood events (e.g., multiple hospitalizations for a chronic medical condition, foster care, abuse, or absent parenting).
3. Although developmental histories are essential (and lengthy) for child psychiatry, they are more focused for adult patients and include the following:
   a. Pregnancy and perinatal complications. A screening question might be, "As far as you know, were there any complications when you were born or while your mother was carrying you? For example, were you born prematurely or did you have to be in a special care nursery?"
   b. Infancy. "Were you told of any serious problems you may have had as an infant, such as head injury, seizures, meningitis, hospitalization, abuse, or other problems?"
   c. School. "In your early years of school, were there any problems, such as fear of going to school (school phobia), being held back, being in special classes, hyperactivity, or learning disabilities?"
      (1) Early phobic behavior may be the first manifestation of an anxiety disorder.
      (2) Hyperactivity and learning disabilities can continue into adult years.
      (3) Being held back a grade can indicate a behavioral or learning problem but also may be the result of a family move or other problem during childhood.

  d. Since adult antisocial personality disorder begins in childhood, ask, "Were you the kind of child who got into trouble a lot?" (See Chapter 17 for fuller discussion of antisocial personality.)
  e. Relations to age 18 years. By the end of high school, a person's pattern of social interactions is generally in place. Therefore, determining the degree of socialization can help with understanding adult problems with social relations.
    (1) Adolescent isolation may be the result of many causes, such as schizoid personality, social phobia, depression, or parental forced isolation.
    (2) The adolescent social baseline would be expected to continue into adult life. Changes from this baseline must be explained.
  f. Abuse history: Nonjudgmental inquiry ("Did you experience sexual, physical, emotional, or verbal abuse?") may be a key in understanding adult posttraumatic symptoms. Patients may choose not to share this information on an initial interview.

SECTION VI: PSYCHOSOCIAL REVIEW

Psychosocial issues are important precipitants of medical visits and affect both physical and mental health.

1. Psychosocial and environmental problems are recorded on Axis IV of DSM-IV (Box 2-3).
2. A productive physician–patient relationship depends on identifying relevant psychosocial issues.
3. Psychosocial impairment and stress are important diagnostic variables in psychiatry.
4. Psychosocial content should include the following:
  a. Income.
    (1) "How do you support yourself?" Money is a critical factor for everyone.

BOX 2-3   Axis IV: Psychosocial and Environmental Problems

Axis IV includes problems in such areas as:
- Educational problems (e.g., problems with grades; discipline problems at school)
- Financial problems (e.g., income unable to meet expenses; significant debt)
- Health insurance (e.g., loss of health insurance coverage; inadequate coverage)
- Legal problems (e.g., arrests, probation, lawsuits)
- Relationship problems (e.g., divorce, separation, marital discord, relationship stresses or dysfunction)
- Work problems (e.g., unemployment; significant stress at work)

    (2) Income sources such as disability or worker's compensation might raise concern about motivation to get better and the possibility that medical symptoms are serving secondary gain.

    (3) Patients on entitlement programs such as General Public Assistance (GPA) or Aid to Families with Dependent Children (AFDC) often require updating of eligibility, which can confound their assessment. A psychiatric symptom may be presented as a basis for a new disability.

b. Work provides structure and is an important source of both gratification and stress.

    (1) Work-related problems may be the cause or the result of psychiatric problems.

    (2) The ability to work also gives insight into adaptive capacities and recovery from illness.

c. Daily activity if not work. If patients are not working, how do they spend their time?

    (1) Lack of structure and involvement contributes to isolation, lack of self-worth, and poor motivation.

    (2) Creating daily structure can be an important intervention. For this reason, structured day programs are set up for the chronically mentally ill, for the elderly, and for patients in the recovery phase of many other disorders.

d. Living arrangements. "With whom do you live?" is an important question, since that person may be a strong influence on the patient's illness and treatment, especially if his or her opinion is different from the clinician's.

e. Social support is an important factor mediating distress. Patients with inadequate or chaotic social support are at higher risk for all types of physical and mental coping problems.

    (1) How much social support is adequate? Counting family or friends is of limited use, because each person has differing needs. The real question is whether the amount available matches the needs.

    (2) Helpful questions are, "Is there someone you can call if you have a problem?" or "Is loneliness a problem?"

    (3) Social supports can involve complex relationships. The identified support may be the very person who is inflicting physical or emotional abuse.

    (4) Make no assumptions about what relationships are like, especially given the high prevalence of domestic violence.

f. Impairment of self-care is a serious stressor as well as a marker of impairment.

    (1) A general screening question is, "How does your condition interfere with taking care of yourself or your daily activities?"

    (2) To inquire about functional skills (and social support), ask, "Who does your grocery shopping? Cooking? Housecleaning? Laundry?"

    (3) On a more basic level of self-care ask, "Are you able to wash yourself? Get out of bed? Dress yourself? Feed yourself?"

g. Stressful events are important determinants of medical help seeking and can exacerbate underlying psychiatric vulnerabilities.
   (1) A screening question would be, "Have any other things been going on that have been stressful for you?"
   (2) Legal issues constitute an important subcategory of stressful events.

5. Global assessment of psychosocial function is recorded as Axis V in the DSM. Box 2-4 gives the Global Assessment of Functioning scale.

SECTION VII: FAMILY HISTORY

Many psychiatric disorders have some genetic contribution. Therefore ask, "Do any nervous conditions run in your family?"

1. Determine whether any first-degree relatives had psychiatric disorders and their treatment responses.

BOX 2-4   Global Assessment of Functioning Scale

Consider psychological, social, and occupational functioning on a hypothetical continuum of mental health to mental illness. Do not include impairment in functioning due to physical (or environmental) limitations.

100 Superior functioning in a wide range of activities; life's problems never seem to get out of hand.

91 Is sought out by others because of his or her many positive qualities. No symptoms.

90 Absent or minimal symptoms (e.g., mild anxiety before an exam), good functioning in all areas, interested and involved in a wide range of activities, socially effective, generally satisfied with life, no more than everyday problems or concerns (e.g., an occasional argument with family members).

80 If symptoms are present, they are transient and expectable reactions to psychosocial stressors (e.g., difficulty concentrating after a family argument). No more than slight impairment in social, occupational, or school functioning (e.g., temporarily falling behind in schoolwork).

70 Some mild symptoms (e.g., depressed mood and mild insomnia) or some difficulty in social, occupational, or school functioning (e.g., occasional truancy or theft within the household), but generally functioning pretty well. Has some meaningful interpersonal relationships.

60 Moderate symptoms (e.g., flat affect and circumstantial speech, occasional panic attacks) or moderate difficulty in social, occupational, or school functioning (e.g., few friends, conflicts with peers or coworkers).

50 Serious symptoms (e.g., suicidal ideation, severe obsessional rituals, frequent shoplifting) or any serious impairment in social, occupational, or school functioning (e.g., no friends, unable to keep a job).

BOX 2-4   Global Assessment of Functioning Scale (*Continued*)

---

40   Some impairment in reality testing or communication (e.g., speech is at times illogical, obscure, or irrelevant) *or* major impairment in several areas, such as work or school, family relations, judgment, thinking, or mood (e.g., depressed man avoids friends, neglects family, and is unable to work; child frequently beats up younger children, is defiant at home, and is failing at school).

30   Behavior is considerably influenced by delusions or hallucinations *or* serious impairment in communication or judgment (e.g., sometimes incoherent, acts grossly inappropriately, suicidal preoccupation) *or* inability to function in almost all areas (e.g., stays in bed all day; no job, home, or friends).

20   Some danger of hurting self or others (e.g., suicide attempts without clear expectation of death; frequently violent; manic excitement) *or* occasionally fails to maintain minimal personal hygiene (e.g., smears feces) *or* gross impairment in communication (e.g., largely incoherent or mute).

10   Persistent danger of severely hurting self or others (e.g., recurrent violence) *or* persistent inability to maintain minimal personal hygiene *or* serious suicidal act with clear expectation of death.

0   Inadequate information.

From American Psychiatric Association. *Diagnostic and Statistical Manual of Mental Disorders*, Text revision, 4th ed. Washington, DC, American Psychiatric Association, 2000, with permission.

2. Family histories also provide clues to important or problematic relationships.
3. Include questions about family medical history because of both the psychological and the biologic impact.
4. Drawing a genogram for the family history is usually helpful. Indicate dates and causes of death, as well as lines showing especially strong or problematic relationships.
5. Family specialists might take several hours for this section of the interview. The small amount of time allocated in the initial interview is for the purpose of identifying potentially important areas that can be revisited later.

SECTION VIII: MEDICAL HISTORY

1. A list of medical problems is essential. Give special consideration to any medical disorders (or treatments) that can affect the central nervous system (see Boxes 3-1 and 3-2), and consider the temporal

relationship between such problems and psychiatric symptoms. Several areas are of direct relevance to psychiatric symptoms.

   a. History of head injury (a risk factor for complex partial seizures, subdural hematomas, and postconcussion syndrome).
   b. Headache (new onset of severe headache raises concern about intracranial pathologic conditions; in addition, migraine may be a psychiatric symptom).
   c. Seizures, including passing out or fainting spells (many psychiatric symptoms can result from complex partial seizures or postictal or interictal phenomena).
   d. Chronic pain is often associated with psychiatric problems, especially depression. Psychiatric problems cannot be assessed without addressing pain.

2. Surgery is important medically and psychologically.
   a. In some instances surgery leads directly to psychiatric symptoms. For example, gastrointestinal surgery might remove part of the intestine where vitamin B_{12} is absorbed.
   b. Cardiovascular surgery can create risks for intraoperative brain hypoxia and later neuropsychological deficits.
   c. Extensive blood loss during surgery can create significant anemia, contributing to delirium or fatigue manifested as depression.

3. Medications and substance use. See Box 3-1 for details of the psychiatric consequences of medications and drugs. The database should include the following:
   a. Drug allergies and reactions. Many reactions that patients report as "allergies" turn out to be side effects, not allergies.
   b. Alcohol use. Because of the prevalence of alcohol abuse, this must be given special attention.
      (1) Screening questions (CAGE questionnaire and Michigan Alcohol Screening Test) are reviewed in Chapter 15.
      (2) Alcohol use patterns: none; not daily, social (one or two drinks); daily (specify quantity); binges (a definite sign of abuse).
   c. Street drugs. The patient might use none or might use narcotics, stimulants, sedatives, or other drugs (such as hallucinogens). If the patient is using alcohol or other drugs, impairment can involve social interactions, emotional symptoms, physical symptoms, and financial consequences.
   d. Tobacco use should be noted and quantified, because nicotine has adverse physical sequelae and can create or mask symptoms involving depression, anxiety, appetite, or energy (see Chapter 18).
   e. Caffeine use is extremely common. Patients vary in sensitivity, but as little as two cups of brewed coffee can cause significant anxiety, palpitations, or insomnia. Caffeine withdrawal is usually associated with fatigue and dull headache.
   f. Is there risk of drug withdrawal? This question must be answered at the time of the interview because of potential serious medical consequences.
   g. All over-the-counter (OTC) drugs and prescribed (Rx) medications should be recorded.

(1) The psychiatric symptoms associated with medications are so numerous that this part of the history must be very thorough.

(2) Ask the patient to bring in all medications.

  (a) Include substances bought at the drugstore or health food store.

  (b) Include recently discontinued medications.

h. Plasma levels can indicate inadequate or toxic levels that may be relevant to psychiatric symptoms.

i. Toxicology screens can be used to assess use of illicit substances.

SECTION IX: PHYSICAL AND NEUROLOGIC EXAMINATION AND VITAL SIGNS

A focused physical and neurologic examination, including vital signs, may be an extremely important part of the initial psychiatric assessment. Further details on the screening value and interpretation of the physical examination can be found in Chapters 3, 4, and 14.

SECTION X: SEXUAL HISTORY

1. Pregnancy history and outcome can be recorded by noting the number of pregnancies, term births, premature births, abortions, and miscarriages. Do not make assumptions that patients have not been pregnant just because they live alone or are unmarried, young, old, or religious.

2. History of sexually transmitted diseases (STDs) can be critical, with the increasing incidence of syphilis and human immunodeficiency virus (HIV) infection.

3. Sexual dysfunction is usually a meaningful problem.

   a. Sexual dysfunction is often correctable. About one third of men referred for impotence have an organic cause (see Chapter 19). Medications are often associated with erectile and ejaculatory disturbances in men and anorgasmia in women.

   b. Because patients are often reluctant to volunteer this information, direct questioning is important. The most basic screening questions include:

     (1) "Are you sexually active?"

     (2) "Are you having any sexual problems or concerns?"

     (3) "Have you ever been a victim of sexual abuse?" (It has been estimated that as many as 30% of adults have experienced sexual abuse during childhood.)

     (4) "Have you been involved in homosexual or bisexual activities?"

4. Menstrual history.

   a. Age at onset of menses (menarche), if delayed or early, can indicate neuroendocrine problems.

   b. Pattern of menses (regular, irregular, or absent) can also reveal neuroendocrine or medical problems.

   c. Date of last menstrual period (LMP) can be a critical question leading to consideration of pregnancy in young women with mysterious psychiatric or medical symptoms.

d. Date of onset of menopause and symptoms can be important to current issues. Inquire about beliefs regarding menopause and its psychosocial impact.

e. Consultation with a gynecology–endocrinology professional may be needed to sort out the facts and fiction.

5. Inquiring about premenstrual syndrome (PMS) can be important because of medical (such as increase in seizures premenstrually) or emotional effects. Assessment is facilitated by having the patient keep a 2- to 3-month diary of symptoms to document any pattern.

2.3 Mental Status Examination

OVERVIEW

The basic components of the mental status examination (MSE) can be summarized as follows:

1. Descriptive and behavioral section (this chapter).
2. Cognitive evaluation (see Chapter 4).
3. Affective evaluation (see Chapters 6 and 8).
4. Anxiety evaluation (see Chapter 9).
5. Psychosis evaluation (see Chapter 12).
6. Personality evaluation (see Chapter 17).

DESCRIPTIVE AND BEHAVIORAL COMPONENT

1. Special (examination) conditions. These factors obviously influence the interview reliability and validity.
   a. Translator. Language differences make assessment difficult, even with a translator. Using family members to translate is generally not a good idea because of issues of bias and confidentiality.
   b. Participants. Other people (students, other staff, family, or friends) might facilitate or impair the interview. Again, issues of confidentiality must be considered.
   c. Setting. Was the interview done in a four-bed room, in the corridor of a busy emergency room, or in some other place that would impair complete and open disclosure?
2. Appearance of the patient. Look for evidence that implies neuropsychiatric impairment. For example, are there signs of a craniotomy? Is there a movement disorder? Is the patient disheveled? Any unusual or inappropriate appearance should be recorded and explained.
3. Participation. Was the patient fully cooperative, hostile, resentful, or suspicious? Any deviation from full cooperation must be taken into account in interpreting findings.
4. Level of consciousness. Unless the patient is fully conscious and alert, the examination cannot be reliably interpreted. It makes little sense to perform a mental status examination on a patient still groggy after being extubated following an overdose. Categories for level of consciousness include:
   a. Within normal limits (WNL).

  b. Decreased. Patients are arousable and might provide brief, poorly sustained interactions. Decreased consciousness may be a result of just being awakened, drugs, or other central nervous system impairment.

  c. Patients in a stupor are more difficult to arouse and are usually incapable of meaningful interaction other than simple verbal and nonverbal responses to strong stimulation. This state of consciousness blends into early stages of coma, which is associated with even less responsiveness.

  d. Fluctuating level of consciousness is a hallmark of delirium (see Chapter 4). Statements during delirium (e.g., "I will not do anything to hurt myself now") might not be reliable.

5. Kinetics. Increased and decreased kinetics (body movements) are nonspecific but important features to note for diagnosis and for monitoring of changes.

  a. Psychomotor agitation or retardation can be seen in mood disorders, anxiety, schizophrenia, and delirium.

  b. Variable kinetics are often seen as part of the behavioral fluctuation occurring in delirium.

6. Affect. Refers to the expression of feelings. Normally people show a broad range of affect (smiling, pensive, sad, angry). Pathologic affect can have the following characteristics:

  a. Pathologic affect may be restricted. A depressed patient might show only a sad affect; a manic patient might show only euphoria; a schizophrenic patient might show no discernible affect (sometimes called *flat*).

  b. Patients with frontal lobe impairment, intoxication, or mild delirium can lose the ability to regulate affect and might show labile affect with rapid fluctuations.

  c. Patients with delirium, intoxication, or frontal lobe impairment might also show inappropriate affect (e.g., laughs at something that should be sad).

  d. In involuntary emotional expression disorder, a patient might laugh or cry for no apparent reason. This can have a number of potential underlying causes including multiple sclerosis, Parkinson's disease, dementia, or stroke.

7. Speech. Descriptions of speech properties help indicate or support a variety of diagnoses.

  a. Loudness may be WNL or:
    (1) Soft as in depression.
    (2) Loud as in patients with mania, hearing impairment, or escalating psychotic episodes.
    (3) Mute as in psychotically depressed patients or schizophrenics.

  b. Rate may be WNL or:
    (1) Slow as in depression or expressive aphasia.
    (2) Fast as in mania and stimulant intoxication.
    (3) Dysarthric as in patients after stroke involving the speech system.
    (4) Pressured as with manic or some brain-damaged patients.

   c. Structure, which refers to the semantic (meaning) and syntactic (grammatical) aspects of language, may be WNL or:
     (1) Vague (the listener has trouble figuring out what the patient is saying because there is so little content) as with dementia, depression, or paranoia.
     (2) Dysphasic (the patient makes word errors or sentence errors) as with stroke involving the language cortex.
     (3) Impoverished as with severe depression, dementia, or brain damage.
     (4) Incoherent as with disorganized schizophrenics, intoxicated patients, disorganized manic patients, or other brain-damaged patients.
     (5) Rapidly changing the subject as usually seen in manic states.
     (6) Tangential as shown by manic or schizophrenic patients.

SUGGESTED READINGS

Goldberg RJ, Faust D, Novack D: Integrating the cognitive mental status examination into the medical interview. *South Med J* 85:491-497, 1992.

Goldberg RJ, Novack DH: The psychosocial review of systems. *Soc Sci Med* 35:261–269, 1992.

Katz S, Ford AB, Moskowitz RW, et al: Studies of illness in the aged: The index of ADL: A standardized measure of biological and psychosocial function. *JAMA* 185:914-919, 1963.

Scheiber SS: The psychiatric interview, psychiatric history, and mental status examination. In Hales RE, Yudofsky SC (eds): *Essentials of Clinical Psychiatry*, 3rd ed. Washington, DC, American Psychiatric Press, 1999, pp 55-86.

Strub RL, Black FW: *The Mental Status Examination in Neurology*, 4th ed. Philadelphia, FA Davis, 2000.

Wise MG, Strub RL: Mental status examination and diagnosis. In Rundell JP, Wise MG (eds): *Textbook of Consultation Liaison Psychiatry*, 1st ed. Washington, DC, American Psychiatric Association Press, 1996, pp 66-87.

Medical Evaluation of Psychiatric Symptoms

3

Richard J. Goldberg

3.1 Medical Causes of Symptoms

HOW MEDICAL DISORDERS PRODUCE PSYCHIATRIC SYMPTOMS

1. Medical problems can produce psychiatric symptoms through nonspecific psychological stress. For example, the stress of entering chemotherapy can trigger a major depression, especially if the patient is vulnerable to affective illness because of previous psychiatric, personal, or family history.
2. Medical problems can produce physical symptoms that mimic a psychiatric disorder. For example, asthma can manifest itself as panic attacks; multiple sclerosis might initially be regarded as a conversion disorder.
3. Structural involvement of the central nervous system (CNS) can cause psychiatric symptoms. The specific psychiatric symptoms are determined by the region and extent of CNS involvement. For example, lung cancer can metastasize to the temporal lobe and cause a mood disorder; frontal lobe involvement can produce impaired executive function or loss of motivation.
4. Pharmacologic effects on the CNS can cause psychiatric symptoms. For example, theophylline can produce anxiety symptoms; dextromethorphan can produce hallucinations; benzodiazepines can produce depressive symptoms.
5. Virtually any psychiatric symptoms may be caused by an underlying medical problem (Table 3-1).

PRINCIPLES OF PSYCHIATRIC EVALUATION

1. Symptoms of disordered mood, thought, or behavior must be considered nonspecific symptoms that require differential diagnosis.
2. It is a mistake to assume that some particular psychosocial situation accounts for psychiatric symptoms without performing a complete evaluation.
3. It is an equally serious mistake to launch into a comprehensive medical diagnostic evaluation not supported by adequate findings from the history or review of systems.
   a. In general, more medically ill patients are more likely to have secondary psychiatric problems. For example, a bedridden cancer patient with recent pelvic surgery who has a panic attack is more likely to have a pulmonary embolism than the onset of a panic disorder.

Table 3-1 **Examples of Medical Causes of Psychiatric Symptoms**	
Psychiatric Symptoms	**Example of Medical Cause**
Delusions	Amphetamine or cocaine
Hallucinations	Delirium tremens, dextromethorphan
Incoherence	Delirium
Catatonia	Neuroleptic malignant syndrome
Flat or inappropriate affect	Frontal lobe CVA
Strange speech	Language cortex CVA
Odd beliefs	Interictal temporal lobe epilepsy
Anxiety	Hyperthyroidism
Depression	Pancreatic cancer
Irritability	Substance abuse

CVA, cerebrovascular accident.

4. History.
   a. Temporal onset. In general, sudden onset of symptoms is more typical of a medical disorder. Schizophrenia and affective disorders usually have a prodromal period. Because the panic attacks of panic disorder have sudden onset, they often suggest some underlying medical problem.
   b. Visual hallucinations are more suggestive of delirium than of schizophrenia or psychotic depression. Ocular disorders, especially in the elderly, can be reported as unusual experiences and mistaken for hallucinations.
   c. History of head injury should raise suspicion of an intracranial pathologic condition.
      (1) The elderly are especially vulnerable to subdural hematomas, which can manifest acutely or as a gradual change in behavior over months.
      (2) Schizophrenics, homeless patients, and substance abusers are at risk for trauma, assault, and head injury.
   d. Migraine headache history should raise consideration of an underlying cerebrovascular etiology for psychiatric symptoms such as acute psychotic symptoms.
      (1) New onset of headache symptoms not typical of a tension headache pattern should suggest the need for a more complete medical evaluation.
      (2) Frontal headache with temporal tenderness should raise the consideration of temporal arteritis, which can produce other psychiatric and constitutional symptoms.
   e. History of a seizure disorder is always relevant for the psychiatric evaluation. Inadequate or excessive plasma levels of anticonvulsant can result in uncontrolled seizure activity, as well as symptoms of medication toxicity such as depression, lethargy, or confusion. In addition, patients with one type of diagnosed seizure (e.g., grand mal seizures) might also have a second type of unrecognized

disorder (such as complex partial seizures) resulting in psychiatric symptoms.
f. Use of medications and substances (Box 3-1).

BOX 3-1   Medications and Substances Causing Psychiatric Symptoms

Analgesics

Narcotic mixed agonist–antagonists: euphoria, dysphoria, derealization
Propoxyphene: euphoria, dysphoria
Salicylates (plasma levels: 25 mg/dL): delirium, anxiety, tinnitus

Anti-AIDS and Antiviral Agents

Acyclovir: hallucinations, confusion, insomnia, hyperacusis
Efavirenz: hallucinations, confusion, anxiety, depression
Ganciclovir: psychosis, confusion
Nevirapine: hallucinations, delirium

Antiarrhythmics

All can cause delirium, excitement, agitation. Procainamide also can cause delusions, depression, or panic.
Disopyramide
Lidocaine
Mexiletine
Procainamide
Quinidine
Tocainide

Antibiotics

Aminoglycosides: toxic psychosis
Cephalothin: delirium, paranoia
Nalidixic acid: delirium
Penicillin (procaine form): psychosis
Sulfonamides: delirium, anorexia
Trimethoprim: psychosis, mutism, depression, anorexia, insomnia, headache

Anticholinergics

Can cause a *peripheral syndrome* consisting of tachycardia; increased temperature; hot, dry, flushed skin; urinary retention; constipation; blurred vision; and dry mouth. These drugs also cause a *central syndrome* consisting of confusion, memory impairment, restlessness, agitation, delirium, hallucinations, and severe anxiety.
Benztropine
Diphenhydramine
Meperidine
Oxybutynin chloride (Ditropan)

Box continued on following page

BOX 3-1   Medications and Substances Causing
Psychiatric Symptoms (Continued)

Propantheline (Pro-Banthine)
Tricyclic antidepressants
Trihexyphenidyl

Anticonvulsants

Anticonvulsants can cause drowsiness, mood change, confusion,
psychosis, and agitation.
Ethosuximide: confusion, paranoia, nightmares
Phenobarbital: depression, confusion, disinhibition
Phenytoin: irritability, depression, visual hallucinations, agitation

Antifungals

Amphotericin-B: delirium, anorexia
5-Flucytosine: confusion, hallucinations
Ketoconazole: headache, dizziness

Antihypertensives

ACE inhibitors: mania, anxiety, psychosis, hallucinations, depression
β-Blockers: depression, insomnia, nightmares, psychosis
Calcium channel blockers (nifedipine, verapamil): irritability, agita-
    tion, depression, hallucinations, panic
Clonidine: depression, hallucinations
Hydralazine: depression, euphoria, psychosis
Methyldopa: depression, lethargy, sedation
Reserpine: depression

Antiinflammatory Agents

Indomethacin: delirium, depression, hallucinations
NSAIDs: depression, anxiety, confusion
Phenylbutazone: anxiety, agitation

Antitubercular Agents

Cycloserine: insomnia, delirium, paranoia, depression
Isoniazid: agitation, hallucinations, depression, euphoria, transient
    memory impairment
Ethambutol: headache, confusion, hallucinations
Rifampin: drowsiness, fatigue, anorexia

Chemotherapy Agents

AZT: headache, restlessness, insomnia, nightmares, agitation
Bleomycin: anorexia
Interferon-α: depression, weakness
Methotrexate: fatigue
Procarbazine: mania, anorexia, confusion
Vinblastine: depression, anorexia, psychosis
Vincristine: hallucinations, weakness

BOX 3-1   Medications and Substances Causing
Psychiatric Symptoms (Continued)

Diuretics

Weakness, apathy, confusion, delirium

Dopaminergics

Dopamine antagonists cause motor symptoms including dyskinesias, dystonias, akinesia, akathisia, and neuroleptic malignant syndrome (see Chapter 12). Dopamine agonists can cause confusion, paranoia, hallucinations, depression, or anxiety.

Dopamine agonists, including amantadine, carbidopa–levodopa (Sinemet), and L-dopa
Dopamine antagonists
Metoclopramide
Neuroleptics

Sedatives and Narcotics

Sedatives and narcotics cause sedation and impaired cognition. Withdrawal can produce delirium, agitation, or confusion, accompanied by tachycardia, fever, mydriasis, sweating, and tremor. Sedatives also occasionally cause disinhibition.

Alcohol
Barbiturates
Benzodiazepines
Narcotics

Serotoninergic Agents

These drugs (SSRIs, tricyclic antidepressants, venlafaxine, nefazodone, trazodone, buspirone, lithium, dexfenfluramine, MAOIs) alone or in combination can result in serotonin syndrome (see Chapter 7).

Steroids

Anabolic steroids: aggression, paranoia, mood disorders
Corticosteroids: mood change, mania, agitation
Oral contraceptives: depression, anxiety, somnolence

Stimulants

Stimulants can cause anxiety, agitation, paranoid psychosis, insomnia, confusion. Withdrawal can cause severe depression.

Amphetamine
Caffeine
Cocaine
Methylphenidate
Theophylline

Box continued on following page

BOX 3-1   **Medications and Substances Causing Psychiatric Symptoms** (*Continued*)

Sympathomimetics

Sympathomimetics can cause anxiety, restlessness, agitation, psychosis, and delirium.
Albuterol
Phentermine
Phenylpropanolamine
Pseudoephedrine

Miscellaneous Drugs

Chloroquine: delirium
Cyclobenzaprine (Flexeril): mania, psychosis
Digitalis: confusion, psychosis, depression
Griseofulvin: depression, delirium
Histamine H_2 receptor blockers: hallucinations, confusion, delirium, depression, paranoia
Hypoglycemic agents: anxiety
Metronidazole: depression, agitation, confusion
Pentamidine: restlessness, headache, dizziness
Quinacrine: delirium

ACE, angiotensin-converting enzyme; AIDS, acquired immunodeficiency syndrome; AZT, azidothymidine (zidovudine); MAOI, monoamine oxidase inhibitor; NSAID, nonsteroidal antiinflammatory drug; SSRI, selective serotonin reuptake inhibitor.

    (1) Obtain a comprehensive list of every substance taken or recently discontinued.
    (2) When in doubt, obtain a toxicology screen. Urine screening is often more useful than plasma screening because drugs and metabolites may be detectable for a longer time.
    (3) If you are unsure whether some medication can cause a psychiatric symptom, look it up!
5. Medical problems that cause psychiatric symptoms (Box 3-2).
  a. Principles.
    (1) Construct a complete medical problem list.
    (2) If any problem could affect the central nervous system (CNS), consider further evaluation.
    (3) The psychiatric symptoms related to medical problems depend on the type of CNS involvement (see Table 3-1).
      (a) Generalized brain impairment results in delirium. Delirium can manifest as agitation, withdrawal, confusion, anxiety, psychosis, or depressive symptoms.
      (b) Focal brain involvement results in specific symptoms determined by location.
      (c) Neurochemical changes (e.g., catecholamine depletion with reserpine) result in specific syndromes.

BOX 3-2   Medical Causes of Psychiatric Symptoms

Metabolic and Endocrine Causes

Addison's disease
Calcium imbalance
Carcinoid syndrome
Cushing's syndrome
Electrolyte abnormalities
Hepatic failure
Hyperparathyroidism
Hyperthyroidism
Hypoglycemia
Hypothyroidism
Hypoxia
Magnesium imbalance
Pheochromocytoma
Porphyria
Renal failure
Serotonin syndrome
Wilson's disease

Electrical Causes

Complex partial seizures
Periictal states (depression, hallucinations)
Postictal states (depression, dissociation, or disinhibition)
Temporal lobe status epilepticus

Neoplastic Causes

Carcinoid syndrome
Carcinoma of the pancreas
Metastatic brain tumors
Primary brain tumors
Remote effects of carcinoma

Drug and Medication Causes

See Box 3-1.

Arterial Causes

Arteriovenous malformations
Hypertensive lacunar state
Inflammation (cranial arteritis, lupus)
Migraine
Multiinfarct states
Subarachnoid bleeds
Subclavian steal syndrome
Thromboembolic phenomena
Transient ischemic attacks

Box continued on following page

BOX 3-2   **Medical Causes of Psychiatric Symptoms**
(*Continued*)

Mechanical Causes

Concussion
Normal pressure hydrocephalus
Subdural or epidural hematoma
Trauma

Infectious Causes

Abscesses
AIDS
Hepatitis
Meningoencephalitis (including tuberculosis, fungal, herpes)
Multifocal leukoencephalopathy
Subacute sclerosing panencephalitis
Syphilis

Nutritional Causes

Folate deficiency
Niacin (vitamin B_3) deficiency
Pyridoxine (vitamin B_6) deficiency
Thiamine (vitamin B_1) deficiency
Vitamin B_{12} deficiency

Degenerative and Neurologic Causes

Aging
Alzheimer's disease
Creutzfeldt–Jakob disease
Heavy metal toxicity
Huntington's disease
Multiple sclerosis
Parkinson's disease
Pick's disease

  b. Systematic evaluation.
    (1) A systematic evaluation decreases errors of omission.
    (2) MEND A MIND, a useful mnemonic for the medical evaluation of psychiatric symptoms, is given in Box 3-3.
  c. Common examples of medical causes of psychiatric symptoms in each category.
    (1) Metabolic: Hyponatremia, hypothyroidism, hypoxia.
    (2) Electrical: Complex partial seizures.
    (3) Neoplastic: Metastatic CNS involvement of lung cancer, breast cancer, multiple myeloma, or AIDS.
    (4) Drugs: See Box 3-1.
    (5) Arterial: Stroke.

BOX 3-3   **MEND A MIND**

A useful mnemonic for the medical evaluation of psychiatric symptoms is MEND A MIND:
Metabolic (including endocrine)
Electrical
Neoplastic
Drug
Arterial
Mechanical
Infectious
Nutritional
Degenerative

(6) Mechanical: Head trauma with concussion, subdural hematoma.
(7) Infectious: CNS involvement in patients with impaired immunocompetence, human immunodeficiency virus (HIV) infection, or fever secondary to any common infection.
(8) Nutritional: Vitamin B_{12}, thiamine, or folate deficiencies.
(9) Degenerative: Alzheimer's disease (AD).

PHYSICAL EXAMINATION

1. Physical examination findings provide important clues to medical causes that underlie psychiatric symptoms. A discussion of these issues is found in Chapter 3.
2. Follow-up and reevaluation of physical examination are especially important when the clinical course is unusual or unresponsive.
3. Underlying medical disorders may be obscured by behavioral symptoms.

3.2 Diagnostic Testing

The use of diagnostic testing must be guided by the history, review of systems, and physical and neurologic examination. There is no set regimen to follow for the routine laboratory evaluation of any psychiatric disorder. However, a routine evaluation has been recommended for the evaluation of dementia (see Chapter 4).

ELECTROENCEPHALOGRAM

1. A waking electroencephalogram (EEG) is useful for documenting the brain's background rhythm. This may be helpful in:
   a. Detecting and documenting mild delirium.
   b. Distinguishing dementia and delirium from depression.
      (1) The background EEG should be normal in depression but is usually slowed in delirium and dementia.
      (2) The EEG may be normal in mild metabolic disorders.
   c. The waking background rhythm decreases with age but usually does not go below 8 Hz without disease.

    d. Slowing by more than 1 Hz per year in an elderly patient suggests a progressive disease process.

    e. Alzheimer's disease usually shows background slowing of less than 8 Hz, along with increased theta (5 to 7 Hz) and delta (1 to 3 Hz) activity and poor organization.

2. A sleep EEG is useful to evaluate possible seizure disorders.

    a. EEGs record only surface electrical activity for a limited time. Therefore a high rate of false-negative results (approximately 40%) occurs even in patients with documented complex and simple partial seizures.

    b. Complex partial seizures may be more accurately diagnosed by EEG (with identification rates approaching 90%) by use of:

      (1) Repeated EEG recordings.

      (2) Sleep deprivation.

      (3) Nasopharyngeal leads.

      (4) Ambulatory monitoring.

      (5) Closed circuit TV monitoring.

    c. The EEG may be useful in distinguishing generalized seizures from nonepileptic seizures, because generalized tonic–clonic seizures are always associated with an abnormal EEG, along with postictal slowing. EEG can also distinguish many partial seizure types from nonepileptic seizures.

3. Ambulatory EEG monitoring can be useful for:

    a. Determining whether some episodic behavioral problems (e.g., atypical panic attacks, episodic psychotic and autonomic symptoms) are caused by seizure activity.

    b. Increasing the yield of routine EEG.

4. Effects of drugs on the EEG. Virtually any psychotropic drug can produce EEG slowing.

    a. The slowing effect of neuroleptics is mild.

    b. Antidepressant slowing is usually also accompanied by some increased fast activity.

    c. At therapeutic doses, benzodiazepines, barbiturates, and stimulants produce increased fast activity.

    d. Lithium (even at therapeutic levels, but more commonly at high levels) can produce high voltage runs of diffuse slow activity.

    e. Tricyclic and neuroleptic agents lower the seizure threshold and can induce paroxysmal activity, with spike or sharp waves. When significant abnormalities occur, the patient should be evaluated for an underlying seizure disorder.

NEUROIMAGING

1. Potential indications. Neuroimaging should not be regarded as a screening test for every psychiatric patient, but it should be considered in the following cases:

    a. Confusion or dementia of unknown cause.

    b. First episode of psychotic disorder of unknown cause.

    c. Movement disorder of uncertain cause.

    d. Anorexia nervosa.

    e. Prolonged catatonia.

    f. First episode of major depression in the elderly.

    g. Personality change after age 50 years.

2. Advantages of magnetic resonance imaging (MRI) over computed tomography (CT) scans.

    a. Better soft tissue contrast.

    b. Multiplanar imaging capability.

    c. Fewer artifacts when imaging the posterior fossa.

    d. Lack of ionizing radiation.

    e. Generally no need for contrast materials, although contrast agents maximize detection of brain metastatic disease. With MRI, a gadolinium-based agent is generally used, which does not have the disadvantages (allergic reactions and nephrotoxicity) of radiographic contrast agents used in CT scanning.

3. Disadvantages of MRI.

    a. Artifacts from excessive patient motion.

    b. Longer scan times.

    c. Claustrophobia. Generally can be managed with anxiolytic agents.

    d. Electromagnetically driven devices and ferromagnetic or metallic objects lead to the following contraindications:

        (1) Cardiac pacemakers in pacer-dependent patients.

        (2) Implanted neurostimulators.

        (3) Cochlear implants.

        (4) Metal in the eye.

        (5) Ferromagnetic aneurysm clips.

    e. Poor bone visualization.

    f. Pregnancy is a relative contraindication, especially in the first trimester. However, the unspecified risks are probably less than the risks of ionizing radiation.

4. Diagnostic indications for MRI. For certain disorders, an MRI is clearly preferable to a CT scan and the cost differential is warranted. These situations in psychiatry include:

    a. Demyelinating disease.

    b. Temporal lobe abnormalities (because artifacts often obscure findings from that region).

    c. Subcortical multiple lacunae or infarcts (often too small to show up on CT scans).

    d. Abnormal endocrine function (better resolution and lack of bone artifact in visualizing the pituitary gland).

    e. Primary and metastatic neoplasms, along with associated features such as edema, vascularity, hemorrhage, and necrosis.

    f. Abscess, encephalitis, meningitis. Early detection of herpes simplex encephalitis is best achieved with MRI. Other infections (often AIDS related) can also be visualized, including toxoplasmosis, lymphoma, cryptococcosis, and neurosyphilis.

    g. Posterior fossa lesions.

    h. Acute stroke, especially ischemic infarcts of the brainstem or cerebellum.

    i. Subacute and chronic brain hemorrhage or hematoma.

    j. Progressive multifocal leukoencephalopathy.

5. Noncontrast CT is the preferred neuroimaging technique in emergency situations and in acute traumatic brain injury.
6. Role of single positron emission computed tomography (SPECT) scans.
   a. SPECT allows imaging of blood flow patterns. Potential uses in psychiatry include evaluation of dementia. The SPECT scan shows a characteristic biparietal hypoperfusion pattern in Alzheimer's disease that can be distinguished from multiinfarct dementia.
   b. Site of a seizure focus.
   c. Cerebral infarct in a patient with recent onset of neurologic findings and no abnormalities on CT or MRI.
   d. Areas of poor perfusion after a stroke or head trauma.
   e. CNS Lyme disease.
   f. Future uses might involve identification of neuroreceptor sites using receptor-binding radiotracers.
7. Role of positron emission tomography (PET) scans.
   a. Interictal seizure focus localization
   b. Differentiating AD from other dementias
   c. Differentiating residual tumor from radiation necrosis
   d. Receptor imaging is being evaluated in research studies.

LUMBAR PUNCTURE

1. Lumbar puncture is indicated to evaluate the following:
   a. Unexplained elevated temperature in a patient with altered mental status, which should be considered CNS infection until proved otherwise. This is especially true for patients with altered immunocompetence from chronic diabetes, cancer, acquired immunodeficiency syndrome (AIDS), immunosuppressive drugs, or steroids.
   b. Possible CNS fungal infection (which has a high false-negative rate).
   c. CNS herpes (associated with increased ferritin levels in cerebrospinal fluid).
   d. Multiple sclerosis (with findings of elevated immunoglobin G [IgG] levels or oligoclonal bands).
   e. Neurosarcoidosis (patient might have lymphatic pleocytosis and elevated angiotensin-converting enzyme [ACE] level).
   f. In AD, lumbar puncture (LP) is not a routine test but should be considered if the patient has atypical features such as rapid progression, fever, meningeal signs, or a positive serologic test for syphilis.
2. LP is contraindicated in:
   a. Infection over the entry site.
   b. Bleeding disorder.
   c. Posterior fossa mass.
   d. Midline shift.

TOXICOLOGY SCREENS

Toxicology screens are useful in the following situations:

1. Assessment of psychiatric symptoms that do not have a clear diagnosis.
2. When doubt exists about possible drug or medication use.
3. If the patient is receiving medications for which levels are available, obtain levels to see if the patient's drug level is toxic or subtherapeutic.
4. Alcohol levels. For interpretation of blood alcohol levels, see Chapter 15.
5. Cocaine levels. Although cocaine has a brief plasma half-life, its metabolite benzoyl ecgonine can be detected in urine for several days.
6. False-positive and false-negative results are possible, depending on technique. When in doubt, talk to the laboratory about suspicion of particular drugs.

THYROID TESTS

Because hypothyroidism can be manifested as depression and hyperthyroidism as anxiety, screening is often indicated.

1. A high-sensitivity thyroid-stimulating hormone (TSH) is sufficient as a screen for both hyperthyroidism and hypothyroidism.
   a. If the TSH level is elevated (indicating possible hypothyroidism), a total or free thyroxine (T_4) level should be obtained.
   b. If the TSH is subnormal (indicating possible hyperthyroidism) follow up with a total or free T_4 and triiodothyronine (T_3).
2. Thyroid testing should be undertaken on a periodic basis (every 6 to 12 months) for patients receiving lithium (see Chapter 8).

GLUCOSE AND GLUCOSE TOLERANCE TESTS

Glucose screening (glucose tolerance test, GTT) should be considered for patients with psychiatric symptoms along with diabetes mellitus, alcoholism, or cirrhosis.

1. Hyperglycemia can cause delirium by creating osmotic imbalances in the brain.
2. Postprandial hypoglycemia is rarely a cause of psychiatric symptoms.
   a. A 5-hour GTT is rarely helpful in evaluating symptoms of anxiety, fatigue, or depression.
   b. A GTT may be relevant in patients after gastric and small intestine surgery with dumping syndrome.
3. Patients receiving excessive insulin have hypoglycemic episodes manifested as anxiety, confusion, agitation, belligerence, or fatigue, which are responsive to glucose infusion.
4. Initial fasting blood glucose (FBG) and periodic follow-up of glucose levels are now indicated for patients treated with the atypical antipsychotic agents.

LIVER FUNCTION TESTS

1. Patients with extensive liver disease caused by malignancy, cirrhosis, or hepatitis are at risk for hepatic encephalopathy if liver function deteriorates further. This disorder is usually marked by generalized slow waves (triphasic waves) on the EEG.
2. Liver function tests (LFTs) are important for patients receiving medications that can cause allergic hepatic responses, such as

carbamazepine, chlorpromazine, or valproic acid, if clinical symptoms such as nausea, abdominal discomfort, or jaundice develop.

ARTERIAL BLOOD GASES

1. Hypoxia. Any cause of brain hypoxia will make a patient feel anxious: congestive heart failure, chronic obstructive pulmonary disease (COPD), pneumonia, cardiac arrhythmia, pulmonary embolism, asthmatic episode, and so on. Therefore assessment of P_{O_2} may be an important part of evaluating acute anxiety symptoms in such patients.
2. Carbon dioxide retention (elevated P_{CO_2}) can result in somnolence, confusion, and impaired attention.
   a. Avoid using benzodiazepines in patients with elevated P_{CO_2}, because they can suppress hypoxic respiratory drive and lead to respiratory depression or arrest.
3. Sleep apnea (see Chapter 11). Oxygen desaturation from sleep apnea can result in a variety of psychiatric symptoms, including daytime sleepiness, fatigue, depression, and cognitive impairment.
   a. Patients at risk often have short, thick necks or snore loudly. However, sleep apnea can occur in patients without these features.
   b. Observing the patient for apneic periods is a first step toward a referral for sleep evaluation.

COMPLETE BLOOD COUNT

The complete blood count (CBC) is relevant to psychiatry in a number of situations:

1. Monitoring for patients taking clozapine.
2. When sore throat or fever develops in patients taking such drugs as carbamazepine, phenothiazine, or mirtazapine.
3. In evaluation of a postsurgical patient with altered mental status who may have had significant operative blood loss.
4. To assess anemia in patients with altered mental status (anemia resulting in fatigue, confusion, anxiety, and depressive symptoms).

BLOOD UREA NITROGEN AND CREATININE

Blood urea nitrogen (BUN) and creatinine are relevant to psychiatry in the following situations:

1. To assess renal function in patients taking drugs that are cleared by the kidneys (e.g., lithium, amantadine, or risperidone).
2. Chronic renal failure. As uremia worsens, psychiatric symptoms become more prominent.
3. As a clue to dehydration and associated orthostasis risk, especially in patients with poor oral intake.

ELECTROLYTES

Electrolytes are relevant to psychiatry in the following situations:

1. Syndrome of inappropriate antidiuretic hormone (SIADH) can be caused by such drugs as lithium, carbamazepine, or the selective serotonin reuptake inhibitors (SSRIs).
2. Hyponatremia from any cause (usually diuretics) can cause delirium.

3. Hypokalemia leads to muscle fatigue and weakness, which many patients identify as symptoms of "depression."
4. For patients taking lithium, anything that significantly alters sodium balance (diuretics, vomiting, diarrhea) will alter lithium levels and can lead to lithium toxicity (see Chapter 8).

CREATINE KINASE

Creatine kinase (CK), an enzyme whose levels are elevated because of muscle damage, is relevant to psychiatry in the following situations:

1. Neuroleptic malignant syndrome (NMS) (see Chapter 12) in which CK elevations (MM fraction) are usually greater than 800 IU/L. Elevations up to (but not above) 800 IU/L can occur after intramuscular injections or struggling in restraints.
2. Fractionation of the CK isoenzymes ensures that the elevation is not caused by the cardiac fraction after a myocardial infarction. Behavioral changes in the elderly may be caused by silent myocardial infarction.
3. High elevations of CK may be found after muscle crush injuries, such as those caused by car accidents.

PORPHYRINS

Porphyria is a rare cause of episodic psychiatric symptoms.

1. Abdominal pain is the usual presenting complaint. Thirty percent to 70% of cases are accompanied by episodic psychiatric symptoms, usually delirium or psychosis.
2. During attacks, qualitative abnormalities of uroporphyrins and coproporphyrins may be observed in the urine. These tests are not useful between attacks.
3. Quantitative urine measurements of aminolevulinic acid (ALA) and porphobilinogen (PBG) may be abnormal between attacks.
4. A more definitive test involves measurement of uroporphyrinogen I synthetase, in which decreased activity can confirm a diagnosis.

COPPER

Wilson's disease is an autosomal recessive genetic disorder that results in abnormal accumulation of copper, leading to hepatic cirrhosis, degeneration of the basal ganglia, neuropsychiatric symptoms, and hemolytic anemia.

1. Screening tests include serum ceruloplasmin and 24-hour urinary copper levels. Ninety percent of patients with Wilson's disease have very low serum ceruloplasmin levels. Twenty-four-hour urinary copper levels are high.
2. Screening for Wilson's disease should be considered in patients with psychiatric symptoms and:
   a. Family history of Wilson's disease.
   b. Unexplained liver disease.
   c. Signs of basal ganglia or frontal lobe disease not otherwise explained.

PREGNANCY TEST

1. Because psychotropic drugs have a number of fetal effects, pregnancy status should be established before medication is prescribed.
2. At times, a mysterious behavioral change in a young woman is caused by an unannounced pregnancy.

VITAMIN B$_{12}$

1. Psychiatric symptoms (anxiety, psychosis, delirium, or dementia) occur in 35% to 85% of patients with vitamin B$_{12}$ deficiency.
   a. The mental manifestation of vitamin B$_{12}$ deficiency can precede the hematologic abnormalities.
   b. The standard lower limit of normal value for vitamin B$_{12}$ is 200 pg/mL, but this may be too low for psychiatric purposes, because psychiatric symptoms can occur with values up to 300 pg/mL.
2. Accompanying physical symptoms are paresthesias and sensory loss (particularly vibration and proprioception leading to ataxia).
3. Vitamin B$_{12}$ deficiency may be present in the absence of classic hypochromic macrocytic anemia.
4. If vitamin B$_{12}$ is deficient, Schilling's test may be performed to differentiate dietary deficiency from impaired absorption resulting from absent intrinsic factor.
5. Methylmalonic acid assay may be helpful in identifying vitamin B$_{12}$ deficiency when the B$_{12}$ level is borderline low.

FOLATE

1. Folate deficiency often accompanies vitamin B$_{12}$ deficiency.
2. Folate levels may also be low in alcoholic patients, patients taking anticonvulsants, pregnant patients, and patients on dialysis.

POLYSOMNOGRAPHY AND SLEEP APNEA

1. Sleep apnea can lead to symptoms of depression, anxiety, panic disorder, and dementia (see Chapter 11).
2. Diagnostic polysomnography (PSG) is performed in a sleep evaluation center and usually includes recordings of EEG, electrocardiogram (ECG), electroculography (EOG; eye movements), and electromyography (EMG; muscle movement), as well as respiratory effort, airflow, snoring, and blood oxygen saturation.

Acknowledgment

I would like to thank Curt LaFrance, MD, for his assistance in reviewing the neuropsychiatric assessment issues.

SUGGESTED READINGS

Alpay M, Park L: Laboratory tests and diagnostic procedures. In Stern TA, Herman JB (eds): *Massachusetts General Hospital Psychiatry Update and Board Preparation*, 2nd ed. New York, McGraw—Hill, 2003, pp 251-265.

Bostwick JM, Philbrick KL: The use of electroencephalography in psychiatry of the medically ill. *Psychiatr Clin North Am* 25:17-25, 2002.

Brown ES, Suppes T: Mood symptoms during corticosteroid therapy: A review. *Harv Rev Psychiatry* 5:239-246, 1998.

Buse JB: Metabolic side effects of antipsychotics: Focus on hyperglycemia and diabetes. *J Clin Psychiatry* 63(suppl 4):37-41, 2002.

Cohen W, Roberts WN, Levenson JL: Psychiatric aspects of SLE. In Lahita RG (ed): *Systemic Lupus Erythematosis*, 4th ed. San Diego, Academic Press, 2004, pp 785-825.

Dougherty DD, Rauch SL: Neuroimaging in psychiatry. In Stern TA, Herman JB (eds): *Massachusetts General Hospital Psychiatry Update and Board Preparation*, 2nd ed. New York, McGraw–Hill, 2003, pp 227-232.

Drugs that may cause psychiatric symptoms. *Med Lett* 44:59-62, 2002.

Giladi N, Treves TA, Paleacu D, et al: Risk factors for dementia, depression and psychosis in long standing Parkinson's disease. *J Neurol Transm* 107:59-71, 2000.

Kornstein SG, Sholar EF, Gardner DG: Endocrine disorders. In Stoudemire A, Fogel BS, Greenberg DB (eds): *Psychiatric Care of the Medical Patient*, 2nd ed. New York, Oxford University Press, 2000, pp 801-819.

Kunkel EJS, Thompson TL, Oyesanmi O: Hematologic disorders. In Stoudemire A, Fogel BS, Greenberg DB (eds): *Psychiatric Care of the Medical Patient*, 2nd ed. New York, Oxford University Press, 2000, pp 835-856.

Levenson JL (Ed): *Textbook of Psychosomatic Medicine*. Arlington, Va, American Psychiatric Publishing, 2005.

Delirium, Dementia, and Other Cognitive Disorders

4

Sandra A. Jacobson

4.1 Delirium

DEFINITION AND IDENTIFICATION

1. Delirium is defined by a disturbed level of consciousness coupled with either change in cognitive function or development of a perceptual disturbance. Symptoms develop acutely and fluctuate over a 24-hour period. By definition, symptoms are secondary to medical illness.

   a. Disturbance of consciousness refers to a reduced clarity of awareness of events in the environment as well as internal states (e.g., pain).

   b. Disturbance of consciousness may be obvious (e.g., falling asleep in midsentence) or subtle (e.g., problems focusing, sustaining, or shifting attention).

   c. Cognitive changes can involve any area of cognitive function but commonly include disorientation, memory problems, visuospatial impairment, and aphasia, at times accompanied by a formal thought disorder, such that the patient appears incoherent.

   d. Perceptual disturbance often takes the form of visual hallucinations, although hallucinations occur in all modalities.

   e. Delirium usually develops over hours to days.

   f. Symptoms of delirium can fluctuate markedly over a 24-hour period, with brief lucid intervals of more normal function interspersed with exacerbations such as sundowning, which often manifest in the evening or nighttime hours.

   g. Medical etiologies of delirium are numerous. The *Diagnostic and Statistical Manual of Mental Disorders* (DSM) divides delirium into five categories:

      (1) Delirium due to a general medical condition.

      (2) Substance-induced delirium.

      (3) Substance-withdrawal delirium.

      (4) Delirium due to multiple etiologies.

      (5) Delirium not otherwise specified (NOS).

   h. In elderly patients, the cause is often multifactorial. A list of medical illnesses commonly associated with delirium is shown in Box 4-1.

2. Some symptoms associated with delirium are not noted in the core criteria. These include:

   a. Delusions (usually persecutory or paranoid), often arising from misperceptions.

   b. Agitation and physical aggression.

BOX 4-1   Medical Illnesses Commonly Associated with Delirium

---

Central Nervous System Insults

Advanced dementia
Encephalitis and meningitis
Primary or metastatic cancer
Seizure (uncontrolled) or postictal state
Stroke
Traumatic brain injury
Uncontrolled hypertension

Postoperative States

Hip fracture repair
Open heart surgery

Systemic Illnesses

Blood gas abnormalities (hypoxemia, hypercarbia)
Congestive heart failure
Fluid or electrolyte derangement
Hepatic insufficiency or failure
Hyperthyroidism (thyrotoxicosis)
Hypoperfusion (myocardial infarction, dysrhythmia, shock)
Infection: pneumonia, urinary tract infection, septicemia
Renal insufficiency or failure
Respiratory insufficiency or failure
Severe burn or trauma
Vitamin B deficiency states (especially thiamine)

---

    c. Nocturnal insomnia, sometimes total, alternating with daytime somnolence.

    d. Motor symptoms (myoclonus, tremor, asterixis, akinesia, bradykinesia, increased tone, extensor plantar responses).

    e. Autonomic instability, which is seen with certain etiologies of delirium such as alcohol and sedative withdrawal. All vital signs may be affected, and diaphoresis, shivering, and pupillary abnormalities may be seen.

3. It is important that delirium is recognized when it appears.

    a. It can be the only sign of life-threatening illness, especially in elders.

    b. It is a marker for severe or developing illness (e.g., infection in a postoperative patient).

    c. Delirious patients present a risk for self-harm (e.g., by self-extubation, falling) or harm to others (aggression toward staff).

    d. Delirious patients are unable to comply with medical orders or to monitor intake (e.g., hydration and swallowing) and output on their own.

    e. Delirious patients are often unable to comprehend medical information, and they require assistance for informed consent.

4. Delirium mimics many other conditions such as depression, anxiety, dementia, paranoia, and personality disorders, among others. Elderly patients with delirium most often appear quiet, withdrawn, and sleepy during the day, but they may be agitated and overtly psychotic at night.

INCIDENCE AND PREVALENCE

1. Delirium is one of the most commonly encountered psychiatric disorders in medical and surgical practice, particularly in geriatrics. It is present in 30% of elderly patients on admission to the hospital, in 50% of patients following hip fracture repair, and in 80% of terminally ill patients.
2. Anything that compromises the brain chronically can increase the risk of delirium: distant traumatic brain injury, undernutrition, dementia, inadequate cerebral perfusion (e.g., from low cardiac output), hypoxemia in chronic obstructive pulmonary disease (COPD), and glucose dysregulation. Other risk factors include extremes of age (babies or the very old) and sensory impairment (blindness, deafness).
3. Patients with moderate to severe dementia are at particular risk for delirium from even minor insults such as constipation, urinary tract infection, or mild dehydration.

PROGNOSIS

1. Delirium is by definition a transient disorder. In young, otherwise healthy patients, delirium usually resolves in a few days if the underlying cause is detected and treated. In elderly patients, some symptoms of delirium persist for several weeks even when the cause is treated.
2. In older patients without dementia, it is important to educate the family about the temporary nature of delirium so that inappropriate plans for nursing home placement are not pursued.
3. Brains already compromised by traumatic brain injury or advanced dementia might not ever return to baseline function after an episode of delirium.

TREATMENT

1. Environmental interventions.
   a. Orientation cues. The patient is reoriented by staff at least once per shift. A calendar and clock are placed in the room.
   b. Activity and mobility are encouraged, as tolerated by the patient.
   c. Sensory aids such as hearing aids or glasses are used and are ensured to function properly.
   d. If possible, continuity of staff from day to day is ensured.
   e. Family and close friends are encouraged to visit quietly. A close family member is encouraged to stay with the patient.
   f. In the absence of a personal caregiver, one-to-one observation involving hospital staff is considered.
   g. Consideration is given to moving the patient closer to the nursing station for better observation.
   h. The patient's room is cleared of sharps and other items that could be harmful.

2. Psychosocial interventions.
   a. The patient and family are reassured, and the family is educated about the temporary nature of delirium.
   b. Staff is educated about the need to observe the patient and to understand that abusive behavior and comments of the patient are not intentional.
3. Pharmacologic interventions.
   a. Two separate treatment algorithms are used: one for alcohol or sedative withdrawal delirium and the other for all other etiologies (see Chapter 15).
   b. Alcohol or sedative withdrawal delirium is treated with a benzodiazepine when vital signs are unstable or when the CIWA-Ar (Clinical Institute Withdrawal Assessment—Alcohol, revised) score is higher than 10. Lorazepam is preferred for elderly patients and for those with hepatic impairment and because it can be given intramuscularly (IM) or intravenously (IV). Chlordiazepoxide (Librium) is sometimes used for convenience because of its longer half-life.
      (1) Lorazepam dosing varies, depending upon severity of withdrawal. Usual start dose is 1 to 2 mg IV/IM/PO q6h standing and 1 to 2 mg IV/IM/PO q2h prn for unstable vital signs or increasing CIWA-Ar score. When the patient stabilizes, lorazepam dose is decreased by 25% every 24 hours to discontinue. Much higher doses of lorazepam may be needed.
      (2) For nonelderly patients without significant hepatic impairment, a more rapid detoxification with chlordiazepoxide (Librium) may be used: 50 to 100 mg PO followed by 50 to 100 mg PO q1-2h until vital signs are normal and the patient is sedated. Librium dosing is then stopped, and the medication slowly self-tapers.
   c. For all other etiologies of delirium, antipsychotics are used when delusions or hallucinations are present or agitation or disorganized behavior present a risk to safety.
      (1) Haloperidol has advantages: It can be used IV; it has little effect on blood pressure, pulse, respiration, or glucose regulation; and it is not as heavily sedating as other medications. Disadvantages: It can cause extrapyramidal symptoms, especially when used orally, and it can cause QTc prolongation when used IV at high doses. Use should be time-limited (preferably < 1 week) to avoid risk of tardive dyskinesia.
         (a) Haloperidol dose for younger patients: 1 to 5 mg IV q8h standing and 1 to 5 mg IV q6h prn for agitation. Electrocardiogram should be checked periodically for QTc changes.
         (b) Haloperidol dose for geriatric patients: 0.25 to 0.5 mg IV q8h standing and 0.25 to 0.5 mg IV q6h prn for agitation.
      (2) Quetiapine has advantages: sedation for agitated patients. Disadvantages: It can cause hypotension and glucose dysregulation, and it is available for oral use only. As with other atypical antipsychotics, quetiapine is associated with increased risk of

mortality in elderly patients with dementia. Actual risk associated with short-term use (as in delirium) is not known.

  (a) Quetiapine dose for younger patients: 25 to 50 mg PO tid standing and 25 to 50 mg PO q6h prn for agitation.

  (b) Quetiapine dose for older patients: 12.5 to 25 mg PO bid to tid standing and 12.5 to 25 mg PO q6h prn for agitation.

  (3) Risperidone can be used at doses from 0.25 to 2 mg PO bid standing and 0.25 to 2 mg PO q6h prn for agitation. Disadvantages: It can cause hypotension and akathisia, even at these suggested doses.

  d. When the interventions detailed above are used, physical restraints are rarely needed.

4.2 Dementia

DEFINITION AND IDENTIFICATION

1. Dementia is a syndrome of acquired intellectual impairment characterized in DSM by persistent deficits in memory (amnesia) and at least one other domain: language (aphasia), motor function (apraxia), recognition (agnosia), or executive function. Some definitions require three domains of impairment for the diagnosis and include personality change as one of the domains.

2. Patients with Pick's disease or frontotemporal dementia may be quite severely affected before memory impairment is manifested. For this reason, not all definitions require the presence of memory impairment for a dementia diagnosis.

3. DSM requires that cognitive deficits be severe enough for impairment in social or occupational functioning to be present. This may be difficult to assess in a setting such as a nursing home.

4. The order in which symptoms become apparent, and their relative severity, depends on etiology.

5. Various psychiatric and behavioral problems are associated with dementia, including disinhibition, sexual inappropriateness, neglect of personal hygiene, disregard for rules of social conduct, agitation, aggression, apathy, depression, irritability, delusions, misidentifications, hallucinations, and sleep disturbances. Suicidality may be present in early stages.

DIFFERENTIAL DIAGNOSIS

1. Delirium is distinguished from dementia by the presence of a disturbance in conscious awareness. In addition, delirium comes on acutely and fluctuates over a 24-hour period.

2. Amnestic disorder is defined by significant impairment in the memory domain only.

3. Age-associated memory impairment is a nonpathologic condition involving subjective report of memory problems without significant abnormalities on objective testing; ability to function socially and occupationally is preserved. The person with age-associated memory impairment might also report some degree of cognitive slowing.

Table 4-1	**Cause of Dementia by Age of Onset**	
Younger than 50 Years	**50 to 70 Years**	**Older than 70 Years**
Traumatic brain injury	Vascular	Alzheimer's disease
HIV–AIDS	Familial Alzheimer's disease	Vascular dementia
Alcohol-related	Brain tumor	Lewy body
Infection	Progressive supranuclear palsy	Medication toxicity
Endocrine disease		Hypoxemia
Pick's disease	Lewy body	Hypoperfusion
	Pick's disease	

Data from Taylor MA: *The Fundamentals of Clinical Neuropsychiatry*. New York, Oxford University Press, 1999.

4. Mild cognitive impairment involves subjective report of memory problems, memory impairment on objective testing that is less severe than that seen in dementia, normal testing in other domains, and preserved ability to function socially and occupationally. This condition can presage the development of dementia in certain persons.
5. Identification of the etiology of dementia is imperative because treatment depends on cause.
6. Not all dementias are irreversible. As an example, cognitive deficits of vitamin B_{12} deficiency may be entirely reversed if the dementia is diagnosed and treated early.
7. Cortical dementia (such as Alzheimer's disease) arises from pathology affecting the cerebral cortex. Subcortical dementia (such as human immunodeficiency virus [HIV]-associated dementia) arises from pathology affecting structures deep to the cortex, both white matter and deep gray.
8. Different etiologies are more common in different age groups (Table 4-1).

SELECTED DISORDERS

1. Alzheimer's disease (AD) is a cortical dementia of insidious onset and slow progression. AD is the most common cause of dementia.
   a. Cognitive difficulties are initially most obvious in recent memory and in word finding, but they ultimately progress to involve all cortical domains. Executive dysfunction and personality changes can occur early.
   b. Neurologic examination is normal until later stages, when sphincter control is lost, limbs become rigid and flexed, and seizures can occur.
   c. Symptoms of apathy, agitation, anxiety, irritability, depression, delusions, and hallucinations occur and most are more common with disease progression.
   d. Laboratory work-up is normal in early stages. Neuroimaging reveals a normal-appearing brain or mild atrophy that could be consistent

with age until the later stages of the disease, when more severe atrophy is seen. Postmortem microscopic examination of the brain shows β-amyloid plaques and neurofibrillary tangles in the cerebral cortex.

2. Vascular dementia is a consequence of significant compromise to the integrity of cerebral vasculature. Onset may be insidious or acute, depending on the cause, and progression may be stepwise. Significant involvement of subcortical domains is the rule, but cortex may be involved.

   a. History is often significant for vascular risk factors: hypertension, hyperlipidemia, diabetes, smoking, sedentary lifestyle, and obesity. History sometimes reveals disorders related to cerebrovascular compromise, such as endocarditis (causing emboli).

   b. Neurologic deficits occur early: problems with ambulation, swallowing (dysphagia), articulation (dysarthria), other cranial nerve findings, and urinary incontinence.

   c. In addition to cognitive signs of memory impairment (poor retrieval) and slowness, symptoms of apathy, poor hygiene, irritability, depression, delusions, and sleep disturbances may be seen.

   d. Laboratory work-up points to risk factors such as high cholesterol. Neuroimaging is by definition abnormal. Magnetic resonance imaging (MRI) is superior to computed tomography (CT) for visualizing ischemic brain disease and should be the procedure of choice unless contraindicated (e.g., metal prosthesis).

3. Dementia with Lewy bodies is a progressive dementia with cognitive symptoms and parkinsonism.

   a. Marked fluctuation of symptoms from day to day is characteristic.

   b. Parkinsonism includes prominent rigidity, akinesia or bradykinesia, and tremor. Tremor is not present in all cases. Postural instability is a frequent problem, and falling is common. The parkinsonism may be labeled "treatment-resistant" because of poor prior response to levodopa therapy. Patients are exquisitely sensitive to the effects of dopamine-blocking medications, particularly high-potency conventional antipsychotics but also atypical antipsychotics.

   c. Associated features include visual hallucinations (sometimes described as Lilliputian figures), delusions, difficult-to-treat depression, and unexplained episodes of loss of consciousness.

4. HIV-associated cognitive impairment can be caused by opportunistic diseases (cytomegalovirus [CMV] encephalitis, cerebral toxoplasmosis, progressive multifocal leukoencephalopathy [PML], cryptococcal meningitis, or central nervous system [CNS] lymphoma), or it can be a consequence of cellular response to HIV infection itself (HIV-associated dementia [HAD]).

   a. The incidence of HAD has declined dramatically with the use of antiretroviral (ARV) therapy.

   b. HAD is seen in later stages of HIV disease, in patients with CD4 counts of less than 200/mm^3.

   c. HAD is a subcortical dementia, with abnormalities in cognition, motor function, and mood. Prominent cognitive difficulties in psychomotor speed and memory are seen, and they may be quantified using an instrument such as the Modified HIV Dementia Scale.

d. Motor abnormalities can include stumbling, slowing of fine repetitive movements (e.g., typing), and parkinsonism. Hyperreflexia and frontal release signs may be present.

e. Apathy and social withdrawal are common in early HAD. Depression is also common and is usually characterized by irritable mood and anhedonia rather than sadness and tearfulness. Neurovegetative symptoms are often seen. Psychosis with paranoia and hallucinations can develop. In late disease (CD4 < 100 cells/mm^3), acquired immunodeficiency syndrome (AIDS) mania can develop, characterized by irritable mood and cognitive slowing, often in the absence of hyperactivity or pressured speech.

f. Treatment of HIV-associated dementia involves optimization of antiretroviral regimens (e.g., addition of protease inhibitors to antiviral agents) with associated lowering of viral loads. There is some evidence that memantine may be useful as a neuroprotective agent. Risperidone and clozapine have shown efficacy in HAD-related psychosis. All antidepressants have shown efficacy, although drugs with anticholinergic effects may be problematic, and St. John's wort should be avoided because of potential interaction with protease inhibitors. First-line antimanic agents (lithium, valproate, and atypical antipsychotics) have shown efficacy in AIDS mania, but they are associated with adverse effects in this population.

EVALUATION OF DEMENTIA

A diagnostic work-up for dementia is given in Box 4-2.

1. History.
   a. Obtain history of cognitive decline in terms of work and social function and of problems with activities of daily living (ADLs) (e.g., accidents, missed appointments, mistakes in keeping checkbook, losing keys, problems with cooking, getting lost on familiar routes, failing to recognize family members).
   b. Note first onset of symptoms and rate and pattern of progression.
   c. Neurologic review of systems (ROS) for dementia diagnosis and differential diagnosis includes trouble walking, urinary incontinence, slurred speech, swallowing problems, stiffness, tremor, slowness, falling, loss of consciousness, weakness, incoordination, seizure, and headache.
   d. Psychiatric ROS for dementia-associated signs and symptoms includes behavioral disinhibition, neglect of personal hygiene, aggression, apathy, depression, irritability, delusions, suicidal ideation, misidentifications, hallucinations, and personality changes.
   e. Other medical problems and current medications that might be contributing to cognitive impairment are reviewed.

2. Examination.
   a. Neurologic examination: cranial nerve dysfunction, weakness, tremor, rigidity, akinesia, myoclonus, asymmetry of reflexes, abnormal reflexes (Babinski's sign, grasp), dysmetria, clumsiness, and ambulation difficulties.

BOX 4-2   Diagnostic Work-up for Dementia

History

First onset of symptoms, rate and pattern of progression
Neurologic and psychiatric review of systems (see text)
Review of other medical problems or medications that might impair
cognitive function

Examination

Neurologic examination: cranial nerve dysfunction, weakness,
tremor, rigidity, akinesia, myoclonus, asymmetry of reflexes,
abnormal reflexes (Babinski's sign, grasp), dysmetria, clumsiness,
and ambulation difficulties
Cognitive screening
Mini Mental State Examination
Mental Alternation Test
Clock-drawing
Timed tasks
Luria hand sequences
Tests of abstract thinking
Neuropsychological testing

Laboratory Evaluation

Routine blood labs: complete blood count, electrolytes, glucose,
blood urea nitrogen, creatinine, liver function tests, thyroid
screening, vitamin B_{12}, and syphilis serology.
Structural neuroimaging: MRI or CT.
Lumbar puncture, EEG, HIV testing, Lyme disease titers (in
endemic areas), apolipoprotein E testing, heavy metal screening
in selected cases.
Functional neuroimaging (SPECT, PET, fMRI) in selected cases.

CT, computed tomography; EEG, electroencephalogram; fMRI, functional magnetic
resonance imaging; HIV, human immunodeficiency virus; MRI, magnetic resonance
imaging; PET, positron emission tomography; SPECT, single-photon emission computed tomography.

b. Cognitive screening: The Mini Mental State Examination
(MMSE) is a screening instrument widely used for this purpose.
The MMSE is most sensitive to cortical impairment. Additional
items to assess for frontal or subcortical impairment include the
Mental Alternation Test, clock-drawing, timed alphabet writing,
Luria hand sequences, and similarities and differences. Specifically
for HIV-associated dementia, the Modified HIV Dementia Scale
may be used.
c. Neuropsychological testing is more extensive and based on more
fully developed norms. It can be helpful to characterize the pattern
and severity of cognitive impairment to clarify the diagnosis, if
there is doubt.

3. Laboratory examination.
   a. Routine blood labs include complete blood count (CBC), electrolytes, glucose, blood urea nitrogen (BUN), creatinine, liver function tests, thyroid screening, vitamin B_{12}, and syphilis serology to rule out reversible causes of dementia.
   b. Structural neuroimaging is required to identify a vascular etiology of dementia and to diagnose dementia secondary to conditions such as tumor or hydrocephalus. Except in cases where acute bleeding is suspected, MRI is preferred because it is much more sensitive than CT to ischemic lesions.
   c. Lumbar puncture is performed in cases where CNS infection or inflammation is suspected or where dementia is rapidly progressive. Cerebrospinal fluid (CSF) tau protein and β-amyloid (1-42) levels can provide additional evidence for or against a diagnosis of AD.
   d. Electroencephalogram (EEG) is performed in patients with a history of seizure, with rapid progression of dementia, or with prolonged confusional state.
   e. HIV testing, Lyme disease titers, and heavy metal screening are done in cases where history shows specific risk.
   f. In cases where the diagnosis remains unclear, functional neuroimaging (single-photon emission computed tomography [SPECT], positron emission tomography [PET], or functional magnetic resonance imaging [fMRI]) may be useful. In addition, apolipoprotein E (ApoE) genotyping can provide additional evidence for or against the diagnosis of AD.

TREATMENT OF PSYCHIATRIC AND BEHAVIORAL PROBLEMS

1. Problematic behavior related to dementia can improve with treatment of core neurotransmitter derangements, using medications such as cholinesterase inhibitors and memantine.
2. Psychosis (delusions, hallucinations) may be treated with any of the following medications: aripiprazole (2.5-5 mg qhs), risperidone (0.25-1 mg qhs or divided bid), olanzapine (2.5-5 mg qhs), or quetiapine (12.5-150 mg, with lower doses given qhs and higher doses divided tid). Conventional antipsychotics may also be used at low doses. Atypical antipsychotics carry some risk of increased mortality in elderly patients, particularly those with dementia; this may apply as well to conventional agents.
3. Depression is treated with environmental enrichment and stress reduction. When pharmacologic treatment is used, selective serotonin reuptake inhibitor (SSRI) antidepressants (e.g., escitalopram, citalopram, sertraline) or dual-acting agents such as venlafaxine, duloxetine, or mirtazapine are used.
4. Mania in the patient with dementia is underdiagnosed. The patient may be irritable and agitated and can suffer from insomnia, delusions, and hallucinations. The syndrome is best treated with an atypical antipsychotic such as those listed in the

earlier point about psychosis. Ultimate doses needed may be higher, although they are reached with the same "start low, go slow" rule. Temporary use of a benzodiazepine such as lorazepam or oxazepam may be helpful. In general, mania in dementia is a shorter-lived syndrome than primary mania, so medications are required for a shorter period.

5. Anxiety can be treated acutely with a benzodiazepine such as lorazepam or oxazepam. For long-term treatment, buspirone can be used at doses ranging from 5 mg bid to 20 mg tid. Alternatives include gabapentin 50 to 300 mg tid or a low dose of an SSRI (e.g., sertraline 12.5 to 25 mg or fluoxetine 2 to 10 mg suspension or capsule).

6. Agitation in dementia ranges from pacing or disruptive vocalization to physical assault. The first step in treatment involves listing and describing target behavior. Consensus guidelines have been developed for treatment and should be consulted. For persistent nonspecific agitation that requires pharmacologic treatment, the following medications are recommended:

   a. SSRI antidepressants: escitalopram 10 to 20 mg daily, citalopram 10 to 30 mg daily.

   b. Trazodone: 12.5 mg bid to 100 mg tid.

   c. Atypical antipsychotics: quetiapine 12.5 mg to 150 mg daily (higher doses divided), risperidone 1 mg daily, aripiprazole 2.5 to 10 mg daily, olanzapine 5 to 10 mg daily. These drugs now carry warnings regarding increased mortality risk in elderly patients, particularly those with dementia.

   d. Other medications reported anecdotally to be effective include propranolol at doses of 10 to 80 mg daily, gabapentin at doses of 300 to 2400 mg daily divided tid, and selegiline 10 mg daily.

   e. Valproate is used despite several controlled studies showing lack of efficacy. For agitation, small doses with serum levels less than 50 μg/mL are used; for aggression, more usual doses with serum levels 50 to 100 μg/mL are used.

7. Sundowning may be treated with an atypical antipsychotic given 1 to 2 hours before the time of usual behavioral disturbance. For example, risperidone 0.5 mg may be given at 2:00 pm and again at bedtime.

8. Inappropriate sexual behavior may be caused by medications (parkinsonism drugs), may be a symptom of mania, or may be associated with neurodegeneration (e.g., with Klüver–Bucy syndrome). In nonbipolar patients, treatment is initiated with an SSRI (fluoxetine 20 mg or citalopram 20 mg daily).

4.3 Amnestic Disorders

DEFINITION AND IDENTIFICATION

1. Isolated memory impairment significant enough to interfere with social or occupational functioning defines an amnestic disorder. By definition, an amnestic disorder is secondary to a general medical condition.

2. An amnestic disorder may be transient ($\leq$1 month) or chronic (>1 month).
3. Substance-induced persisting amnestic disorder by definition persists beyond the time of substance intoxication and withdrawal.

ETIOLOGY

1. Common etiologies include head trauma, thiamine and other vitamin deficiency states, infections such as herpes encephalitis, cerebrovascular insufficiency, and many other conditions that affect the elderly.
2. Substances implicated in substance-induced persisting amnestic disorder include alcohol; sedative, hypnotic, and anxiolytic medication; and other medications or drugs of abuse.

TREATMENT

1. The primary intervention is treatment of the underlying medical condition. Aggressive thiamine replacement or antiviral therapy may be associated with rapid resolution of amnesia.
2. With cerebrovascular insufficiency, one syndrome that is observed is that of transient global amnesia, in which memory impairment occurs in spells lasting minutes to hours. Effective treatment of cerebrovascular disease can result in resolution of such spells.
3. Treatment with cholinesterase inhibitors has been shown effective in reducing amnesia in traumatic brain injury patients, and it may be useful in other etiologies of amnestic disorder.

4.4 Cognitive Mental Status Examination

OVERVIEW

1. Cognitive mental status examination is performed routinely for patients in medical and surgical settings, geriatric patients, those with a history of brain injury or neurologic disease, patients with memory or other cognitive complaints, and in the evaluation of decision-making capacity.
2. Normalizing statements are used to introduce and explain the rationale for the cognitive evaluation. For example, the patient is told that they will be asked a series of questions to see briefly how their brain is functioning in different areas and that this is not a test that can be passed or failed but that it gives a baseline measure to better determine what medication and rehabilitation needs might be.

COMPONENTS OF THE COGNITIVE EXAMINATION

1. Level of consciousness. If level of consciousness is impaired, the remainder of the examination will not likely reflect the patient's baseline function. Consciousness is impaired in delirium, stupor, and coma. If the patient is merely asleep, arousal to full wakefulness should not be difficult.
2. Attention. Inability to focus, sustain, or shift attention also affects all subsequent cognitive testing. Attentional problems might indicate the presence of delirium, dementia, schizophrenia, depression, mania,

anxiety and anxiety disorders, or attention-deficit/hyperactivity disorder (ADHD).

a. Attention is tested on the MMSE using serial 7s, which is confounded by the need to perform the more difficult task of mental calculation. A simpler and sometimes substituted task on the MMSE is spelling "world" backwards (dlrow).

b. A more sensitive test of attention is that of the mental alternation test, which is a brief oral version of Trails B testing. The patient is asked to count from 1 to 10, then to say the alphabet from A to G, then to go back and forth (A-1, B-2, etc.).

3. Language. Impairment in language function (aphasia) provides evidence of cortical dysfunction. Inability to understand language indicates a lesion in the parietal lobe (Wernicke's area) of the dominant hemisphere (usually the left). Inability to speak fluently and to name indicates a more anterior lesion (Broca's area). Inability to repeat involves connecting fibers between Wernicke's and Broca's areas. Language is very well covered by the MMSE, but the instrument is not sensitive to early or subtle impairment, and it does not help to distinguish encoding problems from retrieval problems. Patients with suspected language impairment may be referred for neuropsychological testing, or they may have the MMSE augmented with slightly more difficult tasks.

a. Naming. Ask the patient to name less common objects, such as parts of the watch (stem, crystal) or specific body parts (earlobe, nostril).

b. Verbal fluency. Ask the patient to name as many animals as they can in 60 seconds. (An abnormal score is fewer than 12 words.)

c. Comprehension. Ask the patient to "point to your nose, your foot, and the door to this room, in that order."

d. Repetition. Ask the patient to repeat the sentence, "The beginning movement revealed the composer's intention."

e. Reading. Ask the patient to read a standard paragraph and explain its meaning.

f. Writing. Ask the patient to write a paragraph describing the room.

4. Memory. Several domains of memory are tested, either formally or as part of the interview.

a. Immediate memory is tested by registration of three words on the MMSE. Inattention (because of delirium, ADHD, or severe anxiety) can interfere with this function.

b. After several minutes have elapsed, the free recall of the three words constitutes the test of short-term (verbal) memory. If little time elapses because serial 7s were not attempted, this is an inadequate test of short-term memory. A better test would be registration of five words and free recall of five words after 5 minutes. If a patient is unable to recall the three words of the MMSE, further memory testing is indicated, because this is likely to uncover a significant deficit. Orientation questions on the MMSE (worth 10 points of 30) are also a test of recent or short-term memory.

c. Long-term memory is usually probed by history, but it is important to corroborate history obtained from the patient with that obtained from a family member or other contact. An alternative is to ask about historical events that have occurred in the patient's lifetime.

5. Visuospatial function is tested on the MMSE by the intersecting pentagons task. A more sensitive task is that of clock-drawing, in which the patient is given a large circle and asked to put the numbers on the clock where they belong, and then to draw the hands so the time is "ten after eleven." A patient with a right hemisphere lesion might neglect the whole left side of the clock. A patient with frontal lobe impairment might demonstrate very poor planning in clock construction.

6. Higher cognitive functions include abstraction, reasoning, insight, and judgment. These domains are the focus of interest in the case of an evaluation for decision-making capacity (competence).

   a. Abstraction is tested through use of similarity-and-difference questions or proverbs, the latter being confounded by being more culture-bound. Similarity-and-difference questions include: How are a car and an airplane alike? How are a child and a midget different? An example of a proverb often used in testing is "a stitch in time saves nine."

   b. Reasoning, insight, and judgment are usually tested by asking patients about events pertinent to their own lives and conditions, but it is possible to devise semistandard questions to probe these areas. For example, judgment can be tested by asking patients what they would do if they found a stamped, addressed, and sealed letter on the street, or what they would do if they smelled smoke in a crowded theater.

SUGGESTED READINGS

Alexopoulos GS, Silver JM, Kahn DA, et al: The expert consensus guideline series: Treatment of agitation in older persons with dementia. PDF available for download at http://www.psychguides.com/ecgs1.php (accessed October 2, 2006).

Davis HF, Skolasky RL Jr, Selnes OA, et al: Assessing HIV-associated dementia: Modified HIV dementia scale versus the grooved pegboard. AIDS Read 12:29-38, 2002.

Folstein MF, Folstein SE, McHugh PR: "Mini-mental state." A practical method for grading the cognitive state of patients for the clinician. J Psychiatr Res 12:189-198, 1975.

Mace NL, Rabins PV: The 36-Hour Day. New York: Warner Books, 1999.

McKeith IG, Galasko D, Kosaka K, et al: Consensus guidelines for the clinical and pathologic diagnosis of dementia with Lewy bodies (DLB): Report of the consortium on DLB international workshop. Neurology 47:1113-1124, 1996.

McKhann G, Drachman D, Folstein M, et al: Clinical diagnosis of Alzheimer's disease: Report of the NINCDS-ADRDA Work Group under the auspices of Department of Health and Human Services Task Force on Alzheimer's Disease. Neurology 34:939-944, 1984.

Roman GC, Tatemichi TK, Erkinjuntti T, et al: Vascular dementia: Diagnostic criteria for research studies. Report of the NINDS-AIREN International Workshop. Neurology 43:250-260, 1993.

Alzheimer's Disease: Diagnosis and Treatment

5

Richard J. Goldberg

5.1 Overview

COMMUNICATING WITH ALZHEIMER'S PATIENTS

1. Listen. Talking to someone with cognitive impairment takes patience—it is going to be slower than you are used to.
2. Use simple words and brief phrases. Longer, complex syntax can be confusing.
3. Be aware of tone. Patients can pick up the tone rather than the meaning of the words you use. As a corollary, patients with language impairment might communicate more about their meaning through tone (e.g., sounds sad) than the specific words.
4. Use eye contact and touch. Try to make every contact a meaningful communication. A gentle touch or caring glance can be reassuring even when the meaning of words is lost.

RECOGNITION OF ALZHEIMER'S DISEASE

1. Prevalence. AD is an increasingly common national health problem. The prevalence is approximately 1% at age 60 and doubles every 5 years.
2. Differential diagnosis.
   a. The hallmark of AD is gradual onset of cognitive and functional impairment with continuing decline. Sudden onset of symptoms is incompatible with a diagnosis of AD.
   b. Early onset (prior to age 60), rapid progression, and presence of focal neurologic signs or parkinsonian symptoms should prompt consideration of other diagnoses.
3. Medical evaluation.
   a. Many professional societies have published consensus guidelines regarding the medical work-up indicated for assessing AD. Most would agree on vitamin B_{12} and thyroid-stimulating hormone (TSH) tests.
   b. Other blood tests depend on the clinical status of the patient but would likely include:
      (1) Complete blood count (CBC).
      (2) Blood urea nitrogen (BUN).
      (3) Creatinine (CR).
      (4) Liver function tests (LFTs).
      (5) Calcium.
      (6) Glucose.

BOX 5-1   **Resources**

Alzheimer's Association: For information on local chapters, see http://www.alz.org/Services/LocalChapters.asp.
Alzheimer's Disease Education and Referral Center (ADEAR, a resource of the National Institute on Aging), provides information and publications for professionals, patients, and families: http://www.nia.nih.gov/alzheimers/.

---

    (7) Rapid plasma reagin (RPR).
    (8) Folate.
  c. Neuroimaging. Some guidelines state that neuroimaging (noncontrast head computed tomography [CT] or magnetic resonance imaging [MRI]) is not required to make the clinical diagnosis. Other groups (such as the American Academy of Neurology) state that neuroimaging should be part of the initial assessment or a small percentage of other diagnoses (such as unsuspected tumor) will be missed.
4. The treatment of AD is multidimensional:
  a. Psychoeducational assistance for families and caregivers is extremely important.
  b. Local Alzheimer's Association offices (Box 5-1) can be helpful in providing information and resources.
  c. Behavioral complications such as aggression and psychotic symptoms are common and usually can be managed by a combination of environmental and psychopharmacologic interventions (see later).
  d. The progression of cognitive and functional impairment can be delayed to some extent by pharmacologic agents (see later). Functional impairments that result from AD may be rated using the Functional Activities Questionnaire (Box 5-2).

5.2 Behavioral Symptoms

Prevalence of behavioral symptoms is given in Table 5-1.

1. Physical agitation symptoms.
  a. Physical aggression: hitting, kicking, biting, spitting, throwing things, using weapons, other physical aggression.
  b. Verbal aggression: yelling or screaming, swearing, threatening physical harm, criticizing, scolding, other verbal aggression.
  c. Agitation: pacing, hand wringing, unable to sit or lie still, rapid speech, increased psychomotor activity, repeated expressions of distress, other signs of agitation.
  d. Wandering
2. The Disruptive Behavior Rating Scale (DBRS).
  a. Rates four domains of behavior.
    (1) Physical aggression (e.g., overt behavior such as hitting).
    (2) Verbal aggression (e.g., yelling, threatening, and swearing directed at persons or objects).

BOX 5-2   Functional Activities Questionnaire

Scale

Rate each of the ten areas using the following scale:

0   Normal (or never did but could do now)
1   Has difficulty but does by self (or never did and would have some difficulty now)
2   Requires assistance
3   Dependent

Activities

- Writing checks, paying bills, balancing checkbook.
- Assembling tax records, business affairs, or papers.
- Shopping alone for clothes, household necessities, or groceries.
- Playing a game of skill or working on a hobby.
- Heating water, making a cup of coffee, turning off the stove.
- Preparing a balanced meal.
- Keeping track of current events.
- Paying attention to, understanding, or discussing a television show, book, or magazine.
- Remembering appointments, family occasions, holidays, and medications.
- Traveling out of the neighborhood, driving, or arranging to take buses.

Evaluation

A higher score indicates a poorer level of function with greater impairment. A cutoff point of 9 (dependent in 3 or more activities) is recommended as marking significant functional impairment.

From Pfeffer RI, Kurosaki TT, Harrah CH, et al: *J Gerontol* 37:323-329, 1982.

Table 5-1   Behavioral Symptoms in Alzheimer's Disease

Symptom	Approximate Prevalence (%)
Paranoia	35
Delusions	30
Hallucinations	30
Inappropriate behavior	30
Aggression	25
Sleep disturbances	20
Wandering	20
Depression	10-40

BOX 5-3   The Disruptive Behavior Rating Scale

Although it might not be necessary to use a particular scale, it is extremely important to note target symptoms of behavior problems and document continuous ratings so as to be able to decide on and appropriately document the need for a particular intervention. Potential target symptoms are listed.

0   Insufficient data.
1   Behavior does not occur.
2   Behavior occurs but does not result in intervention.
3   Behavior occurs, resulting in interventions, including the following:

    a Psychotropic medication.
    b Restriction or confinement.
    c Increased observation.
    d Verbal reprimand.

4   Behavior occurs with a major effect (e.g., injury results).
5   Behavior has a severe effect.

---

        (3) Agitation (e.g., pacing, restlessness, repetitive expressions of distress, verbal or physical aggressive behavior not directed at a specific target).
        (4) Wandering (e.g., walking aimlessly in unauthorized areas).
    b. Rating rules. Uses a 5 point scale (Box 5-3).
3. Psychotic symptoms.
    a. Very common, usually in the later stages of the disease.
    b. Consider differential diagnosis:
        (1) Schizophrenia or mood disorder can explain the psychotic symptoms.
        (2) Delusional disorder (might precede the AD).
        (3) Delirium due to some medical problem, medication, or substance.
        (4) Visual disorders such as macular degeneration or cataracts can lead to distortions that account for reports of hallucinations.
        (5) Language impairment can lead to statements that seem bizarre. For example, the patient says "I went to the basement last night" in a site where there is no basement. The person might have a dysphasia and substituted "basement" for "bathroom."
    c. Delusions (occur in 30% to 40% of AD patients) with the following examples:
        (1) People are stealing things. Be sure this is really not happening. This is a vulnerable population.
        (2) Interacting with a dead person.
        (3) Family are impostors.
        (4) Spouse is unfaithful.

     (5) Somatic symptoms.

     (6) Abandonment.

  d. Hallucinations (occur in 15% to 30% of AD patients) with the following examples:

     (1) Seeing or hearing a dead person.

     (2) Seeing or hearing an unfamiliar person.

     (3) Seeing animals.

     (4) Seeing intruders.

     (5) Hearing voices.

     (6) Smelling something.

4. Common medical causes of agitation or psychotic symptoms in AD.

  a. Delirium.

     (1) Central nervous system (CNS). Following a stroke or head injury (consider subdural), metastatic brain disease.

     (2) Infection. Caused by infection with fever, urinary tract infection, pneumonia.

     (3) Repeated hypoxic episodes.

     (4) Significant anemia.

     (5) Metabolic disorders.

       (a) Hypoglycemia.

       (b) Hyponatremia.

  b. Medication effects (Box 5-4).

     (1) Alcohol.

     (2) Anticholinergics.

     (3) Benzodiazepines.

     (4) Caffeine excess.

     (5) Dopamine agonists.

     (6) Narcotics.

     (7) Steroids.

5.3 Medications to Treat Agitation and Psychosis

Medications are listed in Table 5-2; also see Chapters 12 and 14.

There are currently Food and Drug Administration (FDA) approved medications to treat the behavioral or psychotic symptoms that accompany AD. Medication groups used for these symptoms include:

1. Atypical antipsychotics (and conventional neuroleptics)
2. Anticonvulsants
3. Benzodiazepines
4. Trazodone
5. Others:
  a. Hormones
  b. Cholinesterase inhibitors
  c. Memantine
  d. Selective serotonin reuptake inhibitors (SSRIs)

ATYPICAL ANTIPSYCHOTICS

1. The atypical antipsychotics and conventional neuroleptics (e.g., haloperidol) do not have FDA indications to treat the behavioral or

BOX 5-4 Drugs That Produce Agitation

Anticholinergics

Benztropine mesylate (Cogentin)
Diphenhydramine (Benadryl)
Oxybutynin (Ditropan)
Propantheline (Pro-Banthine)
Tricyclics
Trihexyphenidyl (Artane)

Dopaminergics

Bromocriptine
Metoclopramide
Neuroleptic agents
Sinemet
Symmetrel

Sedatives

Alcohol
Barbiturates
Benzodiazepines
Narcotics

Stimulants

Caffeine
Phenylpropanolamine
Pseudoephedrine

Miscellaneous

Digoxin
H_2 antagonists
Phenytoin
Salicylates
Steroids

Table 5-2 Drugs to Treat Agitation in Alzheimer's Disease

Drug Group	Issues in Use
Antipsychotic agents	Extrapyramidal side effects
Benzodiazepines	Sedation
	Cognitive impairment
	Psychomotor impairment
β-Blockers	Hypotension
	Bradycardia
Buspirone	Slow onset
Carbamazepine	Nausea
Lithium	Tremor
	Gastrointestinal upset
	Confusion
Trazodone	Sedation
	Orthostatic hypotension
Valproate	Sedation
	Dizziness
	Tremor

psychological symptoms of AD. However, the atypicals are generally regarded as the treatment of choice when problems are severe and not responsive to other interventions. They include:

a. Aripiprazole (Abilify)
b. Clozapine (Clozaril)
c. Olanzapine (Zyprexa)

    d. Quetiapine (Seroquel)
    e. Risperidone (Risperdal)
    f. Ziprasidone (Geodon)
2. Before using antipsychotics for symptoms accompanying dementia:
    a. Address underlying medical issues.
    b. Address environmental issues.
    c. Document that the symptoms are severe, do not respond to behavioral interventions or re-direction, impair the safety of the patient or others, interfere with the provision of necessary care, and are frequent enough to warrant pharmacologic intervention.
3. Issues in using antipsychotics in AD patients (and elderly patients in general).
    a. Older patients are sensitive to the parkinsonian side effects, and extrapyramidal side effects (EPS) have to be monitored closely because patients might become more incapacitated, especially if they have underlying Parkinson's disease.
        (1) Documentation of Abnormal Involuntary Movement Scale (AIMS) is important (see Chapter 12).
        (2) The atypical antipsychotics are much less likely to produce EPS than the conventional neuroleptics such as haloperidol (see Chapters 12 and 14).
    b. Antipsychotic agents can produce akathisia, resulting in restlessness and agitation (see Chapter 12). Akathisia can be managed by lowering the antipsychotic dose or by giving small doses of β-blockers (propranolol, about 5-10 mg tid) if the patient can tolerate potential bradycardia and hypotension.
    c. Antipsychotic agents should be used at the lowest dose for the shortest time possible.
    d. Table 5-3 summarizes issues involved with their use in patients with AD.
    e. Issues with conventional antipsychotics.
        (1) Thioridazine is no longer an acceptable choice because of associated risk of QT prolongation, especially if it is combined with other medications that prolong its metabolism.
        (2) The high-potency conventional antipsychotics (such as haloperidol, thiothixene, or loxapine) are likely to cause or worsen EPS.
        (3) Haloperidol, even in low doses, is difficult for the elderly to tolerate. Even without obvious dyskinesia, watch for neuroleptized immobility, lack of affect, and withdrawal (which can be mistaken for depression).
        (4) If used for 3 months or more, the conventional antipsychotics carry a high risk of producing tardive dyskinesia, which may be irreversible.
    f. Issues with atypical antipsychotics.
        (1) Metabolic issues. The atypicals, as a class, appear to increase the risk of developing glucose dysregulation and lipid dysregulation.
            (a) When starting an atypical, a baseline measure of glucose should be done, and glucose should be monitored

Table 5-3   **Effects of Antipsychotic Agents for Psychotic Symptoms of Alzheimer's Disease**

Drug	$T_{1/2}$ (h) (mean)	P-450 Substrate	Effect	
			WBC Monitoring	Anticholinergic
Haloperidol (Haldol)	12-36 (16)	2D6, 1A2		
Clozapine (Clozaril)	9-30	2D6, 3A	+	+++
Risperidone (Risperdal)	11-105 (16)	1A2, 2C19, 2C9		+
Olanzapine (Zyprexa)	3-24 (3.6)	2D6, 3A		
Quetiapine (Seroquel)	20-70 (30)	1A2		
Ziprasidone (Geodon)	6	3A4		
Aripiprazole (Abilify)	24-200 (70)	2D6		

WBC, white blood cell.

periodically thereafter (e.g., every 3 months for maintenance patients).

(b) Because patients can develop serious sequelae of glucose dysregulation (e.g., hyperosmolar nonketotic coma), any clinical symptoms suggestive of hyperglycemia should lead to immediate assessment.

(c) When starting an atypical, a baseline lipid panel should be done. Although there are no standard guidelines, patients on maintenance should be periodically reassessed.

(d) Weight gain is generally not as problematic in the elderly as it is in younger patients, especially because frail elderly can benefit from some weight gain.

(2) Cerebrovascular adverse events and death.

(a) Recent data indicate there is a small increased risk for cerebrovascular adverse events and death in elderly dementia patients on atypical antipsychotics. The risk on placebo is in the range of 1% to 3% and on atypicals is approximately double the placebo rate, though still small.

(b) Because of the added risk, atypicals should be used only when behavioral nonpharmacologic interventions do not work, the symptoms in questions are serious, and the patient consents.

(c) It appears that the risk of cerebrovascular adverse events or death with the conventional antipsychotics may be as high as or higher than for the atypical antipsychotics.

Aripiprazole (Abilify)

1. Data are emerging on efficacy in this population.
2. The initial dose is 2.5 mg qd, titrating up to 15 mg/day.
3. Dose-related somnolence is reported.

Clozapine (Clozaril)

1. There is a very low incidence of EPS.
2. Clozapine is helpful in managing psychosis associated with Parkinson's disease without worsening EPS.
3. AD patients and elderly patients might have difficulty tolerating it due to:
   a. High anticholinergic activity
   b. Need for monitoring of white blood cell (WBC) count due to potential for neutropenia and agranulocytosis
   c. Orthostatic hypotension
   d. Sedation
   e. Drooling, which can lead to aspiration
4. Chronic schizophrenics (with or without concurrent dementia) maintained in the community on clozapine and who are tolerating it well continue taking it unless the prescribing psychiatrist is consulted. Schizophrenia in that patient is likely to have been refractory to other antipsychotics.

5. If clozapine is used in an elderly patient, the initial dose should be as low as 6.25 mg/day and raised very gradually.

Olanzapine (Zyprexa)

1. The usual effective dose range is 5 to 10 mg/day.
2. Olanzapine may be associated with initial somnolence.
3. It can cause some abnormal gait.
4. It has some anticholinergic activity, which can make it less suitable for use in AD patients, though the anticholinergic activity is minimal.
5. Formulations:
   a. The orally disintegrating tablet formulation dissolves without swallowing.
   b. An intramuscular (IM) formulation can be used in emergencies.

Quetiapine (Seroquel)

1. Quetiapine requires titration to avoid excess initial sedation.
   a. Starting dose is usually 25 to 50 mg bid.
   b. Dose might need to be titrated up to 100 mg tid.
2. It has a low likelihood of causing EPS, so it can be helpful in patients who have tremor or dyskinesia.

Risperidone (Risperdal)

1. Double blind data support its efficacy in elderly dementia patients with psychosis and agitated behavior.
2. Doses of 0.25 to 0.5 mg bid are usually adequate.
3. EPS is unusual at doses less than 2 mg/day (most elderly nonschizophrenic patients can be managed at or below that dose).
4. Because Risperdal's active metabolite is renally excreted, use lower doses in those with renal failure.
5. Some patients with Parkinson's disease develop tremor. Those patients should be tried on quetiapine or clozapine.
6. Formulations:
   a. Risperidone elixir (odorless and tasteless) is an excellent alternative for patients who are paranoid or in emergency situations as an alternative to IM haloperidol.
   b. The orally disintegrating tablet formulation dissolves without swallowing.
   c. The delayed-release IM formulation (Risperdal Consta) can be helpful in a setting where compliance is a problem once a patient has been confirmed to tolerate the drug and requires maintenance treatment.

Ziprasidone (Geodon)

1. Data on use in the elderly are not extensive.
2. There are some concerns over QTc prolongation in a population such as elderly patients who may have silent myocardial infarctions and underlying cardiac conduction delays. Therefore, obtain an electrocardiogram (ECG) before use.
3. Dosing generally starts at 20 mg qd and goes to 20 mg bid.

Use of Atypicals in Patients with Parkinsonian Symptoms

Any atypical antipsychotic may be used, although quetiapine and clozapine appear to have a lower risk of worsening dyskinesia. Lower the dopamine agonist dose if possible. P450 interactions are listed in Table 5-4.

ANTICONVULSANTS

Anticonvulsants are discussed in Chapter 8 and Box 5-5).

1. General issues.
   a. These drugs may be effective in elderly dementia patients with episodic behavioral agitation or aggression, whether or not they have seizure disorder. The evidence base is less than that for the atypical antipsychotics. Some recent data have questioned efficacy, so this is not a first-line approach.
   b. Start at low doses and gradually build up to usual anticonvulsant plasma levels, even though the plasma level to treat behavioral symptoms is not established.
2. Carbamazepine.
   a. Limiting factors are nausea, diplopia, ataxia, and sedation (also see Chapter 8).

Table 5-4 **Examples of P-450 Interactions with Atypical Antipsychotics**

P-450 family	Inhibitor	Substrate	Inducer
2D6	Fluoxetine	Risperidone	Paroxetine
3A4	Nefazodone	Quetiapine	Phenytoin
	Erythromycin	Ziprasidone	Carbamazepine
	Ketoconazole		
	Diltiazem		
1A2	Fluvoxamine	Clozapine	Smoking
	Ciprofloxacin	Olanzapine	Caffeine

BOX 5-5   Issues in the Use of Anticonvulsants

Carbamazepine
Monitor CBC, LFTs, drug level
Side effects: Nausea, dizziness, ataxia, sedation, pancreatitis, cardiac

Valproate
Monitor LFTs, drug level
Side effects: Nausea, tremor, ataxia

CBC, complete blood count; LFT, liver function test.

  b. Start at 50 to 100 mg tid and obtain a level in 5 days. Based on plasma level, titrate dose upward. Most case reports have used 300 mg/day.
3. Valproic acid.
  a. Limiting factors are nausea, tremor, and occasional increases in LFTs (also see Chapter 8).
  b. Potential for drug interaction is reduced compared with carbamazepine.
  c. Start at 125 mg bid or tid and obtain a level in 5 days, along with aspartate transaminase (AST) and alanine transaminase (ALT). Based on clinical response, titrate dose upward. Effects have been reported with plasma levels ranging from 25 to 90 µg/mL. Behavioral effects are common at around 50 µg/mL.
  d. Divalproex sodium (Depakote) is the preferred agent because of better gastrointestinal (GI) tolerability. The sprinkle formulation can be helpful; and an extended-release (ER) formulation can simplify dosing once a standing dose is established.

BENZODIAZEPINES

Benzodiazepines (see Table 10-1) may be used to treat agitation in elderly AD patients.

1. Limiting factors are sedation, cognitive impairment, ataxia, paradoxical increase in agitation, amnestic effects, tolerance, and withdrawal.
2. Lorazepam in doses of 1 to 2 mg (PO or IM) may be helpful for short-term use to reduce agitation associated with anxiety, for sleep problems, and for muscle tension.
3. Short-acting agents such as alprazolam and oxazepam are preferable because of less likelihood of accumulation with repeated dosages.

TRAZODONE (DESYREL)

1. Trazodone usually has an acute effect on calming an agitated patient with AD in oral doses from 25 to 100 mg.
2. Single doses can sometimes quiet a screaming AD patient who has not been able to tolerate or who has not responded to other medication.
3. In addition to acute sedation, maintenance over 3 to 6 weeks can decrease agitation using doses of 25 to 50 mg tid.
4. Limiting factors are sedation and orthostasis. Orthostasis can be a significant problem when trazodone is used alone or especially when it is combined with other drugs that lower blood pressure (e.g., nitrates, β-blockers) or when it is used in patients with hypovolemia or gait disturbances.

OTHER MEDICATIONS TO TREAT AGITATION

1. Hormonal therapies.
  a. A very small number of published cases reported using estrogen to decrease aggressive physical behavior in elderly men with AD.
    (1) Some patients have been started with conjugated estrogen 0.625 mg/day for 3 to 4 days, then increased to 1.25 mg/day.
    (2) Side effects of estrogen.
      (a) Fluid retention.
      (b) Hypophosphatemia.

    (c) Gynecomastia.
    (d) Decreased libido.
  b. Diethylstilbestrol (DES) 1 to 2 mg/day or medroxyprogesterone acetate (MPA) have been used in other published cases.
2. Acetylcholinesterase inhibitors and memantine (Namenda). These agents have been shown to reduce the likelihood of emergence of behavioral problems. However, once an acute symptom (such as agitation or psychosis) emerges, it is usually necessary to use some other agent, such as an atypical antipsychotic.
3. SSRIs.
  a. SSRIs may be helpful in reducing agitation associated with agitated depression.
  b. SSRIs can reduce episodic crying (emotional incontinence in post-stroke and AD patients.

5.4 Cognitive Symptoms

ELIMINATING FACTORS THAT CONTRIBUTE TO COGNITIVE IMPAIRMENT

1. Examples of drug-induced cognitive impairment.
  a. Anticholinergics. Try to decrease or eliminate oxybutynin (Ditropan), diphenhydramine, tricyclic antidepressants, benztropine mesylate (Cogentin), trihexyphenidyl (Artane).
  b. Benzodiazepines. Try to gradually taper benzodiazepines. Short-acting agents must be reduced gradually to prevent rebound agitation or anxiety.
  c. Digoxin. Levels more than 1.5 g/mL often have behavioral side effects.
  d. Dopamine agonists. Carbidopa–levodopa (Sinemet) and bromocriptine can produce depression, anxiety, or psychotic symptoms.
  e. H_2 blockers. Try to reduce, eliminate, or substitute for H_2 blockers.
  f. Lidocaine can cause agitation and confusion.
  g. Narcotics. Older patients are vulnerable to confusion from narcotics.
  h. Phenytoin. Always check the plasma level to be sure it is not too high (causing confusion) or too low (not adequate to control underlying seizure tendency).
  i. Salicylates. At high levels, salicylates lead to metabolic acidosis and anxious agitation.
  j. Theophylline. Levels 5 µg/mL or higher can cause anxiety, agitation, or confusion.
2. Other causes of cognitive impairment.
  a. Impaired sensory organs.
    (1) Vision. Common problems include macular degeneration, cataracts, incorrect prescription for glasses, and not using glasses.
    (2) Hearing.
      (a) This may be the most common correctable source of confusion.
      (b) Be sure hearing aid is working properly and is used.
  b. Medical and medication causes (see Boxes 3-1 and 3-2).

TREATMENT OF COGNITIVE IMPAIRMENT
Drugs Used to Treat Cognitive Impairment
1. Acetylcholinesterase inhibitors.
    a. Donepezil (Aricept)
    b. Rivastigmine (Exelon)
    c. Galantamine (Reminyl)
    d. Tacrine (Cognex) is rarely used now because of the need to monitor LFTs and problems with GI tolerability.
2. N-methyl-D-aspartate (NMDA) receptor antagonist. Memantine (Namenda)

Treatment
1. There is no current curative treatment.
2. Acetylcholinesterase inhibitors and memantine can:
    a. Delay the progression of cognitive loss.
    b. Help maintain functional status.
    c. Reduce the emergence of behavioral complications.
    d. Reduce time required of caregivers.
3. The effects of acetylcholinesterase inhibitors and memantine may be modest; however, there may be considerable value to individual patients and families of having their disease progression delayed. For example, such a delay can result in delay in nursing home admission.
4. Acetylcholinesterase inhibitors are indicated for the treatment of mild to moderate AD (Mini Mental State Exam [MMSE] range 10 to 24).
    a. There are more similarities than differences among the agents.
    b. They share medical issues:
        (1) Vagotonic effects can cause bradycardia. Use with caution in patients with sick sinus syndrome and other supraventricular cardiac conduction abnormalities.
        (2) Increased gastric acid secretion can lead to GI problems in patients with gastroesophageal reflux disease (GERD) or peptic ulcer disease and in patients on nonsteroidal antiinflammatory drugs (NSAIDs).
        (3) GI side effects include diarrhea, nausea, vomiting.
            (a) GI side effects are usually dose related.
            (b) GI effects can often be managed by lowering the dose and/ or taking longer to titrate up.
        (4) Drug interactions.
            (a) Can interfere with activity of anticholinergic drugs.
            (b) Can augment succinylcholine and bethanechol. Succinylcholine is used as part of electroconvulsive therapy (ECT) anesthesia. There is debate about the clinical relevance of this interaction. Always discuss with the anesthesiologist before ECT.
            (c) Donepezil and galantamine levels may be increased by P450 2D6 inhibitors.
        (5) Dosing.
            (a) Donepezil. Start with 5 mg hs and increase to 10 mg hs after 1 month.

   (b) Rivastigmine. Start with 1.5 mg bid; increase to 3 mg bid
       after 2 weeks, 4.5 mg bid after 2 more weeks, and 6 mg bid
       after 2 more weeks. A slower titration may be needed if GI
       side effects occur.
   (c) Galantamine. Start with 4 mg bid (bid actually means with
       breakfast and dinner in this case, because GI side effects are
       reduced if the drug is taken with meals). Increase to 8 mg
       bid after 1 month. An extended-release formulation
       (Razadyne ER) allows once-daily dosing.
5. Clinical use of memantine (Namenda).
   a. This medication works, in part, by blocking excitatory effects of
      excess glutamate, which can be neurotoxic.
   b. Indication is for moderate to severe AD (MMSE 3 to 14)
   c. Generally well tolerated.
   d. In patients with moderate to severe AD, memantine can reduce
      cognitive decline and maintain activities of daily living.
   e. Combined use with other NMDA agonists such as amantadine,
      ketamine, and dextromethorphan can potentially lead to psychoto-
      mimetic symptoms, although this is rarely reported.
   f. Memantine can be used in combination with donepezil and
      galantamine.
   g. Discontinuation rates are similar to placebo.
   h. Dosing. Start with 5 mg hs; after 1 week go to 5 mg bid; after
      2 weeks go to 5 mg AM and 10 mg hs; after 3 weeks go to 10 mg
      bid.
6. Other agents used to treat cognitive symptoms of AD.
   a. Vitamin E. High doses (1000 IU bid) have been reported to delay
      the progression of cognitive symptoms and also delay time to nurs-
      ing home admission. Recent concerns about safety of high-dose
      vitamin E has put its general use in question.
   b. Monoamine oxidase-B inhibitors: selegiline, L-deprenyl.
   c. Current evidence is not strong enough to support use of NSAIDs,
      estrogen, or gingko.

5.5 Anxiety

Anxiety occurs in 5% to 35% of Alzheimer's disease patients.

1. Etiology.
   a. Anxiety secondary to some medical condition is the most common
      cause (see Boxes 9-2 and 9-5).
   b. Fearful anticipation is common.
   c. Long-standing anxiety (such as generalized anxiety disorder) con-
      tinues into old age.
   d. Anxiety symptoms (panic or obsessive–compulsive) can emerge
      during episodes of depression.
2. Treatment.
   a. Chapter 10 provides details on use of antianxiety agents.
   b. Generalized anxiety (also see Table 10-1).
      (1) Buspirone (BuSpar).

      (a) Buspirone is not sedative and therefore does not produce psychomotor impairment, drowsiness, or cognitive impairment. (see Chapter 10). Starting dose is 5 mg tid.

      (b) Buspirone side effects are uncommon but include nausea, nonvertiginous lightheadedness, and dull headache.

      (c) Antianxiety effect usually takes several weeks.

      (d) There have been rare case reports of serotonin syndrome (see Chapter 7) from the combination of several serotonin-augmenting agents.

    (2) Benzodiazepines.

      (a) Benzodiazepines have liabilities for the elderly, including psychomotor impairments, excessive sedation, and cognitive impairment.

      (b) Always use short-acting benzodiazepines (e.g., lorazepam) in preference to longer-acting agents in elderly patients.

  c. Severe anxiety may require use of low doses of atypical antipsychotics (e.g., risperidone 0.25 mg bid).

  d. OBRA regulations.

    (1) OBRA regulations on the use of benzodiazepines in nursing homes require trying short-acting agents before long-acting agents.

    (2) OBRA regulations on use of hypnotics in nursing homes require the following:

      (a) Document a differential diagnosis.

      (b) Document that the medication improved function.

      (c) Hypnotic medication may not be used for more than 10 days without documenting an attempt to reduce it (this is why clinicians opt to use nonhypnotic medications such as trazodone).

5.6 Depression

1. Significant symptoms of depression occur in 5% to 50% of patients with AD; neurovegetative signs might not be prominent (also see Chapter 5).
   a. Tearful episodes.
   b. Poor appetite and weight loss.
   c. Mood fluctuations.
   d. Apathy, withdrawn behavior.
   e. Social isolation.
   f. Irritability.
   g. Dysphoria.
2. Differential diagnosis.
   a. Major depression. Look for past episodes, because this is a chronic recurrent disease.
   b. Underlying medical issue (see Chapter 3).
   c. Drug-induced depressive syndromes (see Box 6-2).
   d. Dysthymia.
   e. Grief or bereavement.
   f. Post-stroke depression.

    g. Dementia-related apathy.

    h. Dementia-related affective dysregulation (emotional incontinence).

    i. Vascular dementia with executive dysfunction.

3. Use of antidepressants.

    a. Antidepressants are indicated for depression that accompanies AD. Chapter 7 provides detailed information on the use of antidepressants.

    b. Table 5-5 summarizes issues pertinent to their use in AD.

    c. Because pseudodementia is always a possibility, it is wise to err on the side of giving a trial of antidepressants, because often there is little to lose and much to gain.

    d. Tricyclic antidepressants have drawbacks.

       (1) Anticholinergic activity can worsen cognition.

       (2) Orthostasis can lead to falls and fractures.

       (3) Cardiac conduction delay can lead to arrhythmias.

       (4) Inadvertent overdose may be lethal.

    e. SSRIs and other second-generation agents.

       (1) Generally well tolerated.

       (2) Effective in many cases, despite lack of well-controlled evidence.

       (3) Side-effect issues with SSRIs:

          (a) Agitation (somewhat more of an issue with fluoxetine).

          (b) GI side effects and nausea (also see Chapter 7).

          (c) Hyponatremia.

          (d) Initial doses should be conservative. See Chapter 7 for more details.

5.7 Some Common Medical Issues

SLEEP DISTURBANCES

Sleep disturbances are covered in Chapter 11. Common causes in the elderly should be addressed.

1. Caffeine use should always be considered.
2. Environmental causes should be eliminated.
    a. Noise.
    b. Lights.
3. Nocturnal myoclonus (about 15% prevalence).
4. Restless legs (about 5% prevalence).
5. Sleep apnea (affects 25% to 70%).
6. Sedative—hypnotic dependence.
7. Reversed day—night cycle. Easier said than done: Keep the patient from napping during the day. Trial of melatonin agonist may be helpful.

EATING DISTURBANCES

1. Inadequate nutrition is a problem for 20% to 60% of older patients in nursing homes.
2. A serum albumin of less than 3.5 g/dL indicates protein depletion.
3. Drug-induced anorexia.
    a. Digoxin.
    b. NSAIDs.

Table 5-5   Issues in the Use of Antidepressants in Patients with Alzheimer's Disease

Drug	Anticholinergic	Sedation	Activation	Orthostasis	Gastrointestinal	Cardiac Conduction Delay
Bupropion	0	0/+	++	0	0	0
Mirtazapine	0	+++	0	0	0	0
Nefazodone	0	++/+++	0	+	0	0
SSRIs	0	0/++	0/++	0	Nausea	0
Trazodone	0	+++	0	+++	0	0
Tricyclics	++/++++	+/++++		++/++++	Constipation	0
Venlafaxine	0	0/++	0/++	0	Nausea	Increased BP potential

BP, blood pressure; SSRI, selective serotonin reuptake inhibitor.

    c. Theophylline.
    d. Hydrochlorothiazide.
4. Drug-induced hypogeusia (loss of taste).
    a. Allopurinol.
    b. Clindamycin.
    c. Antihistamines.
5. Drug-induced vitamin or mineral deficiencies.
    a. Diuretics can lead to zinc deficiency.
    b. Salicylates can lead to vitamin C deficiency.
    c. Anticonvulsants can lead to vitamin D and folate deficiency.
    d. Tetracycline can lead to calcium or iron deficiency.
    e. Mineral oil can lead to vitamin A or D deficiency.
6. Causes of weight loss in ambulatory geriatric patients.
    a. Unknown: about 25%.
    b. Depression: about 20%.
    c. Cancer: about 15%.
    d. Other gastrointestinal disease: about 10%.
    e. Hyperthyroidism: about 10%.
    f. Secondary to medications: about 10%.
    g. Neurologic abnormalities (AD, cerebrovascular accident [CVA]): about 7%.
    h. Other (tuberculosis, poor eating habits): about 5%.

INCONTINENCE

1. Incontinence occurs in 40% to 60% of older patients in hospitals and nursing homes and 25% in the community.
2. Drug-induced overflow incontinence.
    a. Anticholinergics.
    b. Smooth muscle relaxants, for example, nifedipine.
    c. α-Adrenergic agonists, for example, phenylpropanolamine.
3. Drug-induced urge incontinence.
    a. Diuretics.
    b. Lithium.
    c. Tamoxifen.
    d. Drug-induced oversedation.
    e. Benzodiazepines.
    f. Antipsychotics.
4. Nondrug differential diagnosis of incontinence is summarized by the well-known mnemonic DIAPERS (Box 5-6).

MOBILITY IMPAIRMENT

1. A large number of medical conditions contribute to mobility impairment.
    a. Neurologic diseases.
        (1) CVA.
        (2) Parkinson's disease.
        (3) Normal pressure hydrocephalus.
        (4) Neuropathy.
        (5) Subdural hematomas.
        (6) Vitamin B_{12} deficiency.
        (7) Cervical spondylosis.

BOX 5-6   DIAPERS

Delirium and dementia
Infections
Atrophic vaginitis, urethritis, atonic bladder
Psychiatric disorders (e.g., depression), prostatism
Endocrine abnormalities (diabetes, hypercalcemia, hypothyroidism)
Restricted mobility
Stool impaction (causes up to 10% of incontinence in nursing homes)

    b. Unsuspected fractures.
    c. Arthritis.
    d. Delirium and dementia.
    e. Depression.
    f. Fearfulness.
2. Drug-induced causes of mobility impairment.
    a. Dopamine blockers.
        (1) Neuroleptic agents.
        (2) Metoclopramide.
    b. Hypotension.
        (1) Diuretics.
        (2) Vasodilators.
        (3) Tricyclic antidepressants.
    c. Muscle weakness (steroids).

5.8 Omnibus Budget Reconciliation Act Regulations

Congress enacted legislation to improve the quality of care in nursing homes as part of the 1987 Omnibus Budget Reconciliation Act (OBRA). These guidelines mandate patient assessment and limit psychotropic drug use involving benzodiazepines, neuroleptic agents, and sedative–hypnotics.

1. Guidelines for short-acting benzodiazepines (e.g., lorazepam, oxazepam, alprazolam). If you intend to prescribe one of these drugs, you must document the following:
    a. Differential diagnosis of the symptoms (e.g., consider organic causes, depression, and other causes).
    b. Number and nature of symptoms being treated (if such symptoms are considered secondary to dementia).
    c. That the medication results in some functional improvement.
    d. A gradual reduction of medication after every 4 months, until such reduction attempts have failed twice within a year.
2. Guidelines for the use of long-acting benzodiazepines (diazepam, chlordiazepoxide, clonazepam, and clorazepate). If you plan to use one of these medications, you must document the following:
    a. Failure with a short-acting benzodiazepine.

  b. A differential diagnosis.
  c. Maintenance or improvement in function.
  d. A gradual reduction every 4 months until such attempts have failed twice within a year.
3. Guidelines for the use of hypnotics (flurazepam, estazolam, triazolam, and temazepam). If you intend to prescribe a sleeping pill, you must document the following:
  a. A differential diagnosis.
  b. That the medication results in improved function.
  c. An attempt to reduce the dose if you use the medication for more than 10 days.
4. Guidelines for the use of neuroleptic agents.
  a. OBRA guidelines do not apply to use of neuroleptic agents for psychiatric diagnoses such as schizophrenia or organic psychotic disorders.
  b. You may not prescribe neuroleptic agents for wandering, anxiety, unsociability, uncooperativeness, poor self-care, and agitated behavior that is not a danger.
  c. The guidelines are meant to apply to behavioral control of agitated behavior associated with AD.
  d. If you use a neuroleptic agent in those circumstances, you must document the following.
    (1) Number and content of episodes.
    (2) Failure of other means of control.
    (3) That the symptoms present some danger or functional loss or are of psychotic nature.
    (4) Reassessment of the orders and treatment plan if prn neuroleptic agents are used more than twice in a 7-day period.
    (5) Side effects.
      (a) Tardive dyskinesia.
      (b) Orthostasis.
      (c) Akathisia.
      (d) Parkinsonian symptoms.
      (e) Cognitive or behavioral impairment.
    (6) Gradual dose reduction unless you document two failed attempts to taper within a 1-year period.
    (7) Reasons for exceeding OBRA dose guidelines (examples of dose guidelines include haloperidol (Haldol) 4 mg/day, thioridazine (Mellaril) 75 mg/day, and perphenazine (Trilafon) 8 mg/day. Prescribing outside the guidelines is allowed as long as good clinical reasoning is documented. Simply listing a symptom is not enough.

SUGGESTED READINGS

American Diabetes Association, American Psychiatric Association, American Association of Clinical Endocrinologists, et al: Consensus development conference on antipsychotic drugs and obesity and diabetes. Diabetes Care 27:596-601, 2004.

Cooper AJ: Medroxyprogesterone acetate (MPA) treatment of sexual acting out in men suffering from dementia. J Clin Psychiatry 48:368-370, 1987.

Cummings JL: Use of cholinesterase inhibitors in clinical practice: Evidence-based recommendations. *Am J Geriatr Psychiatry* 11:131-145, 2003.

Knopman DS, DeKosky ST, Cummings JL, et al: Practice parameter: Diagnosis of dementia (an evidence-based review): Report of the Quality Standards Subcommittee of the American Academy of Neurology. *Neurology* 56:1143-1153, 2001.

Mungas D, Weiler P, Franzi C, Henry R: Assessment of disruptive behavior associated with dementia: The disruptive behavior rating scales. *J Geriatr Psychiatry Neurol* 2:196-202, 1989.

Ritchie CW, Ames D, Clayton T, Lai R: Metaanalysis of randomized trials of the efficacy and safety of donepezil, galantamine, and rivastigmine for the treatment of Alzheimer's disease. *Am J Geriatr Psychiatry* 12:358-369, 2004.

Schneider LS, Dagerman K, Insel P: Efficacy and adverse effects of atypical antipsychotics for dementia: Meta-analysis of randomized, placebo-controlled trials. *Am J Geriatr Psychiatry* 14:191-210, 2006.

Schneider LS, Dagerman KS, Insel P: Risk of death with atypical antipsychotic drug treatment for dementia. *JAMA* 294:1934-1943, 2005.

Tariot PN, Farlow MR, Grossberg GT, et al. Memantine treatment in patients with moderate to severe Alzheimer disease already receiving donepezil: A randomized controlled trial. *JAMA* 291:317-324, 2004.

Depression: Identification and Diagnosis

6

Michael A. Posternak
Mark Zimmerman

6.1 General Issues of Identification

1. The term "depression" can mean many different things. Therefore when patients say they are "depressed," it is important to ask, "What do you mean by 'depressed'?"
2. The term "depression" may be used to refer to many things, including the following:
   a. Major depressive disorder (major depression).
   b. Depression secondary to some medical cause.
   c. Adjustment disorder with depressed mood.
   d. Dysthymic disorder (chronic minor depression).
   e. Brief depressive reaction.
   f. Grief.
   g. Bereavement.
   h. Chronic emptiness of the borderline personality.
   i. A component of schizoaffective disorder.
   j. The depressive phase of bipolar disorder.
   k. Boredom, dissatisfaction, loneliness.
   l. Loss of motivation secondary to brain disease (dementia).
3. Because "depression" can mean so many different things, try to be more precise. Start the evaluation by listing "depressive symptoms," as given in Figure 6-1, which presents a summary of the five areas of history pertinent to evaluating depressive symptoms.
   a. Delineation of depressive symptoms themselves and their duration.
   b. Accompanying symptoms (for differential diagnosis).
   c. Possible precipitants and issues (for potential psychotherapy).
   d. Possible medical causes.
   e. Past episodes.

6.2 Strategy for Evaluating Depression

1. Step one.
   a. Consider "depression secondary to a medical cause," which the *Diagnostic and Statistical Manual of Mental Disorders*, fourth edition (DSM-IV), refers to as "mood disorder due to a general medical condition."
   b. Identify and correct (if possible) potential medical causes of depressive symptoms (Boxes 6-1 and 6-2).

Depressive symptoms	Duration
Depressed mood	_____
Decreased energy	_____
Poor concentration	_____
Sleep change	_____
Appetite change	_____
Psychomotor change	_____
Guilt, poor self-esteem	_____
Anhedonia	_____
Suicidality	_____
Chronic pain	_____
Poor functional level	_____
Somatized symptoms	_____

Accompanying symptoms:

Delusions	Panic attacks	Mania
Hallucinations	Generalized anxiety	

Possible precipitants:

_____

_____

Possible medical causes:

_____

_____

Past episodes:

_____

_____

Figure 6-1 Depressive symptoms database.

2. Step two.
   a. Identify psychosocial stressors that warrant attention (see "Psychosocial Review of Systems," Chapter 2).
      (1) Personal or family relationships.
      (2) Work or school problems.
      (3) Living situation.
      (4) Medical status.
      (5) Developmental issues (e.g., retirement).
   b. Decide if psychosocial issues can be addressed by some type of psychotherapy or counseling. If you believe there is a problem that should be addressed because of its relevance to the patient's depressive symptoms, you should state this clearly to the patient and either provide that component of treatment or make an appropriate referral.

BOX 6-1   Examples of Medical Causes of Depressive Symptoms

Autoimmune disorders
- Systemic lupus erythematosus

Cerebrovascular disease
- Stroke

Endocrine disorders
- Hepatic failure
- Hypercalcemia
- Hypercortisolism
- Hyperparathyroidism
- Hyperthyroidism
- Hypocortisolism
- Hypokalemia
- Hypoparathyroidism
- Hypothyroidism
- Renal failure

Epilepsy

Infections
- Hepatitis
- Human immunodeficiency virus
- Mononucleosis

Malignancies
- Gastrointestinal
- Pancreatic

Metabolic disorders
- Diabetes mellitus
- Hypoxia
- Vitamin B_{12} deficiency

Neurologic disorders
- Alzheimer's disease
- Huntington's disease
- Multiple sclerosis
- Parkinson's disease

Sleep apnea

Structural brain disease
- Brain tumor
- Stroke

BOX 6-2   Medications and Substances Causing Depressive Symptoms

Alcohol
Amantadine
Anabolic steroids
Anticholinergic agents
Anticonvulsant agents
Barbiturates
Benzodiazepines
Cimetidine
Clonidine

Corticosteroids
α-Methyldopa
Oral contraceptives
Propranolol
Ranitidine
Reserpine
Sedatives
Stimulant (withdrawal)
Thiazides

---

3. Step three.
   a. Consider the possibility of major depression or other affective disorder.
   b. Use a target symptom approach to decide whether antidepressant medication should be a component of treatment. Treat depressive symptoms with medication if they are severe enough, even if it is impossible to sort out whether they are caused by major

depression, adjustment disorder, or some untreatable underlying medical factors.

6.3 Mood Disorder Resulting from a General Medical Condition

DEFINITION AND IDENTIFICATION

1. In the past, this category was called "organic affective disorder." However, because major depression is an "organic disorder," this terminology has been eliminated. For example, depressive symptoms caused by hypothyroidism are listed as "mood disorder due to hypothyroidism."
2. Box 6-1 lists selected medical causes of depressive symptoms.
3. Box 6-2 lists medications and substances that are associated with depressive symptoms.
4. Potential medical causes should be considered in every patient with depression. The extent of the medical evaluation should be determined by the medical history and review of systems. For example:
   a. In a healthy 28-year-old with depressive symptoms and a negative medical review of systems, an extensive medical work-up is not warranted.
   b. In a patient with a history of lung cancer or breast cancer, the onset of depressive symptoms should raise consideration of a metastatic brain lesion. A careful neurologic and mental status examination should be performed.
   c. Neuroimaging does not play a role in the routine evaluation of depression. However, it may be indicated in patients with an underlying disease that commonly involves the central nervous system (CNS) (e.g., lung cancer, breast cancer, multiple myeloma, and acquired immunodeficiency syndrome [AIDS]).
   d. In elderly patients and in those for whom dementia is a possible diagnosis, a comprehensive dementia evaluation should always be done (see Box 4-2).
   e. Always have a high level of suspicion for the presence of substance abuse, because it has a high comorbidity with depression. Sedative substances, notably alcohol, and stimulant withdrawal are common medical causes of depressive symptoms.
      (1) A definitive diagnosis of major depression cannot be made in the presence of active substance abuse. Diagnose "mood disorder due to [substance]."
      (2) Substance use should be regarded as the primary diagnosis and managed accordingly. Antidepressants can play a role, but they should usually be reserved until after the substance use disorder has been effectively treated.
      (3) Patients in substance abuse programs should have careful assessment for underlying mood disorder that might contribute to relapse.
5. There is no recipe for the medical work-up of depression. The work-up is determined by the specific medical conditions that could affect the CNS.

DIFFERENTIAL DIAGNOSIS

1. Do not assume that depression is necessarily caused by some obvious psychosocial distress.
   a. For example, it would be a mistake to dismiss an evaluation by saying, "Wouldn't you be depressed if you had cancer?" After all, most cancer patients do *not* develop major depression. Certainly, patients with severe medical illness face difficult psychological issues; however, such patients might have depressive symptoms because of hypercalcemia, brain metastases, or severe anemia.
   b. At the same time, it is important not to ignore some of the psychological impact of cancer, which might need to be addressed concurrently with a medical–psychiatric diagnostic evaluation.
2. "Mood disorder due to a general medical condition" deserves consideration in every differential diagnosis of depressive symptoms.

PROGNOSIS

1. Depressive symptoms secondary to some medical cause usually resolve when the underlying medical problem is corrected.
   a. Patients in pain often exhibit depressive symptoms that disappear when the pain is adequately treated.
   b. Patients taking drugs that cause depression (such as alcohol or antihypertensive agents) often recover when that drug is discontinued.
2. Because depressive symptoms can have multifactorial causes, the correction of underlying medical problems (such as mild hypothyroidism) might not resolve all depressive symptoms.
3. If the medical condition has caused permanent neuronal damage (such as with toxic substances), some symptoms might not be resolved.

TREATMENT

1. All potential medical causes of depression should be corrected to the extent possible.
2. In many cases, the relationship between an underlying medical factor and the depressive symptoms cannot be confirmed. For example, if the patient is taking a drug that might cause depression, such as a histamine-2 blocker, the practical approach is to change to some alternative drug.
3. The presence of contributing medical factors does not exclude the need for other dimensions of therapy. For example, a patient with depression secondary to steroids might need antidepressants and certainly might benefit from psychotherapy for issues related to the illness experience.

6.4 Major Depressive Disorder (Major Depression)

DEFINITION AND IDENTIFICATION

1. Major depression was formerly called "endogenous depression."
   a. The distinction between "exogenous" and "endogenous" depression is no longer considered useful.

  b. In the past, "exogenous" implied a less serious, non–biologically based depression that did not require antidepressants. "Endogenous" implied a more serious, biologically based depression. However, many major depressions are triggered by some external event.
  c. Therefore the presence or absence of some identifiable external event is not relevant to making a diagnosis of major depression, although it may be important as an issue to be addressed in treatment.
2. Major depression is defined by the presence of specific symptoms. There is no pathognomonic biological marker for major depression, although its diagnosis implies an underlying psychobiologic disorder.

Criteria for Diagnosis

Criteria for diagnosing an episode of major depression are given in Box 6-3.

1. Five or more of symptoms must be:
   a. Present during the same 2-week period.
   b. Represent a change from previous functioning.
2. At least one of the symptoms must be depressed mood or loss of interest or pleasure.
3. Symptoms that are clearly the result of a medical condition or psychotic process should not be included.
4. The depressive symptoms cannot be caused by some medical condition or bereavement.
5. Depressive symptoms.
   a. Depressed mood (most of the day, nearly every day). It is useful to ask patients, "Have you been feeling sad or discouraged recently?" Some patients might deny being "depressed," considering it a sign of weakness that involves some stigma.
   b. Markedly diminished interest or pleasure in most activities. Ask, "Do you feel that you are not enjoying things as much as you would expect to or as much as you used to?"

BOX 6-3   Diagnostic Criteria for Major Depression

At least five of the following symptoms are present continuously over 2 weeks. One of the symptoms must be either depressed mood or anhedonia.
Depressed mood
Anhedonia
Appetite change or weight change
Sleep disturbance
Psychomotor agitation or retardation
Fatigue
Feeling worthless or guilty
Poor concentration
Suicidal thoughts

    c. Fatigue. Fatigue is one of the most common presenting complaints to primary care physicians. Depression is one of the most common disorders underlying this symptom.

    d. Decreased concentration and indecisiveness. Depression is not just a mood disorder; it is also a cognitive disorder. When the cognitive impairment is prominent, especially in the elderly, clinicians often misdiagnose the problem as dementia (a.k.a. "pseudodementia)." Depression should be strongly considered in evaluations of memory problems.

    e. *Change in sleep pattern.* Sleep problems are another common chief complaint in primary care. Depressed patients might have classic early morning awakening but also might have trouble initiating or maintaining sleep. Ask the patient, "Has there been a change in your usual sleep pattern?" (See Chapter 11 for a review of sleep disorders.)

    f. *Change in appetite.* Depressed patients typically have impaired appetite (which can result in weight loss); however, increased appetite and weight gain are also possible.

    g. *Psychomotor agitation or retardation.* Clinicians might observe hand wringing, restless pacing, or withdrawal and slowed movements as examples of these behavioral aspects of depression.

    h. *Excessive guilt and loss of self-esteem.* Depressed patients frequently magnify their faults and feel excessively and inappropriately guilty about past actions. Ask, "Have you been having a lot of negative thoughts recently, for example, feeling hopeless, worthless, or guilty?"

    i. *Suicidal ideation.*

       (1) Asking about suicidal ideation is a crucial part of every depression evaluation, because patients might not volunteer this information (see Chapter 14 for further discussion of suicide).

       (2) It may be helpful to pursue this topic by an escalating series of questions (Box 6-4).

       (3) Suicidal ideation is not uncommon in depressed patients. The determination of whether more intensive treatment is necessary (such as hospitalization) usually rests on whether the patient is seriously contemplating to carry through with a suicidal act (i.e., has a plan) (see Chapter 14).

       (4) Arrangements must be made for the patient's safety until a psychiatric evaluation takes place or some other competent clinician evaluates the situation.

Screening

1. The single question, "Have you been feeling sad or depressed recently?" can be highly effective in screening for depression. A positive answer should be followed by a more in-depth evaluation.

2. Because of problems in recognition or the reluctance of patients to talk about symptoms, standardized instruments can be useful in screening for depression. Such instruments include both clinician-rated and self-rated instruments.

BOX 6-4   **Interview Protocol for Evaluating Suicidal Ideation**

"You have said you are depressed; could you tell me what that's like for you?"

"Are there times you feel like crying?"

"When you feel that way, what sort of thoughts go through your mind?"

"Do you ever get to the point where you feel that if this is the way things are that it is not worth going on?"

"Have you gone so far as to think of taking your own life?"

"Have you made any plan?"

"Do you have the means to carry out such a plan?"

"Is there anything that would prevent you from carrying out the plan?"

a. Clinician-administered instruments
   (1) The Hamilton Depression Rating Scale (HDRS) is the most commonly used instrument in the United States. It exists in several versions from 17 to 28 items.
   (2) The Montgomery–Asberg Depression Rating Scale (MADRS) is the most commonly used instrument in Europe. It has 10 items.
   (3) The Primary Care Evaluation of Mental Disorders (PRIME-MD) is a screening instrument validated in primary care settings. It also exists in self-report version.
b. Self-rating scales.
   (1) The Beck Depression Inventory (BDI) (included in Fig. 6-2) is one of the most widely used self-rated scales. It contains 21 items. A score of 18 or greater indicates that depression is likely to be present. The score should be interpreted cautiously in medically ill patients because several items are devoted to somatic symptoms.
   (2) The Psychiatric Diagnostic Screening Questionnaire (PDSQ) is a screening instrument validated in psychiatric settings.
   (3) The Inventory for Depressive Symptomatology (IDS) is fast becoming the most widely used self-rating scale for depression, particularly in psychopharmacology trials.
   (4) The Zung Depression Scale (Fig. 6-3) has 20 items measuring the severity of affective and physiologic symptoms of depression. As with the Beck scale, the score should be interpreted cautiously in medically ill patients.
   (5) The Geriatric Depression Scale is a 30-item questionnaire well validated for screening affective status among older adult populations. Problems with validity can occur in patients with dementia. A short form for screening is also useful (Box 6-5).

BECK DEPRESSION INVENTORY, SHORT FORM

Patient is asked to circle how they feel right now.

Instructions: This is a questionnaire. On the questionnaire are groups of statements. Please read the entire group of statements in each category. Then pick out the one statement in that group which best describes the way you feel today, that is, *right now*! Circle the number beside the statement you have chosen. If several statements in the group seem to apply equally well, circle each one.

Be sure to read all the statements in each group before making your choice.

Rating	Feeling	Rating	Feeling
	Sadness		**Social withdrawal**
3	I am so sad or unhappy that I can't stand it.	3	I have lost all of my interest in other people and don't care about them at all.
2	I am blue or sad all the time and I can't snap out of it.	2	I have lost most of my interest in other people and have little feeling for them.
1	I feel sad or blue.	1	I am less interested in other people than I used to be.
0	I do not feel sad.	0	I have not lost interest in other people.
	Pessimism		**Indecisiveness**
3	I feel that the future is hopeless and that things cannot improve.	3	I can't make any decisions at all anymore.
2	I feel I have nothing to look forward to.	2	I have great difficulty in making decisions.
1	I feel discouraged about the future.	1	I try to put off making decisions.
0	I am not particularly pessimistic or discouraged about the future	0	I make decisions about as well as ever.
	Sense of Failure		**Self-image change**
3	I feel I am a complete failure as a person (parent, husband, wife).	3	I feel that I am ugly or repulsive-looking.
2	As I look back on my life, all I can see is a lot of failures.	2	I feel that there are permanent changes in my appearance and they make me look unattractive.
1	I feel I have failed more than the average person.	1	I am worried that I am looking old or unattractive.
0	I do not feel like a failure.	0	I don't feel that I look any worse than I used to.

Figure 6-2   Beck Depression Inventory, Short Form. (From Beck AT, Beck RW: *Postgrad Med* 52(6):81-85, 1972.)

(6) The Clinically Useful Depression Outcome Scale (CUDOS) is a 16-item scale that has been validated to detect remission from depression.

PREVALENCE

1. The community prevalence of major depression is 3% to 5%. The lifetime risk is 5% to 12% for men and 10% to 25% for women. The risk is higher for those with a first-degree relative who has major depression, bipolar disorder, or alcoholism.
2. Prevalence of major depression in the elderly.
   a. Community prevalence of 3% to 5%.
   b. Nursing home prevalence of 15% to 20%.
      (1) Major depression occurs in about 10% to 20% of patients with Alzheimer's disease and following stroke.
3. The prevalence of major depression increases dramatically in patients with medical illness, as shown in Table 6-1.

Rating	Feeling	Rating	Feeling
	Dissatisfaction		**Work Difficulty**
3	I am dissatisfied with everything.	3	I can't do any work at all.
2	I don't get satisfaction out of anything anymore.	2	I have to push myself very hard to do anything.
1	I don't enjoy things the way I used to.	1	It takes extra effort to get started at doing something.
0	I am not particularly dissatisfied.	0	I can work about as well as before.
	Guilt		**Fatigability**
3	I feel as though I am very bad or worthless.	3	I get too tired to do anything.
2	I feel quite guilty.	2	I get tired from doing anything.
1	I feel bad or unworthy a good part of the time.	1	I get tired more easily than I used to.
0	I don't feel particularly guilty.	0	I don't get any more tired than usual.
	Self-dislike		**Anorexia**
3	I hate myself.	3	I have no appetite at all anymore.
2	I am disgusted with myself.	2	My appetite is much worse now.
1	I am disappointed in myself.	1	My appetite is not as good as it used to be.
0	I don't feel disappointed in myself.	0	My appetite is no worse than usual.
	Self-harm		
3	I would kill myself if I had the chance.	3	
2	I have definite plans about committing suicide.	2	
1	I feel I would be better off dead.	1	
0	I don't have any thoughts of harming myself.	0	

Scores	Degree of depression
0-4	None or minimal
5-7	Mild
8-15	Moderate
16+	Severe

Figure 6-2, Cont'd.

4. The prevalence of major depression in primary care practice ranges between 8% and 15%. This makes major depression the number one medical problem in primary care practice.

RECOGNITION

1. There is often a lack of recognition of major depression in primary care practice. Reasons for low recognition include the following:
   a. Patient is reluctant to acknowledge symptoms.
   b. Predominant symptoms mislead the clinician.
      (1) Fatigue may be seen as a medical problem.
      (2) Sleep difficulty may be seen as a primary problem.
      (3) Cognitive symptoms are seen as dementia.
      (4) Somatized symptoms imply a medical problem.
      (5) Chronic pain may be seen as only a physical problem.
      (6) Functional disability may be accepted as inevitable.
      (7) Depression may be seen as a "normal" reaction.
2. Comorbidity.
   a. Anxiety disorders such as obsessive–compulsive disorder, panic disorder, posttraumatic stress disorder (PTSD), and generalized anxiety often coexist with depressive disorders.

	A Little of the Time	Some of the Time	A Good Part of the Time	Most of the Time
1. I feel down-hearted and blue				
2. Morning is when I feel the best				
3. I have crying spells or feel like it				
4. I have trouble sleeping at night				
5. I eat as much as I used to				
6. I still enjoy sex				
7. I notice that I am losing weight				
8. I have trouble with constipation				
9. M heart beats faster than usual				
10. I get tired for no reason				
11. My mind is as clear as it used to be				
12. I find it easy to do the things I used to do				
13. I am restless and can't keep still				
14. I feel hopeful about the future				
15. I am more irritable than usual				
16. I find it easy to make decisions				
17. I feel that I am useful and needed				
18. My life is pretty full				
19. I feel that others would be better off if I were dead				
20. I still enjoy the things I used to do				

Figure 6-3   Self-rating depression scale. (From Zung WW: *Arch Gen Psychiatry* 12:63-70, 1965.)

 b. Substance abuse is a common comorbidity.

 c. Medical illness is commonly comorbid with major depression. Human immunodeficiency virus (HIV), endocrine disease, and severe kidney disease are associated with particularly high rates of depression.

DIAGNOSTIC MODIFIERS FOR MAJOR DEPRESSION

1. Major depression may be a single episode or recurrent.

 a. Psychiatric comorbidity increases the risk of recurrence.

 b. The implications of increased likelihood of relapse with increasing number of episodes involves maintenance treatment.

2. Major depression with psychotic features.

 a. Psychotic symptoms can accompany severe depression, increasing risk for suicide. Typical psychotic symptoms include the following:

  (1) Auditory hallucinations.

  (2) Delusions (fixed, false beliefs), usually paranoid (such as being followed) or somatic delusions (such as being convinced of having AIDS without any supporting evidence).

 b. A question to uncover psychotic symptoms might be, "It is not unusual for someone who is very depressed to hear voices saying unpleasant things (such as, 'You don't deserve to live') or to have disturbing thoughts about your body. Has anything like that happened to you?"

Table 6-1 Prevalence of Depression in Selected Medical Disorders

Disorder	Percent
Alzheimer's disease	15-50
Cancer inpatients	42
Cancer, gastrointestinal	20
Cancer, gynecologic	23
Coronary artery disease	18-26
Cushing's syndrome	67
Diabetes mellitus	15-33
End-stage renal disease	30
Epilepsy	55
HIV positivity	7-15
Huntington's disease	32-41
Multiinfarct dementia	27-60
Multiple sclerosis	6-57
Myocardial infarction	20
Pain (chronic)	32
Parkinson's disease	40
Renal disease	8
Stroke	30-50

BOX 6-5 Five-Item Version of the Geriatric Depression Scale

Are you basically satisfied with your life?
Do you often get bored?
Do you often feel helpless?
Do you prefer to stay at home rather than going out and doing new things?
Do you feel pretty worthless the way you are right now?

More than two positive responses (including "no" to the first question) indicates the need for depression evaluation.

Adapted from Hoyl MT, Alessi CA, Harker JO, et al: *J Am Geriatr Soc* 47:873-878, 1999.

    c. Somatic delusions are not unusual in severely depressed elderly patients.
    d. Treatment of psychotic depressed patients.
      (1) Requires an antipsychotic agent along with an antidepressant.
      (2) Electroconvulsive therapy (ECT) may be a reasonable option if pharmacotherapy is unsuccessful.
3. Major depression with melancholic features.
    a. This modifier is used when the core symptom of the depression is marked anhedonia and lack of reactivity (the patient does not feel

any better when something good happens). In addition, the patient has at least three of the following:
  (1) Distinct quality of mood.
  (2) Depressed mood that is worse in the morning.
  (3) Early morning awakening.
  (4) Notable psychomotor agitation or retardation.
  (5) Significant anorexia or weight loss.
  (6) Excessive or inappropriate guilt.
  b. This subgroup is believed to be better candidates for antidepressant medication and electroconvulsive therapy. They also are less likely to respond to placebo.
4. Major depression with atypical features.
  a. This modifier is used when the essential feature of the depression involves mood reactivity (feeling better when good things happen; e.g., when family comes to visit).
  b. Additional features include the following:
    (1) Significant weight gain or increased appetite.
    (2) Hypersomnia.
    (3) A heavy leaden feeling in the arms or legs.
    (4) A long-standing pattern of being very sensitive to interpersonal rejection (rejection sensitivity).
  c. Atypical features are two to three times more common in women.
  d. These patients often have an earlier onset of their disorder and a more chronic course.
  e. Patients with atypical depression respond preferentially to monoamine oxidase inhibitors (MAOIs) but should be given trials of selective serotonin reuptake inhibitors (SSRIs) first due to safety concerns in using MAOIs.
5. Major depression with postpartum onset.
  a. This modifier is applied when the episode of major depression occurs within 4 weeks of delivery.
  b. In general, the symptoms and response to treatment of postpartum depression do not differ from other nonpostpartum depressions.
  c. The *maternity blues* are defined as feeling sad, often with periods of spontaneous crying, which occur 3 to 7 days postpartum and resolve spontaneously.
  d. The incidence of postpartum depression is 10%.
  e. Without treatment, postpartum depression adversely affects the patient, spouse, and infant.
  f. Postpartum depression with psychotic features occurs in about 0.1% of new mothers.
  g. There is a high risk of recurrence (30% to 50%) in a subsequent postpartum period.
6. Major depression with a seasonal pattern.
  a. This modifier is applied when there is a regular pattern of association between some time of year and the onset and the remission of depression.
  b. Typically, illness begins in autumn or spring.
  c. Carbohydrate craving and weight gain are often associated with the depression.

d. Sleep disturbance is usually hypersomnia.
e. Many of these patients also have nonseasonal depressions.
f. There are no definitive data in these areas, although prevalence is definitely higher the farther one lives from the equator.
g. Differential diagnosis.
 (1) Bipolar disorder without a clear seasonal pattern.
 (2) Recurrent depression without a clear seasonal pattern.
 (3) Recurrent psychiatric symptoms triggered by seasonal events (such as seasonal pattern of layoff from work).
h. Treatments.
 (1) Bright light stimulation at dawn or dusk has been reported to help people with winter depression.
 (2) There is no single agreed-upon approach to the dose or duration of light that is most effective. Treatments often consist of about 2 hours of bright full-spectrum light.
  (a) Some studies have demonstrated a superiority for morning light treatment.
  (b) No ophthalmologic problems have been demonstrated in patients using bright-light treatment for 5 to 8 years.
 (3) Antidepressant medication is often necessary in conjunction with light treatment.

DIFFERENTIAL DIAGNOSIS

1. Schizoaffective disorder.
 a. This disorder should be considered in patients with psychotic features accompanying depression, because in schizoaffective disorder, a major depressive episode occurs concurrently with psychotic features.
 b. However, there are times when the psychotic symptoms occur in the absence of mood symptoms.
2. Bipolar disorder with depression.
 a. The diagnosis of a major depressive episode is the same for patients with bipolar disorder as it is for unipolar depression. Bipolar disorder is diagnosed when there is a prior history of mania (bipolar I) or hypomania (bipolar II).
 b. In any patient with major depression, ask about manic or hypomanic episodes to determine if the patient is bipolar. Screening questions might be the following:
  (1) "Have there been times when you felt the opposite of depressed, that is, euphoric, or irritable, clearly different from your normal self?" Many people report frequent and at times dramatic fluctuations in mood. The diagnosis of bipolar disorder should only be made, however, if the patient's affect is clearly distinct from baseline and lasts at least 4 to 7 days. Other diagnoses should be considered if the patient does not clearly report both an increased level of energy and a decreased need for sleep.
  (2) "Have there been times when you stayed up all night, spent a lot of money, or acted socially in a way you later regretted?"

c. Bipolar depressed patients usually require a mood stabilizer (see Chapter 8) for prophylaxis against future manic episodes. There is controversy in the field as to whether antidepressant therapy increases the risk of mania. If an antidepressant is used, however, it is clearly prudent to also use a mood stabilizer.

3. Mood disorder due to a general medical condition should always be considered (see previous section).

4. Adjustment disorder with depressed mood (see next section).
   a. The presence of a precipitating event does not affect the diagnosis of major depression. Many major depressions have an identifiable precipitant and respond to medication no differently from those that do not.
   b. Adjustment disorders.
      (1) Do not meet the full criteria for major depression.
      (2) Occur in relation to a specific stress.
      (3) Last less than 6 months once the stress has terminated.

5. Because bereavement is believed to be a natural reaction to the loss of a loved one, the diagnosis of major depression is not made *unless* the symptoms are unusually severe or last much longer than would normally be expected. The duration of bereavement may be culturally determined, and it is problematic to diagnose a depressive disorder before the prescribed bereavement phase has been completed.

6. Dysthymia (see later section).

7. Borderline personality disorder with chronic emptiness, depressed mood, and suicidal ideation (see Chapter 17).

PROGNOSIS FOR MAJOR DEPRESSION

1. Untreated, episodes of major depression last on average about 6 to 9 months.

2. Some cases of major depression are episodic and recurrent. After a single episode, there is about a 50% chance of a second episode. After a second episode, there is about a 70% chance of a third. After three or four episodes, the likelihood of recurrence seems so high that long-term (i.e., 5 years to lifetime) medication therapy is recommended.

3. The prognosis worsens the longer the depression has been present. Nevertheless, the overwhelming majority of patients do recover.

4. Without treatment, major depression is a serious illness that affects quality of life to the same extent as chronic medical illnesses. In addition, depression increases the risk of cardiac disease and stroke, and there is a definite increased risk of suicide.

5. Treatment has a significant positive effect, with 70% or more of major depression responding to adequate treatment.

TREATMENT

Three forms of effective treatment of major depression are psychotherapy, antidepressant medication, and ECT.

1. Psychotherapy.
   a. Several forms of psychotherapy have research evidence to confirm that the response of patients with moderate levels of major

depression is equivalent to antidepressants. Among the most studied psychotherapies are the following:

(1) Cognitive behavior therapy. In this form of therapy, a patient is helped to identify and alter repetitive, distorted, maladaptive ways of thinking that create depressive responses.

(2) Interpersonal psychotherapy. This therapy focuses on interpersonal relationships, exploring decisions that are made, and developing new insight.

b. Should you use medication or psychotherapy?

(1) In most cases, both are equally effective. This should be emphasized to patients when considering the alternatives. Patients whose symptoms interfere with participation in talking therapy should start medication first.

(2) Patients with milder symptoms who seem willing to talk about their problems should be started with psychotherapy, reserving medication for an inadequate response.

(3) Between these extremes, the two treatments can be used conjointly.

(4) As a generalization, psychotherapy addresses problems, medication addresses symptoms.

(5) Psychotherapy may be the primary treatment for:

(a) The 5% to 10% of patients who refuse to take medication.

(b) The 10% to 15% of patients who discontinue or cannot tolerate medications.

(c) Those for whom medication may not be appropriate, for example:

(i) During pregnancy or lactation.

(ii) With major surgery or acute medical conditions.

(iii) With recent myocardial infarction.

(6) The choice of medication or psychotherapy is sometimes determined mostly by the preference of the patient and the availability and affordability of therapists.

2. Antidepressant medication (see Chapter 7).

3. ECT indications and use are presented in Chapter 16.

6.5 Adjustment Disorder with Depressed Mood

DEFINITION AND IDENTIFICATION

1. Excessive reaction to some identifiable life stress, occurring within 3 weeks of a stressor and lasting less than 6 months following the termination of the stressor.

2. It is also possible for adjustment disorders to be characterized by depression alone, by anxiety alone, or by mixed anxious and depressed mood.

3. In addition, conduct problems can develop during an adjustment disorder.

PREVALENCE

1. No one is immune from brief depressive reactions. These transient self-limited feelings generally remain separate from the medical care

system; however, in many cases they contribute to use of medical resources.
2. Brief depressive reactions are common during the course of serious medical illness.

DIFFERENTIAL DIAGNOSIS

See the "Differential Diagnosis" section for major depressive disorder (previous section).

PROGNOSIS

Adjustment disorders are generally self-limited; however, they do have the potential to become unresolved, chronic disorders. It is not unusual, for example, to find unresolved grief reactions manifesting as chronic medical symptoms.

TREATMENT

1. Adjustment disorders should be treated by some form of time-limited therapy that focuses on the precipitant and the development of more adaptive coping responses.
2. Anxiolytics or antidepressants can be used as an adjunct to the psychotherapy if the symptoms are severe or if the patient is not psychologically minded.
3. Some patients transform their distress into a somatic symptom. In those cases, the physician should educate the patient about the connection between the underlying distress and the resulting physical symptom (see Chapter 13 for a review of acute somatization).

6.6 Dysthymic Disorder

DEFINITION AND IDENTIFICATION

Dysthymia refers to chronic depressive symptoms that do not become severe enough to meet criteria for major depression and are present for at least 2 years.

1. Depressed mood is present for most of the day.
2. Depressed mood is present most, but not all, days.
3. Depressed mood has not been absent for more than 2 months during the 2 years.
4. Depressive symptoms have not met the severity of number criteria to qualify for major depression.

PREVALENCE

1. The community-based prevalence of dysthymia is 4.5% to 10.5%, and it is more common in women than men. Lifetime prevalence is approximately 6%.
2. Dysthymic patients are at increased risk for poor general health, and they frequently use medical services.

DIFFERENTIAL DIAGNOSIS

1. Adjustment disorder. No specific stressor is identified as the precipitant of dysthymia.
2. Chronic sense of emptiness and anhedonia that can accompany borderline personality disorder (see Chapter 17).

3. Chronic major depression (symptom number and severity are greater than with dysthymia).
4. Dysthymia can coexist with other psychiatric disorders. "Double depression" is sometimes used to refer to an episode of major depression superimposed on dysthymia.

PROGNOSIS

Dysthymia is, by definition, a chronic condition.

TREATMENT

Dysthymia should be treated the same as major depression (i.e., with an appropriate combination of psychotherapy and antidepressants). However, antidepressants might take longer to work, and 8- to 12-week trials are recommended.

6.7 Mixed Anxiety and Depression

DEFINITION AND IDENTIFICATION

1. DSM-IV includes this category as an area for further study, although it seems to be a common clinical presentation.
2. Mixed anxiety and depression is a state of general distress characterized by:
   a. At least 1 month of persistent dysphoric mood, accompanied by the following:
      (1) Difficulty concentrating.
      (2) Sleep disturbance.
      (3) Fatigue.
      (4) Irritability.
      (5) Worry.
      (6) Crying readily.
      (7) Hypervigilance.
      (8) Negative anticipation.
      (9) Pessimism.
      (10) Low self-esteem.
   b. The patient has both anxious and depressive symptoms, with neither of sufficient number or severity to qualify for a separate anxiety or depressive disorder (Fig. 6-4).

PREVALENCE

Mixed anxiety and depression had been thought to be one of the most common psychiatric presentations in primary care practice, with a prevalence estimated to be at least 5%, although a large study found a low prevalence.

1. These patients have significant functional disability and high rates of medical utilization.
2. There is often a history of prior psychiatric diagnosis and treatment.

DIFFERENTIAL DIAGNOSIS

1. Primary depressive disorders with some anxiety symptoms. Symptoms of anxiety are present in more than 70% of cases of major depression.

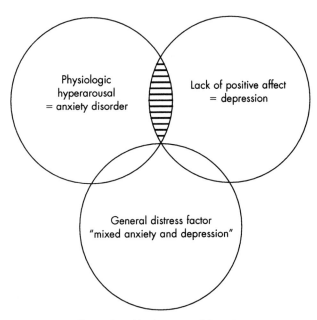

Figure 6-4   Mixed anxiety and depression.

2. Primary anxiety disorders with some depressive symptoms. More than half the cases of generalized anxiety or panic disorder have significant depressive symptoms.
3. Adjustment disorder with mixed anxiety and depression.
4. Coexistence of an anxiety and a depressive disorder.

PROGNOSIS

The natural course is not well known at this time.

TREATMENT

1. Because data on the natural history are limited, treatment effects are also not well known. This is another area of significant interest in primary care in terms of effects on illness behavior, use of medical resources, functional impairment, and response to psychotropic medication or supportive counseling.
2. If symptoms are clinically significant, it would be reasonable to give the patient a trial of the following:
   a. Any antidepressant from Table 7-1, because all antidepressants also have antianxiety properties.
   b. Buspirone, because the azapirone group has both antianxiety and antidepressant activity.

6.8 Premenstrual Dysphoric Disorder

DEFINITION AND IDENTIFICATION

1. Premenstrual dysphoric disorder (PMDD) is listed as an area for further study in the DSM-IV.
2. PMDD was called late luteal phase dysphoric disorder in DSM-III.
3. PMDD can be distinguished from premenstrual syndrome (PMS). PMS is reserved for milder physical symptoms (which are experienced by at least 75% of women with a regular menstrual cycle), such as the following:
   a. Breast tenderness.
   b. Bloating.
   c. Headache.
   d. Minor mood changes.

PREVALENCE

PMDD is much less common than PMS.

1. It affects 3% to 8% of menstruating women.
2. Most common time of occurrence is late 20s and early 30s.

DIAGNOSIS

PMDD diagnostic criteria include the following:

1. Symptoms present in most menstrual cycles over the past year.
2. Symptoms begin during the last week of the luteal phase, begin to remit during the first few days of the follicular phase, and are absent in the week after menses.
3. One of the symptoms involves:
   a. Depressed mood.
   b. Marked anxiety or tension.
   c. Marked affective lability.
   d. Anger, irritability, increased interpersonal conflicts.
4. Other symptoms can include:
   a. Decreased interest in usual activities.
   b. Difficulty concentrating.
   c. Lack of energy.
   d. Overeating.
   e. Sleep difficulty (too much or too little).
   f. Feeling out of control or overwhelmed.
   g. Other physical symptoms of PMS.

DIFFERENTIAL DIAGNOSIS

Differential diagnosis includes premenstrual magnification of an underlying mood or anxiety disorder.

TREATMENT

PMDD has been linked to serotonin dysregulation.

1. Lifestyle and stress management.
   a. Elimination or reduction of the following:
      (1) Caffeine.
      (2) Alcohol.

      (3) Tobacco.
  b. Diet change to include frequent high-protein, low–refined sugar meals.
  c. Decrease in excess sodium in the diet.
  d. Weight reduction to within 20% of ideal weight.
  e. Regular exercise.
  f. Stress management or self-regulation (see Chapter 10).
  g. Identification and counseling for stressful life events or situations.
2. Psychotropic medication.
  a. Antidepressants. Medications that raise serotonin levels have been helpful. Most studies of clomipramine or the SSRIs have shown positive results in reducing symptoms. Dosing strategies involve either continuous dosing starting at a low dose or:
    (1) Phased dosing beginning around midcycle.
    (2) Many experts recommend starting with continuous dosing and then switching to phased dosing if the patient responds.
  b. Alprazolam has been shown to be helpful in reducing anxiety and irritability.
3. Hormonal therapy.
4. Oophorectomy as a last resort.

6.9 Minor Depression (Subthreshold Depression)

1. The validity of a diagnostic category of minor depression is of great interest because of the number of patients who present with the following:
  a. At least 2 weeks of depressed mood or anhedonia (the same core symptoms as for major depression).
  b. Fewer than five of the other symptoms that are needed to diagnose major depression.
2. The DSM-IV lists this as an area for further study.
3. In primary care, the major questions are whether subthreshold depression responds to antidepressants, how much it is associated with functional impairment, and how it affects use of medical services.

SUGGESTED READINGS

Afari N, Buchwald D: Chronic fatigue syndrome: A review. Am J Psychiatry 160(2):221-236, 2003.
Beck AT, Guth D, Steer RA, Ball R: Screening for major depression disorders in medical inpatients with the Beck Depression Inventory for Primary Care. Behav Res Ther 35(8):785-791, 1997.
Judd LL, Paulus MJ, Schettler PJ, et al: Does incomplete recovery from first lifetime major depressive episode herald a chronic course of illness? Am J Psychiatry 157(9):1501-1504, 2000.
Judd LL, Rapaport MH, Yonkers KA, et al: Randomized, placebo-controlled trial of fluoxetine for acute treatment of minor depressive disorder. Am J Psychiatry 161(10):1864-1871, 2004.
Mahoney J, Drinka TJ, Abler R, et al: Screening for depression: Single question versus GDS. J Am Ger Soc 42:1006-1008, 1994.

Melartin TK, Rytsala HJ, Leskela US, et al: Severity and comorbidity predict episode duration and recurrence of DSM-IV major depressive disorder. *J Clin Psychiatry* 65(6):810-819, 2004.

Mueller TI, Keller MB, Leon AC, et al: Recovery after 5 years of unremitting major depressive disorder. *Arch Gen Psychiatry* 53(9):794-799, 1996.

Partonen T, Lonnqvist J: Seasonal affective disorder. *Lancet* 352(9137):1369-1374, 1998.

Roose SP: Treatment of depression in patients with heart disease. *Biol Psychiatry* 54(3):262-268, 2003.

Ross LE, Steiner M: A biopsychosocial approach to premenstrual dysphoric disorder. *Psychiatr Clin North Am* 26(3):529-546, 2003.

Rush AJ, Gullion CM, Basco MR, et al: The Inventory of Depressive Symptomatology (IDS): Psychometric properties. *Psychol Med* 26(3):477-486, 1996.

Schrag A: Psychiatric aspects of Parkinson's disease—an update. *J Neurol* 251(7):795-804, 2004.

Weisberg RB, Maki KM, Culpepper L, Keller MB: Is anyone really M.A.D.?: The occurrence and course of mixed anxiety–depressive disorder in a sample of primary care patients. *J Nerv Ment Dis* 193:223-230, 2005.

Yesavage JA, Brink TL, Rose TL, et al: Development and validation of a geriatric depression screening scale: A preliminary report. *J Psychiatr Res* 17:37-49, 1983.

Zimmerman M, Mattia JI: A self-report scale to help make psychiatric diagnoses: The Psychiatric Diagnostic Screening Questionnaire. *Arch Gen Psychiatry* 58(8):787-794, 2001.

Zimmerman M, Posternak M, Chelminski I: Using a self-report depression scale to identify remission in depressed outpatients. *Am J Psychiatry* 161(10):1911-1913, 2004.

Zung WK: A self-rating depression scale. *Arch Gen Psychiatry* 12:63-70, 1965.

Antidepressants

Michael A. Posternak
Mark Zimmerman

7.1 Overview

WHEN TO USE ANTIDEPRESSANTS

1. Antidepressants are indicated primarily for treatment of depressive symptoms of:
   a. Major depression.
   b. Depressed phase of bipolar disorder.
2. Other uses of antidepressants.
   a. Depressive symptoms secondary to some medical disorder (assuming the medical cause is being addressed).
   b. Dysthymia.
   c. Anxiety disorders.
      (1) Obsessive–compulsive disorder (OCD).
      (2) Panic disorder.
      (3) Generalized anxiety disorder (GAD), especially with mixed depressive symptoms.
      (4) Posttraumatic stress disorder.
      (5) Social phobia.
   d. Adjunctive use for pain control (e.g., diabetic neuropathy).
   e. Premenstrual dysphoric disorder (PMDD).
   f. Seasonal affective disorder (SAD).
   g. Postpartum depression.
   h. Insomnia.
   i. Smoking cessation (bupropion).

GENERAL GUIDELINES FOR USING ANTIDEPRESSANTS

1. When antidepressants are properly used, 50% to 70% of patients with major depression should respond, assuming:
   a. The diagnosis of depression is correct.
   b. Adequate dose and duration are used.
   c. The patient can tolerate the medication. Side effects and noncompliance are not uncommon.
2. Patients who respond should receive medication for at least 6 months, longer (or continuously) for chronic, relapsing symptoms.
3. Doses used by many clinicians are too low.
   a. Plasma levels are available for most of the commonly used tricyclic antidepressants (TCAs).

b. Many patients respond to lower doses of selective serotonin reuptake inhibitors (SSRIs), such as 10–20 mg fluoxetine, 10–20 mg paroxetine, 50 mg sertraline, 20 mg citalopram, or 10 mg escitalopram. For patients who do not respond, however, doses should be increased to the maximum recommended dose, if tolerated. Blood levels have not been found to be useful for SSRIs.

c. Venlafaxine and nefazodone have linear dose–response relationships (doses should be increased in nonresponders).

4. Response rate can often be improved by combinations of medication or augmentation strategies. Before any combination is started, adequate trial(s) of single drugs should be confirmed.

PRINCIPLES OF USING ANTIDEPRESSANTS

1. A good trial of an antidepressant generally means:
   a. Using the medication at a therapeutic level for at least 4 to 8 weeks.
   b. Avoiding premature changes, which result in a series of inadequate trials.
   c. Recognizing that response can take longer than 4 weeks. In some trials with SSRIs in the elderly, responses have been noted to occur as late as 10 weeks.

2. If the patient cannot tolerate the medication due to side effects, consider lowering the dose. If the lower dose would be considered ineffective, document that and switch to another medication.

3. When switching antidepressants, be aware of the following:
   a. Drugs with long half-lives (such as fluoxetine) can be stopped immediately.
   b. Drugs with short half-lives (e.g., paroxetine and venlafaxine) might cause withdrawal symptoms associated with sudden discontinuation and should be tapered. Decrease the dose by 25% per day over 4 days. Some patients require 2 weeks or longer to taper.
   c. When switching medications, be aware that drugs with long half-lives (such as fluoxetine) can remain present for about 3 weeks.
   d. An adequate washout period (about 4 to 5 half-lives) is necessary when switching to a monoamine oxidase inhibitor (MAOI) (usually 2 weeks, though fluoxetine requires 5 weeks).
   e. When switching to another antidepressant from an MAOI, allow at least 2 weeks.
   f. SSRI (including venlafaxine) withdrawal symptoms include the following:
      (1) Dizziness.
      (2) Lightheadedness.
      (3) Vertigo.
      (4) Paresthesias.
      (5) Flu-like symptoms.
      (6) Gastrointestinal activation.
      (7) Insomnia.
      (8) Sweating.

4. If the patient does not respond to a well-administered trial of a single medication:
   a. Reconfirm the diagnosis.

b. Consider whether psychotherapy is needed to address factors that may be interfering.
   (1) Unresolved secondary gain (e.g., disability issue).
   (2) Ongoing family disagreements.
   (3) Unaddressed psychological conflict.
   (4) Unaddressed psychosocial stressors.
c. Consider extending the trial longer, especially if some benefit is noted.
d. Document the details of an adequate trial in the medical record.
e. Options for continued treatment.
   (1) Optimization. Be sure that the drug being used is at the highest recommended dosage that is tolerated.
   (2) Substitution. Switch to another antidepressant.
   (3) Augmentation or combination (approximately equal efficacy to substitution).
      (a) Lithium. Of the controlled trials of lithium augmentation, half show superiority of lithium over placebo. Recommended dosage is 900 mg/day and blood levels are usually not necessary.
      (b) Triiodothyronine (T_3): about half the patients responded in a 2- to 4-week trial. For unclear reasons, T_3 appears to be more effective than T_4 (e.g., Synthroid). The usual dosage for T_3 augmentation is 25 to 50 μg/day.
      (c) Combining two antidepressants is probably the most popular augmentation strategy. For partial responders, a second antidepressant with a different mechanism of action can be added (e.g., adding bupropion or mirtazapine to an SSRI).
      (d) Stimulants such as methylphenidate and dextroamphetamine are also useful augmenters, especially for patients with lethargy or poor concentration. One advantage of this strategy is that the benefits of stimulants are usually apparent very quickly.
      (e) Atypical antipsychotics (e.g., olanzapine, risperidone) may be helpful for patients who are agitated or severely anxious. There is a small risk of tardive dyskinesia to be considered for maintenance treatment.
      (f) Patients who do not respond to two good trials of antidepressants and whose symptoms are severe may be considered for a second opinion or for electroconvulsive therapy (ECT). For a review of ECT, see Chapter 16.
5. If the patient does respond to an antidepressant:
   a. For an initial episode of major depression, treat for at least 6 to 9 months before considering a taper.
   b. For patients with three or more episodes, consider indefinite maintenance therapy.

7.2 Specific Issues in Using Antidepressants

1. Table 7-1 does not list MAOIs or stimulants (such as methylphenidate), which are discussed later in this chapter.

Table 7-1 Antidepressant Profiles

| | Chemistry | | | Adverse Effects | | | | | | | |
Drug	Half-life (h)	Dose Range (mg)	Therapeutic Level (ng/mL)	Anticholinergic	Sedation	Activation	Hypotension	His Bundle	GI	Seizures
Tricyclics										
Amitriptyiline (Elavil)	20-46	100-300	75-175	4	3	0	3	+	0	+
Clomipramine (Anafranil)	20-40	50-250		4	4	0	3	+	0	+
Desipramine (Norpramin)	10-32	100-300	100-160	2	1-2	2	2	+	0	+
Doxepin (Sinequan)	8-47	100-300		3	4	0	2	+	0	+
Imipramine (Tofranil)	4-34	100-300	>265	3	4	1	3	+	0	+
Nortriptyline (Pamelor)	18-88	50-150	50-150	2	2	0	1	+	0	+
Protriptyline (Vivactil)	53-124	10-60		4	1	3	2	+	0	+
Trimipramine (Surmontil)	9	100-300		3	3	0	3	+	0	+
SSRIs										
Citalopram	33	20-40		0	1	1-2	0	0	1	0
Escitalopram	30	10-20		0	1	1-2	0	0	1	0

Table continued on following page

Table 7-1 **Antidepressant Profiles** *(Continued)*

	Chemistry			Adverse Effects						
Drug	Half-life (h)	Dose Range (mg)	Therapeutic Level (ng/mL)	Anticholinergic	Sedation	Activation	Hypotension	His Bundle	GI	Seizures
Fluoxetine (Prozac)	2 days	20-40		0	0	1-2	0	0	1-2	+
Paroxetine (Paxil)	7 days*	20-40		1	1	1-2	0	0	2	0
Sertraline (Zoloft)	26	50-200		0	0	1-2	0	0	2	+
SNRIs										
Duloxetine	8-17	20-60		0	1	1-2	0	0	1-2	?
Venlafaxine (Effexor-XR)	9-11	150-450		0	1	1-2	0	0	1-2	+
5-HT₂ + SRI										
Nefazodone (Serzone)	4	300-600		0	3	0	1	0	1	0
Trazodone (Desyrel)	18-30*	100-600		0	3	0	2	0	0	+
Other Antidepressants										
Bupropion (Wellbutrin)	8-24	150-450		1	0	3	0	0	0	++
Mirtazapine (Remeron)	20-40	15-45		1	4	0	2	0	0	?

* Data for active metabolite.

Ratings are from "very sedating" at "4" to "not sedating" at "0"; higher numbers indicate more activating drugs; + indicates delayed conduction; HT, hydroxytryptamine; SNRI, serotonin and norepinephrine reuptake inhibitor; SRI, serotonin reuptake inhibitor; SSRI, selective serotonin reuptake inhibitor.

2. The first section of Table 7-1 lists the TCAs (first-generation antidepressants). The lower sections contain the nontricyclic, second-generation antidepressants.

CHOOSING WHICH ANTIDEPRESSANT TO USE

1. There is no clear efficacy advantage to any of these antidepressants (the one exception to this is the use of MAOI for atypical depression) (Tables 7-2 and 7-3).
2. Past patient response and response of first-degree relatives can predict response.
3. Cost may be an important consideration. TCAs, although significantly cheaper per pill than newer antidepressants, might not offer a cost advantage to society due to the associated costs of blood draws, electrocardiograms (ECGs), and potential medical complications.
4. Overdose danger. Several weeks' supply of TCAs can be lethal in overdose due to potential seizures and cardiac arrhythmias. The newer antidepressants are almost never lethal in overdose.

SIDE EFFECTS

Anticholinergic

1. Some medications such as amitriptyline have high anticholinergic activity (indicated by a "4" in Table 7-1), whereas a number of the others, indicated by a "0," have none.
2. Try to minimize anticholinergic activity because of its adverse affects. Anticholinergic agents are contraindicated in patients with narrow angle glaucoma.
   a. Dry mouth can be a nuisance and can predispose to stomatitis (patients can suck on sugarless mints).
   b. Blurred vision.
   c. Urinary retention is a greater risk with prostatic enlargement or spinal cord problems.
   d. Constipation is a common effect that can require stool softeners. In patients on narcotics or with recent gastrointestinal (GI) surgery, anticholinergics can lead to paralytic ileus.
   e. Confusion or impaired memory, especially in older patients.
3. Anticholinergic effects are additive with other drugs, including:
   a. Benztropine (Cogentin).
   b. Diphenhydramine (Benadryl).
   c. Meperidine (Demerol).
   d. Oxybutynin (Ditropan).
   e. Propantheline (Pro-Banthine).
   f. Trihexyphenidyl (Artane).
4. If anticholinergic symptoms develop, consider a lower dose or another antidepressant.
   a. Anticholinergic side effects can often be counteracted by using bethanechol (Urecholine).
   b. Bethanechol should be started in small doses (5-10 mg tid). Patients should be observed for GI hyperactivity and cardiac rhythm disturbances.

Table 7-2 Neuroreceptor Effects of Antidepressants

Drug	Serotonin Reuptake Inhibition	Norepinephrine Reuptake Inhibition	5-HT$_2$ Antagonist	Cholinergic Antagonist	Histamine Antagonist	Alpha$_1$- Antagonist	Alpha$_2$- Antagonist	Dopamine Uptake Inhibitor
TCAs	+/++++	+/+++		++/+++	++/+++	++		
SSRIs	++++	0/+		+ (paroxetine)				+ (sertraline)
Venlafaxine	+++	0/++						
Duloxetine	+++	+++	+					
Bupropion	0/+	+++						+
Mirtazapine	0	0		+/++	++		++	
Possible clinical consequences	GI disturbances, sexual dysfunction, extrapyramidal symptoms	Tremor, tachycardia, erectile and ejaculatory dysfunction	Decreases sexual dysfunction, decreases sleep disturbances	Blurred vision, dry mouth, sinus tachycardia, constipation, urinary retention, memory dysfunction	Sedation, drowsiness, potentiates other sedatives, weight gain	Hypotension, dizziness, reflex tachycardia	Enhances central NE and 5-HT function	Psychomotor activation, antiparkinsonian effects

5-HT, serotonin; SSRI, selective serotonin reuptake inhibitor; TCA, tricyclic antidepressant.

Table 7-3 Adverse Effects Associated with Second-Generation Antidepressants

Drug	Anorexia	Diarrhea	Dizziness	Dry Mouth	Fatigue	Insomnia	Nausea	Nervousness	Sexual Dysfunction	Somnolence	Sweating	Tremor	Weight Gain	Pregnancy Category
Bupropion	+					++		+	++/+++		+	+		C
Citalopram, escitalopram		+	++	+		+	++	+	++		+			B
Duloxetine				+			+	+	++	At low doses	+			C
Fluoxetine	+	+	?	+		+	+	+	+++	+		+		B
Mirtazapine				++	+/++				++	++			++	C
Paroxetine		+	+	+	+	+	++	++	+++	+	++	+	+	B
Sertraline		++	+	+		+	++	+	+++		++	+		B
Venlafaxine		++	+	+		+	+	+	0/+		+			B

Drug adverse effects greater than those of placebo are indicated as follows: ++++, >30%; +++, >15%; ++, >10%; +, >5%.

5. All factors being equal, use of anticholinergic medications for elderly and medically ill patients should be avoided.

Sedation

Sedation is caused by central histamine receptor blockade or serotonin effects (5-HT_2 blockage). Ratings in Table 7-1 are from "very sedating" at "4" to "not sedating" at "0."

1. If a patient is agitated, restless, insomniac, or anxious, sedation might be helpful.
2. Patients who are anergic, hypersomnic, and concerned about oversedation should not be given a sedating medication as first choice.
3. Tolerance to sedation can take place over the first 10 to 14 days. Starting at a low dose and gradually titrating up can prevent initial sedation.
4. Antidepressant-induced sedation and asthenia might respond to methylphenidate starting at 5 mg in the morning and gradually increased if necessary to 20 mg bid.
5. Modafinil and amantadine are being explored for use in this area

Activation

Higher numbers indicate more activating drugs in Table 7-1.

1. Patients who are anergic, withdrawn, and hypersomnic might benefit from being started on a more activating medication.
2. Activation can consist of a sense of increased energy and alertness but can also consist of dysphoric agitation, tremulousness, anxiety, restlessness (akathisia), and insomnia. Patients sensitive to dysphoric arousal should not be continued on a drug that causes it or should have the dose lowered.
3. With activated patients, consider alternative diagnoses such as:
   a. Switching into manic episode.
   b. Early serotonin syndrome.
4. Activation can sometimes be improved by:
   a. Lowering the dose.
   b. Adding a benzodiazepine.
   c. Using a β-blocker if akathisia develops.

Orthostatic Hypotension

Orthostatic hypotension is a result of peripheral α-adrenergic blockade as well as a central brainstem mechanism.

1. Risk factors for orthostasis.
   a. Depleted intravascular volumes.
   b. Prolonged bedrest.
   c. Old age.
   d. Autonomic disorders.
   e. Labile autonomic system (in young women).
   f. Pretreatment orthostasis.
   g. Concurrent treatment with other medications that lower blood pressure (e.g., antihypertensives and β-blockers).
2. Orthostasis can lead to falls and injuries such as hip fracture.

3. Ask about lightheadedness and obtain orthostatic blood pressure readings.

Cardiac Conduction Delay

A "+" in Table 7-1 indicates delayed conduction through the intraventricular portion of the His bundle.

1. Patients older than 40 years or with a history of cardiac disease should have an ECG before a TCA is initiated.
2. TCAs should be avoided with preexisting conduction problems.
3. The TCAs also have quinidine-like effects.
4. Summary information on cardiac issues pertaining to antidepressants is shown in Table 7-4. Documented cardiac effects in patients taking fluoxetine are shown in Box 7-1.

Gastrointestinal

1. Nausea and GI activation are the most common side effects of the SSRIs. Up to 25% have nausea, and another 10% to 15% have diarrhea. Paroxetine is associated with the highest rates of nausea, and sertraline is associated with the highest rates of diarrhea. Only about 5% of patients need to discontinue because of these side effects.
   a. If nausea develops, try to lower the dose for about a week. This usually allows the patient to develop tolerance to this side effect.
   b. It is possible to treat SSRI-induced nausea with a 5-HT_3 antagonist (such as 8 mg ondansetron orally.) Mirtazapine may also be considered, as it is associated with 5-HT_3 antagonism as well.
   c. Cisapride (Propulsid) has also been reported to counteract antidepressant-induced nausea (doses are usually 10 mg qid). This drug should not be used with fluoxetine or nefazodone because it is a P450 3A4 substrate and can be cardiotoxic at high plasma levels.
2. The TCAs decrease gastroesophageal sphincter tone, leading to symptoms of reflux.

Seizures

1. TCA antidepressants tend to lower seizure threshold. This is not a reason to avoid their use in epileptic patients as long as the patient is receiving adequate doses of anticonvulsants.
2. Patients who develop a first seizure on antidepressants need a full seizure evaluation.
3. The SSRIs and other second-generation drugs do not seem to lower seizure threshold.
4. Bupropion probably conveys the highest risk of seizures in doses higher than 300 mg/dL, and it should be avoided in anyone with a history of seizures or eating disorders (eating disorders are associated with metabolic disturbances that lower the seizure threshold).

Suicide

As of mid-2006, the Food and Drug Administration (FDA) has suggested a link might exist between antidepressant therapy and increased risk of suicide *only in children*, although fluoxetine was not found to be associated with an increased risk. Patients should be reassured that

Table 7-4 **Cardiac Issues with Antidepressants**

Drug	Myocardial Depression	Orthostatic Hypotension	Arrhythmias	Conduction Delay	Drug Interactions
Bupropion (Wellbutrin)	0	0	"0"	"0"	"0"
Nefazodone (Serzone)	0	0	0	0	0[†]
SSRIs*	0	0	Very rare	Very rare	0[†]
TCAs	Toxic	+	Quinidine-like; withdrawal tachycardia	+	Clonidine, guanethidine, nitrates, quinidine
Venlafaxine	0	0	"0"	0	0

*Also see Box 7-1.
[†]SSRIs can interfere with metabolism of drugs dependent on the P450 system.
Note: "0" indicates little experience in patients with cardiac disease. Therefore document why, follow electrolytes and blood levels, and monitor.

BOX 7-1   **Cardiac Effects in Patients Receiving Fluoxetine**

In more than 3 million patients receiving fluoxetine up to 1991, there have been:
60 cases of bradycardia
54 ventricular arrhythmias
34 atrial arrhythmias
26 cases of heart block
24 cases of congestive heart failure
42 other arrhythmias

there is *no* evidence supporting an increased risk of suicide in adults and that depression itself left untreated *is* associated with an increased risk of suicide.

Sexual

Sexual side effects (anorgasmia, impaired erection, or decreased sex drive) are common reasons for noncompliance, but patients may be unaware of these effects or reluctant to discuss them. Therefore, clinicians should always inquire directly about their presence.

1. Incidence.
   a. Up to at least 50% of patients receiving SSRIs or venlafaxine.
   b. About 10% to 20% (placebo levels) for nefazodone, mirtazapine, and bupropion.
   c. Sexual side effects with TCAs are higher than with nefazodone, mirtazapine, and bupropion, but they are lower than with SSRIs.
2. Treatment.
   a. Attempting to lower the dose is usually the best first option in patients who have responded well to an antidepressant.
   b. Sildenafil (Viagra), tadalafil (Cialis), or verdenafil (Levitra) provide the most effective treatment for counteracting sexual side effects
   c. For drugs with a short half-life, a "drug holiday" (i.e., stop the drug on Thursday, have sex on the weekend, and restart the drug on Monday) can be tried, though this can increase noncompliance.
   d. Switch to bupropion, mirtazapine, or nefazodone.
      (1) When switching from fluoxetine to nefazodone, wait 2 weeks to prevent activating side effects.
      (2) When switching from other drugs, an immediate cross-over is possible.

PHARMACOKINETICS

1. Elimination half-life of the parent compound or the active metabolite or both.
   a. Most of the antidepressants can be given once a day.
   b. Norfluoxetine, the active metabolite of fluoxetine, has an elimination half-life of about 7 days. This may be an advantage for compliance and a disadvantage for elimination of side effects or drug interactions.

       c. Fluoxetine now exists in a once-a-week formulation as well (Serafim). This may be appropriate for some patients who have difficulty remembering to take medication.

2. Oral dose range needed to obtain a therapeutic response shows wide intraindividual variation. Starting dose is usually 50% to 100% of the lower number in the "oral dose range" column (see Table 7-1). Patients started too quickly on higher doses have higher rates of side effects.

       a. In general, the patient's dose should be moved up into the midrange of the oral dose range over the first few weeks.

       b. If a patient does not respond at a midrange dose over 3 to 4 weeks, move up to the top range number.

3. Plasma therapeutic levels are listed in Table 7-1 for four medications that have supporting data.

       a. For these drugs, levels can be used as an adjunct in monitoring treatment. For example, start the patient on 25 mg of nortriptyline and measure the plasma level about 5 days later. If the level is below the therapeutic window (i.e., less than 50 ng/mL), the oral dose could be raised to 50 mg hs. Another plasma level can be obtained 5 days later. If that level is within the therapeutic range, that oral dose can be maintained for 3 to 4 weeks to provide a good clinical trial.

       b. In general, the SSRIs have fairly flat dose—response curves.

       c. Venlafaxine and nefazodone have linear dose—response curves.

ANTIDEPRESSANTS IN PREGNANCY AND BREAST-FEEDING

1. It is preferable to avoid psychotropics during pregnancy and lactation. Psychotherapy or close monitoring should be considered. However, antidepressants may be preferable in those with a history of severe depression and suicidality. Depression itself may have more deleterious effects on the fetus than medications, and the risk of suicide must also be weighed.

2. During pregnancy, the current preferred agent is fluoxetine (based on its having the most data available of any of the newer medications). Preliminary evidence also supports the safety of citalopram, paroxetine, and sertraline.

3. During breast-feeding, nortriptyline, paroxetine, and sertraline are associated with the lowest drug levels present in breast milk.

4. TCAs.

       a. TCAs can be associated with short-term withdrawal effects in the newborn.

       b. TCAs appear to have little potential for teratogenicity.

       c. The more anticholinergic agents can produce fetal tachyarrhythmias.

5. ECT is another option for pregnant patients. There is no evidence that ECT poses a significant risk to the fetus, provided the procedure is adequately monitored (see Chapter 16).

7.3 Tricyclic Antidepressants

1. TCAs may be less well tolerated than second-generation agents (except for fewer sexual side effects).

2. Several (including amitriptyline and desipramine) are useful for chronic pain (see Chapter 15 on analgesic augmenters).
3. Clomipramine has an FDA indication for OCD due to its strong serotoninergic activity.
4. Dosage.
   a. For drugs with established therapeutic plasma levels (amitriptyline, nortriptyline, desipramine, imipramine), titrate oral dose to achieve desired plasma level. Generally, starting on 50 mg hs makes sense. Plasma levels can be checked about every 5 days.
      (1) Plasma level information is not definitive and serves only as a guideline.
      (2) For drugs without known plasma levels, start with low doses and gradually increase until the patient responds or cannot tolerate side effects.
5. Drug interactions are listed in Box 7-2.

7.4 Second-Generation Antidepressants

SELECTIVE SEROTONIN REUPTAKE INHIBITORS

1. SSRIs are usually better tolerated than the TCAs.
2. See Table 7-3 for a summary of side effects.
3. See Chapter 20 for P450 interactions.
4. Fluoxetine (Prozac) dosage.
   a. Most patients respond well to 20 mg daily, given in the morning.
   b. Watch for onset of side effects several weeks into treatment (because of long half-life), such as tremulousness, activation, and insomnia, especially in older patients.
   c. Some patients require doses beyond 40 mg/day, but there is no way to predict who will need higher doses. Some patients who appear to respond to higher doses may actually be responding because they have been receiving medication for a longer time.
   d. Because of activation-induced insomnia, some patients need trazodone (50 to 100 mg hs).
   e. An enteric-coated version of fluoxetine is now available that is dosed once a week. This can be an advantage for patients who have difficulty remembering to take medicine every day. One 90-mg pill per week is comparable to 20 mg/day of fluoxetine.
5. Sertraline (Zoloft) dosage.
   a. Most patients do well receiving 50 to 75 mg daily. Dose range is generally between 25 mg (in the elderly) to 150 mg/day.
   b. There seems to be a lower tendency to activation with sertraline than with fluoxetine.
   c. This drug uncommonly causes clinically significant effects on the P450 system.
6. Paroxetine (Paxil) dosage.
   a. Effective dose range is 10 to 40 mg/day (10 mg is a reasonable starting dose for older patients, 20 mg for others).
   b. Withdrawal syndrome. Because of the short half-life, paroxetine should be tapered, because immediate discontinuation can lead to flulike symptoms.

BOX 7-2   Drug Interactions with Tricyclic Antidepressants

Drugs That Potentiate Hypotension

α-Adrenergic blocking agents
Prazosin

Drugs That Can Cause Increased Blood Pressure

Sympathomimetics

Drugs Whose Antihypertensive Effects May Be Decreased

Clonidine
Guanethidine
Reserpine

Drugs That Raise Antidepressant Levels

Cimetidine
Disulfiram
Methylphenidate

Drugs That Lower Antidepressant Levels

Alcohol
Barbiturates
Oral contraceptives
Phenytoin (Dilantin)

Drugs That Can Prolong Cardiac Conduction

Carbamazepine
Phenothiazines

Drugs That Augment Quinidine-like Effects

Quinidine
Type 1A antiarrhythmics

Drugs That Augment Anticholinergic Effects

Benztropine (Cogentin)
Diphenhydramine (Benadryl)
Meperidine (Demerol)
Oxybutynin (Ditropan)
Propantheline (Pro-Banthine)
Trihexyphenidyl (Artane)

---

    c. Paroxetine has a controlled-release (CR) formulation with the same half-life but a lower peak plasma level.

    d. Paroxetine is associated with the highest rates of weight gain, sedation, and withdrawal effects among the SSRIs.

7. Citalopram (Celexa) and escitalopram (Lexapro) dosage.

    a. Effective dosage of citalopram is 20 to 40 mg/day (20 mg is a reasonable starting dose).

  b. Escitalopram is the *S*-enantiomer of citalopram, which provides the clinical activity of citalopram molecule. Effective dosage is 10 to 20 mg/day (10 mg as starting dose).
    (1) This "purified" form of citalopram is thought to be effective at a lower dose range. Its starting dose is 10 mg qd and the usual dose range is 10 to 30 mg/day.
    (2) Escitalopram may have a faster onset of action than citalopram and less sedation.
8. Loss of drug effect after several months has been noted with the SSRIs ("tachyphylaxis"). The first approach would be to raise the dose. A second approach would be to augment the SSRI or switch to another antidepressant.
9. Other differences among the SSRIs.
  a. Half-life. Fluoxetine is 5 days; sertraline and paroxetine are 1 day.
    (1) A 5-day half-life can be an advantage, because missed doses will not result in much fluctuation in plasma level.
    (2) A 5-day half-life can be a disadvantage because of the lengthy plasma-elimination period.
  b. Paroxetine is the only SSRI with some anticholinergic activity. This may be a disadvantage in older patients.
  c. Fluoxetine and paroxetine have the most potential to inhibit the P450 2D6 system. Citalopram and escitalopram are least likely to be involved in P450 interactions. This is relevant for patients on multiple medications. Fluoxetine also inhibits the P450 3A4 and P450 2C9 families (see Chapter 20).
  d. Patients who do not tolerate one SSRI are often able to tolerate another SSRI.
  e. Patients who do not respond to one SSRI might respond to another SSRI.

SEROTONIN AND NOREPINEPHRINE REUPTAKE INHIBITORS

1. Venlafaxine (Effexor and Effexor XR)
  a. Venlafaxine, in doses less than about 125 mg/day, is primarily a serotonin reuptake inhibitor. At doses more than 125 mg/day it inhibits both norepinephrine and serotonin reuptake and is therefore classified as a serotonin and norepinephrine (NE) reuptake inhibitor (SNRI).
  b. Unlike the TCAs, which also inhibit reuptake of both NE and 5-hydroxytryptamine (5-HT), venlafaxine lacks anticholinergic, antihistaminergic, and antiadrenergic effects.
  c. Its side-effect profile resembles that of the SSRIs, with the most reported effects being nausea (dose dependent), sedation, and dry mouth. Sweating is also seen at times.
  d. The parent compound has a 3- to 4-hour elimination half-life, and the active metabolite (O-desmethyl-venlafaxine) has a 9- to 11-hour half-life, with similar pharmacodynamics.
  e. The effective oral dose appears to be between 75 and 375 mg/day divided in two doses. Elderly, frail, or medically ill patients can be

started on 25 mg bid. Use of the extended release (XR) formulation reduces side effects and allows for once-daily dosing.

f. Venlafaxine has a linear dose—response relationship, and in patients who do not respond, doses should be gradually increased up to a limit of 300 mg/day. Most moderately depressed outpatients respond at doses of 37.5 to 50 mg bid. More severely depressed patients can require doses 100 mg bid or more. Frail geriatric patients are often best started with doses of 12.5 mg bid.

g. At doses higher than 225 mg/day, a small fraction of patients (5% to 10%) experience a dose-dependent increase in supine diastolic blood pressure (SDBP).

  (1) Age, sex, renal or hepatic function, and baseline blood pressure do not predict who will develop increased SDBP.

  (2) Blood pressure elevations generally occur within the first 2 months of dose stabilization. Therefore, patients on doses of 225 mg/day should have blood pressure readings on follow-up visits.

h. Because venlafaxine affects both NE and 5-HT, it is often considered to be a good choice for patients who have failed on serotoninergic agents.

i. Venlafaxine does not inhibit the P450 system (but it is a P450 2D6 substrate and its active metabolite is a P450 3A4 substrate).

j. Some studies have shown superior efficacy compared with SSRIs for hospitalized patients with severe major depression. Due to its dual reuptake mechanism of action, some meta-analyses suggest that venlafaxine can lead to higher remission rates than SSRIs, with lower rates of tachyphylaxis.

2. Duloxetine (Cymbalta)

a. Pharmacology. Duloxetine is a dual uptake inhibitor of both norepinephrine and serotonin.

b. Pharmacokinetics. Elimination half-life is 8 to 17 hours. Metabolites are not active.

  (1) Not recommended for patients with end-stage renal disease (mild renal dysfunction is not a problem).

  (2) Not recommended for patients with any hepatic insufficiency.

c. P450 issues. Substrate for both 2D6 and 1A2 systems. Moderate inhibitor of 2D6.

d. Data on efficacy have been established in four double-blind, placebo-controlled trials in outpatients with major depression. Duloxetine may be especially helpful for depressed patients with somatic (e.g., pain) complaints.

e. Medical issues in use.

  (1) Contraindicated in patients with uncontrolled narrow-angle glaucoma (due to mydriasis).

  (2) Not known how concurrent proton pump inhibitors affect absorption.

  (3) Pregnancy category C.

f. Side effects (differing from placebo).

  (1) Nausea, dry mouth, constipation.

      (2) Sweating.
      (3) Insomnia.
      (4) Sexual dysfunction.
   g. Dosing.
      (1) Start at 30 mg qd and increase to 60 mg after 1 week
      (2) Dose range is between 20 mg and 60 mg

OTHER SECOND-GENERATION ANTIDEPRESSANTS

1. Bupropion (Wellbutrin).
   a. Bupropion has a side-effect profile similar to profiles for stimulants (anorexia, insomnia, agitation, tremor) and is a reasonable choice for many patients, especially those who need some activation.
   b. It has a greater tendency to produce seizures than the other drugs (incidence of about 4 out of 1000 persons) when used in higher doses ($\geq$300 mg/day).
   c. According to some reports, bupropion may be less likely than other antidepressants to cause a switch from depression into mania in patients prone to bipolar disorder.
   d. Bupropion is now available in a sustained release (SR) preparation for twice-a-day dosing and an XR preparation for once-a-day dosing.
   e. Wellbutrin is the same as Zyban and is an effective adjunctive treatment for smoking cessation.
   f. Bupropion is largely devoid of sexual side effects and weight gain and may be a good choice for patients who wish to avoid these side effects.
2. Trazodone (Desyrel).
   a. Trazodone has good hypnotic properties in doses of 50 to 100 mg.
   b. It may be too sedating because the antidepressant dose is often more than 200 mg/day.
   c. It may cause priapism in a few men. Though priapism is rare, patients should be informed of the possible side effect and instructed to go to the emergency department if they develop a painful erection lasting several hours. Make sure to document this discussion in the chart as well.
   d. Trazodone is often used in low doses as a medication to reduce agitation in patients with dementia (see Chapter 5).
3. Nefazodone.
   a. A generic formulation is available.
   b. Nefazodone may be a reasonable choice for prior responders and for those who do not tolerate other antidepressants. Potential liver toxicity is a black box warning for this drug and should be discussed with the patient and documented. Brand-name nefazodone (Serzone) is off the market due to concerns of possible liver toxicity.
   c. Nefazodone acts as a 5-HT$_2$ antagonist and a serotonin uptake inhibitor, similar to trazodone.
   d. Unlike other antidepressants, it does not suppress rapid eye movement activity. Although the SSRIs tend to cause some increase in light stage sleep and increased frequency of awakening, nefazodone causes decrease in light stage sleep and decreased frequency of awakenings.

  e. It has a placebo level of sexual side effects.
  f. It is a P450 3A4 inhibitor.
  g. Metabolites.
      (1) Hydroxynefazodone has a half-life of 3 to 4 hours and has the same pharmacokinetics and pharmacodynamics as the parent compound.
      (2) Triazoledione has a half-life of 18 to 33 hours and is a selective 5-HT$_{2A}$ inhibitor.
      (3) Meta-chlorophenylpiperazine (mCPP) (half-life of 4 to 9 hours) is a potent 5-HT$_{2c}$ agonist which may lead to increased anxiety. Because mCPP is a P450 2D6 substrate, its concentration may be increased by coprescribed SSRIs.
  h. Starting doses are recommended as 100 mg bid for 7 days, with an increase to 150 mg bid. However, older, frail, or medically ill patients should be started at 50 mg bid and increased more slowly if tolerated. Higher starting doses may result in excessive sedation.
  i. Visual trails are an unusual side effect (seen in about 2% of patients) and may be reported as "double vision" or even hallucinations.
  j. Nefazodone does not potentiate the sedative—hypnotic effects of alcohol.
4. Mirtazapine (Remeron).
  a. Neuropharmacology.
      (1) Mirtazapine enhances central noradrenergic and serotoninergic activity.
      (2) It acts as an agonist at central presynaptic α_2-adrenergic inhibitory autoreceptors.
      (3) It acts as antagonist of 5-HT$_2$ and 5-HT$_3$ receptors.
      (4) It is a potent histamine (H$_1$) receptor antagonist, which explains its sedating properties.
      (5) It is a peripheral α_1-adrenergic antagonist and is associated with orthostatic hypotension.
      (6) It has minimal anticholinergic activity.
  b. Pharmacokinetics.
      (1) Half-life of 20 to 40 hours.
      (2) P450 2D6 and 1A2 substrate to form an 8-hydroxy metabolite and 3A4 substrate to form desmethyl and n-oxide metabolites which are three or four times less active than the parent compound.
      (3) Elderly patients and patients with hepatic dysfunction have delayed clearance.
  c. Clinical use.
      (1) Studies have been primarily on moderately depressed outpatients. Mirtazapine is especially useful in depressed patients who have weight loss and/or insomnia.
      (2) In premarketing clinical trials, two of the 2796 subjects developed agranulocytosis, and a third patient developed severe neutropenia. These effects resolved after mirtazapine was stopped. Therefore if a patient develops sore throat, fever, stomatitis, or other signs of infection, mirtazapine should be stopped and white blood cell count checked.

(3) Initial dose should be 15 mg at bedtime because of significant sedative side effects. Dose can be increased up to 45 mg/day. Older patients can be started on 7.5 mg hs.

(4) Because of reports of lowering white blood cell counts, care should be exercised in using this drug in those on other medications that suppress white blood cell production (such as carbamazepine).

d. Side effects. See Table 7-1.

e. Mirtazapine also exists in an orange-flavored dissolvable tablet (Mirtazapine Sol-tab). This may be useful for patients unable to swallow tablets.

7.5 Uncommon (But Important) Medical Complications of the SSRIs and SNRIs

SYNDROME OF INAPPROPRIATE ANTIDIURETIC HORMONE SECRETION (SIADH)

1. Continuous scattered case reports have described SIADH associated with the use of SSRIs. It is important to monitor serum sodium levels in elderly patients receiving SSRIs if behavioral symptoms develop that might be consistent with hyponatremia. SIADH has also been reported as a component of mood disorders in patients not receiving psychotropic medications.

2. Definition. Reduced ability to excrete water, resulting in extracellular dilution and hyponatremia.

3. SSRI mechanism for inducing SIADH is unknown.

4. Clinical symptoms.
   a. Generally do not occur until the sodium level falls below 130 mmol/L, and many patients do not manifest significant symptoms until the sodium level falls below 125 mmol/L.
   b. Onset of symptoms can occur as early as 2 days after starting an SSRI, or they can emerge after many months.
   c. Typical signs and symptoms.
      (1) Headache.
      (2) Confusion.
      (3) Generalized weakness.
      (4) Decreased appetite.
      (5) General malaise.
      (6) Somnolence.
      (7) Coma.
      (8) Seizures.
      (9) Transient focal neurologic signs.
      (10) Abnormal electroencephalogram (EEG).

5. Laboratory findings.
   a. Although patients with SIADH are hyponatremic, they do not manifest edema, hypotension, azotemia, or dehydration.
   b. Because of increased intravascular volume, it is not unusual to find decreases in chloride, blood urea nitrogen (BUN), creatinine, and uric acid.

    c. Hypokalemia is not typical of SIADH but has been reported.

    d. Serum osmolalities are typically low, and case reports show values ranging from 242 to 272 mOsm/kg. Urine sodium levels are typically elevated (> 30 mEq/L), ranging in case reports from 46 to 102 mEq/L.

6. Medical differential diagnosis.

    a. Malignant tumors (especially of lung, duodenum, and pancreas).

    b. Intracranial disorders (e.g., meningitis, trauma, brain abscess, encephalitis, hemorrhage, hydrocephalus).

    c. Infectious diseases (pneumonia, tuberculosis).

    d. Congestive heart failure.

    e. Hypothyroidism.

    f. Liver cirrhosis.

    g. Postoperative states (e.g., surgical stress, positive-pressure ventilation).

    h. Lung diseases (e.g., pneumonia, tuberculosis, emphysema).

    i. Elderly patients are often on thiazide diuretics. SIADH associated with diuretics is generally accompanied by hypokalemia (unlike SIADH associated with SSRIs), alkalosis, and normal or increased serum creatinine and BUN.

    j. Psychogenic polydipsia. Pure polydipsia (in the absence of SIADH) rarely leads to hyponatremia. A triad of symptoms consisting of acute psychosis, massive water ingestion, and SIADH has been reported. Psychogenic polydipsia has also been reported as a feature of schizophrenia and primary affective disorders.

7. Other medications associated with SIADH.

    a. Antipsychotic agents.

    b. Carbamazepine.

    c. Chlorpropamide.

    d. Clofibrate.

    e. Cyclophosphamide.

    f. MAOIs.

    g. Narcotics.

    h. Nicotine.

    i. Oxytocin.

    j. Phenothiazines.

    k. Thiazide diuretics.

    l. Tricyclic antidepressants.

    m. Vasopressin.

    n. Vincristine.

8. Medical management.

    a. Symptoms improve following correction of the electrolyte disturbance, through elimination of the causative agent and restriction of fluid intake.

    b. Mild forms clear up with fluid restriction.

    c. Severe cases might require furosemide diuresis and electrolyte replacement.

    d. Caution should be used in correcting hyponatremia too quickly, because this could result in central pontine demyelination.

e. Typical fluid restriction limits intake to about 1000 mL/day. Return of serum sodium to normal has ranged from 48 hours to 6 weeks after the discontinuation of fluoxetine.

f. Some patients can be restarted on an SSRI without a recurrence of SIADH.

EXTRAPYRAMIDAL SIDE EFFECTS

1. Scattered case reports have described the onset of extrapyramidal side effects (EPS) associated with SSRIs. EPS emergence may be facilitated by SSRIs in patients receiving dopamine receptor–blocking drugs.

2. Epidemiology. EPS occur in about 1 out of 1000 patients treated with SSRIs.

3. Akathisia. SSRIs are known to induce psychological and motor activation, which can appear similar to akathisia associated with antipsychotics.

   a. Akathisia can occur with one dose or within the first week of treatment.

   b. Akathisia has an incidence of up to 20%.

4. Management.

   a. Initial strategy is dose reduction or elimination of the medication.

   b. Low-dose β-blockers (such as propranolol in doses of 5 to 10 mg tid) or clonazepam (in doses of approximately 0.5 mg tid).

5. SSRI mechanisms for inducing EPS.

   a. Indirect inhibition of the dopamine system.

   b. Inhibition of P450 2D6 system, which is responsible for the metabolism of many antipsychotics.

BLEEDING COMPLICATIONS

1. Scattered case reports. One study found the risk of GI bleeding was 3.6 times higher in patients taking SSRIs. This risk was enhanced in the presence of nonsteroidal antiinflammatory drugs (NSAIDs) and aspirin, and it returned to normal once the SSRI was stopped.

2. SSRI mechanism for producing bleeding complications. SSRIs block serotonin uptake into platelets and can impair aggregation and prolong bleeding time.

3. Laboratory findings associated with SSRI-induced bleeding.

   a. Platelet counts are normal.

   b. Prothrombin and partial thromboplastin times are normal.

   c. Bleeding time is prolonged.

   d. Platelet aggregation in response to adenosine diphosphate (ADP) and epinephrine is decreased.

4. Medical management. When in doubt about the clinical impact of bleeding as a possible drug-induced side effect, the SSRI should be stopped and appropriate consultation requested.

CARDIAC ARRHYTHMIAS

1. Given the huge number of patients exposed to SSRIs, there are extremely few reported cases of associated cardiac arrhythmias.

2. Some caution may be needed with severe heart disease (such as bradycardic disorders) or tachyarrhythmias with a tendency to atrial fibrillation. Care should also be exercised in coprescribing SSRIs with β-blockers or type IC antiarrhythmics.

3. Prevalence.
   a. In the first 1.2 million patients exposed to fluoxetine, there were reports of 10 cases of atrial fibrillation, 2 of atrial flutter, 23 of bradycardia, and 2 of atrioventricular block.
   b. ECG studies of patients without cardiovascular disease have not demonstrated any significant abnormalities associated with SSRIs.
   c. SSRI and cardiovascular drug interactions. SSRIs might contribute to the development of cardiac dysfunction through drug interactions mediated through the P450 system.
      (1) SSRIs might lead to bradycardia by impairment of metabolism of β-blockers. Fluoxetine might impair the metabolism of propranolol, metoprolol, and timolol.
      (2) The P450 2D6 system is also responsible for the metabolism of type IC antiarrhythmics such as encainide, flecainide, mexiletine, and propafenone.

SEROTONIN SYNDROME

1. Clinical symptoms. The diagnosis of serotonin syndrome should be considered when at least three of the symptoms from Box 7-3 emerge in the context of the use of serotoninergic agents.

2. Medications causing serotonin syndrome (Box 7-4).
   a. It seems unlikely that a patient would develop serotonin syndrome from an SSRI alone.
   b. There is a potential for serotonin syndrome associated with the use of SSRIs and weight loss medications.
      (1) Combining fluoxetine and phentermine can cause physical and psychic activation with stomach cramps, palpitations, and tremors.
      (2) This interaction may be from 2D6 inhibition of phentermine metabolism or from combined serotonin activity.

3. Medical differential diagnosis.

BOX 7-3   Symptoms of Serotonin Syndrome

Agitation	Incoordination
Diaphoresis	Insomnia
Diarrhea	Mental status changes
Dizziness	(confusion or hypomania)
Drowsiness	Myoclonus
Fever	Nausea or vomiting
Hyperreflexia	Shivering
Hypertension	Tremor

BOX 7-4   **Drugs Reported to Cause Serotonin Syndrome**

Alone

Dextromethorphan
MAOIs
SSRIs

In Combination

MAOIs PLUS

Meperidine
Tricyclics
L-Tryptophan

SSRIs PLUS

Carbamazepine
Dexfenfluramine
Lithium
MAOIs
Pentazocine
Phentermine
L-Tryptophan

MAOI, monoamine oxidase inhibitor; SSRI, selective serotonin reuptake inhibitor.

   a. Serotonin syndrome can be confused with neuroleptic malignant syndrome (NMS), because several of the most common clinical features overlap.
      (1) The major clinical feature distinguishing NMS from serotonin syndrome is EPS (usually severe rigidity) in NMS as opposed to myoclonus, which occurs in serotonin syndrome.
      (2) Elevated creatine phosphokinase (CPK), which is typical for NMS, is not present in serotonin syndrome.
   b. Other medical problems to consider are found in Box 7-5.
4. Medical management.
   a. Symptoms generally abate within 24 hours after discontinuation of the causative agent(s).
   b. β-Blockers block 5-HT receptors and can inhibit serotonin syndrome caused by L-tryptophan and MAOIs.
   c. Clonazepam can be helpful in relieving serotonin syndrome–related myoclonus.

7.6 Stimulants as Antidepressants

1. Indications.
   a. Stimulants should not be considered first-line drugs for the treatment of depression.
   b. Potential indications. Geriatric and medically ill patients (such as acquired immunodeficiency syndrome [AIDS] patients) with depressive symptoms involving withdrawn behavior, lack of motivation and energy, and depressed mood.
2. Clinical use. Methylphenidate (more commonly) and dextroamphetamine are used.
   a. Patients are usually started on 5 mg orally in the morning. When a response is seen, it is often apparent within 24 hours. If there is no response, the dose may be raised daily by 5-mg increments up to 20 mg. If no response at 20 mg, consider the trial failed.
   b. Because the effect may be short lived, a second dose may need to be given at noon.

BOX 7-5   Differential Diagnosis of Serotonin Syndrome

CNS Disorders

Central hyperthermia (postsurgical or traumatic)
Collagen vascular disorders
Infections: viral encephalitis, postinfectious encephalitis, HIV, tetanus, and other bacterial, fungal, or parasitic agents
Neuroleptic malignant syndrome
Tumors
Vascular or neoplastic lesions

Systemic Disorders

Heat stroke
Infections
Systemic lupus erythematosus

Drugs

Alcohol or sedative withdrawal
Anesthetics
Anticholinergics
Dopamine antagonists
Psychedelics
Salicylates
Stimulants
Toxins (CO, strychnine, phenols)

CNS, central nervous system; HIV, human immunodeficiency virus.

    c. Both methylphenidate and dextroamphetamine now exist in long-acting once-a-day formulations.
3. Side effects.
    a. In general, these doses are well tolerated. Only about 15% of patients have side effects, which include the following:
        (1) Overstimulation without antidepressant effect.
        (2) Anxiety.
        (3) Confusion.
        (4) Paranoia.
        (5) Tachycardia (unusual).
        (6) Appetite disturbance (unusual).
4. Medical issues in clinical use. These drugs have been used safely in a variety of medically ill patients, though caution should be used in patients with a history of cardiac disease.

7.7 Monoamine Oxidase Inhibitors

1. Indications.
    a. Treatment-resistant major depression.
    b. Treatment-resistant panic disorder.

Table 7-5	**Dosing of Monoamine Oxidase Inhibitors**	
Drug	**Starting Dose**	**Daily Dose**
Phenelzine (Nardil)	15 mg at 9 AM, 1 PM	45-90 mg
Selegiline (Eldepryl)	10 mg at 9 AM	10-30 mg
Selegiline transdermal patch (ENSAM) (selective for MAO-B)	6 mg patch	6-18 mg
Tranylcypromine (Parnate)	10 mg at 9 AM, 1 PM	20-40 mg

    c. Treatment-resistant mixed anxiety and depression.
    d. Treatment-resistant depression in patients with bipolar disorder.
    e. Dysthymia not responsive to other antidepressants.
    f. "Atypical" depression (defined as depression characterized by anxiety, somatization, feeling better in the morning and worse as day goes on, hyperphagia, hypersomnia, weight gain, sensitivity to rejection).

2. Available MAOIs with the daily dose and starting dose are listed in Table 7-5.
3. Effective dose.
    a. Greater than 80% MAOI must be reached for a clinical effect. This usually requires a dose of 60 mg/day of phenelzine or 40 mg/day of tranylcypromine. Start with 15 mg orally for phenelzine (10 mg for Parnate) and increase by that dose increment every 7 days until reaching 45 mg and 30 mg, respectively.
    b. Three to five weeks at a therapeutic dose is necessary to judge response.
    c. A transdermal selegiline (an irreversible MAOI) system has been recently approved that substantially avoids inhibition of intestinal and liver MAO-A and MAO-B enzymes, making it potentially safer than traditional MAOIs. A recent placebo-controlled study comprising almost 300 subjects found modest, but significant benefit compared with placebo in the absence of a tyramine-restricted diet. An MAOI diet is not needed when prescribing the 6 mg patch, but it is still necessary for higher dosages.
4. Side effects.
    a. Orthostatic hypotension is a common limiting factor (10% to 15%).
        (1) Ensure adequate hydration.
        (2) Use support stockings.
        (3) Try to eliminate other hypotensive agents.
    b. Weight gain (carbohydrate craving or edema).
    c. Insomnia. Low doses of trazodone (50 to 100 mg hs) or benzodiazepine hypnotics may be helpful in counteracting this side effect.

    d. Sexual dysfunction (anorgasmia).

    e. Pyridoxine deficiency can develop with phenelzine, producing paresthesias. Treatment (which some clinicians feel should be supplied prophylactically) is vitamin B_6 100 to 400 mg/day.

    f. Hypertensive crisis is a rare (incidence 0.5% with mortality 0.001%) but potentially life-threatening reaction that is usually associated with mixing MAOIs with a pressor medication or food with high tyramine content (Box 7-6).

       (1) Medications and food to avoid when using MAOIs (see Box 7-6). Patients should be competent and willing to follow restrictions. Review the list with the patient.

       (2) Some clinicians give nifedipine capsules (10 mg) for patients to take orally if they sense a hypertensive reaction (usually noted as a pounding headache). Patients should bite the capsule and swallow the contents. This recommendation remains controversial.

       (3) Patients who think they are having a hypertensive crisis should go to an emergency deparmtnent. Phentolamine 5 mg IV or nifedipine is usually given.

5. Drug interactions are numerous (see Box 7-6). Look up every drug before a patient takes it.

    a. MAOIs increase intracellular catecholamine stores. Therefore indirect-acting sympathomimetics, which release these stores, are contraindicated.

       (1) Indirect-acting agents include cocaine, amphetamines, methylphenidate, pseudoephedrine, ephedrine, and phenylpropanolamine.

       (2) Many over-the-counter cold remedies contain these agents.

       (3) Because intracellular dopamine is also increased, carbidopa—levodopa (Sinemet) can cause hypertension with MAOIs. Direct-acting dopamine agonists are safer. Selegiline is safe to combine with dopamine agonists in doses of about 10 mg/day.

    b. Direct-acting sympathomimetics can be used safely. This includes bronchodilators (inhalers are safer than oral drugs).

    c. Combining MAOIs with serotonin-augmenting drugs (e.g., TCAs, SSRIs, trazodone, or buspirone) can produce serotonin syndrome. Discontinue MAOIs for 2 weeks before switching to another antidepressant. Clinical features of serotonin syndrome are listed earlier.

    d. MAOIs and anesthesia.

       (1) A 2-week washout before elective general anesthesia would be ideal, but it is definitely not necessary.

       (2) Curare should be avoided because of its indirect sympathomimetic effect.

       (3) For hypotension, volume expansion or direct-acting sympathomimetics (e.g., norepinephrine) should be used instead of indirect-acting agents such as metaraminol.

       (4) Droperidol should be avoided because of reports of cardiac and respiratory depression with MAOIs.

BOX 7-6   Food and Medication to Avoid by Patients Receiving Orally Administered MAOIs

Foods to Avoid

Avocados (if overripe)
Banana peel
Bean curd (fermented)
Broad beans
Caviar
Cheese* (cottage, cream, and skim mozzarella and ricotta in moderate amounts are permissible)
Chocolate (in large amounts)
Fava beans*
Figs (overripe)
Fish, pickled or salted (safe if fresh)
Ginseng
Licorice
Liqueurs
Liver* (safe if fresh)
Meats, aged or processed*
Miso soup
Protein (powdered supplements)
Sauerkraut*
Sausage
Shrimp paste
Soy sauce*
Wines (especially Chianti)
Yeast extracts*

Drugs to Avoid

DRUGS THAT INCREASE BLOOD PRESSURE WITH MAOIs
Aminophylline
Amphetamines
Caffeine
Carbamazepine
Cocaine
Cyclic antidepressants
Cyclobenzaprine
Direct-acting sympathomimetics
Epinephrine
Ephedrine
Guanethidine
Isoproterenol
Levodopa
Methyldopa
Metaraminol
Methylphenidate
Phenylethylamine
Phenylpropanolamine
Pseudoephedrine
Theophylline
Tyramine

DRUGS THAT LOWER BLOOD PRESSURE WITH MAOIs
Calcium channel blockers
Diuretics
Hypoglycemic agents
Prazosin
Propranolol

DRUGS WITH PROLONGED (INCREASED) ACTIVITY WITH MAOIs
Anticholinergics
Anticoagulants
Succinylcholine

DRUGS THAT CAN CAUSE SEROTONIN SYNDROME WITH MAOIs
Buspirone
Cyclic antidepressants
Meperidine
SSRIs
Tryptophan

OTHER DRUGS TO AVOID WITH MAOIs
Aldomet
Clonidine
Guanethidine
Reserpine

*These foods have the highest tyramine content and the most potential for interaction.
MAOI, monoamine oxidase inhibitor; SSRI, selective serotonin reuptake inhibitor.

SUGGESTED READINGS

Amsterdam JD: A double-blind, placebo-controlled trial of the safety and efficacy of selegiline transdermal system without dietary restrictions in patients with major depressive disorder. J Clin Psychiatry 64(2):208-214, 2003.

Bielski RJ, Ventura D, Chang CC: A double-blind comparison of escitalopram and venlafaxine extended release in the treatment of major depressive disorder. J Clin Psychiatry 65(9):1190-1196, 2004.

Dalton SO, Johansen C, Mellemkjaer L, et al: Use of selective serotonin reuptake inhibitors and risk of upper gastrointestinal tract bleeding: A population-based cohort study. Arch Intern Med 163(1):59-64, 2003.

Dennis CL, Stewart DE: Treatment of postpartum depression, part 1: A critical review of biological interventions. J Clin Psychiatry 65(9):1242-1251, 2004.

Dennis CL: Treatment of postpartum depression, part 2: A critical review of nonbiological interventions. J Clin Psychiatry 65(9):1252-1265, 2004.

Laine K, Heikkinen T, Ekblad U, Kero P: Effects of exposure to selective serotonin reuptake inhibitors during pregnancy on serotonergic symptoms in newborns and cord blood monoamine and prolactin concentrations. Arch Gen Psychiatry 60(7):726, 2003.

Leon AC, Keller MB, Warshaw MG, et al: Prospective study of fluoxetine treatment and suicidal behavior in affectively ill subjects. Am J Psychiatry 156(2):195-201, 1999.

Nonacs R, Cohen LS: Depression during pregnancy: Diagnosis and treatment options. J Clin Psychiatry 63(Suppl 7):24-30, 2002.

Posternak MA, Zimmerman M: Switching versus augmentation: A prospective, naturalistic comparison in depressed, treatment-resistant patients. J Clin Psychiatry 62(4):221-224, 2001.

Rosen RC, Lane RM, Menza M: Effects of SSRIs on sexual function: A critical review. J Clin Psychopharmacol 19(1):67-85, 1999.

Schwartz TL, Azhar N, Cole K, et al: An open-label study of adjunctive modafinil in patients with sedation related to serotonergic antidepressant therapy. J Clin Psychiatry 65(9):1223-1227, 2004.

Thase ME, Entsuah AR, Rudolph RL: Remission rates during treatment with venlafaxine or selective serotonin reuptake inhibitors. Br J Psychiatry 178:234-241, 2001.

Walkup JT, Sambamoorthi U, Crystal S: Use of newer antiretroviral treatments among HIV-infected Medicaid beneficiaries with serious mental illness. J Clin Psychiatry 65(9):1180-1189, 2004.

Weissman AM, Levy BT, Hartz AJ, et al: Pooled analysis of antidepressant levels in lactating mothers, breast milk, and nursing infants. Am J Psychiatry 161(6):1066-1078, 2004.

Wender PH, Wolf LE, Wasserstein J: Adults with ADHD. An overview. Ann N Y Acad Sci 931:1-16, 2001.

Zimmerman M, Posternak M, Friedman M, et al: Which factors influence psychiatrists' selection of antidepressants? Am J Psychiatry 161(7):1285-1289, 2004.

Bipolar Disorder and Mood-Stabilizing Drugs

8

Christine J. Truman

8.1 Bipolar Disorder

1. *Bipolar I disorder* refers to patients who have had one or more manic or mixed episodes (for definitions of manic and mixed episodes, see the next section).
   a. Patients may also have had one or more major depressive episodes.
   b. Manic episodes caused by drugs or medical diagnoses do not count.
   c. Clinical features of bipolar I disorder.
      (1) Usually a lifelong illness with a variable, episodic course.
      (2) Between 10% and 15% of adolescents with a major depressive episode will develop bipolar disorder.
      (3) Equal prevalence in men and women and across cultures and ethnic groups.
      (4) Women with bipolar disorder are at high risk for a subsequent episode during the postpartum period.
      (5) Bipolar I disorder has a strong genetic component; family history is important.
      (6) Approximately 10% to 15% of patients with bipolar I disorder eventually commit suicide.
      (7) Bipolar I disorder is a recurrent disorder. More than 90% of those with a single episode go on to additional episodes.
      (8) From 50% to 60% of manic episodes occur just before or just after a major depressive episode.
      (9) The interval between manic episodes tends to decrease with age.
      (10) Community prevalence is 0.4% to 1.6%.
2. *Bipolar II disorder* is defined as one or more major depressive episodes with at least one hypomanic episode (for definition, see the next section)
   a. Hypomanic episodes caused by drugs or medical diagnoses do not count toward the diagnosis.
   b. Clinical features of bipolar II disorder.
      (1) Approximately 10% to 15% of patients with bipolar II disorder eventually commit suicide.
      (2) Risk of completed suicide may be higher in bipolar II than bipolar I disorder.
      (3) More common in women than men.
      (4) Increased risk of recurrence in postpartum period.

(5) From 60% to 70% of hypomanic episodes occur just before or after a major depressive episode.
(6) From 5% to 15% of bipolar II patients have multiple mood episodes within a given year. This feature is defined as *rapid cycling*.
(7) Strong genetic component.
(8) Lifetime prevalence of bipolar II disorder is 0.5%.
(9) With mild hypomanic episodes, clinical history may only suggest recurrent unipolar depression.
3. *Cyclothymia* refers to patients whose mood swings are not severe enough to qualify as bipolar disorder.
4. *Rapid cycling* refers to patients who alternate highs and lows frequently (as often as every few weeks or days but at least four times per year).
    a. About 10% of patients with bipolar illness are rapid cyclers.
    b. Rapid cycling is more common in women than in men.

8.2 Manic, Hypomanic, Mixed, Cyclothymic, and Rapid Cycling Episodes

DEFINITIONS
1. Manic episode.
    a. A manic episode is a distinct period of abnormally and persistently elevated, expansive, or irritable mood lasting at least 1 week (or any duration if severe enough to require hospitalization).
    b. During the period of mood disturbance, at least three of the following symptoms have persisted (four if the mood is only irritable):
        (1) Inflated self-esteem or grandiosity.
        (2) Decreased need for sleep.
        (3) More talkative or pressured speech.
        (4) Racing thoughts or flight of ideas.
        (5) Distractibility.
        (6) Physical agitation (or increased work, social, or sexual activity).
        (7) Poor judgment about activities (e.g., buying sprees).
    c. The mood disturbance must be significant enough to cause work or social impairment, hospitalization, or concern over harmfulness.
    d. Bipolar patients might have delusions or hallucinations during the period of mood disturbance, but not at other times.
2. Hypomanic episode.
    a. A hypomanic episode is a distinct period of abnormally and persistently elevated, expansive, or irritable mood lasting at least 4 days.
    b. During the period of mood disturbance, at least three of the following symptoms have persisted (four if the mood is only irritable):
        (1) Inflated self-esteem or grandiosity.
        (2) Decreased need for sleep.
        (3) More talkative or pressured speech.
        (4) Racing thoughts or flight of ideas.
        (5) Distractibility.
        (6) Physical agitation (or increased work, social, or sexual activity).
        (7) Poor judgment about activities (e.g., buying sprees).

BOX 8-1   Medical Causes of Mania

Medications and Drugs	*Medical Disorders*
Antidepressants	Brain infections
AZT	Brain trauma
Bromide	Brain tumors
Bronchodilators	Dialysis dementia
Caffeine	Electrical trauma
Cocaine	Epilepsy
Dopamine agonists	HIV infection
Isoniazid	Hyperbaric diving
Procarbazine	Hyperthyroidism
Pseudoephedrine	Open heart surgery
Steroids	Sleep deprivation
Stimulants	Stroke
	Vitamin B_{12} deficiency

AZT, zidovudine (azidothymidine); HIV, human immunodeficiency virus.

---

    c. The mood disturbance *is not severe enough to cause marked impairment* in work or social function, is not serious enough to require admission, and has no psychotic features.

    d. It is not due to drugs or medical disorder (Box 8-1).

3. Mixed episode. Criteria are met for *both manic episode and major depressive episode* during a 1-week period.

4. Cyclothymic disorder: At least 2 years of numerous periods of hypomanic symptoms *and* numerous periods of depressive symptoms that do not meet criteria for major depression.

5. Rapid cycling episodes: At least four episodes of mood disturbance in a 12-month period that meet criteria for major depressive, manic, mixed, or hypomanic episodes.

DIFFERENTIAL DIAGNOSIS OF MANIC SYMPTOMS

1. Psychotic disorders. Acute manic illness may seem indistinguishable from schizophrenia or other psychotic disorders. Both disorders can manifest with agitated, paranoid, irritable, or psychotic symptoms. These disorders are distinguished by the following:

    a. Absence of prominent mood symptoms in psychotic disorders.

    b. Family history (these diseases tend to segregate genetically).

    c. Previous history (manic–depressive illness is episodic, with higher functioning between episodes and absence of psychosis between episodes).

2. Temporal lobe epilepsy sometimes manifests as episodic mood disturbance.

    a. Many drugs used to treat complex partial seizures (e.g., carbamazepine, lamotrigine, valproate) also treat bipolar disorder.

    b. Patients with episodic mood disturbance and risk factors for complex partial seizures should have an electroencephalogram (EEG), especially if the presentation is atypical. The following are risk factors for temporal lobe epilepsy:

(1) Family history of epilepsy.
(2) Previous head injury.
(3) Febrile convulsions in childhood.
(4) Presence of another type of seizure disorder.
(5) Presence of cancer that could metastasize to the brain.
(6) Central nervous system infections.
(7) Risk factors for human immunodeficiency virus (HIV) infection.

3. Stimulant abuse can produce periods of manic behavior followed by severe depressive withdrawals.
4. Alcohol (or sedative) abuse can produce "depression" during the sedative phase and "mania" during the withdrawal delirium. Attempts to self-medicate underlying mood disorders can lead to alcohol or other substance abuse, which then confuses the diagnosis.
5. Attention-deficit/hyperactivity disorder (ADHD) in adults can manifest as restlessness and distractibility, but there is not a manic mood component.
6. Brief psychotic disorder can appear as a manic episode, but the episode is brief, may be temporally related to a stressor, usually has no elevated mood component, and rarely has a recurrent course.
7. Manic disorder due to a general medical condition can result from the following:
   a. Lesions of the frontal, limbic, or temporal lobes, most often right-sided lesions.
   b. Metabolic or endocrine conditions (e.g., vitamin B_{12} deficiency, hypo- and hyperthyroidism, hypo- and hyperparathyroidism).
   c. Viral or other infections (e.g., HIV, hepatitis, mononucleosis).
   d. Medications.
      (1) Levodopa.
      (2) Antidepressants.
      (3) Corticosteroids.
      (4) Decongestants with phenylephrine.
      (5) Sympathomimetics or bronchodilators.
      (6) Theophylline or albuterol.
      (7) Interferon.
8. First onset of mania after age 40 is more likely to be associated with general medical factors including stroke or other central nervous system (CNS) lesions.

OVERVIEW OF TREATMENTS
General Issues for Acute Mania

Pharmacologic treatments for acute mania are summarized in Tables 8-1 and 8-2.

1. Acute mania is best approached as a behavioral emergency (see Chapter 14).
2. American Psychiatric Association (APA) and expert consensus guidelines recommend first-line pharmacologic treatment with a

Table 8-1 **Atypical Antipsychotics for Acute Mania**

Medication	Starting Dose (mg/day)	Target Dose (mg/day)	Final Dose (mg/day)	IM Available
Aripiprazole (Abilify)	15	15-30	30	—
Olanzapine (Zyprexa)	15	10-30	25	Equivalent dosing
Quetiapine (Seroquel)	150	300-800	700	—
Risperidone (Risperdal)	2.5	2.5-6	7	—
Ziprasidone (Geodon)	80	80-180	160	IM equivalent to half of oral dose

IM, intramuscular.

Table 8-2   Other Medications for Acute Mania

Agent	Rapid Loading Guideline	Nonrapid Initial Titration	Target Dose (mg/day)	Therapeutic Level
Carbamazepine		400-800 mg/day divided tid or qid	400-1200	4-12 µg/mL
Divalproex (Depakote)	20-30 mg/kg divided bid or tid	15-20 mg/kg divided bid or tid	1000-2000	50-125 µg/mL
Lithium		300 mg tid	300-1800	0.7-1.2 mEq/L
Oxcarbazepine		150 mg qd, then increase 150 mg qod	1200-1600	10-35 µg/mL

mood stabilizer (lithium or divalproex) alone or with an antipsychotic.

3. Divalproex and lithium are the preferred first-line mood stabilizers for acute mania. Carbamazepine is a second-line alternative.

4. For mania with psychotic features, a mood stabilizer plus an antipsychotic or an antipsychotic alone is recommended.

5. Preferred antipsychotic medications for use as first-line treatments for mania (alone or in combination strategies) include olanzapine, risperidone, and quetiapine. Second-line options include aripiprazole and ziprasidone.

6. Divalproex may be orally loaded (20 mg/kg in divided bid or tid dosing).

7. Adjunctive use of a sedating benzodiazepine such as clonazepam 1 to 2 mg prn may be helpful in controlling acute agitation.

8. Oxcarbazepine may be an acceptable alternative second-line mood stabilizer.

9. For mixed episodes, valproate may be preferable to lithium.

10. When possible, antidepressants should be tapered and discontinued.

11. For breakthrough episodes despite maintenance treatment, initial therapy should focus on optimizing doses of existing medications.

12. Electroconvulsive therapy (ECT) is used in rare circumstances to control a severe manic episode that is treatment resistant or mixed or to treat patients who are acutely suicidal or pregnant or whose condition is medically complex.

General Issues for Bipolar Depression

1. Bipolar depression generally responds to tricyclic, selective serotonin reuptake inhibitor (SSRI), monoamine oxidase inhibitor (MAOI), bupropion, and other antidepressants effective in treating unipolar depression.

2. Concern about the possibility of inducing cycling or switch into mania or mixed episodes often limits the use of conventional antidepressants in the treatment of bipolar depression.

3. Due to concern for inducing cycling or switches, antidepressant monotherapy is not a recommended treatment for bipolar I depression. An alternative for more severely ill patients is simultaneous initiation of an antidepressant and lithium or valproate, along with close clinical monitoring.

4. APA and expert consensus guidelines recommend lithium or lamotrigine alone as first-line treatments. Alternatives include lithium plus lamotrigine or lithium and divalproex plus an antidepressant.

5. For acute depressive episodes that do not respond to optimal doses of first-line treatments, consider adding the alternative first-line treatment (lithium or lamotrigine) or a newer antidepressant (SSRI, bupropion, venlafaxine) or an MAOI.

6. Combination treatment with an atypical antipsychotic medication is recommended for depressive episodes with psychotic features.

7. ECT is used for severe or refractory episodes, when life life-threatening suicidality or psychosis is present, or for severe depression during pregnancy.

8. Consensus guidelines support the use of adjunctive psychotherapy (interpersonal, cognitive behavior, or family-focused therapy) in combination with medication as a first-line treatment for nonpsychotic bipolar depression.
9. For "breakthrough" episodes despite maintenance treatment, initial therapy should focus on optimizing doses of maintenance medications.
10. Novel treatment strategies being investigated for the treatment of bipolar depression include atypical antipsychotics (in particular, olanzapine and quetiapine) alone or in combination with antidepressants.

General Issues for Maintenance Treatment of Bipolar Disorder

1. Following an acute episode, bipolar patients remain at high risk for relapse for up to 6 months.
2. The long-term objective of maintenance treatment is to prevent the recurrence of mood episodes.
3. APA guidelines note that the best empirical evidence supports the use of lithium and valproate for maintenance treatment, with alternatives including lamotrigine, carbamazepine, and oxcarbazepine.
4. First-line agents for reducing the recurrence of depressive episodes include lithium and lamotrigine.
5. First-line agents for reducing the recurrence of manic episodes include lithium, divalproex, olanzapine, and clozapine. Second-line options include aripiprazole, ziprasidone, quetiapine, carbamazepine. and risperidone.
6. Medication(s) that resolved the acute episode are often continued in the maintenance phase.
7. The need for ongoing antidepressant or antipsychotic medication treatment should be reevaluated during the maintenance phase while weighing the risks of treatment as well as the severity and frequency of symptoms.
8. Psychotherapy or psychosocial interventions (e.g., support groups) that focus on illness management and interpersonal difficulties are often beneficial during the maintenance phase of illness.

8.3 Lithium

1. Indications.
   a. Lithium continues to be a first-line treatment for acute mania, for reducing both manic and depressive recurrence, and for acute bipolar depression.
   b. Lithium alone is effective in about 60% to 80% of patients with classic bipolar disorder but may be less effective in patients with mixed or rapid cycling bipolar disorders.
   c. Lithium can treat acute mania. It is difficult to rapidly load patients due to toxicity; therefore, in the acute phase it usually requires supplementation with neuroleptic agents, benzodiazepines, or both (see Chapter 14).

BOX 8-2   Drugs That Alter Lithium Levels

Drugs That Increase Lithium Levels

ACE inhibitors
Enalapril
Erythromycin
Indomethacin and NSAIDs
Metronidazole
Potassium-sparing diuretics
Spironolactone
Thiazide diuretics
Tetracycline
Triamterene

Drugs That Decrease Lithium Levels

Acetazolamide
Aminophylline
Osmotic diuretics
Theophylline

Treatments That Have Increased Toxicity When Prescribed with Lithium

Calcium channel blockers
Clozapine
Digoxin
Electroconvulsive therapy
Haloperidol
α-Methyldopa
Serotoninergic antidepressants
Succinylcholine

ACE, angiotensin-converting enzyme; NSAID, nonsteroidal antiinflammatory drug.

---

    d. By current APA guidelines, lithium monotherapy remains a first-line treatment for acute bipolar depression and maintenance treatment of bipolar disorder.

2. Pharmacology.

    a. Lithium is minimally protein bound.

    b. It is excreted by the kidney unchanged and has an elimination half-life of about 24 hours.

       (1) Baseline renal laboratory tests should be performed before initiating lithium therapy.

       (2) Excretion is controlled by osmotic factors and relies on renal sufficiency. Lithium toxicity can develop in the context of restricted sodium intake, diarrhea, vomiting, volume depletion, or diuretic use.

3. Drug interactions. Drugs that increase and decrease lithium levels are listed in Box 8-2.

4. Clinical use.
   a. Formulations.
      (1) Lithium is available in multiple preparations (lithium carbonate capsules and tablets, lithium citrate, and slow-release forms).
      (2) Sustained-release forms (Lithobid and Eskalith CR) may improve compliance (by allowing once- or twice-daily dosing) and minimize plasma level fluctuations.
   b. Laboratory monitoring.
      (1) Baseline assessments.
         (a) Medical history, renal function tests (blood urea nitrogen [BUN], creatinine [Cr]), and thyroid function tests (TFT).
         (b) Women of childbearing age should have a pregnancy test.
         (c) Patients older than 40 years or with a history of cardiac disease should have an electrocardiogram (ECG).
      (2) First 6 months of treatment. Renal function test every 2 to 3 months, TFT 1 or 2 times
      (3) After 6 months of treatment. Renal function test and TFT every 6 to 12 months
   c. Dosage.
      (1) Start with divided doses (e.g., 300 mg lithium carbonate tid). Steady state is reached in 4 to 5 days.
      (2) Lithium levels should be obtained in the morning (about 12 hours after the night dose) before the first morning dose.
      (3) Target dose estimate is based on 15 mg/kg (7.5 mg/lb), with a typical target level of 0.7 to 1.2 mEq/L.
      (4) Adjust the oral dose based on the first level. Increase incrementally and repeat the level in another 4 or 5 days.
         (a) This process can be repeated until a therapeutic level is achieved.
         (b) Once a therapeutic level is achieved, it can be checked in another month or so, and then every 3 to 6 months. Once established, a level remains steady unless there is a drug reaction or a change in renal function or sodium.
      (5) Manic patients with partial responses should have levels raised to approach 1.2 to 1.4 mEq/L. Response to lithium alone in acute mania is generally not seen for at least 7 days and can take 2 to 3 weeks.
      (6) Elderly patients should be monitored closely with attention to medical comorbidity, neurotoxicity, and concomitant medications. However, response and therapeutic blood levels are often similar to those in younger adults.
   d. Side effects.
      (1) Fine tremor (usually dose related) is not uncommon (about 4% to 65%).
         (a) May be treated with β-blockers (e.g., propranolol 10 to 20 mg qid).
         (b) More severe tremor suggests toxicity.

(2) Nephrogenic diabetes insipidus, with resulting polyuria and polydipsia.
  (a) Due to unresponsiveness of kidney to antidiuretic hormone.
  (b) Occurs in approximately 10% of patients on long-term lithium therapy.
  (c) May be corrected by amiloride (10 to 20 mg/day) or thiazide diuretics.
(3) Hypothyroidism can develop (approximately 3% to 14%).
  (a) May be more common in women and those older than 50 years.
  (b) Baseline and periodic TFT monitoring is important in clinical management.
(4) Weight gain may be partially related to increased thirst and increased consumption of caloric beverages.
(5) Gastrointestinal discomfort is not uncommon. At toxic levels, patients develop nausea, vomiting, and diarrhea. Gastrointestinal side effects may be lessened by taking lithium with meals or by use of the slow-release preparation.
(6) Cardiac effects include sinus bradycardia, sinus node dysfunction, occasional T-wave changes, and rare cases of atrioventricular block.
  (a) Cardiac disease does not preclude lithium use in the presence of clinical indications.
  (b) ECG and dose monitoring should be used in patients older than 50 years or with known cardiac disease.
(7) Leukocytosis without a left shift.
(8) Teratogenicity.
  (a) Lithium is considered a first-line treatment for bipolar disorder during pregnancy.
  (b) As with any treatment, the risks and benefits of lithium use must be carefully assessed in the context of pregnancy or breast-feeding.
  (c) Recent data suggest that lithium exposure during pregnancy is less harmful than previously believed in the 1970s.
  (d) The risk of Ebstein's anomaly, a surgically treatable cardiac malformation, from first-trimester lithium exposure has been estimated to be 0.05% to 0.1%. This is approximately 10 to 20 times the risk in the general population.
  (e) Divalproex carries up to a 5% prevalence of neural tube defects or other neurologic problems.

8.4 Valproic Acid

1. Indications.
  a. Approved by the Food and Drug Administration (FDA) for the treatment of acute mania associated with bipolar disorder. May be orally loaded.
  b. First-line treatment for acute mania and for reducing recurrence of mania.

   c. May be more effective than lithium for mixed mania and rapid-cycling bipolar disorder. May also be superior to lithium for patients with a history of nonresponse to lithium, irritable subtype of mania, and a high number of lifetime episodes.

2. Pharmacology.
   a. Highly protein bound.
      (1) Toxic effects can occur if the drug is displaced from binding sites, because only the unbound portion crosses the blood–brain barrier.
      (2) Aspirin (highly protein bound) can raise total and free valproate levels.
   b. All oral preparations are rapidly absorbed. Peak serum concentrations vary by preparation and occur between 2 and 8 hours.
   c. Elimination half-life is about 12 to 16 hours
   d. Metabolized primarily through the liver by glucuronidation and a mitochondrial pathway.

3. Drug interactions.
   a. Inhibits drug oxidation (does not induce hepatic microsomal enzymes) and increases serum concentrations of:
      (1) Phenobarbital.
      (2) Phenytoin.
      (3) Tricyclic antidepressants.
   b. Metabolism of valproate is induced by:
      (1) Carbamazepine.
      (2) Phenobarbital.
      (3) Phenytoin.
      (4) Primidone.
   c. Monitor levels closely when coprescribing with drugs that are highly protein bound. Patients can show toxicity even at therapeutic plasma levels.
   d. Protein binding is increased by low-fat diets and decreased by high-fat diets.
   e. Concurrent use of other drugs excreted by glucuronide conjugation (e.g., lamotrigine) raises valproate levels. Requires lamotrigine to be started at lower doses (usually 25 mg qod) and increased more cautiously.

4. Clinical use.
   a. Formulations.
      (1) Available in the United States in five oral preparations (including sprinkle capsules), a sodium valproate intravenous preparation, and a suppository form for rectal administration.
      (2) Extended-release (ER) form of divalproex provides once-daily dosing and can reduce the side-effect profile.
   b. Laboratory monitoring. Pretreatment medical evaluation should include the following:
      (1) Complete blood count (CBC) including platelet count.
      (2) Liver function tests (LFTs). Fatal hepatotoxicity has been confined to children younger than 10 years taking multiple antiepileptic drugs.

   c. Dosing.
     (1) Usually started at dose of 15 to 20 mg/kg in divided doses (bid-tid).
     (2) Most outpatients are started at 250 mg tid.
     (3) Rapid oral loading of inpatients is possible using an initial dose of 20 to 30 mg/kg divided bid or tid.
     (4) Monitor trough plasma level after 2 to 4 days and increase the oral dose to achieve target trough serum levels of 45 to 125 µg/mL. Higher serum levels (>100 µg/mL) are associated with more adverse effects but without much greater clinical response.
     (5) Because of a wider therapeutic margin, close monitoring of serum levels is not as critical as with lithium. Levels every 3 to 6 months are generally adequate for monitoring unless there is a change in adverse effects or clinical status.
   d. Contraindications to use of valproic acid.
     (1) Hepatic dysfunction.
     (2) Blood dyscrasia.
5. Side effects.
   a. Generally well tolerated.
   b. Nausea, vomiting, and gastrointestinal irritation are common dose-related side effects that can be reduced or minimized by using the enteric coated form (divalproex sodium [Depakote]).
   c. Tremor and sedation are the most common neurologic side effects (might reduce over time).
   d. Hepatic reactions.
     (1) Benign, often transient, increase in LFTs occur in up to 40% of patients.
      (a) Drug should be discontinued if the LFTs rise above two times the limit of normal.
      (b) LFTs should be monitored regularly (e.g., every 2 to 3 weeks for the first 2 to 3 months, then every 6 months thereafter).
     (2) A more severe form of hepatic reaction is rare. Patients should be advised to report symptoms such as abdominal swelling, jaundice, nausea, vomiting, or edema.
     (3) Serum ammonia levels may rise, but specific monitoring is not warranted in the absence of clinical signs of hyperammonemia (changes in mental status: cognitive slowing, confusion, stupor, fatigue, lethargy, somnolence, coma).
   e. Increased appetite and weight gain (likely dose dependent).
   f. Alopecia (may be transient; zinc and selenium supplements may be helpful).
   g. Polycystic ovary syndrome develops in up to 10% of women with bipolar disorder who take valproate.
   h. Thrombocytopenia.
     (1) Dose dependent.
     (2) Counts above 150,000/mm^3 are rarely associated with bleeding.
     (3) Patients should be advised to report any easy bruisability.

   i. Pancreatitis is rare.
   j. Teratogenecity.
      (1) When valproic acid is taken during pregnancy, neural tube
          defects in 1% to 5% have been reported.
      (2) Multivitamins with trace metals and folic acid might reduce
          teratogenicity.
   k. Mild, asymptomatic leukopenia is usually reversible with dose
      reduction or discontinuation.

8.5 Carbamazepine

1. Indications.
   a. Although carbamazepine is FDA approved only for the treatment of
      seizures and trigeminal neuralgia, there is substantial clinical and
      clinical trial evidence supporting the efficacy of carbamazepine in
      the treatment of acute mania.
   b. There is also considerable evidence supporting the use of carba-
      mazepine for prophylaxis of episodes in bipolar disorder.
   c. A few controlled studies exist suggesting acute antidepressant
      efficacy.
   d. Carbamazepine can be used in stabilizing episodically aggressive
      behavior (see Chapter 5).
   e. Carbatrol, a sustained-release carbamazepine formulation, has not
      been adequately studied to date for the treatment of bipolar
      disorder.
   f. Although carbamazepine is largely considered problematic due to
      side-effect profile and drug—drug interactions, the APA guidelines
      consider it an alternative agent in the management of bipolar
      disorder.
2. Pharmacology.
   a. Protein binding of carbamazepine is 75%.
      (1) Only the unbound form crosses the blood—brain barrier.
      (2) Medically ill patients with low albumin can become more
          toxic.
      (3) Plasma levels measure bound and unbound portions.
   b. Extensive metabolism.
      (1) Primarily through the P450 system to active metabolite
          carbamazepine-10,11-epoxide via CYP450 3A3/4 (less
          contributions via P450 2C8 and aromatic hydroxylation by
          P450 1A2).
      (2) Autoinduction (approximately 2 to 4 weeks into treatment via
          P450 3A3/4 pathway) decreases half-life from initially 24 hours
          to 8 hours.
3. Drug interactions (carbamazepine induces P450 enzymes, especially
   the 3A3 and 3A4 family) (Box 8-3).
   a. Carbamazepine is well known for induction of metabolic enzymes
      (P450 system) decreasing the serum concentration of itself as well
      as other medications.
   b. Carbamazepine metabolism can be inhibited by other P450 enzyme
      inhibitors, resulting in increases in serum carbamazepine levels and

---

BOX 8-3   Drugs That Alter Carbamazepine Levels

Drugs That Lead to Increased Carbamazepine Levels (Includes Drugs That Inhibit P450 Enzymes, Especially the 3A4 Family)

Acetazolamide
Antidepressants (fluoxetine, fluvoxamine, nefazodone)
Antimicrobials (isoniazid, quinupristin/dalfopristin)
Calcium channel blockers (diltiazem, verapamil)
Cimetidine
Danazol
Hypolipidemics (gemfibrozil, nicotinamide)
Macrolide antibiotics (erythromycin, clarithromycin, etc.)
Omeprazole
D-Propoxyphene
Valproate (increases 10,11-epoxide)

Drugs with Most Significantly Decreased Serum Levels due to Carbamazepine or Oxcarbazepine

Alprazolam
Buprenorphine
Clonazepam
Dihydropyridine calcium channel blockers
Hormonal contraceptives
Lamotrigine
Paclitaxel
Repaglinide

---

possible toxicity. Caution is advised with other CYP 3A3/4 inhibitors.

c. Metabolism of the active metabolite (10,11-epoxide) can be inhibited by valproic acid, resulting in increased serum metabolite concentrations (without measurable increase in carbamazepine levels), resulting in intoxication. Valproic acid also can induce displacement of carbamazepine protein binding and produce increased free carbamazepine levels.

4. Clinical use.
   a. Formulations and dosing.
      (1) Carbamazepine is available in suspension, chewable tablets, nonchewable tablets, and sustained-release formulations.
      (2) Also available in generic formulations; some differences have been observed between the bioavailability of proprietary and generic formulations.
      (3) In the inpatient setting, carbamazepine is commonly started at 400 to 800 mg/day and adjusted by 200 mg/day every 2 to 4 days, based on clinical efficacy. Typical doses are 800 to 1600 mg/day in divided tid or qid dosing. Titration is based more on side effects than on blood levels.

          (4) Typical blood levels are 4 to 12 µg/mL.
             (a) The first therapeutic level should be drawn about 4 days after starting.
             (b) Efficacy for seizures or mood disorders does not appear to be tightly related to blood levels.
          (5) Loading-dose strategies and rapid titration of carbamazepine dose are typically limited by increased adverse effects (neurotoxicity and gastrointestinal disturbances) associated with rapid titration.
          (6) Lack of clinical antimanic response after 7 to 10 days suggests that alternative or augmentation strategies should be considered.
     b. Laboratory monitoring.
          (1) Baseline: CBC with differential and platelets, hepatic function (LFTs).
          (2) Periodic LFTs, CBC, and blood levels as clinically indicated.
5. Side effects.
     a. Relative contraindications to carbamazepine.
          (1) Cardiac arrhythmias.
          (2) Significant renal or hepatic impairment.
          (3) History of blood dyscrasia.
     b. Common initial side effects, often brief or dose-dependent and minimized with gradual titration, include:
          (1) Sedation.
          (2) Nausea.
          (3) Tremor.
          (4) Ataxia.
          (5) Double vision.
     c. Antidiuretic action by a direct effect on renal tubules can result in hyponatremia, manifesting as water intoxication or seizures.
     d. Leukopenia. Low leukocyte counts, usually not below 3000/mm^3, transiently occur in about 10% of patients and persist in about 3%. Usually benign.
     e. Aplastic anemia (1 in 10,000 to 1 in 100,000 patients).
          (1) Patients should be instructed to immediately report fever, sore throat, oral ulcers, or easy bruising or bleeding.
          (2) Discontinue carbamazepine for white blood cell (WBC) count less than 3000/mm^3 or absolute neutrophil count less than 1000 to 1500/mm^3.
          (3) Routine blood monitoring is not indicated.
          (4) Extreme caution should be used in combining carbamazepine with other drugs that suppress WBC production, such as clozapine.
     f. Hepatitis (rare).
          (1) About 5% of patients show a mild increase in alanine aminotransferase (ALT) and aspartate aminotransferase (AST). It is usually not necessary to discontinue the drug unless the elevations are two to three times normal.
          (2) Serious, life-threatening hepatic reactions occur in only 1 out of 10,000 persons.

(3) Routine monitoring is not indicated. Patients should be told to report symptoms such as anorexia, nausea or vomiting, or abdominal pain.

(4) Underlying liver disease is a relative contraindication.

g. Rash occurs in 10% to 15% with rare Stevens–Johnson syndrome. Because this can develop into a serious problem, carbamazepine should be discontinued and the patient assessed for any rash more significant than a simple macular rash.

h. Cardiac conduction may be slowed. Initial ECG should be done to check for preexisting atrioventricular delay, which can contraindicate the use of carbamazepine.

i. Teratogenicity.

(1) 3% risk of spina bifida. May be reduced with folate supplementation.

(2) Also associated with low birth weight, craniofacial abnormalities.

(3) For rare patients, with severe disorders, the benefits of treating with carbamazepine can outweigh the risks compared to other options for treatment.

(4) Carbamazepine is present in breast milk; patients should be discouraged from breast-feeding when taking carbamazepine.

j. Thrombocytopenia can occur. Unless the platelet count drops below $100,000/\text{mm}^3$, only close monitoring, not discontinuation, is necessary.

k. Weight gain may be less common than with lithium or valproic acid.

l. Thyroid.

(1) Can lower serum thyroxine (T_4) and free T_4 index; decrease in triiodothyronine is less common.

(2) Clinical hypothyroidism is rare.

8.6 Oxcarbazepine

1. Indications.

a. Oxcarbazepine (a keto-derivative of carbamazepine), though less well studied, appears to have efficacy for acute mania and might have a better side-effect profile.

b. Similar to carbamazepine, at present oxcarbazepine only has FDA indication for treating seizures.

2. Pharmacology.

a. Oxcarbazepine is 60% protein bound.

b. Metabolism is complex, as with carbamazepine.

(1) Unlike carbamazepine, oxcarbazepine does not induce its own metabolism.

(2) Causes less heteroinduction than carbamazepine.

3. Drug interactions.

a. Less problematic than carbamazepine due to less heteroinduction.

b. Modest P450 3A3/4 inducer, and might reduce serum concentrations of some medications (see Box 8-3).

    c. Metabolism is not inhibited by valproic acid; therefore, coadminis-tration does not cause toxicity.

4. Clinical use: formulations and dosing.
   a. Available in suspension and tablets. No extended-release formula-tions are available.
   b. Commonly started at 150 mg/day and increased every other day by 150 mg/day. Typical doses are 1200 to 1600 mg/day divided bid or tid.
   c. For patients treated with carbamazepine, equivalent doses of oxcar-bazepine are often 1.2 to 1.5 times the carbamazepine dose.
   d. Serum concentration for epilepsy ranges from 10 to 35 µg/mL. For bipolar disorder, dose is titrated to clinical response.

5. Side effects.
   a. Often better tolerated than carbamazepine.
   b. Most commonly involve the CNS.
      (1) Dizziness.
      (2) Sedation.
      (3) Fatigue.
   c. Rash can occur.
   d. Unlike carbamazepine, not associated with blood dyscrasias.
   e. Mild increase in AST or ALT.
   f. Hyponatremia.
      (1) Occurs more commonly than with carbamazepine.
      (2) Most often is clinically insignificant.
   g. Induces female hormone metabolism. Can decrease efficacy of hor-monal contraceptives.
   h. Teratogenicity.
      (1) Not yet associated with congenital malformations in humans, possibly due to inadequate number of exposures to date.
      (2) Present in breast milk.

8.7 Lamotrigine

1. Indications.
   a. First-line treatment for acute bipolar depression and for mainte-nance treatment and prevention of recurrence of depression.
   b. Also has demonstrated efficacy in preventing mood episodes in patients with rapid-cycling bipolar disorder.

2. Pharmacology.
   a. Rapid oral absorption with peak concentrations in 2 to 3 hours. Half-life approximately 27 hours.
   b. Only 55% protein bound, does not compete significantly for bind-ing sites.
   c. Competitively metabolized by hepatic glucuronidation.
   d. Elimination half-life may be doubled in renal failure.

3. Drug interactions.
   a. Due to competitive hepatic metabolism, addition to the following enzyme inducers reduces lamotrigine concentration by 40% to 50%:
      (1) Carbamazepine.

    (2) Phenytoin.

    (3) Phenobarbital.

  b. Addition of enzyme inhibitors, such as valproate, increases half-life up to 2 to 3 times.

  c. Oral contraceptives containing ethinyl estradiol can reduce lamotrigine levels.

4. Dosing.

  a. For monotherapy, dosing commonly begins with 25 mg qd for 2 weeks, then is increased to 50 mg qd for 2 weeks. Target dose is 50 to 200 mg qd. May be divided bid.

  b. For addition of lamotrigine to valproate, cut dose in half. Begin at 25 mg qod for 2 weeks, then increase to 25 mg qd for 2 weeks, then increase by 25 to 50 mg/day every 1 to 2 weeks.

  c. For addition in the presence of an enzyme inducer (carbamazepine), double the dose. Begin at 50 mg qd for 2 weeks, then increase to 100 mg/day for 2 weeks.

5. Side effects.

  a. Commonly include dizziness, headache, nausea, emesis, diplopia, ataxia.

  b. Rash: Lamotrigine has been associated with serious rash, including Stevens–Johnson syndrome and toxic epidermal necrolysis.

    (1) Rates of nonserious rash are less than 10%; rates of serious rash are less than 1%.

    (2) Slow titration reduces risk.

    (3) Risk is highest early in treatment (but can occur any time). Early in treatment, patients with a rash should hold the next dose and seek medical attention.

    (4) Patients should be warned about rash and told to contact physician if a rash develops.

    (5) Worrisome rashes are accompanied by fever or sore throat, are diffuse or widespread, and involve prominent facial or mucosal involvement.

8.8 Atypical Antipsychotics

1. Many atypical antipsychotics have indications for the treatment of acute mania as single agent or acute mania when combined with a mood stabilizer. See Chapter 12 for general information).

2. Olanzapine has an indication for maintenance treatment.

3. Olanzapine–fluoxetine combination has an indication for treating acute bipolar depression.

4. Table 8-1 contains information on formulations and dosing.

8.9 Benzodiazepines

Benzodiazepines have a role as adjunctive medications in acute mania. When additional sedation is required during titration with some other medication, prn doses of lorazepam 1 to 2 mg or clonazepam 0.5 to 1 mg may be helpful.

8.10 Nonmedication Dimensions of Treatment

1. Patients are often helped by understanding the underlying medical basis of their illness, removing much of the stigma and self-deprecation.
2. Societies for manic–depressive patients function as information sources and support groups.
3. Mood hygiene.
   a. Maintain stable sleeping pattern.
   b. Avoid extremes in work or recreation.
   c. Identify warning signs of episodes with caregivers and treatment providers.

8.11 Electroconvulsive Therapy

1. ECT may be used at any time during bipolar illness (see Chapter 16).
2. ECT can be particularly effective for patients whose symptoms resist treatment, for those who are acutely suicidal, pregnant, or psychotic, and for patients whose problems are medically complex.
3. Lithium should be discontinued during ECT because of potential neurotoxicity, interactions with succinylcholine, and production of cardiac arrhythmias.

SUGGESTED READINGS

American Psychiatric Association: *Diagnostic and Statistical Manual of Mental Disorders*, 4th ed, text revision. Washington, DC, American Psychiatric Association, 2000.
Goodwin FK, Fireman B, Simon GE, et al: Suicide risk in bipolar disorder during treatment with lithium and divalproex. *JAMA* 290(11):1467-1473, 2003.
Goodwin FK, Jamison KR: *Manic–Depressive Illness*. New York, Oxford University Press, 1990.
Hirschfeld RMA, Keck PE Jr, Kramer M, et al: Rapid anti-manic effect of risperidone monotherapy: A 3-week multicenter, double-blind, placebo-controlled trial. *Am J Psychiatry* 161:1057-1065, 2004.
Joffe H, Cohen LS, Suppes T, et al: Valproate induces oligomenorrhea with hyper-androgenism in women with bipolar disorder. Poster presented at the Endocrine Society 86th Annual Meeting, New Orleans, La, June 16-19, 2004.
Judd LL, Akiskal HS: The prevalence and disability of bipolar spectrum disorders in the US population: Re-analysis of the ECA database taking into account sub-threshold cases. *J Affect Disord* 73(1-2):123-131, 2003.
Keck PE Jr, McElroy SL, Tugrul KC, Bennett JA: Valproate oral loading in the treatment of acute mania. *J Clin Psychiatry* 54(8):305-308, 1993.
Keck PE, Perlis RH, Otto MW, Carpenter D, Ross R, Docherty JP: The expert consensus guideline series: Treatment of bipolar disorder 2004. *Postgrad Med Special Report* 1-20, 2004.
McElroy SL, Keck PE, Pope HG, Hudson JL: Valproate in psychiatric disorders: Literature review and clinical guidelines. *J Clin Psychiatry* 50:23-29, 1989.
Pellock JM, Willmore LJ: A rational guide to routine blood monitoring in patients receiving antiepileptic drugs. *Neurology* 41:961-964, 1991.
Pope HG, McElroy SL, Keck PE, Hudson JL: Valproate in the treatment of acute mania: A placebo-controlled study. *Arch Gen Psychiatry* 48:62-68, 1991.

Schatzberg AF, Nemeroff CB (eds): *The American Psychiatric Publishing Textbook of Psychopharmacology*, 3rd ed. Arlington, Va, American Psychiatric Publishing, 2004.

Vestergaard P, Amdisen AS, Schou M: Clinically significant side effects of lithium treatment: A survey of 237 patients in long-term treatment. *Acta Psychiatr Scand* 62:193-200, 1980.

Wang PO, Ketter TA: Clinical use of carbamazepine for bipolar disorder. Expert Opin Pharmacother 6(16): 2887-2902, 2005.

Zajecka J: Pharmacology, pharmacokinetics, and safety issues of mood-stabilizing agents. *Psychiatric Ann* 23(2):79-85, 1993.

Anxiety Disorders: Diagnosis and Management

9

Richard J. Goldberg
Donn Posner

9.1 Overview and Background

1. Anxiety is not necessarily a problem. It can be a positive motivating factor.
2. Anxiety becomes a problem when:
   a. It interferes with adaptive behavior.
   b. It causes disruptive physical symptoms.
   c. It exceeds a tolerable level.
3. Anxious patients are likely to present to nonpsychiatric physicians with somatic complaints or substance use disorders (Box 9-1).

9.2 Diagnostic Approach to Anxiety Symptoms

1. Step one: medical assessment. Do not assume that anxiety is explained by the patient's psychosocial situation. Review the medical problem list, history, and substance use.
   a. See Box 9-2 for medical causes of anxiety symptoms.
      (1) When anxiety is judged to be the direct physiologic outcome of some medical condition, the diagnosis is "anxiety disorder due to _____ [that condition]."
      (2) If the medical condition causes delirium and the anxiety occurs as a component of the delirium, then "delirium" is an adequate single diagnosis.
   b. See Box 9-3 for drugs that cause anxiety symptoms.
      (1) When the anxiety is judged to be the direct physiologic outcome of some substance, the diagnosis is "substance-induced anxiety disorder."
      (2) Anxiety secondary to substance-induced intoxication or withdrawal is diagnosed as "substance intoxication or substance withdrawal." The diagnosis of substance-induced anxiety would more likely be used for prominent anxiety secondary to theophylline use, for example.
      (3) For anxiety secondary to delirium, "delirium" is an adequate single diagnosis.
2. Step two: psychosocial assessment. Always ask, "Why do you think you are so anxious?" The patient might identify some problem that should be addressed by counseling or therapy. For example, if a stressful marriage underlies anxiety, marriage therapy is probably indicated.

BOX 9-1 Physical Symptoms of Anxiety

Autonomic

Dry mouth
Headaches
Hot flushes
Sweating

Cardiovascular

Chest pain
Faintness
Palpitations
Tachycardia

Gastrointestinal

Abdominal pain
Irritable bowel
Nausea
Swallowing

Genitourinary

Frequency
Menstrual problems
Sexual dysfunction
Urgency

Musculoskeletal

Aches and pains
Fatigue
Stiffness
Twitching

Neurologic

Dizziness
Numbness or tingling
Tremor
Visual disturbance
Weakness

Respiratory

Chest pressure
Choking
Dyspnea
Sighing

---

3. Step three: self-regulation and behavioral therapy. Consider whether the patient could benefit from some form of self-regulation or behavioral therapy such as relaxation exercises, breathing exercises, or meditation.
4. Step four: medication could be used to lessen symptom severity. Therapy treats problems; medication treats symptoms. Medication may be an important adjunct to psychotherapies (such as cognitive behavior therapy) or self-regulation treatments if the patient continues to have significant somatic symptoms.

9.3 Panic Disorder

DEFINITION AND IDENTIFICATION

1. Panic disorder is basically defined as:
   a. The presence (or history) of recurrent unexpected panic attacks that do not have an underlying medical etiology.
   b. At least one of the attacks is followed by:
      (1) Persistent concern about having another attack.
      (2) Worry about what might happen as the result of an attack (e.g., losing control, having a heart attack).
      (3) A significant change in behavior related to the attack.

BOX 9-2   **Medical Causes of Anxiety**

Cardiovascular

Angina pectoris
Arrhythmias
Congestive heart failure
Hypertension
Hypotension
Mitral valve prolapse

Endocrine

Carcinoid syndrome
Hypercortisolemia
Hyperthyroidism
Hypoglycemia
Pheochromocytoma

Metabolic

Hypercalcemia
Hyperkalemia
Hyponatremia
Porphyria

Neurologic

Akathisia
Complex partial seizures
Delirium
Essential tremor
Otoneurologic disorders
Parkinson's disease
Postconcussion syndrome

Respiratory

Asthma
Chronic obstructive pulmonary disease
Hypoxia
Pulmonary edema
Pulmonary embolism

---

    c. Panic attacks can occur outside of panic disorder.
      (1) Social or specific phobia, in which the panic attack is triggered by some specific feared situation.
      (2) Obsessive–compulsive disorder, in which the panic attack is triggered by exposure to some disturbing situation (such as exposure to a dirty toilet in a patient with a cleanliness obsession).
      (3) Posttraumatic stress disorder, in which the panic attack is triggered by the reminder of a past traumatic event.
      (4) Separation anxiety disorder, in which the panic attack is triggered as a response to being away from home or friends.
    d. Panic attacks as part of panic disorder can occur in the middle of the night and wake a patient from sleep.
2. A panic attack (which by itself is not a disorder) is defined as an episode of extreme anxiety that often comes on suddenly (it may be uncued or arise out of extreme worry, obsessions, specific fears, etc.) and is characterized by a number of typical somatic and psychological features. See Box 9-4 for the criteria for a panic attack.
3. Panic attack patients often believe they are having a medical crisis and seek emergency care.
4. Not every panic attack is part of panic disorder. Panic attacks may be a result of other medical or psychiatric conditions.
5. Agoraphobia often is part of panic disorder. Some patients become fearful of being in certain locations or situations and start to avoid those.

BOX 9-3   Drugs That Cause Anxiety

Anticholinergics

Benztropine (Cogentin)
Diphenhydramine (Benadryl)
Oxybutynin (Ditropan)
Propantheline (Pro-Banthine)
Trihexyphenidyl (Artane)

Antidepressants

Atamoxetine
Bupropion
Selective serotonin reuptake inhibitors
Tricyclic agents
Venlafaxine

Dopaminergics

Amantadine
Bromocriptine
Carbidopa–levodopa (Sinemet)
Levodopa
Metoclopramide

Drug Withdrawal

Alcohol
Barbiturates
Benzodiazepines
Narcotics
Sedatives

Stimulants

Aminophylline
Amphetamine
Caffeine
Cocaine
Methylphenidate
Theophylline

Sympathomimetics

Ephedrine
Epinephrine
Neuroleptic agents
Phentermine
Phenylpropanolamine
Pseudoephedrine

Miscellaneous

Baclofen
Cycloserine
Hallucinogens
Indomethacin
Meperidine (Demerol)

BOX 9-4   Panic Attack Criteria

Panic attack is defined as a discrete period of intense fear or discomfort, starting abruptly and reaching a peak within 10 minutes, with at least four of the following symptoms:

Chest pain or discomfort
Chills or hot flushes
Choking
Dizziness or faintness
Fear of dying
Fear of going crazy
Feeling unreal or detached
   from oneself

Nausea or abdominal distress
Palpitations, tachycardia
Paresthesias
Shaking or trembling
Shortness of breath
Sweating

PREVALENCE

1. Panic disorder has a prevalence in the general population of 1% to 3.5%. The highest occurrence is in young women and the average onset is in the early 20s. Forty percent of patients have onset after age 30 years.
   a. In older and medically ill patients, suspect an underlying medical cause for a panic attack.
   b. About 30% to 40% of patients with panic disorder also have agoraphobia.
   c. Up to 35% of the general population experience infrequent panic attacks.
2. Because of the medical symptoms of panic attacks, these patients tend to cluster in medical practices, where there is a prevalence of 0.4% to 9%.
   a. The use of primary care services by patients with panic attacks is about three times that for other patients.
   b. The prevalence in cardiology, gastroenterology, or neurology is probably about four times the community prevalence. Typical presentations include:
      (1) Cardiovascular symptoms (up to 40% of patients with panic disorder).
         (a) Atypical chest pain.
         (b) Tachycardia.
         (c) Irregular heartbeat.
      (2) Neurologic symptoms (up to 40% of patients).
         (a) Headache.
         (b) Dizziness, vertigo.
         (c) Syncope.
         (d) Pseudoseizures.
      (3) Gastrointestinal symptoms (up to 30%), such as epigastric pain.
      (4) Although dyspnea is present in almost all patients with panic disorder, it is often not the presenting complaint.
3. Panic disorder often occurs concurrently with other psychiatric disorders. About 15% of patients with major depression have concurrent panic disorder.
4. Panic disorder appears to have a genetic component, with a substantially greater risk for first-degree relatives.

DIFFERENTIAL DIAGNOSIS

1. Medical disorders or substance-induced anxiety presenting as panic attacks should always be considered, especially in older patients (Boxes 9-2, 9-3, and 9-5). However, millions of dollars each year are spent for unnecessary medical care for undiagnosed panic disorder.
2. Major depression. Panic attacks often emerge in the context of a major depression. Treating the depression often resolves the panic attacks.
3. Other psychiatric disorders with panic attacks.
   a. Posttraumatic stress disorder.
   b. Borderline personality disorder.
   c. Delirium.

> **BOX 9-5   Some Common Medical Causes of Panic Attacks**
>
> Allergies   Nocturnal apneic events
> Hyperthyroidism   Otoneurologic disorders
> Hypoglycemia   Structural lesions of the brain
> Irritable bowel syndrome   Temporal lobe epilepsy
> Mitral valve prolapse

   d. Decompensating schizophrenia.
   e. Separation anxiety.
   f. Social anxiety.

COURSE AND PROGNOSIS

1. Panic disorder appears to be an episodic disorder that can emerge, disappear, and reemerge years later.
   a. After a period of stability (of at least several months) patients may be able to taper (slowly) treatment and remain symptom-free for extended periods.
   b. There are more difficult cases where the disorder recurs following attempts to discontinue medication. Relapse can be diminished by combining cognitive behavior therapy (CBT) with medications.
2. Do not underestimate the impact of panic disorder.
   a. Symptoms are frightening and disabling.
   b. Secondary substance abuse is not uncommon.
   c. In some cases, the associated agoraphobia becomes chronic.
   d. Some panic sufferers become suicidal.

TREATMENTS

1. Overall, panic disorder is responsive to psychopharmacology and CBT. Medication can abolish panic attacks of any etiology; therefore the success of medication does not imply the absence of some underlying medical cause.
2. Psychopharmacology. Panic disorder responds to several drug groups including benzodiazepines (especially alprazolam and clonazepam) and antidepressants, including tricyclics, selective serotonin reuptake inhibitors (SSRIs), and monoamine oxidase inhibitors (MAOIs).
   a. Benzodiazepines. Among the benzodiazepines, alprazolam (Xanax) and clonazepam (Klonopin) appear to have the most potent anti-panic effects. Further details of using benzodiazepines may be found in Chapter 10.
      (1) Alprazolam (Xanax).
         (a) Alprazolam is effective at abolishing panic attacks, often at fairly low doses (e.g., 0.25 or 0.5 mg tid, or once-daily dosing with Xanax XR), although higher doses may be needed.

(b) Some patients ask for or require increasing doses or frequencies of alprazolam. For this type of patient, it may be helpful to cross over to clonazepam (because of its longer half-life) on a 2:1 ratio (i.e., 1 mg of alprazolam to 0.5 mg of clonazepam).

(c) It can be quite difficult to taper off alprazolam. If it is discontinued too rapidly, there can be withdrawal seizures (if the daily dose is about 6 mg/day or more), rebound anxiety, or rebound panic attacks. Tapering should be done slowly, by 0.5 mg/week until reaching 1 mg/day, then by 0.25 mg/week.

(2) Clonazepam (Klonopin).

(a) Clonazepam appears to be an effective antipanic medication in doses about half that of alprazolam.

(b) It can be taken twice a day rather than four times, as is necessary with alprazolam (see Chapter 10).

(c) Many patients find clonazepam too sedating, especially in the first 2 weeks of use before some tolerance develops to the sedation.

b. Antidepressants.

(1) Imipramine, often in low doses (such as 25 mg/day) can effectively treat panic disorder.

(2) This effect is not unique to imipramine and appears to be a property of other tricyclic antidepressants including desipramine.

(3) All the SSRIs as well as venlafaxine can treat panic disorder effectively. Starting doses should be 10 mg of fluoxetine, 10 mg of paroxetine, or 25 mg of sertraline. If there is inadequate response after 1 week, the dose can be doubled. Further dose increases are necessary in some cases. See Table 9-1 for current Food and Drug Administration (FDA) indications.

(4) For some patients, it may be helpful to start the SSRI and alprazolam simultaneously, because the benzodiazepine can have some more immediate effects. After 1 week the benzodiazepine can be tapered and treatment can be continued with only the SSRI.

(5) Chapter 7 describes the side effects of antidepressants.

(6) Some patients with panic disorder (about 10% to 15%) develop a dysphoric agitated response to antidepressants. Such patients are reluctant to try antidepressants again, although they would probably tolerate very tiny doses (such as 10 mg of imipramine or 2.5 mg of fluoxetine). These patients usually end up taking benzodiazepines.

3. CBT. Several studies have demonstrated that CBT can be as effective as medication in the treatment of panic disorder.

a. CBT involves two components.

(1) In the cognitive component, the patient learns to identify cues that can trigger panic attacks and to apply some alternate way of dealing with the situation.

Table 9-1 **Psychopharmacology for Generalized Anxiety Disorder**			
Agent	**Starting Dose**	**Target dose (mg/day)**	**Pregnancy Risk**
Anticonvulsants			
Tiagabine (Gabatril)	2 mg bid	2-16	C
Azapirones			
Buspirone (Buspar)	5 mg bid	10-60	B
Benzodiazepines			
Clonazepam (Klonopin)	0.25 mg bid	0.5-2.0	D
Lorazepam (Ativan)	0.5 mg bid	1-4	D
Selective Serotonin Reuptake Inhibitors			
Citalopram (Celexa)	10 mg/day	10-40	C
Escitalopram (Lexapro)	10 mg/day	10-20	C
Paroxetine (Paxil)	10 mg/day	10-40	C
Sertraline (Zoloft)	25 mg/day	50-200	C
Serotonin–Norepinephrine Reuptake Inhibitors			
Venlafaxine XR	37.5 mg/day	75-225	C
Tricyclics			
Imipramine (Tofranil)	10 mg/day	50-200	D
Nortriptyline (Pamelor)	10 mg/day	20-150	D

(2) In the exposure component the patient is made to confront the feared object or situation. This can be done all at once (flooding), or can be achieved gradually in a hierarchical fashion. With panic disorder, an important type of exposure is interoceptive, in which the patient is made to repeatedly re-experience the sensations of panic, but in controlled settings. This can be achieved by exercises such as hyperventilating, spinning, straw breathing, etc.
  b. This treatment usually requires referral to a therapist specially trained in this technique.
4. Treatment of comorbidities. When panic attacks are treated and the patient remains functionally impaired, there may be coexisting problems.
  a. Agoraphobia (which can require behavioral therapy).

b. Generalized anxiety disorder (which can require a second medication, such as buspirone, or further CBT).
c. Depression (requiring a higher dose or additional antidepressants or further CBT).
d. Anticipatory anxiety. After experiencing panic attacks, patients become fearful of a recurrence. This component often requires some behavioral therapy to desensitize the patient.

9.4 Obsessive–Compulsive Disorder

DEFINITION AND IDENTIFICATION

1. Obsessions are recurrent thoughts, ideas, or images that intrude into conscious awareness and are perceived as senseless and intrusive.
2. Compulsions are urges or impulses for repetitive intentional behavior, performed in a stereotyped manner, in order to attempt to reduce anxiety. Some typical compulsions involve touching, counting, arranging, or cleaning.
3. Obsessive–compulsive disorder (OCD) patients come to a physician's office in a number of disguised presentations.
   a. Dermatologic presentations of compulsive hand washing or skin picking.
   b. Some forms of "hypochondriasis" or chronic pain.
4. Patients might not reveal their OCD behavior unless specifically asked. Screening questions for OCD include the following:
   a. "Are there certain thoughts that go through your mind over and over that you can't seem to get rid of?"
   b. "Is there any behavior or habit that you feel compelled to repeat?"
5. Many people have obsessive–compulsive (OC) behavior that is not sufficiently severe to qualify as a disorder. When the behavior is less severe, it would be more accurate to say such people have OC personality features or "traits" (see Chapter 17).

PREVALENCE

1. OCD has a community prevalence of about 2% and a lifetime prevalence of 2.5%.
2. There is a higher incidence of OCD in first-degree relatives of patients with OCD.

DIFFERENTIAL DIAGNOSIS

1. Schizophrenia. Patients with severe OCD might appear psychotic, be misdiagnosed as schizophrenic, and be given neuroleptic agents because of the extreme and seemingly bizarre practices associated with their illness.
2. Major depression. About 15% of patients with major depression have OCD. When patients with obsessive–compulsive (OC) traits develop major depression, these traits can become magnified, misleading the clinician into diagnosing OCD as the primary disorder.
3. Dementia. When patients with underlying OC traits become demented, their underlying traits may become magnified.

4. Gilles de la Tourette's syndrome. From 30% to 50% of these patients have OC symptoms. Tourette's patients have characteristic recurrent involuntary movements, vocal tics, or both.
5. Personality change resulting from some medical condition. Some neurologic problems, such as stroke or temporal lobe epilepsy, can produce compulsive, repetitive behaviors.
6. Phobic disorders. Phobias typically show symptoms only in relation to a specific object. At times, these two disorders may be difficult to distinguish (for example, fear of fire may lead to stove checking).
7. Body dysmorphic disorder, in which preoccupations are limited to physical appearance, can be difficult to distinguish from OCD (see Chapter 13).
8. Trichotillomania (recurrent compulsive pulling out of hair).
9. Excessive worry is a characteristic of generalized anxiety disorder, although generally the worries pertain to realistic problems. These can be hard to distinguish.
10. If the recurrent thoughts are exclusively related to fears of having a disease, the more appropriate diagnosis is hypochondriasis (which may be a form of OCD).

COURSE AND PROGNOSIS
1. OCD tends to be a chronic disorder, although many patients experience remissions, often for extended periods.
2. Recovery takes place in about 50% of patients.
3. OCD can begin in childhood, but it is usually first noted in adolescence or in the 20s.

TREATMENTS
1. Psychopharmacology. Drugs that augment serotonin function are effective in decreasing OCD symptoms.
   a. Clomipramine is a tricyclic antidepressant with potent serotonin reuptake blocking activity.
      (1) Side effects are listed in Table 7-1.
         (a) Sedation and anticholinergic effects are difficult for some patients to tolerate.
         (b) There is a high incidence of anorgasmia.
      (2) Relatively high doses (such as 250 mg/day) are often necessary.
   b. The SSRIs are effective. For details on use, refer to Chapter 7.
      (1) For OCD, higher doses than those used to treat depression are often necessary. For example, it may be necessary to go as high as 80 mg of fluoxetine, 80 mg of paroxetine, or 200 mg of sertraline.
      (2) Fluvoxamine (Luvox) is another SSRI that, in the United States, is marketed with an indication for the treatment of OCD.
   c. Augmenters.
      (1) If OCD symptoms partially respond to one medication, there may be further improvement by augmenting with buspirone (starting with doses of 5 mg tid and increasing to 20 mg tid).

      (2) For patients with coexisting mood disorder, augmenting with lithium may be helpful.

      (3) For patients with a significant anxiety component, augmenting with a benzodiazepine may be helpful.

      (4) For severe cases, it may be helpful to attempt augmentation with the atypical neuroleptic agents (see Chapter 12).

2. Psychological and behavioral therapies.

   a. OCD patients can be helped by specific behavioral interventions. Exposure and response prevention is used in some severe cases, where it may be necessary to get control of the entire environment for sufficient response prevention. There are a few inpatient behavioral units in this country for this purpose.

   b. Psychotherapy focused on trying to achieve some underlying psychological understanding and resolution by reasoning is usually not helpful.

   c. Family therapy may be needed along with medication to help change the patient's habit patterns associated with this disorder.

3. For severe, unremitting cases, psychosurgery, involving stereotactic limbic leukotomy (with lesions in the orbitomedial frontal areas) has been used with success.

9.5 Generalized Anxiety Disorder

DEFINITION AND IDENTIFICATION

1. Generalized anxiety disorder (GAD) is defined as:

   a. Excessive anxiety and worry most of the time over a period of at least 6 months.

   b. Other symptoms include the following:

      (1) Restlessness.

      (2) Fatigue.

      (3) Difficulty concentrating.

      (4) Irritability.

      (5) Muscle tension.

      (6) Sleep problems.

2. Patients with GAD often go to primary care physicians complaining of somatic symptoms (see Box 9-1).

3. The significance of GAD should not be underestimated. Such patients are in distress and tend to have both social and vocational impairment.

COURSE AND PREVALENCE

1. GAD appears to have a community prevalence of about 3% to 4% and a lifetime prevalence of 5%.

2. Because these patients often have somatic symptoms, the prevalence in medical practices may be as high as 10% to 15%.

3. Many patients with GAD report that symptoms have been present for their lifetime. When generalized anxiety is noted in childhood, it is called *overanxious disorder of childhood*.

4. The course is usually chronic and fluctuating, becoming worse during periods of stress.
5. The risk of GAD among adolescents who smoke is 5 to 6 times higher than in nonsmokers.

DIFFERENTIAL DIAGNOSIS

1. Normative anxiety.
2. Medical disorders. Symptoms of generalized anxiety may be a result of some underlying medical condition or drug (see Boxes 9-2 and 9-3).
3. Worry that is only associated with another anxiety disorder (e.g., worry about social interaction, about having a panic attack).
4. Depression is often accompanied with ruminative worry, but if the worry is only in the context of the depressive episode then GAD is not diagnosed.
5. Comorbidities.
   a. Major depression is the most common coexisting condition and is present in almost two thirds of GAD patients.
   b. Panic disorder co-occurs in about 25%.
   c. Alcohol abuse co-occurs in more than one third. Patients with GAD often attempt to self-medicate with alcohol or other sedatives. Unfortunately, these "treatments" only lead to substance abuse with secondary depressive symptoms and increased anxiety during withdrawal.
   d. Patients with GAD with coexisting medical illnesses have more impairment and seek more medical attention.
6. Somatoform disorders. Patients with GAD may focus on physical symptoms and make repeated medical visits for evaluation or reassurance. Some of these patients may appear to be hypochondriacal or present as persistent somatizers. Sometimes no clear distinction between somatization and GAD exists (see Chapter 13).

PROGNOSIS

1. GAD usually is noted to emerge in the early 20s and tends to be a lifelong disorder.
2. Because GAD tends to be a chronic, often lifelong disorder, it may need to be treated chronically. Unfortunately, as patients age and become demented, they have less ability to manage their anxiety.
3. It is unlikely that GAD can be completely abolished by treatment. It is more realistic to think of treatment as decreasing symptom intensity.

TREATMENTS

1. Psychopharmacology. GAD symptoms can be reduced with benzodiazepines, azapirones (see Chapter 10 for more details), or antidepressants (see Table 9-1).
   a. Benzodiazepines are generally helpful in low to moderate doses such as diazepam 2 to 5 mg tid or the equivalent (Table 10-1 lists benzodiazepine conversions).
      (1) Some patients are helped by maintenance benzodiazepines and do not abuse them.
      (2) Benzodiazepines may be more effective initially but not in the long term.

b. The azapirone buspirone (BuSpar) is generally effective in doses of between 20 and 40 mg/day. A good starting dose is 15 mg bid (10 mg bid in older patients and those with brain damage).

c. Antidepressants.

(1) Tricyclics. Imipramine can help reduce symptoms by about 50%. GAD patients are sensitive to developing jitteriness and insomnia, so the initial dose should be low (e.g., 25 mg/day). Anticholinergic side effects might limit treatment.

(2) SSRIs and serotonin and norepinephrine reuptake inhibitors (SNRIs) have efficacy similar to tricyclics.

(a) Starting doses should be low to minimize initial restlessness.

(b) SSRIs and SNRIs with FDA approval for GAD are listed in Table 9-1.

d. Duration of treatment. GAD tends to be a long-standing disorder, requiring years of maintenance. It is worthwhile to consider periodic tapering of medication to ensure that the patient still needs it.

e. Expected treatment response. Response to medication is likely to be partial; nevertheless, "taking the edge off" can significantly improve patients' quality of life.

2. Psychotherapies.

a. Relaxation (self-regulation) therapies, if practiced sufficiently, can decrease symptoms of GAD. However, this therapy can require professional training and continued booster sessions. See Chapter 10 for a review. Exercise and/or certain forms of yoga should be encouraged.

b. CBT. Teaching patients to challenge their overestimated and catastrophic thoughts and expand flexible thinking can be helpful. Worry exposure, in which the patient is taught to isolate the worry to specific times and places, slow their thoughts, and work through the worry, can also be helpful.

c. Supportive psychotherapy is usually not helpful in resolving GAD. However, focused therapy aimed at managing episodic stressful situations may be important.

9.6 Phobias

DEFINITION AND IDENTIFICATION

1. A phobia is defined as a persistent, irrational fear of a clearly definable object or situation that interferes with normal behavior.

2. Three major groups of phobias.

a. Agoraphobia without panic disorder.

b. Social phobia.

c. Simple phobia (e.g., fear of animals, heights, water, needles, airplanes, elevators).

AGORAPHOBIA

1. Identification. Agoraphobia is manifested as a fear of experiencing distressful or embarrassing symptoms if one leaves home.

2. Onset is usually between ages 20 and 40 years. Agoraphobia is more common in women.
3. Comorbidity. Agoraphobia often accompanies panic disorder and should be considered secondary to that disorder when they occur together. Agoraphobia should be considered as a possible diagnosis in any reclusive patient.
4. Differential diagnosis.
   a. Major depression (withdrawn behavior).
   b. Schizophrenia (reclusive behavior).
   c. Social phobia (avoidant behavior).
   d. Panic disorder (fear that going outside will precipitate an attack).
5. Treatment. Combinations of behavioral treatment (see discussion of CBT under "Panic Disorder"), supportive psychotherapy, and antianxiety medication are often helpful and should be integrated.

SOCIAL PHOBIA

1. Identification. Social phobics have specific (e.g., public speaking) or general (embarrassment) fears of being with people, manifesting as extreme anxiety in those contexts.
2. Differential diagnosis.
   a. Normative anxiety (e.g., some nondisabling anxiety of public speaking, stage fright, shyness).
   b. Avoidant personality disorder (a more severe form of generalized social phobia) manifests as a generalized avoidance of social situations, not limited to particular circumstances.
   c. Patients with delusions or hallucinations (e.g., schizophrenia, delirium, dementia) appear to show phobic behavior based on their psychotic determinants of behavior.
   d. Depressed patients often feel they want to avoid being with people.
   e. Panic disorder with agoraphobia (in which situations are avoided because of fear of triggering a panic disorder as in the past).
   f. Schizoid personalities avoid social situations because they are disinterested, not because of fearfulness.
3. Course and prevalence.
   a. Lifetime prevalence is approximately 10%. This disorder seems to be generally overlooked as a diagnosis.
   b. Usual onset is in midteenage years, emerging out of a childhood history of social inhibition.
   c. Usual course is continuous, with some attenuation or even remission in adulthood.
   d. There appears to be a familial pattern.
4. Treatment.
   a. Social phobia symptoms may be helped by benzodiazepines in low doses, antidepressants, or MAOIs. A trial of SSRIs is probably the best first approach in terms of risk-to-benefit ratio.
   b. Anxiety reduction through exposure and practice is often the preferred approach to treatment and can be quite successful. Assertiveness training is also quite useful.
   c. Chapter 10 presents a review of the use of β-blockers for performance anxiety. For example, 20 to 40 mg of propranolol

about 45 minutes before the performance can abolish the autonomic symptoms of anxiety (such as tremulousness, sweating, tachycardia) that augment the person's fear and escalate the anxiety.

SIMPLE PHOBIA

1. Identification. Common simple phobias include fear of snakes, heights, crossing bridges, darkness, flying, and needles.
   a. These phobias generally come to medical attention only when interfering with work or activity.
   b. Two phobias that affect medical care include needle phobia and claustrophobia (in patients requiring magnetic resonance imaging [MRI] or radiation therapy).
   c. Simple phobias are almost ubiquitous in the general population. They may be persistent or have a limited course.
2. Differential diagnosis.
   a. Normative anxiety.
   b. Major depression (with emergent phobia).
   c. Psychosis. Patients with delusions or hallucinations (e.g., schizophrenia, delirium, dementia) appear to show phobic behavior based on their psychosis.
   d. Posttraumatic stress disorder.
   e. OCD. Fears of contamination can interfere with normal activities and appear to be phobic behavior.
3. Treatment.
   a. Behavioral therapy involves a combination of relaxation and gradual exposure. In general, psychologists with special training in behavioral therapy are most effective at providing these treatments.
   b. If the phobic behavior occurs as a component of another disorder (such as agoraphobia associated with panic disorder), the accompanying disorder should be treated simultaneously.
   c. Needle phobia usually responds to a few sessions of behavioral therapy.
   d. Claustrophobia for MRI usually responds to low-dose benzodiazepines (e.g., 5 to 10 mg diazepam [Valium]) or behavioral therapy, or both.

9.7 Adjustment Disorder with Anxiety

DEFINITION AND IDENTIFICATION

An adjustment disorder with anxiety is defined as an excessive reaction to an identifiable stressor.

1. The symptoms emerge within 3 months of the identifiable stressor.
2. The symptoms do not persist for more than 6 months after the stressor (or the consequences of the stressor) has terminated.
3. An adjustment disorder can become chronic if the disturbance lasts for more than 6 months.

PREVALENCE

Adjustment reactions are common in the general population and especially in the medically ill, who are confronted with many new, frightening, and uncomfortable situations.

DIFFERENTIAL DIAGNOSIS

1. Normative anxiety.
2. Personality disorder.
3. Posttraumatic stress disorder is characterized by the history of some extreme traumatic stressor as well as a more specific constellation of symptoms (see later section).
4. Psychological factors affecting medical condition (PFAMC). In this disorder, specific kinds of behavior or other psychological factors exacerbate some medical disorder. In an adjustment disorder, it is the other way around (i.e., the medical disorder leads to problem behavior or psychologic symptoms).
5. Bereavement is a specific category for what is essentially an adjustment problem following the death of a loved one.
6. Normal reaction to stress. A behavior is not a disorder if it does not lead to significant distress or impairment.

TREATMENT

Adjustment disorders require psychotherapeutic attention to the underlying stress and how it is perceived and managed by the patient. Relaxation training and increased exercise can be helpful. Medication can play an adjunctive role, but it will not be sufficient to resolve the underlying problem.

9.8 Acute Stress Disorder

DEFINITION

1. Acute stress disorder (ASD) is anxiety precipitated by an exposure to or memory of some past traumatic situation. Stressors causing ASD are severe and outside the range of normal experience (such as rape, assault, or traffic accidents).
2. The symptoms occur within 4 weeks of the traumatic event and last for at least a few days and possibly up to 4 weeks. If the symptom lasts longer than 1 month, the diagnosis evolves into posttraumatic stress disorder.
3. Symptoms associated with acute stress disorder include the following:
   a. Numbing or detachment from emotions.
   b. Feeling in a daze.
   c. Derealization.
   d. Depersonalization.
   e. Dissociative amnesia (i.e., not recalling some aspect of the trauma).

DIFFERENTIAL DIAGNOSIS

1. V codes are used in the *Diagnostic and Statistical Manual of Mental Disorders* (DSM) system to refer to problems that do not qualify as disorders, often because they represent normative life responses.

a. No person goes through life without reactive anxiety. Most people find ways either to tolerate such anxiety or to relieve it through personal formulas that reduce it or distract them from it. Common stresses include the following (see Chapter 2 for psychosocial review of systems):
   (1) Mental or physical disorders.
   (2) Family problems.
   (3) Relationship problems.
   (4) Abuse.
   (5) Work or school problems.
b. Situational anxiety responses to psychosocial stress are among the leading precipitants of physician visits. It is for this reason that the medical evaluation should always include some questions about current life stresses (see Chapter 2).
c. Psychosocial stress. A fairly minimal amount of interviewing is usually necessary to determine the psychosocial context underlying an anxiety reaction (see Chapter 2).
   (1) Often it is only necessary to ask, "What do you think is making you so anxious?"
   (2) Because of the increasing awareness of and willingness to discuss the problem, issues of sexual or physical abuse should be considered in patients presenting with acute anxiety symptoms.
2. Panic attacks. Brief anxiety reactions may be confused with panic attacks, but anxiety reactions are not as extreme and do not have the full cluster of symptoms of panic attacks (see Box 9-4).
3. Medical causes of acute anxiety.
   a. Anxiety may be the outcome of some underlying medical problem (see Boxes 9-2 and 9-3), such as an asthma attack, cardiac arrhythmia, or drug or medication reaction.
   b. Repeated anxiety symptoms with no other apparent explanation should increase suspicion of some underlying medical cause.
4. Anxiety as an aspect of another psychiatric disorder. Repeated anxiety symptoms without an apparent cause should raise suspicion of some underlying psychiatric disorder including the following:
   a. An affective disorder with accompanying anxiety.
   b. An anxiety disorder such as OCD or posttraumatic stress disorder.
   c. Substance abuse.

PROGNOSIS

Episodes of acute anxiety are self-limited, although they can be extremely uncomfortable for the patient.

TREATMENT

1. A thorough review of the traumatic event, in the context of emotional safety, is probably the single most important approach to this problem. However, patients should not be pushed beyond what they feel comfortable addressing.

2. Reassurance that patients are not medically ill and not "losing their mind," along with some structured problem solving, is generally sufficient.
3. If the underlying cause is continuing and the patient is in extreme distress, short-term use of an anxiolytic may be helpful.
   a. Diazepam 5 to 10 mg orally. If it is necessary to give a drug intramuscularly, lorazepam 1 to 2 mg may be used.
   b. In the medically ill patient or in patients who should avoid benzodiazepines, low-dose atypical antipsychotic agents can be helpful (such as risperidone 0.25 mg bid or quetiapine 25 mg bid-tid).
   c. Commonly employed anxiety-reduction strategies are helpful and adaptive (such as exercise programs and social support).

9.9 Posttraumatic Stress Disorder

DEFINITION AND IDENTIFICATION

1. Posttraumatic stress disorder (PTSD) is recurrent anxiety precipitated by an exposure to or memory of some past traumatic situation. Stressors causing PTSD are severe and outside the range of normal experience (such as rape, assault, or traffic accidents).
2. Diagnostic criteria for PTSD.
   a. History of traumatic experience.
   b. Re-experience of the traumatic event.
      (1) Intrusive memories.
      (2) Disturbing dreams or nightmares.
      (3) Flashbacks.
      (4) Psychological or physical distress caused by reminders of the event.
   c. Numbing and avoidance of things associated with the trauma.
   d. Other symptoms include the following:
      (1) Sleep problems.
      (2) Irritability.
      (3) Trouble concentrating.
      (4) Hypervigilance.
      (5) Easy startling (hyperarousal).

PREVALENCE

1. PTSD has an estimated prevalence of about 1% in the general population, but it is obviously higher (up to 20%) in people who have been exposed to traumatic life events such as war, rape, or catastrophes.
   a. More than 20 years after the Vietnam War, about 15% of Vietnam veterans continue to suffer from PTSD.
   b. About 15% of psychiatric inpatients have some form of PTSD as a comorbidity.
   c. About 5% to 6% of men and 10% to 14% of women have PTSD at some point in their lives.
   d. Occurs in 14% of those experiencing sudden, unexpected loss of a loved one and in more than 50% of rape victims.
2. Unfortunately, as a consequence of an increasingly violent society, we might see more PTSD.

DIFFERENTIAL DIAGNOSIS

1. In psychotic disorders, intrusive disturbing thoughts are not limited to a single uncomfortable event for the patient.
2. Cognitive deficits (of concentration and memory) in PTSD can resemble dementia.
3. Impulsive, irritable, or aggressive behavior in personality disorders have a history that predates the traumatic event.
4. Substance abuse should always be sought because it is not uncommon in PTSD patients as a way of coping with their symptoms. (This is a complication, not a differential.)
5. The anxiety associated with PTSD and reliving trauma can reach the level of a panic attack, but only uncued attacks are suggestive of panic disorder.
6. The stressor and anxiety of an adjustment disorder are generally less severe.
7. The recurrent thoughts in OCD are not a result of a severe traumatic event.
8. Fabrication, malingering, factitious symptoms.

PROGNOSIS

1. Early intervention can help lessen the duration and severity of the resulting anxiety disorder.
2. Acute forms of PTSD, which come and go in 6 months or less, have a good prognosis for remaining in remission.
3. Chronic, remitting forms can be quite difficult to resolve and can require ongoing support and episodic interventions.

TREATMENTS

1. Support groups have been helpful for many patients.
2. Psychotherapeutic support can help decrease symptom frequency and severity. PTSD usually requires some form of therapy (such as imaginal exposure) designed for the specific trauma. It is probably best to seek out a therapist who has some experience dealing with the specific problem. Therapy often consists of a component of slowly coming into contact with the traumatic experience and reintegrating it into the present with some combination of support and desensitization.
3. Psychopharmacology. Most psychotropics have been tried to treat symptoms of PTSD. The groups showing the most promise are the antidepressants.
   a. Tricyclic antidepressants: Several double-blind studies of tricyclic agents have found them to be modestly successful in reducing overall symptoms.
   b. SSRIs are first-line treatment. FDA-approved agents include sertraline (Zoloft) and paroxetine (Paxil).
   c. Approach to nonresponders and partial responders to SSRIs:
      (1) Augment or switch to venlafaxine (Effexor-XR).
      (2) Trial of divalproex (Depakote).
   d. Atypical antipsychotics may be tried in unresponsive cases.

e. Benzodiazepines. Alprazolam or clonazepam appear not to be better than placebo.

SUGGESTED READINGS

Barlow DH, Gorman JM, Shear MK, Woods SW: Cognitive-behavioral therapy, imipramine, or their combination for panic disorder: A randomized controlled trial. JAMA 283(19):2529-2536, 2000.

Brunello N, Davidson JR, Deahl M, et al: Posttraumatic stress disorder: Diagnosis and epidemiology, comorbidity and social consequences, biology and treatment. Neuropsychobiology 43(3):150-162, 2001.

Fricchione G: Generalized anxiety disorder. N Engl J Med 351:675-682, 2004.

Glass RM: Panic disorder—it's real and it's treatable. JAMA 283(19):2573-2574, 2000.

Hirschfeld RMA: Panic disorder: Diagnosis, epidemiology, and clinical course. J Clin Psychiatry 57(Suppl 10):3-8, 1996.

Kessler RC, McGonagle KA, Zhao S: Lifetime and 12-month prevalence of DSM-III-R psychiatric disorders in the United States. Arch Gen Psychiatry 51(1):8-19, 1994.

Kessler RC, Sonnega A, Bromet E, et al: Post-traumatic stress disorder in the National Comorbidity Survey. Arch Gen Psychiatry 52(12):1048-1060, 1995.

Kushner MG, Abrams K, Borchardt C: The relationship between anxiety disorders and alcohol use disorders: A review of major perspectives and findings. Clin Psychol Rev 29(2):149-171, 2000.

Lepine JP: The epidemiology of anxiety disorders: Prevalence and societal costs. J Clin Psychiatry 63(Suppl 14):4-8, 2002.

Shear MK, Brown TA, Barlow DH, et al: Multicenter collaborative panic disorder severity scale. Am J Psychiatry 154(11):1571-1575, 1997.

Ursano RJ, Bell C, Eth S, et al: Practice guideline for the treatment of patients with acute stress disorder and posttraumatic stress disorder. Am J Psychiatry 161(11 Suppl):3-31, 2004.

Yehuda R: Post-traumatic stress disorder. N Engl J Med 346(2):108-114, 2002.

Treatment of Anxiety: Medications and Therapies

10

Richard J. Goldberg
Donn Posner
Mark Zimmerman

10.1 Benzodiazepines

INDICATIONS

1. Benzodiazepines (BZs) for anxiety disorders.
   a. Panic disorder.
      (1) Alprazolam and clonazepam are most commonly used for their antipanic activity. For panic attacks, alprazolam in a dose as low as 0.25 mg tid is often helpful, although some patients require 2 mg tid or more. A sustained-release formulation of alprazolam is available as Xanax-XR.
      (2) Diazepam also appears to be effective for reducing panic attacks, but its use is associated with more side effects.
      (3) Approximate diazepam to alprazolam conversion ratio is 10:1.
   b. Generalized anxiety. All BZs have a positive effect on generalized anxiety disorder (Table 10-1; also see the azapirone section in this chapter). A broad range of oral doses seems necessary for different patients (e.g., diazepam 2.5-10 mg tid).
   c. Acute anxiety. BZs are appropriate for acute or short-term anxiety when the anxiety cannot be relieved by reassurance and the reason for the anxiety meets the following conditions:
      (1) The reason can be identified.
      (2) Is considered time-limited, for example, a patient awaiting a cardiac catheterization who is extremely anxious and cannot control anxiety despite reassurance. Prescribe, for example, lorazepam 0.5 mg bid or tid or diazepam 2 to 5 mg bid or tid.
2. Other indications for BZs.
   a. Short-term use as hypnotics (see Chapter 11).
   b. Musculoskeletal disorders (diazepam is approved for the treatment of muscle spasm).
   c. Seizure disorders (intravenous diazepam remains one of the drugs of choice for terminating repetitive grand mal seizures; lorazepam and clonazepam are also used as anticonvulsants).
   d. Treatment of sedative-withdrawal syndromes (see Chapter 15).
   e. Anesthesia (midazolam is commonly used as a preoperative adjunct).
   f. Restless legs syndrome.

Table 10-1   Benzodiazepines

Drug	Plasma peak (h)	Half-life (h)	Active metabolites	Metabolite Half-life (h)	Dose Equivalent	Duration
Alprazolam (Xanax)	1-2	12-15	Alpha-hydroxy-alprazolam	6	0.5	Short
Chlordiazepoxide (Librium)	1-4	7-28	Desmethylchlordiazepoxide Demoxepam Desmethyldiazepam Oxazepam	5-30 14-95 25-100 3-24	12.5	Long
Clonazepam (Klonopin)	1-2	18-56	None		0.25	Long
Clorazepate (Tranxene)	1-2		Desmethyldiazepam Oxazepam	25-100 3-24	7.5	Long
Diazepam (Valium)	0.5-2	20-50	Desmethyldiazepam Oxazepam	25-100 3-24	5	Long
Lorazepam (Ativan)	1-3 IM	10-24	None		1	Short
Midazolam IM (Versed), IV	0.5	1-6	1-Hydroxymethylmidazolam		1-3	Short
Oxazepam (Serax)	1-4	3-24	None		15	Short

PHARMACOKINETICS

1. Absorption.
   a. The onset of action of orally administered BZs is largely determined by gastrointestinal (GI) absorption. Diazepam and clorazepate are the two most rapidly absorbed, although all BZs are well absorbed orally.
   b. Lorazepam and midazolam are the only BZs reliably absorbed from intramuscular (IM) sites. Diazepam and chlordiazepoxide IM absorption is erratic.
   c. Sublingual absorption. Lorazepam, alprazolam, and triazolam are compounded to allow sublingual absorption. Tablets should be placed under the tongue and allowed to dissolve passively. This may be an alternative for patients who are receiving nothing by mouth (NPO). Absorption is slightly faster than oral rates. Clonazepam is also available in an oral wafer formulation for sublingual use.
   d. Diazepam, lorazepam, and midazolam are used intravenously (IV) in some emergency situations, such as agitated delirium or laryngeal dystonia (from neuroleptic agents) that does not respond to anticholinergic agents. Lorazepam 1 to 2 mg given slowly IV is a reasonable dose. Intravenous benzodiazepines should be pushed slowly to minimize the risk of respiratory depression and should not be used unless there is immediate resuscitation capability available.

2. Distribution.
   a. All BZs are highly lipophilic and rapidly cross the blood–brain barrier.
   b. The BZs that are the most lipophilic (diazepam and clorazepate) have a shorter duration of clinical activity because they are rapidly redistributed to peripheral sites. Even though diazepam has a lengthy plasma elimination half-life, it has a relatively short duration of clinical activity.

3. Metabolism.
   a. All BZs are metabolized by the liver, involving either oxidation or glucuronide conjugation. Oxidation can be impaired by conditions including advanced age and hepatic cirrhosis or by other drugs (such as cimetidine, estrogens, or isoniazid).
   b. BZs can be classified as long-acting or short-acting (Box 10-1).
   c. The long-acting drugs tend to have active metabolites with elimination half-lives of about 4 days.
      (1) Long-acting BZs, if suddenly discontinued, do not have medically serious withdrawal symptoms and tend to self-taper. Therefore, you can load a patient in delirium tremens (DTs) with chlordiazepoxide or diazepam and stop the BZs after a day (see Chapter 15).
      (2) Long-acting BZs tend to accumulate with repeated doses, especially in the elderly or those with hepatic impairment.
   d. The short-acting BZs, which are quickly eliminated, have the potential to produce serious withdrawal reactions, including seizures. At moderate or high doses, clinically important withdrawal symptoms are common.

BOX 10-1   Benzodiazepine Metabolism

Oxidative, Long-Acting

Clorazepate
Chlordiazepoxide
Diazepam

Conjugative, Short-Acting

Alprazolam
Estazolam*
Lorazepam
Oxazepam
Temazepam*
Zolpidem*

---

*Used primarily as hypnotics; see Chapter 11.

SIDE EFFECTS

1. Psychomotor impairment and drowsiness.
   a. Symptoms consist of muscle weakness, ataxia, dysarthria, vertigo, somnolence, and confusion.
   b. Older patients are especially susceptible to psychomotor impairment and falls.
   c. Psychomotor impairment creates risk for car accidents, machinery accidents, or falls, especially if patients are also taking other sedative drugs or alcohol.
   d. Although patients develop tolerance to these psychomotor side effects after 3 to 4 weeks, they apparently do not develop tolerance to the anxiolytic side effects.
2. BZs augment the sedative side effects of other sedatives, including narcotics, barbiturates, and alcohol.
3. Cognitive impairment. BZs impair memory in two ways.
   a. Acute anterograde amnesia, usually associated with IV use but also with high-dose, high-potency BZs taken orally, as well as with relatively low doses of ultra-short-acting agents (e.g., traveler's amnesia).
   b. Impaired long-term memory from interference with memory consolidation is most often a problem in the elderly.
4. Depression of hypoxic respiratory drive.
   a. The respiratory-depressant effect of BZs is most marked in patients with CO_2 retention. Therefore BZs should not be used in patients with pulmonary disease without checking blood gas for elevated P_{CO_2}.
   b. This problem is most marked when BZs are given intravenously with other respiratory depressants such as narcotics.
5. Depressive symptoms may be produced or increased.
6. Depersonalization, paranoia, and confusion are reported with triazolam, generally at doses of 0.5 mg or more.

7. Paradoxical effects resulting in disinhibition, agitation, or aggression appear rarely, usually in patients with preexisting personality disorders, substance abusers, and underlying delirium or dementia. To manage BZ-induced dyscontrol, haloperidol 5 mg IM may be effective.

ISSUES OF ABUSE

1. BZs are potentially drugs of abuse.
2. It is extremely rare that the average person is turned into a drug abuser by a brief exposure to BZs.
3. Addiction-prone personalities are more likely to become addicted to BZs. Other than for medically indicated short-term use, BZs should be prescribed cautiously, if at all, for such patients. See Chapter 15 for further discussion of medication and drug abuse issues.
4. When the patient taking BZs asks for higher doses more frequently.
   a. Some patients actually need higher doses than commonly prescribed. However, when a patient seems to require doses beyond the customary range, the physician should consider the potential for abuse.
   b. Look for other signs of abuse.
      (1) Multiple prescribers.
      (2) Lost pills.
      (3) Emergency room visits for medication.
      (4) A pattern of running out too soon.
      (5) Concurrent abuse of other substances.
      (6) Lack of legitimate diagnosis to warrant medication.
      (7) Buying drugs on the street.
      (8) Adverse behavioral consequences.
   c. Eliminate multiple prescribers.
5. Patients legitimately maintained with BZs for generalized anxiety should not be considered abusers.

DISCONTINUING BENZODIAZEPINES AND WITHDRAWAL ISSUES

1. When to discontinue BZs.
   a. If the patient is abusing the drug.
   b. If the drug is causing significant side effects.
   c. If the underlying disorder may no longer be present. For example, panic disorder is likely to be episodic; therefore, after about 4 to 6 months of stability, consider a gradual taper of the drug.
2. How to discontinue BZs.
   a. The long-acting drugs "self-taper." Although a patient taking diazepam 30 mg/day might feel anxious or somewhat uncomfortable about stopping "cold turkey," there will be no serious medical consequences.
   b. The short-acting drugs should be tapered to avoid sedative withdrawal symptoms.
3. Symptoms of BZ withdrawal are listed in Box 10-2.
4. Risk of withdrawal symptoms increases with the following:
   a. Higher doses.

BOX 10-2   **Benzodiazepine Withdrawal Symptoms**

Anorexia
Anxiety
Blurred vision
Dizziness
Headache
Hyperthermia
Hypotension
Insomnia
Muscle irritability
Psychosis
Tinnitus
Tremor

 b. Duration of use (risk of withdrawal may be present within 1 week of continuous use).
 c. Shorter plasma elimination half-life.
5. Treatment of withdrawal.
 a. Typical treatment involves giving a BZ or a cross-tolerant sedative in sufficient amount to eliminate the withdrawal symptoms. Then the drug is gradually withdrawn on a more controlled schedule.
 b. Details of treatment of BZ and sedative withdrawal are described in Chapter 15.
 c. Autonomic symptoms, if intense, can be controlled with β-blockers.

DRUG INTERACTIONS

The BZs have relatively few drug interactions. Relevant interactions include the following:

1. Augmentation of other central nervous system (CNS) sedatives (such as alcohol, narcotics, antihistamines).
2. Drugs that increase benzodiazepine levels include:
 a. Cimetidine.
 b. Disulfiram.
 c. Fluoxetine.
 d. Isoniazid.
 e. Low-dose estrogen-containing oral contraceptives.
 f. There is a report that erythromycin inhibits triazolam metabolism.
3. Drugs whose levels may be increased by BZs include:
 a. Coumadin.
 b. Digoxin.
 c. Phenytoin.
4. Drugs that can impair or delay BZ absorption include:
 a. Antacids.
 b. Anticholinergics.
5. Drugs that decrease BZ levels include carbamazepine (and possibly other anticonvulsants).

OVERDOSE

1. Patients can ingest extremely large doses of BZs without dying.
2. Deaths from BZs alone are extremely rare, but death can occur when BZs are mixed with other sedatives such as alcohol or barbiturates.
3. Flumazenil (Mazicon) is a BZ receptor antagonist that can reverse excessive sedation and psychomotor impairment.

USE DURING PREGNANCY

1. Reports that use of diazepam during the first trimester is associated with increased risk of cleft palate and dysmorphism have not been fully substantiated. However, there is not good evidence to establish the safety of BZs during pregnancy. Diazepam use in pregnancy has been associated with the following:
   a. Floppy baby syndrome (hypotonia, lethargy, sucking difficulties).
   b. Withdrawal syndrome (tremors, irritability, vigorous sucking, hypertonicity).
2. For treating agitation and anxiety after the second trimester, tricyclic antidepressants and diazepam both appear relatively safe and preferable to neuroleptic agents.

DIFFERENCES AMONG THE BENZODIAZEPINES

1. Alprazolam (Xanax and Xanax XR).
   a. Antipanic properties are very good. It is often effective within 24 hours. Effective doses may be as little as 0.25 mg or 0.5 mg tid (if a patient does not respond, the dose can be doubled). Usually, patients do not require more than 6 mg/day.
   b. Alprazolam is an unusual BZ because of some reports of antidepressant effects. Although not indicated as a first-line antidepressant, alprazolam may be helpful in mixed anxiety—depression states.
   c. It is often difficult to discontinue alprazolam. Tapering must be done slowly (often decreasing by as little as 0.25 mg a week) to avoid rebound anxiety or withdrawal.
   d. Some patients request an increase in dose or frequency to maintain an effect. This can raise concern about potential abuse. In such cases, consider crossing the patient over to longer-acting clonazepam.
      (1) Add up the total alprazolam dose and convert to one half that amount of clonazepam. Give the clonazepam twice a day.
      (2) During the first 7 days, small doses of alprazolam can be used as needed. If more medication is needed after 7 days, clonazepam can be increased by 0.25 to 0.5 mg a week.
2. Chlordiazepoxide (Librium).
   a. Often used to prevent or treat sedative withdrawal syndromes, such as DTs, in doses of approximately 50 mg q3h.
   b. Should be given orally, because it is not well absorbed intramuscularly. Details on treating DTs are presented in Chapter 15.
3. Clonazepam (Klonopin).
   a. Indicated for the treatment of akinetic, myoclonic, and absence-type seizures.

  b. An effective antipanic drug, often in doses as low as 0.25 mg bid. Some patients require about 1 mg tid.
  c. Sedation is the most problematic side effect.
  d. Clonazepam nonspecifically slows down and sedates agitated manic patients. Unfortunately, it is only available in oral form.
  e. Active manic patients might require doses of 2 mg tid or qid. (Chapter 14 presents a review of the treatment of behavioral emergencies.)
  f. Effective in the treatment of restless legs syndrome.
4. Diazepam (Valium).
  a. Indicated for treatment of status epilepticus and recurrent convulsive seizures.
  b. Effective anxiolytic for short-term and acute use. The patient or family member who needs to be "calmed down" might do well taking diazepam 5 mg given orally as needed.
  c. Diazepam is often preferred by sedative abusers, possibly because of its rapid brain uptake.
  d. Not well absorbed from IM sites.
5. Lorazepam (Ativan) and oxazepam (Serax).
  a. Short-acting BZs with no active metabolites.
  b. Metabolism does not depend on hepatic P450 system; therefore plasma levels are not altered by other medications, aging, or liver disease.
  c. Lorazepam is well absorbed IM, a useful property in medically ill patients, agitated patients, and patients with DTs (e.g., 2 mg lorazepam IM can substitute for 50 mg of chlordiazepoxide or 10 mg of diazepam). See Chapter 14 for more details on its use in emergency situations.
6. See Chapter 11 for use of BZs as hypnotics.

10.2 Azapirones

1. The azapirones, a group of nonsedating anxiolytics, are represented by buspirone (BuSpar).
2. Indications.
  a. Generalized anxiety disorder.
  b. General anxiety with accompanying depressive symptoms.
3. Other clinical applications include treatment of aggression. This drug group can reduce the frequency and severity of episodic aggression in some populations with brain damage (such as developmentally disabled and demented persons).
4. Clinical use.
  a. The antianxiety dose range is between 20 and 40 mg/day, with a usual starting dose of 10 mg tid.
    (1) In patients with brain damage (e.g., from stroke, Parkinson's disease, Alzheimer's disease, and developmental disabilities), the starting dose should be 5 mg tid because of increased likelihood of side effects.
    (2) Many patients can be managed using twice-daily doses.

    b. An adequate clinical trial requires about 1 month. If response is inadequate, increase the dose by increments of 5 to 10 mg every few weeks to a maximum of 20 mg tid.

    c. Response lag time of several weeks is usual. Patients should be educated and supported through the first few weeks.

      (1) For the patient who does not want to wait several weeks, try reasoning that their disorder has been present for a long time.

      (2) If this does not work, two drugs can be started at one time, for example, lorazepam 0.5 mg tid and buspirone 10 mg tid. For the CO_2 retainer, try a low-dose atypical antipsychotic and buspirone 10 mg tid. After about 3 weeks, the BZ or antipsychotic agent can be stopped.

5. Side effects (5% to 10% incidence).

    a. Dizzy or lightheaded feeling. This is often dose related and may be reduced by dividing the dose.

    b. Dull headache.

    c. Nervousness (different from the underlying anxiety).

6. Drug interactions.

    a. Do not use with monoamine oxidase inhibitors (MAOIs).

    b. Can increase haloperidol levels.

10.3 Comparison of Benzodiazepines and Azapirones

Azapirones and benzodiazepines are compared in Table 10-2.

1. The basic differences between these two drug groups.

    a. Indications. Azapirones are indicated only for generalized anxiety and unlike BZs are not effective for acute anxiety or panic disorder.

    b. The azapirones lack the sedative side effects of the BZs, such as the following:

      (1) Psychomotor impairment and drowsiness. Patients are less likely to get into accidents. Elderly patients are less likely to fall.

      (2) Augmentation of other sedatives. As a nonsedating anxiolytic, buspirone may be useful in patients who should avoid additional sedation.

        (a) Medical patients receiving narcotics for chronic pain (e.g., patients with cancer).

        (b) Epileptics taking phenobarbital or a BZ.

        (c) Patients at risk for abusing alcohol.

    c. Because the azapirones lack cognitive impairment, they are preferable for elderly patients with generalized anxiety.

    d. Azapirones lack abuse potential. This may be a consideration for patients with a history of addiction.

    e. Azapirones do not cause respiratory depression and are safe in patients with CO_2 retention.

    f. The azapirones are not cross-tolerant with other sedatives and cannot be used to cover the physiologic withdrawal symptoms from alcohol or other sedatives.

Table 10-2 **Comparison of Benzodiazepines and Azapirones**

Features	Benzodiazepines	Azapirones
Uses		
Acute anxiety	Yes	No
General anxiety	Yes	Yes
Panic attacks	Yes	No
Sedative Effects		
Drowsiness	Yes	No
Psychomotor impairment	Yes	No
Sedative augmentation	Yes	No
Other Effects		
Abuse potential	Yes	No
Cognitive effects	Yes	No
Respiratory depression	Yes	No

10.4 Antidepressants for Anxiety

1. Tricyclics for panic disorder.
   a. Antipanic effects of imipramine have been noted for more than 30 years. Typical doses range from a starting dose of 25 mg/day, gradually increased to much higher doses such as 250 mg/day, required by some patients.
   b. Clomipramine (which has greater potency for serotonin reuptake inhibition than imipramine) is more effective than imipramine for treating panic attacks. Typical doses range from a starting dose of 50 mg/day gradually raised to as much as 250 mg/day, which is required by some patients.
   c. Because of fewer side effects, selective serotonin reuptake inhibitors (SSRIs) are preferred to tricyclic agents for treating panic disorder.
2. SSRIs for panic disorder.
   a. Fluoxetine.
      (1) May be associated with more anxiety, nervousness, and agitation in the initial weeks than other SSRIs.
      (2) Between 10% and 40% of panic patients might not be able to tolerate doses as low as 10 mg/day without an increase in anxiety symptoms.
         (a) These patients may be able to tolerate and benefit from 2.5 mg/day (in liquid form).
         (b) Starting doses should not be more than 10 mg/day.
   b. Sertraline is demonstrated to be effective in reducing panic attacks in doses ranging from a starting dose of 25 mg/day up to 200 mg/day required by some patients.
   c. Paroxetine.
      (1) Although paroxetine is more selective at blocking serotonin reuptake than the other SSRIs, this has not translated into demonstrated superior efficacy.
      (2) Paroxetine has been shown to be effective for panic disorder in doses from a starting dose of 10 mg/day up to 60 mg/day required by some patients.

        (3) The controlled-release (CR) formulation results in less nausea.
            Dosing begins at 12.5 mg/day.
   d. Citalopram and escitalopram are both effective.
3. Other antidepressants for panic disorder.
   a. Venlafaxine (Effexor XR).
   b. Trazodone and nefazodone have both shown efficacy in panic disorder (although there is not a Food and Drug Administration [FDA] indication).
4. Antidepressants for the treatment of other anxiety disorders. See Chapter 7 for a review of the use of antidepressants for disorders including posttraumatic stress disorder (PTSD), premenstrual dysphoric disorder (PMDD), social phobia, generalized anxiety, and obsessive–compulsive disorder (OCD).

10.5 Other Sedative–Hypnotics

1. Antihistamines, such as diphenhydramine (Benadryl) or hydroxyzine (Vistaril), are sometimes used to treat anxiety; however, they have no specific antianxiety properties. Patients feel less anxious because of sedative effects. In addition, these drugs have significant anticholinergic activity.
2. Barbiturates have basically no role in treating anxiety because of rapid tolerance, need for increased doses, abuse potential, lack of safety at high doses, overdose lethality, and many drug interactions.
3. Meprobamate (Miltown, Equanil) was the anxiolytic of choice during the 1950s, but it has little place in the armamentarium today because it is not as effective as the other choices.
4. Antipsychotics may be useful for anxiety in medically ill patients requiring a rapid response and in those who cannot tolerate BZs because of respiratory disease.
   a. In the anxious delirious patient, low-dose antipsychotic agents such as perphenazine (Trilafon) 2 mg bid or tid, haloperidol (Haldol) 1 mg bid, or risperidone (Risperdal) 0.5 mg bid, for example, may be helpful.
   b. Because of the risk of tardive dyskinesia, these drugs should be used for as short a time as possible (e.g., less than 3 months).
5. β-Blockers.
   a. The best use of β-blockers for anxiety involves their use to prevent performance anxiety. Propranolol 20 to 40 mg given 45 to 75 minutes before a performance can decrease symptoms of anxiety. Propranolol is well absorbed orally and has a half-life of about 3 hours.
   b. Nadolol and atenolol, although they do not cross the blood–brain barrier, also appear to be effective in these situations.
   c. These drugs are not indicated as maintenance therapy for anxiety disorders.
   d. They should not be used in patients with heart failure, depression, delirium, asthma, and hypoglycemia.
6. The antidepressant drug group has a variety of antianxiety effects (Table 10-3).

Table 10-3 Antidepressants: FDA Indications for Anxiety Disorders

Drug	GAD	OCD	Panic Disorder	PTSD	Social Phobia
Bupropion (Wellbutrin-XL)					
Escitalopram (Lexapro)	Yes				Coming
Fluoxetine (Prozac)		Yes	Yes		
Fluvoxamine (Luvox)		Yes			
Mirtazapine (Remeron)					
Nefazodone (Serzone)					
Paroxetine (Paxil)	Yes	Yes	Yes	Yes	Yes
Sertraline (Zoloft)		Yes	Yes	Yes	Yes
Venlafaxine (Effexor-XR)	Yes				Yes

GAD, generalized anxiety disorder; OCD, obsessive–compulsive disorder; PTSD, posttraumatic stress disorder.

10.6 Cognitive Behavior Therapy

1. Cognitive behavior therapy (CBT) has been shown to be highly effective in the treatment of a wide variety of anxiety disorders, both in combination with medications and as a stand-alone therapy.
2. Combination therapy can improve relapse rates once medication is tapered.
3. CBT usually requires referral to a specifically trained therapist.
4. CBT addresses physical, cognitive, and behavioral systems.

PHYSICAL INTERVENTIONS

Physical interventions address physical hyperarousal that accompanies anxiety. These include:

1. Progressive muscle relaxation (PMR) (Box 10-3).
2. Diaphragmatic breathing training, which is especially useful in patients suspected of hyperventilating or in patients who cannot tolerate other forms of more intensive relaxation training.
3. Mindfulness meditation (Box 10-4).
4. Some considerations before starting any relaxation training.
   a. Discuss the training beforehand to elicit any questions, misconceptions, or concerns.
   b. Although tape-recorded or printed instructions can be used, an initial session with the clinician can be important to make sure the patient is doing it correctly and in establishing a positive alliance.

BOX 10-3   Basic Instructions for Progressive Muscle Relaxation

1. Select a comfortable sitting or reclining position.
2. Loosen any tight clothing.
3. Take a deep breath, hold it momentarily, and exhale as fully as possible.
4. Tense toes and feet (curl the toes, turn the feet in and out). Hold the tension, become aware of the tension, then relax toes and feet.
5. Tense lower legs, knees, and thighs. Hold the tension, become aware of the tension, and then relax legs.
6. Tense buttocks. Hold and become aware of the tension, then relax.
7. Tense fingers and hands. Hold the tension, become aware of the tension, then relax.
8. Tense lower arms, elbows, and upper arms. Hold the tension, become aware of it, then relax.
9. Tense abdomen. Hold the tension, become aware of it, then relax.
10. Tense chest. Hold the tension, relax. Take a deep breath, hold it momentarily, then slowly exhale.
11. Tense the lower back. Hold the tension, become aware of it, then relax.
12. Tense the upper back. Hold the tension, become aware of it, then relax.
13. Tense the shoulders. Hold the tension, be aware of the tension, then relax and let your shoulders droop down.
14. Tense the neck in front and back. Hold the tension, become aware of it, then relax.
15. Now clench the teeth until tension in the facial muscles is felt. Become aware of it, then relax, letting the jaw drop slightly.
16. Now wrinkle the forehead. Become aware of the tension on the top and back of the head, then relax, and let the eyes relax.
17. Continue sitting for a few minutes, feeling the relaxation flowing throughout the body. Know the difference between muscles that are tense and muscles that are relaxed. Scan for any muscle groups that remain tense. Increase the tension, then relax them.
18. Now stretch, feeling renewed and refreshed, and continue usual activities.

---

c. Establish a comfortable, quiet setting, without interruptions.
d. The patient should be encouraged to practice at home every day for greatest effectiveness. The best practice time is when the patient is most calm, can afford to make mistakes, and can concentrate best.

BOX 10-4   Basic Mindfulness Meditation Exercise

The therapists can read the instructions to the client in a slow and soft fashion.

1. Get in a comfortable position in your chair. Sit upright with your feet flat on the floor, your arms and legs uncrossed, and your hands resting in your lap. Allow your eyes to close gently. [Pause 10 seconds.] Take a couple of gentle breaths: in ... and out—in ... and out. Notice the sound and feel of your own breath as you breathe in [pause] and out. [Pause 10 seconds.]

2. Now turn your attention to being inside this room. Notice any sounds that occur inside the room [pause] and outside. [Pause 10 seconds.] Notice how you are sitting in your chair. [Pause 10 seconds]. Focus on the place where your body touches the chair. What are the sensations there? How does it feel to sit where you sit? [Pause 10 seconds.] Next, notice the places where your body touches itself. [Pause 10 seconds.] Notice the spot where your hands touch your legs. How do your feet feel in the position that they are in? [Pause 10 seconds.] What sensations can you notice in the rest of your body? If you feel any sensations in your body, just notice them and acknowledge their presence. [Pause 10 seconds.] Also notice how they may, by themselves, change or shift from moment to moment. Do not try to change them. [Pause 10 seconds.]

3. Now let yourself be in this room. See if you can feel the investment of you and me in this room—what we are here for. [Pause 10 seconds.] If you are thinking this sounds weird, just notice that and come back to the sense of integrity in this room. Be aware of the value that you and I are serving by being here. [Pause 10 seconds.] See if you can allow yourself to be present with what you are afraid of. Notice any doubts, reservations, fears, and worries. [Pause 10 seconds.] See if you can just notice them, acknowledge their presence, and make some space for them. [Pause 10 seconds.] You don't need to make them go away or work on them. [Pause 10 seconds.] Now see if for just a moment you can be present with your values and commitments. Why are you here? Where do you want to go? What do you want to do? [Pause 10 seconds.]

4. When you are ready, let go of those thoughts and gradually widen your attention to take in the sounds around you [pause 10 seconds] and slowly open your eyes with the intention to bring this awareness to the present moment and the rest of the day.

From Eifert GH, Forsyth JP: *Acceptance and Commitment Therapy for Anxiety Disorders.* Oakland, Calif, New Harbinger Publications, 2005.

5. Contraindications for these techniques.
   a. Dementia or delirium.
   b. Psychosis.
   c. Patients with an obsessive need for control.
   d. Some patients with panic disorder become anxious with relaxation induction and might respond better to diaphragmatic breathing control training.

COGNITIVE INTERVENTIONS

Cognitive interventions are aimed at changing faulty and overly negative thoughts, beliefs, and attributions that are often associated with anxiety. These can be categorized as follows:

1. *Education* consists of didactic information (such as description of how the fight-or-flight reflex works physiologically or the normalcy of having anxiety under certain stressful situations). Workbooks or self-help manuals may be helpful.
2. *Cognitive restructuring* is helping the patient to reassess faulty beliefs and/or attributions about the likelihood and catastrophic nature of the negative outcomes their anxiety causes them to predict. This type of restructuring is often best accomplished using the Socratic method, in which patients are encouraged to recognize for themselves how their own thoughts magnify their anxiety. Some of the most common distortions are:
   a. *All or none thinking.* Seeing things in only black-and-white terms with no room for shades of gray (e.g., "My speech failed because I didn't deliver it smoothly").
   b. *Overgeneralization.* Seeing a single negative event as a never-ending pattern (e.g., "I got rejected once, so I will probably always be rejected").
   c. *Disqualifying the positive.* Rejecting evidence of positive experience because for some reason it doesn't count (e.g., " I didn't die from that last panic attack because I was lucky to be near an emergency room").
   d. *Mind reading.* Arbitrarily assuming that you know what someone is thinking (e.g., "My boss must think I'm stupid").
   e. *Fortune telling.* Anticipating that things will turn out badly as if it is already an established fact (e.g., "If I give this talk, I will freeze").
   f. *Emotional reasoning.* Assuming your negative belief is true because it just feels true (e.g., "I just know that everything is going to go wrong").
   g. *Should statements.* Allowing oneself to be governed by a series of unwritten rules about what should or must be done (e.g., "I should always be perfect," "I must never lose control").
3. *Thought monitoring* encourages the patient to identify which of the distortions operate in their life and then to examine evidence that inevitably refutes the assumptions.

BEHAVIOR INTERVENTIONS

Behavior interventions are aimed at having the patient face their most feared thoughts, objects, or situations in a way that allows them to interact with these stimuli more normally and with less or no anxiety. There are two approaches.

1. *Desensitization* involves a process of reciprocal inhibition (a classical conditioning paradigm) in which the patient first achieves a state of relaxation, and then faces the feared stimuli until they feel their anxiety getting too high. Then they remove themselves from the situation until the state of relaxation is re-established. This process is repeated until the feared object elicits feelings of calm rather than anxiety. This is usually done by using imagery (systematic desensitization), or real objects or situations (in vivo desensitization). The process can start with the most feared object (implosion) or proceed in a hierarchical fashion from the least fear provoking stimulus to the most (gradual desensitization).

2. *Exposure* involves facing the situation and remaining exposed until the patient's anxiety is reduced. Exposure can be done with imagery (imaginal exposure) or with real settings or objects (in vivo exposure). Exposure can be hierarchical or gradual. Both desensitization and exposure have been shown to be effective, though data support exposure as the technique of choice.

3. Examples of exposure with different anxiety disorders.

   a. Panic disorder. Interoceptive exposure involves regular exercises such as hyperventilation, spinning in chairs, or breathing through straws. These exercises elicit symptoms similar to those the patient has when panicking and thus help the patient to see that such symptoms do not always have to suggest death, loss of control, or impending doom, thus diminishing fear over time.

   b. Agoraphobia. Gradual exposure to feared settings can be very effective, but again it is the fear of fear that is to be extinguished more so than the fear of the situation itself.

   c. Specific phobias. The feared object can be almost anything, and the fear is specific to the object (dogs, heights, snakes, driving, etc.), not the sensation of fear itself. Exposure here must entail directly confronting the feared object, usually in a graded hierarchy.

   d. OCD. The behavioral treatment involves *exposure and response prevention* because the patient engages in exposure to the feared stimulus and must also be prevented from undoing the exposure by checking, cleaning, counting, and so on. For example, someone obsessed with contamination must be made to touch numerous "dirty" surfaces and at the same time be prevented from washing their hands.

   e. PTSD. In this case, some of the exposure must be done through imagination and not in vivo. Patients can be encouraged to write down the story of their trauma and eventually read the story into a tape recorder so that later this can be played back repeatedly until the patient's anxiety level, while listening, drops.

   f. Social anxiety. The concern here is to prevent the exposure from being cognitively processed incorrectly by the patient. Ultimately, it is the repeated attempts at social discourse, not just showing up and being quiet, over fairly long periods of time, that will extinguish the fear of how others are judging the patient.

  g. Generalized anxiety disorder. Here again exposure is focused on worry and is largely done in imagination. *Worry time* should help the patient to stop pushing away their worries and to actually imagine their worst fears, and then try to imagine how they would actually handle these situations. In a sense, for the first time they are answering the question "what if ..." rather than just asking it and then trying to block it out.

4. Some considerations before starting.

  a. CBT work requires a significant amount of training on the part of the clinician.

  b. When considering how long a patient should stay in a particular exposure exercise, it is often best to consider the amount of anxiety reduction and not absolute time.

  c. Given the last point, it becomes clear that exposure can be fairly time intensive and is usually best accomplished by scheduling the time in, rather than by fitting it in as a last or quick activity of the day.

  d. One of the variables that can determine the level of hierarchy (e.g., particular highway or elevator, day or night, how crowded) can be whether the patient goes alone or with someone. Group therapy can be particularly useful for arranging partners for exposure exercises. Eventually as the patient improves and moves up the hierarchy, they should be encouraged to engage in the exposure alone, but accompanying the patient early in the treatment can be very useful for getting started.

SUGGESTED READINGS

Ballenger JC: Treatment of anxiety disorders to remission. *J Clin Psychiatry* 62(Suppl 12):5-9, 2001.

Barlow DH: Anxiety and Its Disorders: The Nature and Treatment of Anxiety and Panic, 2nd ed. New York, Guilford Press, 2001.

Eifert GH, Forsyth JP: *Acceptance and Commitment Therapy for Anxiety Disorders.* Oakland, Calif, New Harbinger Publications, 2005.

Foa EB, Liebowitz MR, Kozak MJ, et al: Randomized, placebo-controlled trial of exposure and ritual prevention, clomipramine, and their combination in the treatment of obsessive–compulsive disorder. *Am J Psychiatry* 162(1):151-161, 2005.

Otto MW, Smits JA, Reese HE: Cognitive-behavioral therapy for the treatment of anxiety disorders. *J Clin Psychiatry* 65(Suppl 5):34-41, 2004.

Yonkers KA, Bruce SE, Dyck IR, Keller MB: Chronicity, relapse, and illness—course of panic disorder, social phobia, and generalized anxiety disorder: Findings in men and women from 8 years of follow-up. *Depress Anxiety* 17(3):173-179, 2003.

Sleep Problems and the Use of Hypnotics

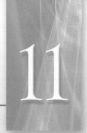

11

Richard P. Millman

11.1 Overview

1. Up to 40% percent of American adults complain of excessive sleepiness. The major causes include insufficient sleep, shift work, and obstructive sleep apnea (OSA).
2. Twelve percent of adults have chronic insomnia. Intermittent insomnia occurs in an additional 25% to 30%.
3. Physicians tend to disregard or minimize sleep complaints in their patients.

11.2 Evaluation of Sleep Problems

1. History. A sleep history is often ignored in primary care and psychiatric evaluations. Elements of sleep history (with patient and bed partner if possible) are:
   a. Timing of bedtime on workdays and weekends (for shift workers: on workdays and off days).
   b. Time to fall asleep initially.
      (1) Dozing on and off might suggest an organic disorder such as OSA.
      (2) Being wide awake suggests a psychological problem or discomfort (e.g., restless legs).
   c. When the problem started and how frequently it occurs.
   d. Number of awakenings per night and what triggers them. Does the patient have trouble falling back to sleep and how often does this occur?
   e. Time of getting up on workday and on nonworkday.
   f. How the patient feels upon awakening (e.g., rested, tired, stiff, headache).
   g. Presence of snoring. Snoring with obstructive sleep apnea (as opposed to primary snoring) is very loud, occurs in any position, and can be heard down the hall.
   h. Presence of observed apneas during sleep, or awakenings with a choking sensation not associated with gastroesophageal reflux disease (GERD) or postnasal drip.
   i. Other areas to question:
      (1) Presence of restless leg symptoms.
      (2) Breathing problems (may be related to sleep apnea, cardiopulmonary disease, or nasal obstruction).

BOX 11-1   **Epworth Sleepiness Scale**

Use the sleepiness score to indicate the chance of dozing in each situation.
Epworth Sleepiness Score

0 = Would never doze
1 = Slight chance of dozing
2 = Moderate chance of dozing
3 = High chance of dozing

Situation: Chance of Dozing

Sitting and reading: ___
Watching TV: ___
Sitting inactive in a public place (e.g., a theater/meeting): ___
As a passenger in a car for an hour without a break: ___
Lying down to rest in the afternoon when circumstances permit:___
Sitting and talking to someone: ___
Sitting quietly after lunch without alcohol: ___
In a car, while stopped for a few minutes in traffic: ___
Total: ___

---

     (3) Nightmares.
     (4) Pain or headaches.
     (5) Nocturia.
     (6) GERD, which can manifest as choking arousals.
     (7) Hot flushes.
     (8) Panic attacks (panic disorder can manifest as nighttime attacks).
     (9) Sleepwalking, night terrors, sleep eating, or dream enactment.
  j. Daytime alertness or level of fatigue. Daytime inappropriate napping or dozing. The level of daytime sleepiness may be assessed with the Epworth Sleepiness Scale (presented in Box 11-1). A normal score is less than 10.
  k. Problems with memory or attention and concentration during the daytime.
  l. Problems with coping, irritability, anxiety, or depressive symptoms during the day.
  m. History of depression, anxiety, psychosis, or any other psychiatric disorder (as a possible primary cause of the sleep problem).
  n. Medication (see section 11.6).
  o. Alcohol and drug use.
  p. Medical history. About one third of men with hypertension, for example, are likely to have undiagnosed sleep apnea.
2. Sleep log. Ask the patient to keep 2-week log of sleep and wake times, medications, substances, eating, activity, and symptoms.

3. Physical examination is most helpful in OSA. Anatomic findings that can indicate a possible narrowed pharyngeal airway that will collapse during sleep include:
    a. A thick neck due to upper-body obesity. Men with a 17-inch neck or larger have been shown to be at an increased risk for OSA.
    b. Nasal obstruction.
    c. Retrognathia.
    d. Enlarged tonsils.
    e. A deep-set palate and long uvula.
4. Objective sleep studies.
    a. Guidelines for referral to a specialist.
        (1) Failure to respond to treatment.
        (2) Suspicion of a primary sleep disorder such as OSA or periodic limb movements during sleep.
        (3) Sorting out etiology in a complex or refractory case.
    b. Full polysomnography at night involves monitoring two electroencephalogram (EEG) leads, two ocular leads, and a submental electromyographic (EMG) lead to measure sleep states and arousals. Respiration is assessed using nasal and oral thermistors, a nasal pressure transducer, snoring monitors, chest and abdominal bands, and continuous pulse oximetry. Typically, studies also monitor electrocardiogram (ECG) and bilateral tibialis EMG. Newer equipment provides instantaneous onscreen video monitoring.
    c. Multiple sleep latency testing (MSLT) can be performed the day after polysomnography. Patients wear the sleep stage monitors noted in point b. They are put into bed every 2 hours to see how quickly they fall asleep. Pathologic sleepiness is present if the patient falls asleep in a mean latency of 5 to 6 minutes over the five naps that constitute the test. Narcoleptic patients typically fall into rapid eye movement (REM) sleep in at least two out of five naps, but this is not a specific finding.

11.3 Hypersomnia

1. Insufficient sleep is probably the major cause of daytime sleepiness in all ages starting with adolescence.
    a. Adolescents and young adults are major offenders.
        (1) They need 9 to 10 hours of sleep.
        (2) The lack of sleep affects daytime performance and mood.
        (3) Insufficient sleep has been associated with increased motor vehicle accidents in 16- to 24-year-olds.
    b. After age 25 years, adults need 7.5 to 8 hours of sleep.
    c. It is a myth that the elderly need less sleep.
    d. The association of medical mistakes with lack of sleep among residents has led to new rules restricting the number of hours a resident in training can work.
2. Shift-work sleep disorder.
    a. Worst affected are those working third shift or rotating shifts.

    b. The disorder can manifest as marked difficulty sleeping during the day after getting off of work.

    c. The patient might have significant sleepiness at work or driving home from work in the early morning hours.

3. Obstructive sleep apnea syndrome.

    a. Identification and definition.

        (1) Involves repetitive collapse of the pharynx during sleep resulting in no (apnea) or minimal (hypopnea) airflow despite continued respiratory effort. Events last 10 seconds or longer, resulting in multiple episodes of hypoxemia and multiple brief awakenings (of which patient is not aware). In adults, OSA is defined as more than five apneas and hypopneas per hour of sleep.

        (2) Sleep disruption can also result from being awakened by bed partners or nocturia due to an increase in production of atrial natriuretic factor.

        (3) Patients with sleep apnea rarely present with a chief complaint of insomnia.

        (4) The patient or bed partner might complain of very loud snoring or apneas.

        (5) Symptoms secondary to OSA.

            (a) Excessive daytime sleepiness (associated with motor vehicle accidents).

            (b) Cognitive impairment.

            (c) Depressive symptoms.

            (d) Personality changes.

            (e) Impotence.

        (6) Risk factors include male gender, upper body obesity, upper airway anatomic abnormalities, nasal obstruction, evening alcohol ingestion, hypothyroidism, a family history of OSA, and advancing age. Recent data have demonstrated that OSA is increased in diabetes mellitus.

        (7) Earlier studies have demonstrated that OSA is as common as asthma in middle-aged adults. The incidence will most likely increase as the population becomes heavier.

    b. Consequences of sleep apnea.

        (1) Poor performance at work and at home.

        (2) Injury or death due to falling asleep while driving or at work.

        (3) Nocturnal (as well as daytime) hypertension.

        (4) Increase in myocardial infarction, pulmonary hypertension, cardiac arrhythmias, and death.

    c. Diagnosis is made using all-night polysomnography.

    d. Treatment.

        (1) If apnea only occurs in the supine position, the patient can be conditioned to sleep on a side.

        (2) Weight loss.

        (3) Avoidance of evening alcohol and benzodiazepines because these agents cause pharyngeal muscle relaxation and promote airway collapse during sleep.

    (4) Medications or nasal strips to keep the nose open.

    (5) Positive airway pressure (PAP) is the mainstay of treatment. Compliance has improved with heated in-line humidification and different types of flow-delivery systems.

    (6) Adjustable oral appliances may be useful in patients with mild to moderate cases who do not tolerate PAP.

    (7) Pharyngeal surgery for select patients.

    (8) At present, there are no effective OSA medications, though modafanil might help those with persistent sleepiness despite adequate treatment (see later).

4. Narcolepsy.

  a. Narcolepsy can be a serious, lifelong disabling disorder related to central nervous system hypocretin (orexin) deficiency.

  b. Onset is usually during teens or twenties.

  c. Narcolepsy has a genetic component; chances of disorder in offspring are about 1 in 20.

  d. Prevalence is estimated at 0.02% to 0.1%.

  e. Symptoms (may be widely variable, only 10% have all).

    (1) Excessive daytime sleepiness with irresistible sleep attacks.

    (2) Cataplexy (sudden muscle weakness in response to intense emotional stimulus) is diagnostic.

    (3) Disrupted nighttime sleep with multiple awakenings.

    (4) Sleep paralysis. The patient is aware of an inability to move despite wanting to. This usually occurs on waking up (hypnopompic) or falling asleep (hypnagogic).

    (5) Hypnagogic hallucinations.

    (6) Automatic behavior (doing things with reduced awareness, often resulting in a period of little recollection of activity).

  f. Diagnosis.

    (1) The clear-cut presence of cataplexy.

    (2) Multiple sleep latency test. In narcolepsy, sleep onset is usually in the range of only 5 minutes, and REM sleep can occur in two or more naps. This pattern is nonspecific, and other conditions, such as insufficient sleep, have this pattern

  g. Treatment.

    (1) Global stimulants can help to restore alertness and decrease daytime sleepiness.

      (a) Dextroamphetamine in doses up to 60 to 90 mg/day.

      (b) Methylphenidate in doses up to 60 to 90 mg/day.

      (c) Both these medications are available in short-acting and sustained-release forms.

    (2) Modafanil (Provigil) has an unclear mechanism of action.

      (a) Shown to improve wakefulness in narcolepsy, idiopathic hypersomnia, and OSA patients who remain sleepy despite effective nasal continuous PAP (CPAP). The drug has also been shown to be effective to keep awake persons who work third shift. It has been found useful for treating the fatigue associated with multiple sclerosis.

(b) Usual dose is up to 400 mg in the morning, but it can also be given as 200 mg in the morning and at noon. Typically a third-shift worker takes 200 mg at the beginning of their shift.

(3) Cataplexy, sleep paralysis, and hypnagogic hallucinations may be reduced by medications that suppress REM activity, such as tricyclic antidepressants and selective serotonin reuptake inhibitors (SSRIs).

(4) Sodium oxybate (Xyrem), which is structurally similar to γ-hydroxybutyric acid, has been approved to treat narcolepsy. It is given as a liquid at bedtime and again in the middle of the night. It induces such a deep sleep that it has been shown to decrease daytime sleepiness and cataplexy.

(5) Preventive naps can reduce the total dose of stimulant required.

5. Idiopathic hypersomnia.
   a. Excessive sleepiness, occurring almost daily.
   b. Nighttime sleep is usually normal (8 to 12 hours' duration).
   c. The patient often takes long naps or falls asleep unintentionally during the day.
   d. On MSLT testing the patient may be pathologically sleepy, and there is no REM sleep during the naps. These patients also have none of the other symptoms consistent with narcolepsy.
   e. Treatment is typically the stimulant drugs noted earlier.

11.4 Insomnia

1. Primary insomnia.
   a. It also has been called "psychophysiologic," "learned," "idiopathic," or "conditioned" insomnia.
   b. Criteria include:
      (1) Difficulty initiating or maintaining sleep.
      (2) Resulting daytime fatigue, distress, or impairment in functioning.
   c. It often starts with some increased arousal or anxiety and then becomes conditioned.
   d. It is maintained by bad habits and sleep-incompatible behavior such as worrying before bedtime, working in bed, arguing in bed, exercising too late, or eating too late.
   e. Treatment.
      (1) Approach to improving sleep hygiene (Box 11-2).
      (2) Behavioral approaches using a combination such as sleep restriction, stimulus control, and relaxation may be very effective.

2. Sleep state misperception.
   a. The patient might have a fixed and inaccurate or unrealistic idea of how much sleep is necessary.
   b. Education can help, especially by pointing out that there are minimal effects on daytime behavior. Sleep hygiene interventions can also help.

BOX 11-2   **Improving Sleep Hygiene**

- Go to sleep and get up at the same time every day.
- Discontinue possibly offending drugs.
- Maintain regular mealtimes with a small dinner, and avoid eating after dinner.
- Maintain a predictable evening routine.
- Avoid overstimulation from exercise, disturbing reading, television, arguing with family, or work projects.
- Exercise daily, but not too late at night.
- Avoid daytime naps.
- Learn some relaxation method (see Chapter 10) and practice it near bedtime.
- Create a sleep-promoting environment by cutting down on noise, light, and other disruptive factors.

    c. These patients warrant an all-night sleep study to exclude sleep apnea or periodic limb movements.

3. Circadian rhythm sleep disorders.

    a. These involve misalignment between biologic circadian rhythms and external conditions.

    b. Treatment usually involves some manipulation of cues to regulate sleep timing.

    c. Diagnosis is based primarily on history.

    d. Delayed sleep phase.

      (1) Mismatch of endogenous sleep cycle with external schedule demands.

        (a) "Night owls" who become most alert and awake just at the time they are expected to go to sleep at night. They experience sleep-onset insomnia, have no problems sleeping through the night and have morning hypersomnia if they have to get up too early.

        (b) Very common in adolescents, and this can result in tardiness to school and behavioral problems. It is exacerbated by early school start times.

      (2) Treatment.

        (a) Behavioral therapy involves pushing bedtime later and later until the right times are established.

        (b) Melatonin prior to bedtime.

        (c) Morning bright light therapy.

        (d) All treatments can fail if the adolescent does not maintain a rigid bedtime and wake-up time, even on weekends.

    e. Advanced sleep phase syndrome.

      (1) People (usually older patients) who experience hypersomnolence in early evening and middle of night arousal.

(2) Treatment involves slowly pushing bedtime later to the desired time.
 f. Jet lag resulting from shifts in time zones.
4. Periodic limb movement disorders.
 a. Periodic limb movements during sleep.
  (1) Consists of 1- to 3-second muscle twitches in the legs and feet, which occur every 20 to 40 seconds during sleep (usually in non-REM phase).
  (2) The patient might have a history of kicking off bed covers or disrupting a bed partner's sleep, but leg movements might go unnoticed.
  (3) It can occur in children and has been associated with attention deficit disorder.
  (4) It may be asymptomatic (periodic limb movements without associated arousals should not be treated).
  (5) The patient might present with insomnia or excessive daytime sleepiness.
  (6) Treatment.
   (a) Dopaminergic agents such as pramipexole (Mirapex) or ropinirole (Requip). Doses should be given at bedtime and slowly titrated.
   (b) Opioids such as hydrocodone (Vicodin) only at bedtime.
 b. Restless legs syndrome.
  (1) A sleep-onset disorder.
  (2) Patients shift legs because of feelings of vague discomfort.
  (3) Associated medical conditions include uremia, anemia, pregnancy, and periodic limb movements during sleep.
  (4) Associated medication use includes neuroleptic agents, antidepressants, lithium, diuretics, and narcotics withdrawal.
  (5) Treatment includes the same medications used for periodic limb movements (see earlier).
5. Sleep disorders associated with medical conditions.
 a. The following common disorders are associated with sleep difficulty. The sleep problem usually resolves when the primary medical condition is treated.
  (1) Congestive heart failure.
  (2) Asthma.
  (3) Chronic obstructive pulmonary disease (COPD).
  (4) Incontinence (including diuretic induced).
  (5) GERD.
  (6) Uremia and chronic renal failure.
  (7) Hyperthyroidism.
  (8) Estrogen deficiency.
 b. The following usually need treatment with sedating agents in addition to treatment of the underlying condition because poor sleep exacerbates the underlying condition:
  (1) Fibromyalgia.
  (2) Chronic pain.
  (3) Chronic headaches.

11.5 Sleep Disorders Related to Another Mental Disorder

1. Major depression and dysthymia. Insomnia is a common presentation of affective disorders.
   a. Sleep disturbance is a component of 90% of major depression, with sleep fragmentation and early onset and overall increase in REM sleep.
   b. Patients with depression often present with insomnia, although hypersomnolence occurs in some patients.
2. Schizophrenia (during acute phase).
3. Panic disorder (nighttime panic attacks occur).
4. Generalized anxiety (interferes with sleep onset).
5. Obsessive–compulsive disorder (rumination or nighttime rituals).
6. Posttraumatic stress disorder (repetitive dreams).
7. Delirium (sundowning and sleep–wake dysregulation).
8. Dementia (increased awakenings, daytime napping).
9. Parkinson's disease (sleep disturbance in 75%, with increased awakenings and decreased REM and delta sleep).
10. Kleine–Levin syndrome (a rare form of periodic hypersomnolence) accompanied by hyperphagia, hypersexuality, mood disturbance, and hallucinations. Most often occurs in boys in late adolescence.

11.6 Sleep Disorders Associated with Medications

1. All stimulants including caffeine, theophylline, amphetamines, cocaine, methylphenidate, pseudoephedrine, phenylpropanolamine, nicotine, over-the-counter nasal decongestants and appetite suppressants, and β-adrenergic agonists.
2. Dopamine agonists.
3. All sedatives (because of withdrawal arousal).
   a. Alcohol (when used to initiate sleep, there is often rebound alerting after 4 to 5 hours).
      (1) In moderate doses, alcohol initially shortens sleep latency in the first half of the night, but it causes more frequent arousals, with fragmentation of sleep, later in the night.
      (2) Alcohol also increases the frequency of upper airway obstruction, increasing the potential for sleep apnea.
   b. Barbiturates.
   c. Benzodiazepines.
4. Other drugs.
   a. Steroids.
   b. α-Methyldopa.
   c. Propranolol.
   d. Oral contraceptives.
   e. Thyroid hormone.

   f. Neuroleptic agents (produce akathisia).
   g. Metoclopramide (akathisia).
   h. Reserpine.
   i. Tricyclic antidepressants (during withdrawal because of REM rebound).
   j. Antidepressants (bupropion, SSRIs, desipramine, monoamine oxidase inhibitors [MAOIs], protriptyline).

11.7 Parasomnias

The parasomnias are abnormal behavior or physiologic events that occur during sleep.

1. Sleepwalking.
   a. Between 10% and 30% of children have sleepwalking episodes, which are considered pathologic only if they persist into adulthood.
   b. Sleepwalking begins during slow-wave sleep (non-REM, stage 3 or 4); therefore it most often occurs during the first third of the night.
   c. The sleepwalker:
      (1) Has a blank, staring face.
      (2) Is unresponsive to communication (some limited speech and responses are possible).
      (3) Is awakened only with great difficulty.
      (4) Has amnesia on awakening.
      (5) Has no impairment within a few minutes of awakening.
   d. The episode may be as brief as simply sitting up in bed or prolonged enough to go to another building.
   e. Sleepwalking can involve specific behavior such as sleep eating or sleep sex.
   f. It usually occurs in adults who sleepwalked as children or have a strong family history of sleepwalking. It can be triggered by stress, sleep deprivation, or sleep fragmentation from disorders such as sleep apnea.
   g. Intervention involves insuring safety, avoidance of alcohol or drug use, and potential stress management. Patients who are potentially going to injure themselves or others might need clonazepam.
2. Night terrors.
   a. Abrupt awakening (with a panicky scream) that occurs during the first third of the night during stage 3 to 4 non-REM sleep.
   b. Intense fear and autonomic arousal lasting 1 to 10 minutes.
   c. Unresponsive to being comforted during the episode.
   d. Unlike nightmares, the patient does not recall any dream content, although fragmentary images may be reported.
   e. Amnesia for the episode.
      (1) Episodes may be worsened by alcohol, substances, fatigue, stress, anxiety, and sleep deprivation.
      (2) Usually occurs in childhood and resolves spontaneously by adolescence, but can begin during adulthood and become chronic.

3. Nightmares.
   a. Occur in about 10% to 50% of children and 5% to 10% of adults during REM sleep.
   b. Patient wakes and is frightened with recall of the threatening nightmare.
   c. Patient becomes alert and oriented on awakening (unlike the confusion associated with waking from night terror).
   d. Nightmares may be precipitated by withdrawal from drugs that suppress REM activity (e.g., tricyclic antidepressants and SSRIs).
   e. Associated with certain drugs (propranolol, reserpine, thioridazine).
   f. Most common in personality disorders or during stressful periods. Can accompany severe premenstrual syndrome and posttraumatic stress disorder.
   g. Treatment involves psychotherapy and potentially REM reduction with low-dose amitriptyline (50 to 75 mg hs).
4. REM sleep behavior disorder.
   a. Unlike the typical hypotonia seen in REM sleep, in patients with this disorder, REM sleep motor paralysis is absent.
   b. Patients might act out their dreams, occasionally causing injury.
   c. It is usually associated with vivid violent dream recall.
   d. It usually responds to clonazepam 1 to 2 mg qhs.

11.8 Hypnotic Drugs

1. Sedative–hypnotics.
   a. These drugs are generally underused. They should be used aggressively along with sleep hygiene in acute insomnia to prevent the progression to chronic insomnia. Chronic insomnia can develop in some patients in 3 to 4 weeks.
   b. Sedative–hypnotics may be used intermittently in chronic primary insomnia.
   c. They may be used chronically when a comorbid condition worsens sleep and when the insomnia exacerbates the chronic condition (e.g., in those with underlying psychiatric disorders, chronic pain, headaches, or fibromyalgia).
   d. Some patients on PAP therapy for OSA need nightly sedation to tolerate the device.
   e. Shift workers can benefit from a hypnotic in the morning after getting off of a night shift.
2. Over-the-counter medications.
   a. Melatonin.
      (1) Not effective for insomnia.
      (2) Best used for circadian rhythm disorders.
      (3) Therapeutic dose is unknown, but synthetic is preferred for safety concerns.
   b. Diphenhydramine and hydroxyzine.
      (1) Very long acting; can cause residual daytime sedation.
      (2) Can be excitatory in some patients.
      (3) Prominent anticholinergic side effects.

       (4) Contraindicated in nursing home patients due to well-described cognitive dysfunction and an increased incidence of falls. Use with caution in healthy elderly.

3. Sedating antidepressants. A recent National Institutes of Health Conference did not recommend these agents as treatment for insomnia.

  a. Amitriptyline (Elavil) and other tricyclics are sometimes used as hypnotics.

     (1) For patients with chronic pain and headaches.

     (2) Start at a low dose, such as amitriptyline 10 to 25 mg, and slowly titrate. Best given 1 to 1.5 hours before bedtime.

     (3) Significant side effects including anticholinergic activity, orthostasis, and cardiac conduction delays.

  b. Trazodone.

     (1) Long-acting sedating agent.

     (2) In doses of 50 to 100 mg, trazodone may be an effective hypnotic. It appears to increase stages 3 and 4 sleep (restorative sleep) and does not interfere with REM sleep.

     (3) Can induce orthostasis.

     (4) Should be given 1 to 1.5 hours before bedtime to reduce daytime sedation.

  c. Mirtazapine (Remeron).

     (1) Sedating agent at doses of 7.5 to 30 mg (more sedating at lower doses).

     (2) Minimal anticholinergic and serotoninergic side effects.

     (3) Major problems are increased appetite and weight gain.

  d. Antipsychotics alone (with no other indication) are generally not appropriate hypnotic agents.

4. Benzodiazepines.

  a. Bind to γ-aminobutyric acid (GABA)-A receptors, facilitating the action of GABA. All benzodiazepines cause muscle relaxation and decrease anxiety before sedation occurs.

  b. Even though some benzodiazepines have been classified as anxiolytics and some as hypnotics, all are potentially sedating.

  c. Benzodiazepines are indicated only for short-term use because of the high chance of tolerance.

  d. Benzodiazepines prolong the first two stages of sleep and shorten stages 3 and 4 and REM sleep.

  e. Diazepam (Valium), flurazepam (Dalmane), and chlordiazepoxide (Librium) have extremely long half-lives and have been associated with increased falls and subsequent fractures in the elderly.

  f. Temazepam (Restoril) and lorazepam (Ativan) are intermediate-acting agents, but they might still have some residual effects on cognition the next morning.

  g. Triazolam (Halcion) has a rapid elimination that can provoke a middle of the night rebound wakefulness. It has also been reported to cause agitation, antegrade amnesia, and paranoia.

5. Newer drugs modulating GABA-A receptor activity selectively induce a normal sleep pattern with no effect on stages 3 or 4 sleep or REM

sleep. These agents induce sedation before triggering muscle relaxation and anxiolytic effects. With any of these agents, the medications should be taken and the patient should immediately try to go to sleep to avoid a "drunk" state.

a. Zaleplon (Sonata) is chemically unrelated to the benzodiazepines as well as the other drugs in this class.
   (1) Rapid onset.
   (2) Short duration of action.
   (3) Dose is 10 mg, and it does not have to be reduced in the elderly. Dose should be cut in half in the presence of liver disease.
   (4) Indicated for patients with purely initiation insomnia with no problems staying asleep.
   (5) Zaleplon is the only medication available for patients who intermittently wake up in the middle of the night and cannot fall back to sleep. As long as the patient is going to be in bed for an additional 3 hours, this medication may be taken in the middle of the night and it will cause no daytime dysfunction.
b. Zolpidem (Ambien and Ambien CR) is also chemically unrelated to the benzodiazepines.
   (1) Rapid onset.
   (2) Longer half-life than zaleplon. Normal half-life is about 2.5 hours for the immediate-acting agent (Ambien) and 2.8 hours for the mixture of immediate and slow release preparation (Ambien CR) (longer in elderly and patients with liver disease). These drugs may be used for patients with initiation and maintenance insomnia or for patients who fall asleep without difficulty but have frequent awakenings in the middle of the night.
   (3) Side effects are dose related. If the dose is pushed up to 20 mg or higher for the immediate-release preparation, it becomes more like a benzodiazepine.
      (a) Sensory distortion experiences have been rarely reported.
      (b) In usual hypnotic doses (10 mg), zolpidem does not appear to cause any respiratory depression in patients with advanced COPD.
      (c) Does not show muscle relaxant or anticonvulsant activity at usual dose levels.
      (d) Sleepwalking and sleep eating have been described with the immediate-acting preparation, and this is an indication to stop the medication.
   (4) Usual dose is 10 mg (5 mg for elderly or debilitated patients or patients with hepatic disease) for Ambien and 12.5 mg (6.25 mg for at-risk patients) for Ambien CR.
   (5) Clinical trials did not show evidence of withdrawal syndrome or rebound insomnia on discontinuation of this agent or zaleplon.
   (6) Studies showed no indication of the development of tolerance over 12 weeks (one study showed no development of tolerance up to 1 year). Ambien CR does not have any restrictions for duration of use as do the earlier agents, Ambien and Sonata.

c. Eszoplicone (Lunesta).
   (1) Brand new agent also binding at the GABA receptor, which is different structurally from the benzodiazepines and the other agents in this class. It is the S isomer of a much longer acting drug zoplicone, which is used in Europe.
   (2) Has longer half-life of 6 hours to prevent early morning awakenings, so patients should allow 8 hours in bed.
   (3) Potential concern is early morning sleepiness in patients who are not getting sufficient sleep.
   (4) Manufacturer obtained an indication for long-term use.
   (5) Doses are 1 mg, 2 mg, and 3 mg. As with the other agents, the lowest dose is recommended in the elderly and in patients with liver disease. A dose of 2 mg may be used in patients with purely initiation problems, but 3 mg is the standard dose for patients with difficulty maintaining sleep.
   (6) Ramalteon (Rozerem) is a new agent with high affinity for melatonin MT_1 and MT_2 receptors. A dose of 8 mg can be used in patients with sleep-onset problems. It probably will not work in patients who have been on stronger sedative–hypnotics.

SUGGESTED READINGS

Agostini JV, Leo-Summers LS, Inouye SK: Cognitive and other adverse effects of diphenhydramine use in hospitalized older patients. Arch Intern Med 161:2091-2097, 2001.

Aslan S, Isik E, Cosar B: The effects of mirtazapine on sleep: A placebo controlled, double-blind study in young healthy volunteers. Sleep 25:677-679, 2002.

Chesson AL, Anderson WM, Littner M, et al: Practice parameters for the nonpharmacologic treatment of chronic insomnia. An American Academy of Sleep Medicine report. Standards of Practice Committee of the American Academy of Sleep Medicine. Sleep 22:1128-1156, 1999.

Cote KA, Moldofsky H: Sleep, daytime symptoms, and cognitive performance in patients with fibromyalgia. J Rheumatol 27:2014-2023, 1997.

Dinges DF, Weaver TE: Effects of modafinil on sustained attention performance and quality of life in OSA patients with residual sleepiness while being treated with nCPAP. Sleep Med 4:393-402, 2003.

Edinger JD, Wohlgemuth WK, Radtke RA, et al: Cognitive behavior therapy for treatment of chronic primary insomnia. JAMA 285:1856-1864, 2001.

Hening W, Allen R, Earley C, et al: The treatment of restless legs syndrome and periodic limb movement disorder. An American Academy of Sleep Medicine review. Sleep 22:970-999, 1999.

James SP, Mendelson WB: The use of trazodone as a hypnotic: A critical review. J Clin Psychiatry 65:752-755, 2004.

Jamieson AO, Zammit GK, Rosenberg RS, et al: Zolpidem reduces the sleep disturbance of jet lag. Sleep Med 2:423-430, 2001.

Kingshott RN, Vennelle M, Coleman EL, et al: Randomized, double-blind, placebo-controlled crossover trial of modafinil in the treatment of residual excessive daytime sleepiness in the sleep apnea/hypopnea syndrome. Am J Respir Crit Care Med 163:918-923, 2001.

Krystal AD, Walsh JK, Laska E, et al: Sustained efficacy of eszoplicone over 6 months of nightly treatment: Results of a randomized, double-blind, placebo-controlled study in adults with chronic insomnia. Sleep 26:793-799, 2003.

Littner M, Johnson SF, McCall WV, et al: Practice parameters for the treatment of narcolepsy: An update for 2000. *Sleep* 24:451-466, 2001.

Littner MR, Kushida C, Anderson WM, et al: Practice parameters for the dopaminergic treatment of restless legs syndrome and periodic limb movement disorders. *Sleep* 27:557-583, 2004.

Millman RP, Rosenberg CL, Kramer NR: Oral appliances in the treatment of snoring and sleep apnea. *Clin Chest Med* 19:69-75, 1998.

Modofsky H, Broughton RJ, Hill JD: A randomized trial of the long-term, continued efficacy and safety of modafinil in narcolepsy. *Sleep Med* 1:109-116, 2000.

Morin C: Cognitive-behavioral approaches to the treatment of insomnia. *J Clin Psychiatry* 65(Suppl 16):33-40, 2004.

Patel SR, White DP, Malhotra A, et al: Continuous positive airway pressure therapy for treating sleepiness in a diverse population with obstructive sleep apnea. *Arch Intern Med* 163:565-571, 2003.

Roth T, Stubbs C, Walsh JK: Ramelteon (TAK-375), a selective MT_1/MT_2-receptor agonist, reduces latency to persistent sleep in a model of transient insomnia related to a novel sleep environment. *Sleep* 28:303-307, 2005.

Sateia MJ, Doghramji K, Hauri PJ, Morin CM: Evaluation of chronic insomnia. *Sleep* 23:243-308, 2000.

Thorpy M: Current concepts in the etiology, diagnosis and treatment of narcolepsy. *Sleep Med* 2:5-17, 2001.

Vermeeren A, Danjou PE, O'Hanlon JF: Residual effects of evening and middle-of-the-night administration of zaleplon 10 and 20 mg on memory and actual driving performance. *Hum Psychopharmacol Clin Exp* 13:S98-S107, 1998.

Walsh JK, Randazzo AC, Stone KL, Schweitzer PK: Modafinil improves alertness, vigilance, and executive function during simulated night shifts. *Sleep* 27:434-439, 2004.

Young T: Epidemiology of daytime sleepiness: Definitions, symptomatology, and prevalence. *J Clin Psychiatry* 65(Suppl 16):12-16, 2004.

Psychotic Symptoms, Schizophrenia, and Antipsychotic Agents

12

Moataz M. Ragheb

12.1 Identification of Psychotic Symptoms

1. Psychosis is a general disturbance of thinking with inability to distinguish reality from fantasy and impaired reality testing, with the creation of a new reality.
2. Every mental status examination must include questions about psychotic symptoms.
3. Patients might not reveal psychotic symptoms without specific questioning.
4. Mental status examination for psychotic symptoms (Box 12-1).

DELUSIONS

Delusions are false, unshakable ideas or beliefs that are out of keeping with the patient's educational, cultural, and social background. They are held with extraordinary conviction and subjective certainty despite refuting evidence. Typical delusions include:

1. Somatic delusions are common in major depression in the elderly. Screening questions include:
   a. "Do you believe something is wrong with your body?"
   b. If the patient complains of a somatic symptom, "What do you think may be causing that problem?"
2. Paranoid (persecutory and reference) delusions. Beliefs of being followed, persecuted, poisoned, or in some way singled out as special.
   a. Typical of many schizophrenics.
   b. Common secondary to stimulant (e.g., amphetamine, cocaine) abuse.
   c. Common in Alzheimer's disease.
   d. Screening questions may include the following:
      (1) "Do you feel uncomfortable around people? Why is that?"
      (2) "Do you feel that people are out to get you or might have something to do with your problems?"
   e. Denial of paranoid delusions does not mean they are absent. It may be important to record that the patient seems guarded and appears paranoid.
   f. Other common delusions include:
      (1) Grandiosity.
      (2) Someone is stealing from patient.
      (3) A dead person is present.
      (4) Family members replaced by impostors (Capgras' syndrome).

BOX 12-1   Psychosis Symptoms for Mental Status Examination

Disorganization

Motor behavior
Speech (verbal behavior)

Perception

Auditory hallucinations: command, commenting
Visual hallucinations
Other

Thought Content

Delusions: somatic, paranoid, other
Thought insertion, withdrawal, broadcasting

Thought Process (Formal Thought Disorder)

Illogical reasoning
Impaired abstraction
Incoherence
Loose association
Neologism
Thought blocking

---

  (5) Spouse infidelity.
  (6) Abandonment.
  (7) Guilt and worthlessness (in depression).
 g. Before deciding that someone is delusional, consider whether the alleged issues are actually true or are culturally acceptable. This is especially important in nonbizarre delusions.

HALLUCINATIONS

Hallucinations are false sensory perceptions not associated with real external stimuli.

1. Auditory hallucinations.
 a. Often present in schizophrenics, especially commenting on the patient's behavior.
 b. Also common in major depression (see Chapter 6).
 c. Screening questions.
  (1) "Are you hearing voices?" (may be too abrupt for patients to reveal their symptoms).
  (2) An alternative question is, "It is not unusual for someone who is very depressed or distressed to hear voices saying disturbing things, such as, 'You are a bad person or a person who does not deserve to live.' Are you experiencing anything like that?"
 d. Command hallucinations, telling patients to hurt themselves or others, are very dangerous.
 e. As psychotic patients improve, "voices" may become less bothersome and then become less distinct before disappearing.

2. Visual hallucinations.
   a. A hallmark of delirium, most common secondary to a medical disorder.
   b. Screening questions.
      (1) "Are you sometimes having difficulty telling whether you are awake or dreaming?"
      (2) "It is not unusual for someone withdrawing from medication to have strange visions of things not really there. Are you having any symptoms like that?"
   c. It may be necessary to infer the presence of visual hallucinations from behavior (e.g., looking over shoulder, use of ear plugs, picking invisible objects).
   d. In the elderly and others with visual disorders (e.g., macular degeneration or cataracts), visual misinterpretations may be mistaken for hallucinations.
   e. In those with language problems or limited intelligence, some statements may be misinterpreted as describing a hallucination.
3. Olfactory hallucinations.
   a. Warrant consideration of a temporal lobe abnormality.
   b. Olfactory hallucinations of depressed or schizophrenic patients are generally bizarre.
4. Tactile hallucinations are sensations of something crawling on the skin.
   a. Most commonly seen during drug withdrawal (cocaine bugs) or as a symptom of complex partial seizures.
   b. Rare in other primary psychiatric diagnoses.
   c. Grossly disorganized behavior, thinking, or speech.

12.2 Differential Diagnosis of Psychotic Symptoms

1. Underlying medical conditions can create psychotic symptoms (see Boxes 3-1 and 3-2). This category should always be the first consideration. Chapter 14 reviews the history and physical examination relevant to identifying these underlying medical problems.
2. Psychotic depression is sometimes misdiagnosed as schizophrenia, but it has different treatment and prognosis. Depressed mood may be noted in schizophrenics (or schizoaffective patients), but in affective disorder, the psychotic symptoms occur only in the context of the severe depression.
3. Schizoaffective disorder manifests with symptoms that meet criteria for major depression and schizophrenia. When in doubt, the patient should be treated for both the mood and schizophrenic disorder to avoid neglecting one treatable component (Box 12-2).
4. Mania as part of bipolar disorder (see Chapter 8) or secondary to some medical problem can be difficult to distinguish from schizophrenia, especially during an acute presentation. When in doubt, err on the side of mania, because it is more treatable.
5. Patients with brief psychotic disorder can look like schizophrenics, except that brief psychotic disorder usually occurs in relation to some traumatic event and its duration is between 1 day and 1 month.

BOX 12-2   Diagnosis of Schizoaffective Disorder: Basic Elements

An uninterrupted period with either a major depressive, manic, or mixed episode concurrent with symptoms meeting criteria for schizophrenia

Delusions or hallucinations for at least 2 weeks during this period in the absence of prominent mood symptoms

Symptoms are not due to a substance or a general medical condition

For complete diagnostic criteria, please refer to *Diagnostic and Statistical Manual of Mental Disorders*, 4th ed, text revision. Washington, DC, American Psychiatric Association, 2000.

BOX 12-3   Diagnosis of Delusional Disorder: Basic Elements

Nonbizarre delusions of at least 1 month's duration.

Symptoms do not meet criteria for schizophrenia.

Apart from the delusion(s), functioning is not significantly impaired and behavior is not obviously bizarre.

Symptoms are not due to a substance or general medical condition.

Types include erotomanic, grandiose, jealous, persecutory, somatic, mixed, and unspecified.

For complete diagnostic criteria, please refer to *Diagnostic and Statistical Manual of Mental Disorders*, 4th ed, text revision. Washington, DC, American Psychiatric Association, 2000.

6. Schizophreniform disorder consists of psychotic symptoms lasting longer than 1 month but less than 6 months. This diagnosis is usually made when schizophrenia is the suspected diagnosis but the duration has been less than 6 months.

7. Delusional disorder consists of an isolated delusional belief. This disorder usually emerges in middle or late life and is usually not responsive to neuroleptic agents (or other treatments). More treatable disorders that appear as delusions include body dysmorphic disorder or obsessive–compulsive disorder (OCD) (Box 12-3).

8. Personality disorder (schizotypal) is characterized by odd beliefs (including ideas of reference, suspiciousness, or peculiar behavior) and interpersonal difficulties, without psychotic (persistent delusions or hallucinations) or disorganized behavioral criteria for schizophrenia.

9. OCD can manifest as bizarre behavior, obsessions, or both, leading to misdiagnosis and treatment with antipsychotics instead of anti-OCD drugs (see Chapter 9).

10. Autism consists of onset of disturbances in social interaction, social communication, or imaginative play before age 3. Most of these

---

BOX 12-4   Diagnosis of Schizophrenia: Basic Elements

Characteristic symptoms include at least two of the following during a 1-month period (less if successfully treated):
- Delusions
- Hallucinations
- Disorganized speech (e.g., frequent derailment or incoherence)
- Grossly disorganized or catatonic behavior
- Negative symptoms, i.e., flat affect, limited speech or motivation

Social or occupational dysfunction

Continuous signs for at least 6 months, including at least 1 month of symptoms along with prodromal or residual symptoms

Schizoaffective and mood disorder are ruled out

The disturbance is not due to a substance or general medical condition

---

For complete diagnostic criteria, please refer to *Diagnostic and Statistical Manual of Mental Disorders*, 4th ed, text revision. Washington, DC, American Psychiatric Association, 2000.

patients show further behavioral deterioration during adolescence involving multiple psychological functions. Autism is not characterized by delusions or hallucinations.
11. Mentally retarded patients might behave strangely and talk in ways that seem psychotic.
12. Malingering with psychotic symptoms usually involves patients with personality disorders seeking some secondary gain (see Chapter 13).
13. Schizophrenia. After other possibilities listed above are considered, psychotic symptoms may be attributable to schizophrenia (Box 12-4).

12.3 Schizophrenia

Schizophrenia is the most costly mental illness in the United States, accounting for 2.5% of annual health care expenditures.

DEFINITION AND IDENTIFICATION

Accurate diagnosis has enormous implications for short- and long-term treatment planning. Diagnosis is a process, not a one-time event.

1. Three criteria must be met (beyond the exclusion of other disorders).
   a. Characteristic symptoms. Two or more of the following must be present for a significant portion of time during a 1-month period (this 1-month period may be less if symptoms were successfully treated).
      (1) Delusions.
      (2) Hallucinations.
      (3) Disorganized speech (e.g., incoherence).
      (4) Grossly disorganized or catatonic behavior.
      (5) Negative symptoms (e.g., flattened affect, lack of motivation).

b. Social or occupational dysfunction. There should be notable problems with work, school, interpersonal relations, or self-care (below the patient's baseline level of function).

c. Duration. Continuous signs of the disturbance persist for at least 6 months (including at least 1 month of characteristic symptoms). This 6-month period can include prodromal or residual symptoms such as social withdrawal or odd beliefs short of being fully delusional.

EPIDEMIOLOGY AND RISK FACTORS

1. Peak incidence of onset is between the late teens and mid-30s. However, onset can occur in succeeding decades, including into the 70s (but less than 1% of all schizophrenia begins after age 65).

2. Lifetime prevalence is approximately 1% and appears to be the same for men and women, but it increases about tenfold if a parent, sibling, or child is affected.

3. Annual incidence rate is estimated to be approximately 1 per 10,000 population per year.

4. Risk factors:
   a. Winter birth.
   b. Obstetric complications.
   c. Advanced paternal age.
   d. Lower socioeconomic status.
   e. Environmental stress.
   f. Single marital status.
   g. Premorbid schizoid, paranoid, or eccentric personality.
   h. A family setting characterized by high emotional expression in the form of criticism, hostility, and emotional overinvolvement *does not* increase the risk of developing schizophrenia. It increases risk of relapse in schizophrenic patients.

CLINICAL FEATURES

Schizophrenia has been traditionally described as a primary disorder of thinking, although emotional and cognitive disturbances are often present.

1. Abnormalities of thinking.
   a. Abnormalities of thought content.
      (1) Being controlled by outside forces.
      (2) Thoughts can be overheard.
      (3) Thoughts are being inserted.
   b. Abnormalities of thought process (formal thought disorder).
      (1) Loose association.
      (2) Incoherence.
      (3) Neologisms (made-up words).
      (4) Thought blocking.
      (5) Impaired abstraction ability (concrete thinking).
      (6) Illogical reasoning.
2. Abnormalities of verbal behavior (speech).
   a. Perseveration.
   b. Echolalia (repeating heard words).

    c. Poverty of speech.

    d. Mutism.

3. Abnormalities of motor behavior.

    a. Repetitive behavior (stereotypy).

    b. Echopraxia (imitating movements).

    c. Mannerisms and grimacing.

    d. Negativism.

    e. Prolonged motor hyperactivity.

    f. Catatonia (posturing, rigidity, stupor, excitement).

4. Abnormalities of perception.

    a. Hallucinations (usually auditory).

    b. Illusions (distorted perceptions).

5. Abnormalities of affect.

    a. Flat or blunt affect (indifference).

    b. Inappropriate affect.

    c. Anhedonia.

    d. Unusual fears.

6. Abnormalities of ego functions.

    a. Lack of reality testing.

    b. Lack of behavioral self-control.

    c. Distorted interpersonal behavior.

    d. Impaired sense of self (identity, individuality, boundaries).

7. Volitional symptoms (loss of interest, initiative, drive, and ambition).

8. Other symptoms.

    a. Deterioration of grooming and self-hygiene.

    b. Lack of insight.

    c. Impaired judgment.

9. Intelligence and basic cognitive functions, such as memory, orientation, and attention, are usually intact, except in the active psychotic, disorganized phase.

10. Positive and negative symptoms.

    a. Positive symptoms include delusions, hallucinations, disorganized thinking and behavior.

    b. Negative symptoms include poverty of speech, affective blunting, anhedonia, apathy, and avolition.

      (1) *Secondary* negative symptoms are those that occur due to positive symptoms, adverse effects of antipsychotics such as extrapyramidal symptoms (EPS), comorbid depression or anxiety, demoralization, or environmental deprivation. Treatment of the causes should improve secondary negative symptoms.

      (2) *Primary* negative (deficit state) symptoms represent a core feature of the illness. They persist after treatment of positive symptoms, depression, and EPS. There are no treatments with proven efficacy for primary negative symptoms.

NATURAL HISTORY AND COURSE

1. Schizophrenia can be viewed as a disorder that develops in three phases.

    a. The *premorbid phase* encompasses a period of normative function.

    b. During the *prodromal phase* the person experiences substantial functional impairment and nonspecific symptoms such as sleep

disturbance, anxiety, irritability, depressed mood, poor concentration, fatigue, and social withdrawal.
   c. The *psychotic phase* typically begins during adolescence or early adulthood. The onset may be abrupt but is usually insidious.
2. The most common course involves acute exacerbations of psychosis, with increasing residual dysfunction between episodes. About 10% to 15% experience one episode only and another 10% to 15% remain chronically severely psychotic. The psychotic phase of the illness progresses through three phases.
   a. The *acute phase* is a period of florid psychotic symptoms, often with more severe negative symptoms as well.
   b. The *stabilization phase* is the period when acute symptoms decrease in severity, often lasting for 6 or more months after the acute phase.
   c. The *stable phase* is the period when symptoms are less severe or in remission.
3. Good outcome is associated with the following (poor outcome with the opposite occurrence):
   a. Female, married.
   b. Family history of affective disorders.
   c. No family history of schizophrenia.
   d. Good premorbid social and academic functioning.
   e. High IQ.
   f. Acute onset, with precipitating stress in midlife.
   g. Presence of affective component.
   h. Minimal comorbidity.
   i. Paranoid subtype with predominantly positive symptoms and less disorganization.
   j. Supportive extended family and social network.
4. Although a return to full premorbid functioning is possible, residual impairment often increases with repeated acute episodes. Residual symptoms can become attenuated late in the course of the disease ("burnout").
5. The "conventional" or typical antipsychotic medications (with the possible exception of thioridazine hydrochloride [Mellaril]) reduce the positive symptoms more than the negative symptoms.
6. Atypical antipsychotic agents, such as clozapine, risperidone, olanzapine, ziprasidone, and aripiprazole, generally treat both positive and *secondary* negative symptoms. Clozapine (and some of the other atypicals) may be effective in 30% to 60% of cases refractory to conventional antipsychotics.

COMORBIDITY AND MORTALITY

1. Psychiatric and substance abuse comorbidity.
   a. Substance use disorders.
      (1) Excluding nicotine, nearly 50% of patients with schizophrenia have comorbid substance abuse or dependence. Most commonly used are alcohol, cannabis, and cocaine.
      (2) Smoking has been estimated to have 50% to 75% prevalence in schizophrenia. Nicotine increases the metabolism of antipsychotics, and patients may be using it to decrease EPS.

Some studies have suggested it decreases positive symptoms as well.

(3) A comprehensive integrated treatment model is used to address schizophrenia and substance abuse.

b. Depression.

(1) Depressive symptoms are common during all phases of schizophrenia.

(2) Atypical antipsychotics are more effective for depression than typical antipsychotics.

(3) Antidepressants may be needed as an adjunct in severe cases of depression.

c. Other psychiatric disorders such as OCD, posttraumatic stress disorder (PTSD), and social phobia are more common in schizophrenia than in the general population.

2. General medical comorbidity.

a. Schizophrenic patients have higher incidence of medical comorbidities than the general population.

(1) Excluding suicide, age-adjusted mortality rate is twice as high in schizophrenia.

(2) Respiratory, cardiovascular, and infectious diseases, as well as diabetes, are especially prevalent.

(3) Possible contributing factors include diabetes, smoking, substance abuse, obesity, lack of exercise, institutionalization, effects of medications (EPS, tardive dyskinesia [TD], hyperprolactinemia, weight gain, hyperglycemia, hyperlipidemia, and cardiac arrhythmias), and limited access to primary care.

(4) For unclear reasons, rheumatoid arthritis rarely occurs in schizophrenic patients.

b. Careful attention to these comorbidities is essential during initial assessment and at appropriate intervals thereafter.

3. Suicide.

a. Suicide is the leading cause of premature death among patients with schizophrenia; 30% attempt it, and 4% to 10% die by suicide.

b. General risk factors include male sex, white race, single marital status, social isolation, unemployment, a family history of suicide, previous suicide attempts, substance use disorders, depression or hopelessness, and a significant recent adverse life event.

c. Specific risk factors for suicide in schizophrenia are young age, high socioeconomic status background, high IQ with a high level of premorbid scholastic achievement, high aspirations and expectations, early age at onset or first hospitalization, a chronic and deteriorating course with many relapses, greater insight into the illness, severe depression, and increased paranoid behavior.

d. Suicide should be considered and screened for at all stages of the illness. Patient and family members should be advised to look for warning signs.

e. Clozapine has the greatest therapeutic effect on suicidal behavior in schizophrenia, reducing the rate by 75% to 85%.

12.4 Antipsychotic Agents Used to Treat Schizophrenia and Other Psychotic Disorders

OVERVIEW

1. Table 12-1 provides a summary of the antipsychotic agents in general use.
2. Antipsychotic agents can be identified as being either first generation (FGA; typical or conventional) or second generation (SGA; atypical).
   a. The typical agents include those introduced before clozapine in the early 1990s. Typical antipsychotics are characterized by a relatively high tendency to produce EPS and a relatively poor effect on negative symptoms.
   b. Atypical agents have different neuroreceptor profiles with different affinities for dopamine receptors and different effects on serotonin receptors (Table 12-2). They have lower rates of EPS, significantly reduced risk of TD, and potential efficacy for both positive and negative symptoms (Table 12-3).

Intramuscular Antipsychotics

Haloperidol, ziprasidone, and olanzapine are available in intramuscular (IM) formulation (Table 12-4). Although they are often used in other conditions, only acute schizophrenia and bipolar mania have Food and Drug Administration (FDA) indication. Intravenous (IV) haloperidol has been used in treating delirium, but it does not have FDA approval.

Depot Antipsychotics

Depot preparations are available for treating chronic schizophrenia and other psychotic conditions where compliance is a problem.

1. Before starting a depot preparation, the patient should be stabilized on the lowest effective dose of the oral preparation.
2. Usual dose conversion:
   a. 10 mg/day oral fluphenazine = 12.5 to 25 mg (0.5 mL to 1 mL) of depot fluphenazine decanoate every 2 to 3 weeks. Oral supplementation is needed for several weeks.
   b. A loading-dose strategy for depot haloperidol (Haldol decanoate) has been suggested:
      (1) An initial loading dose that is 20 times the oral maintenance dose is given.
      (2) If this dose is more than 100 mg, it should be given in divided injection 3 to 7 days apart.
      (3) Subsequent doses are decreased monthly to about 10 times the oral. Usual maintenance dose is 50 to 100 mg every 2 to 4 weeks.
      (4) In this method, oral supplementation may be discontinued 2 weeks after the second injection dose.
   c. Long-acting risperidone (Risperdal Consta)
      (1) Dose 25 to 50 mg IM every 2 weeks.
      (2) If the patient is already taking oral risperidone, continue a supplemental oral dose for 3 weeks.

Table 12-1 **Commonly Used Antipsychotic Medications**

Antipsychotic Medication	Recommended Dose Range (mg/day)*	Chlorpromazine Equivalents (mg/day)†
First-Generation (Typical) Agents		
Phenothiazines		
Chlorpromazine (Thorazine)	300-1000	100
Fluphenazine (Prolixin)	5-20	2
Mesoridazine (Serentil)	150-400	50
Perphenazine (Trilafon)	16-64	10
Thioridazine (Mellaril)	300-800	100
Trifluoperazine (Stelazine)	15-50	5
Butyrophenone		
Haloperidol (Haldol)	5-20	2
Others		
Loxapine (Loxitane)	30-100	10
Molindone (Moban)	30-100	10
Thiothixene (Navane)	15-50	5
Second-Generation (Atypical) Agents		
Aripiprazole (Abilify)	10-30	
Clozapine (Clozaril)	150-600	
Olanzapine (Zyprexa)	10-30	
Quetiapine (Seroquel)	300-800	
Risperidone (Risperdal)	2-8	
Ziprasidone (Geodon)	120-200	

*Dose range recommendations are adapted from Lehman AF, Kreyenbuhl J, Buchanan RW, et al. *Schizophr Bull* 30(2):193-217, 2004.
†Chlorpromazine equivalents represent the approximate dose equivalent to 100 mg of chlorpromazine (relative potency). Chlorpromazine equivalents are not relevant to the second-generation antipsychotics; therefore, no chlorpromazine equivalents are indicated for these agents.

    (3) If patient is taking another oral antipsychotic, test for hypersensitivity before giving the injection. Then supplement with the oral antipsychotic for 3 weeks.
  d. Typical doses are lower for elderly or debilitated patients.

Pharmacokinetics of Antipsychotics

In general, there is a large variability in pharmacokinetic parameters, with up to a 30-fold or greater difference in blood levels resulting from similar oral doses.

1. Absorption. Oral absorption is somewhat variable (30 to 60 minutes) and may be impaired by antacids, calcium-rich food, caffeine, and nicotine.
  a. Oral elixirs are better absorbed than capsules or tablets and offer a good alternative to IM injections, with comparable onset of action (15 to 30 minutes).

Table 12-2 Receptor Affinities of the Atypical Antipsychotics

Drugs	Dopamine Receptors				Serotonin Receptors				Other Receptors				
	D_1	D_2	D_3	D_4	5-HT_{1a}	5-HT_{2a}	5-HT_3	Muscarinic-1	α_1	α_2	H_1	NE
Aripiprazole	+	PA	0	++	PA	+	?	0	+	0	+	?
Clozapine	++	0	?	+	++	+++	++	+++	++	++	+++	?
Haloperidol	++	+++	+++	+++	0	+++	0	0	+	+	0	0
Olanzapine	++	+	+	?	0	++	++	++	+	+	+++	+
Quetiapine	+	0	+	+	0	+	+	0	+++	++	++	?
Risperidone	++	+++	?	+	+	++	0	0	+++	+++	+	0
Ziprasidone	+	0	+	?	+++	++++	?	0	+++	0	+	+++

H_1, histamine-1 receptor; 5-HT, serotonin; NE, norepinephrine; PA, partial agonist.
Key: 0, minimal activity; +, weak activity; ++, moderate activity; +++, strong activity; ++++, very strong activity; ?, insufficient data.

Table 12-3 Adverse and Therapeutic Effects of the Atypical Antipsychotics

Effects	Dopamine Receptors				Serotonin Receptors			Muscarinic-1	Other Receptors			
	D₁	D₂	D₃	D₄	5-HT₁ₐ	5-HT₂ₐ	5-HT₃		α1	α2	H₁	NE
Therapeutic	—	Treats positive symptoms	—	—	Enhances cognition Augments antidepressants	Treats negative symptoms Mitigates EPS	Mitigates nausea (antagonists)	Mitigates EPS	Unknown	Unknown	Sedation Treats nausea, vomiting, hiccups	—
Adverse	—	EPS, dystonia, akathisia, TD, increased prolactin (galactorrhea, amenorrhea, impotence)	—	—	Increased feeding (agonists)	Sexual dysfunction	Nausea, colic (agonist)	Blurred vision, cognitive impairment, dry mouth, tachycardia, constipation, urinary retention	Postural hypotension, dizziness, QTc prolongation, incontinence	Retrograde ejaculation, priapism, blocks antihypertensive effects of clonidine and methyldopa	Sedation, drowsiness, weight gain	—

EPS, extrapyramidal symptoms; H₁, histamine-1 receptor; 5-HT, serotonin; NE, norepinephrine; TD, tardive dyskinesia.

Table 12-4 **Intramuscular Antipsychotics**

Drug	Initial dose (mg)	Frequency (h)	Maximum daily dose (mg)	ECG Precautions
Haloperidol	1-5	2-4	20-30	Monitor ECG for QTc prolongation, watch for dystonia
Ziprasidone	10-20	2-4	40	Monitor ECG for QTc prolongation
Olanzapine	5-10	2-4	40	None

    b. All agents are highly lipophilic, leading to increased volume of distribution.

    c. Steady state is reached in a period four to five times the drug's half-life; depot preparations can take 3 to 6 months to reach steady state.

    d. Ziprasidone is best taken with food; food increases its bioavailability.

2. Distribution.

    a. All are highly protein bound; drugs like phenytoin, valproic acid, and digoxin can displace bound antipsychotics, leading to short-term elevation in serum levels.

    b. Lipophilic property allows a large amount of these drugs to be stored in body tissues (fat, liver, lung, kidney), which prevents effective removal via hemodialysis in case of overdose. It also allows them to readily cross the placenta to the fetus in pregnancy.

    c. Aripiprazole takes about 2 weeks to reach a steady state, which can delay clinical response. Up to 4 weeks can pass before aripiprazole reaches its full effect. Dose increases should not be made before 2 weeks of continuous therapy.

3. Metabolism and excretion. All antipsychotic agents undergo hepatic metabolism, mostly through the cytochrome P450 system (Table 12-5).

    a. All typical antipsychotics, risperidone, and aripiprazole have active metabolites, which is another reason it has not been possible to obtain a meaningful correlation between plasma levels and clinical response in most of them. Haloperidol and clozapine are the only two exceptions.

    b. Except for ziprasidone and quetiapine, all antipsychotics have a long elimination half-life, allowing once-daily doses following stabilization.

    c. Clozapine reaches higher plasma levels with similar oral doses in women than in men.

    d. Caffeine in high amounts can raise the clozapine level.

    e. Cytochrome P450 (Table 12-6; also refer to Chapter 20).

        (1) 2D6, 3A4, and 1A2 are the P450 enzymes responsible for metabolism of antipsychotics.

        (2) 2D6 is the only enzyme that has genetic polymorphism, with alleles identified that are responsible for a weaker enzyme

Table 12-5 Antipsychotics: Pharmacokinetics, Dosing, and Formulations

| | | Pharmacokinetics | | | | Dosing | | |
Drug	Formulation	$T_{1/2}$ (h)*	Active Metabolites	Time to Peak Conc. (h)	Typical Starting (mg)	Typical Maintenance (mg)	Depot (mg)	Cost per Month (est)
Aripiprazole (no generic available)	Tab: 5, 10, 15, 20, 30 mg	>75	Dehydroaripiprazole	3-5	5-10	15-20	NA	$375 (15 mg/day)
Clozapine (generic available)	Tab: 12.5, 25, 100 mg ODT (FazaClo): 25, 100 mg	10-100	None	3	25	300-600	NA	$90 (generic) $300 (brand) (300 mg/day)
Fluphenazine (generic available)	Tab: 1, 2.5, 5, 10 mg Elixir: 2.5, 5 mg/mL IM: 2.5 mg/mL Depot (decanoate): 25 mg/mL; 1-mL vials	13-33	Oxide, 7,8-OH	3	1-2	5-20	12.5-50	$145 (25 mg/day)

Haloperidol (generic available)	Tab: 0.5, 1, 2, 5, 10, 20 mg Elixir: 1, 2 mg/mL IM: 5 mg/mL; 1 mL amp, 10 mL vial Depot (decanoate): 50 mg/mL; 50-, 100-mg vials	12-36	Reduced form	3	1-2	5-10	50-100	$50 (10 mg/day)
Risperidone (no generic available)	Tab: 0.25, 0.5, 1, 2, 3, 4 mg ODT (M-Tab): 0.5, 1, 2-mg Elixir: 1 mg/mL Depot (consta): 25-, 37.5-, 50-mg dose-pack vials	6-24	9-OH (renal)	1.5	0.5-1	2-3	25-50	$250 (3 mg/day)

Table continued on following page.

Table 12-5 **Antipsychotics: Pharmacokinetics, Dosing, and Formulations** *(Continued)*

		Pharmacokinetics			Dosing			
Drug	Formulation	T$_{1/2}$ (h)*	Active Metabolites	Time to Peak Conc. (h)	Typical Starting (mg)	Typical Maintenance (mg)	Depot (mg)	Cost per Month (est)
Olanzapine (no generic available)	Tab: 2.5, 5, 7.5, 10, 15, 20 mg ODT (Zydis): 5, 10, 15, 20 mg IM: 5 mg/mL; 10-mg single-use vial	20-70	None	5	5	10-15	NA	$525 (15 mg/day)
Quetiapine (no generic available)	Tab: 25, 100, 200, 300 mg	4-10	None	1.5	25-100	300-800	NA	$310 (400 mg/day)
Ziprasidone (no generic available)	Cap: 20, 40, 60, 80 mg 20 mg/mL; 20-mg single-use vial	3-10	None	4	20-40 bid	40-80 bid	NA	$325 (30 mg/day)

amp, ampule; cap, capsule; conc, concentration; est, estimated; IM, intramuscular injection; NA, not applicable; ODT, orally disintegrating tablet; tab, tablet.
*The half-life of a drug is the amount of time required for the plasma drug concentration to decrease by one-half. Half-life can be used to determine the appropriate dosing interval. The half-life of a drug does not include the half-life of its active metabolites.

Table 12-6 Cytochrome P450 System and Antipsychotics

P450 Isoform	Substrate	Inhibitor (Increases Level)	Inducer (Decreases Level)	Frequency of Poor Metabolizers	Frequency of Ultraextensive Metabolizers
1A2	Clozapine Haloperidol Olanzapine	Caffeine Cimetidine Ciprofloxacin Fluvoxamine Mexiletine	Charcoal-broiled beef Cigarette smoke Cruciferous vegetables Marijuana smoke Omeprazole	None	None
2D6	Haloperidol Risperidone Thioridazine	Cimetidine Fluoxetine Paroxetine Quinidine Sertraline (dose specific)	None documented in vivo	5%-14% of whites 3% of blacks 70% of Asians	1%-5% of European whites 20%-30% of Arabs and Ethiopians
3A4	Haloperidol Pimozide Quetiapine Ziprasidone	Diltiazem Erythromycin Grapefruit juice Indinavir Ketoconazole Methadone Nefazodone Ritonavir	Carbamazepine Phenobarbital Phenytoin Rifampin St. John's wort	None	None

(poor and intermediate metabolizers) in some patients, and multiplication of functional alleles (extensive and ultraextensive metabolizers). Table 12-6 illustrates ethnic variability of this polymorphism.

- (a) Variability in 2D6 activity might explain why some patients need higher doses and others are very sensitive to side effects.
- (b) 2D6 activity is slightly lower in women than in men.
- (c) Only 2D6 enzyme *inhibitors* have clinical value; no significant 2D6 inducers are known.

(3) 1A2 has only a few inhibitors but many important *inducers*.

(4) 3A4 has significant *inhibitor* drug and dietary items, and only a few important inducers.

(5) Cigarette smoke induces P450-1A2 and can reduce plasma levels of haloperidol, olanzapine, and clozapine. This warrants special attention on inpatient units that do not allow smoking and when patients are quitting.

f. Plasma levels.

(1) There are no established therapeutic plasma levels for most antipsychotics.

(2) Haloperidol might have a therapeutic window between about 3 and 15 ng/mL, a level generally reached with oral doses at or below 20 mg/day.

(3) Clozapine concentrations of 350 ng/mL or greater have been considered evidence of an adequate trial in nonresponders.

g. Special populations.

(1) Geriatric patients metabolize most antipsychotics less efficiently and are more sensitive to side effects than younger adults. In general, elderly patients should be prescribed lower doses with slower titration. Exceptions are ziprasidone and aripiprazole, which do not need dose adjustment.

(2) Hepatic or renal impairment requires reduction of the dose of most antipsychotics except clozapine, ziprasidone, and aripiprazole.

Pharmacodynamics of Antipsychotics

Tables 12-2 and 12-3 illustrate affinities of antipsychotics to neuroreceptors and their relevant clinical effect.

1. Risperidone acts as a typical antipsychotic in doses higher than about 6 mg/day(or above 2 mg/day in frail or elderly patients).

2. Ziprasidone has significant norepinephrine reuptake inhibitor activity, which is hypothesized to partly account for its effect on negative and depressive symptoms. This also adds a risk of manic switch if the drug is used in bipolar depression, which has been reported in several case reports as of mid-2006.

Drug Interactions

1. Pharmacokinetics (see earlier section).

2. Pharmacodynamics. Drugs with similar or antagonistic activity can modify clinical effects (Table 12-7).

Table 12-7 Antipsychotic Pharmacodynamic Drug Interactions

Agents	Effect	Examples of Antipsychotics Involved
Anticholinergics	Worsen anticholinergic side effects	Chlorpromazine, thioridazine, clozapine
Antihypertensives	Worsen orthostasis	Clozapine, thioridazine, quetiapine
CNS depressants (alcohol, benzodiazepines, barbiturates)	Worsen sedative effect	Clozapine, olanzapine, low-potency typicals
Potassium- and magnesium-depleting drugs and drugs that prolong QTc (amiodarone, quinidine, gatiflocaxin)	Increase incidence of arrhythmias	Ziprasidone, pimozide, chlorpromazine, thioridazine

CNS, central nervous system.

CLINICAL GUIDELINES FOR ANTIPSYCHOTIC TREATMENT OF SCHIZOPHRENIA

1. Because schizophrenia is a chronic illness that influences virtually all aspects of life of affected persons, treatment planning has three goals.
   a. Reduce or eliminate symptoms.
   b. Maximize quality of life and adaptive functioning.
   c. Promote and maintain recovery from the debilitating effects of illness to the maximum extent possible.
2. Medications make up one component of the treatment. Other aspects of care are equally important.
3. Initial assessment in the acute phase.
   a. Psychiatric examination to establish diagnosis and assess risk of aggression and suicide.
   b. History and full physical and neurologic examination (as much as acute condition permits), relevant lab studies and radiologic evaluation to detect comorbid general medical conditions (Box 12-5).
   c. Start building therapeutic alliance and collaborate with family members.
   d. Decide on treatment setting (inpatient, outpatient, partial hospital program, Program for Assertive Community Treatment [PACT]).
4. Choosing an antipsychotic agent.
   a. To simplify decision making, the American Psychiatric Association (APA) practice guideline for schizophrenia divides antipsychotics into four general groups (Table 12-8).
   b. The best guidance for selecting an antipsychotic is the patient's previous experience, including symptom response and adverse reactions.
   c. With the exception of clozapine, all antipsychotics have similar efficacy in treating positive symptoms.
   d. With few exceptions, SGAs should be first line because of their favorable side-effect profile and superior efficacy in treating negative, mood, and cognitive symptoms.
   e. No evidence supports efficacy of one SGA over another. Prior response and side-effect profile tailored for individual patient needs and comorbidities dictate the choice (Tables 12-8 and 12-9).
      (1) Clozapine is the treatment of choice in patients with resistant illness, TD, persistent suicidal behavior, or hostile behavior.
      (2) Elderly patients and patients with dementia, Parkinson's disease, mental retardation, or structural brain pathology are at particularly high risk for EPS. Medications with few or no EPS (e.g., quetiapine) are recommended. Dosing should start low and be titrated slowly.
      (3) For patients with osteopenia or osteoporosis and women with breast cancer or menstrual, or fertility problems, a drug with minimal or no effect on prolactin is clinically indicated (e.g., aripiprazole, which actually suppresses prolactin release).
      (4) In patients at risk for diabetes, hypertension, or myocardial ischemia or in obese patients, risk should be weighed against benefit on an individual basis. Medications that have less effect

BOX 12-5   Suggested Physical and Laboratory Assessments for Patients with Schizophrenia

Assessments to Monitor Physical Status and Detect Concomitant Physical Conditions

Vital signs: pulse, blood pressure, temperature

Body weight, height, BMI

Hematology: CBC

Blood chemistries: electrolytes, renal function tests (BUN-to-creatinine ratio), liver function tests, thyroid function tests

Infectious diseases: syphilis, hepatitis C, HIV (if clinically indicated)

Pregnancy (consider in women of childbearing potential)

Toxicology: Drug toxicology screen, heavy metal screen (if clinically indicated)

Imaging: EEG, brain imaging (CT or MRI [MRI preferred]) (if clinically indicated)

Assessments Related to Other Specific Side Effects of Treatment

Diabetes*: screen for risk factors; fasting blood glucose†

Hyperlipidemia: lipid panel

QTc prolongation: ECG and serum potassium before treatment with thioridazine, mesoridazine, or pimozide; ECG before treatment with ziprasidone in the presence of cardiac risk factors‡

Hyperprolactinemia

Extrapyramidal side effects, akathisia

Tardive dyskinesia: clinical assessment of abnormal involuntary movements

Cataracts: clinical history to assess for changes in distance vision or blurred vision; ocular examination including slit-lamp examination for patients treated with antipsychotics associated with an increased risk of cataracts

---

BMI, body mass index; BUN, blood urea nitrogen; CBC, complete blood count; CT, computed tomography; ECG, electrocardiogram; EEG, electroencephalogram; HIV, human immunodeficiency virus; MRI, magnetic resonance imaging.

*Factors that indicate an increased risk for undiagnosed diabetes include a BMI greater than 25, a first-degree relative with diabetes, habitual physical inactivity, being a member of a high-risk ethnic population (African American, Latin American, Native American, Asian American, Pacific Islander), having delivered a baby heavier than 9 lb or having had gestational diabetes, hypertension, a high-density lipoprotein cholesterol level <35 mg/dL and/or a triglyceride level >250 mg/dL, history of abnormal findings on the glucose tolerance test or an abnormal level of fasting blood glucose, and history of vascular disease. Symptoms of possible diabetes include frequent urination, excessive thirst, extreme hunger, unusual weight loss, increased fatigue, irritability, and blurred vision.

†As an alternative to measurement of fasting blood glucose, a hemoglobin A1c level may be obtained. An abnormal value (fasting blood glucose >110 mg/dL or hemoglobin A1c >6.1%) suggests a need for medical consultation. More frequent monitoring may be indicated in the presence of weight change, symptoms of diabetes, or a random measure of blood glucose >200 mg/dL.

‡In this context, cardiac risk factors include known heart disease, a personal history of syncope, a family history of sudden death at an early age (younger than 40 years, especially if both parents had sudden death), or prolonged QTc syndrome.

Table 12-8 **Choice of Medication in the Acute Phase of Schizophrenia**

Patient Profile	First-Generation Agents	Risperidone, Olanzapine, Quetiapine, Ziprasidone, or Aripiprazole	Clozapine	Long-Acting Injectable Antipsychotic Agents
First episode	Yes	Yes	No	No
Persistent suicidal ideation or behavior	Yes	Yes	Yes	Yes
Persistent hostility and aggressive behavior	Yes	Yes	Yes	Yes
Tardive dyskinesia	Yes	Yes, but less than first generation, and may decrease tardive dyskinesia when already present	Yes	
History of sensitivity to extrapyramidal side effects	No	Yes, except higher doses of risperidone	Yes	
History of sensitivity to prolactin elevation	No	Yes, except risperidone	Yes	
History of sensitivity to weight gain, hyperglycemia, or hyperlipidemia	Mixed	Ziprasidone or aripiprazole favored	No	
Repeated nonadherence to pharmacologic treatment				Yes

Table 12-9   Selected Side Effects of Commonly Used Antipsychotic Medications

Medication	EPS, TD	Prolactin Elevation	Weight Gain	Glucose Abnormalities	Lipid Abnormalities	QTc Prolongation	Sedation	Hypotension	Anticholinergic Side Effects
Aripiprazole*	0†	0	0	0	0	0	+	0	0
Clozapine‡	0†	0	++	++	++	0	+++	++	++
Fluphenazine	+++	+++	+	0	0	0	++	0	0
Haloperidol	+++	+++	+	0	0	0/Dose dependent	++	0	0
Olanzapine	0†	0	+++	+++	+++	0	++	+	+†
Perphenazine	++	++	++	+?	+?	0	++	+	0
Risperidone	+/Dose dependent	+++	++	++	++	+	++	+++	0
Quetiapine*	0†	0	++	++	++	0	++	++	0
Thioridazine	+	++	++	+?	+?	+++	++	++	+‡
Ziprasidone	0†	+	0	0	0	++	0	0	0

EPS, extrapyramidal symptoms; TD, tardive dyskinesia.

0, No risk or rarely causes side effects at therapeutic dose; +, mild or occasionally causes side effects at therapeutic dose; ++, sometimes causes side effects at therapeutic dose; +++, often causes side effects at therapeutic dose; ?, data too limited to rate with confidence.

*Also causes nausea and headache.
†Also causes agranulocytosis, seizures, and myocarditis.
‡Possible exception of akathisia.
*Also carries warning about potential development of cataracts.

on weight and blood lipids and are less hyperglycemic are indicated (e.g., ziprasidone, aripiprazole).

   (5) Patients at risk for orthostatic hypotension (elderly patients and patients with peripheral vascular disease, diabetic neuropathy, or debilitating diseases) should use medications with low affinity for α-adrenergic receptors (e.g., olanzapine).

   (6) Patients with QT syndrome, bradycardia, electrolyte imbalance, heart failure, or recent myocardial infarction should not be treated with drugs that further prolong QT interval or increase the risk of torsades de pointes (e.g., thioridazine, droperidol, ziprasidone, and pimozide).

   (7) In patients with benign prostatic hyperplasia or glaucoma, medications with higher anticholinergic activity (olanzapine, clozapine) are less desirable.

5. Management of acute agitation (also see Chapter 14).

   a. Haloperidol, ziprasidone, and olanzapine are available for IM use and have an FDA indication for treatment of acute agitation in schizophrenia and bipolar mania.

   b. Studies have shown equal efficacy, less need for frequent doses, less need for adjunctive benzodiazepines, and fewer adverse effects with ziprasidone and olanzapine.

   c. Table 12-4 illustrates typical doses and precautions. A second dose may be needed after 2 to 24 hours with the two atypicals.

6. Response and resistance.

   a. No patient characteristics predict response to a particular antipsychotic agent.

   b. Full therapeutic benefits take several weeks to realize, but symptoms can begin to improve as early as the first week after starting treatment, and more than 50% of improvement in positive symptoms occurs in the first 3 to 4 weeks.

   c. Standardized rating scales (Positive and Negative Syndrome Scale [PANSS], Brief Psychiatric Rating Scale [BPRS]) are helpful in gauging response to treatment.

   d. From 10% to 30% of patients have little or no response to antipsychotics, and up to an additional 30% have only partial response.

   e. Resistance is defined as little or no symptomatic response to at least two antipsychotic trials of an adequate duration (at least 6 weeks) and adequate dose.

   f. It is crucial to make sure that the patient has been taking the right dose of the medications for an adequate period. Lack of adherence to treatment can be easily mistaken for resistance.

   g. Clozapine is the standard treatment for resistant patients; a few other agents have been used for augmentation with little or no evidence of benefit.

7. Treatment continuation in stabilization and stable phase.

   a. The patient should be monitored and maintained on the same medication and same dose for at least 6 months.

   b. Only 10% to 15% of patients have one episode in their lifetime. The decision to discontinue medication should involve discussing with the patient and family members the risks of long-term use of drugs versus risk of relapse.

c. If a decision is made to discontinue the medication, dose reduction should be very gradual (10% per month), and both the patient and the family should be educated about early signs of relapse.

d. For a patient maintained on an FGA, the maintenance dose should be the lowest effective dose. Studies have shown lower medication doses to be as effective as higher doses and more promoting of adherence.

e. Dose adjustments should be made slowly and carefully as well.

f. Depot antipsychotics are useful in patient with poor adherence to medications (see later).

g. Continuous treatment appears to be more effective than intermittent treatment of emergent symptoms in preventing relapse (hence, intramuscular depot forms have an advantage).

ADVERSE EFFECTS OF ANTIPSYCHOTICS
Neurologic

Extrapyramidal Symptoms

Extrapyramidal symptoms are the major potential neurologic side effects of the typical antipsychotics. EPS can have an acute onset (acute dystonia, medication-induced parkinsonism, and akathisia) or chronic onset, including tardive dyskinesia and tardive dystonia.

1. EPS occur in 50% to 75% of patients taking typical antipsychotics. Neurologically vulnerable populations, such as the elderly or those with Parkinson's disease, might not be able to tolerate even very low doses of potent D_2 blockers such as haloperidol.

2. The atypical agents are characterized by lower rates of EPS.
   a. Clozapine is the only antipsychotic with no incidence of EPS.
   b. Risperidone has a low rate of EPS in doses less than 4 mg/day. It has dose-related EPS at doses greater than 6 mg/day.
   c. Except for akathisia, other atypicals have EPS incidence that is similar to placebo.

3. Acute dystonic reactions.
   a. Reactions include:
      (1) Torticollis (neck rotation).
      (2) Oculogyric crisis (eyes turn upward). This can also occur later in treatment.
      (3) Opisthotonus (back arching).
      (4) Lingual.
      (5) Laryngeal (very rare, life-threatening).
   b. Acute dystonia can result from one dose of any dopamine D_2 blocking agent, but it is more commonly seen with high-potency typical antipsychotics, especially when administered IM. Ten percent of patients on those drugs develop dystonia. Most cases develop within the first 3 days of treatment. Young muscular male patients and recent cocaine users are especially at risk.
   c. Treatment (IM or IV).
      (1) Benztropine (Cogentin) 2 mg.

(2) Diphenhydramine (Benadryl) 50 mg.
(3) Repeat doses in about 20 minutes if needed.
(4) If no response, try lorazepam 1 mg IM (or IV).
(5) With laryngeal symptoms, give doses closer together. Very rarely, tracheotomy is required.
d. Prevention.
(1) Young muscular men are at highest risk of acute dystonia (with an incidence of about 40%) and should be treated prophylactically when given high-potency typical antipsychotics (such as haloperidol).
(2) Add 2 mg of benztropine (Cogentin) to the initial haloperidol dose (compatible in the same syringe if given IM).
(3) It is usually sufficient to repeat the benztropine only once every 24 hours.
4. Medication-induced parkinsonism is the most common EPS with typical antipsychotics.
a. It develops within days or weeks of initiating treatment and is characterized by the same symptoms as idiopathic Parkinson's (rigidity, tremors, bradykinesia, and akinesia). Bradykinesia and akinesia need to be distinguished from negative symptoms and depression.
b. Treatment. Decrease the antipsychotic dose or switch to an atypical. Adding an anticholinergic (such as benztropine 1 to 2 mg qd) or a dopamine agonist (such as amantadine 50 to 100 mg bid; Table 12-10) are other options. However, the anticholinergics have additional side effects, and the dopamine agonists carry a risk of exacerbating psychosis.
5. Akathisia.
a. Identification.
(1) Incidence is 20% to 40% for patients taking antipsychotic agents (less common with the atypical antipsychotics).
(2) May be subjective only, with the patient complaining only of an uncomfortable inner feeling (like a motor running).
(3) More often, patients are restless.
(4) Akathisia can be so distressing that patients jump out of a window to try to escape the terrible feelings.
(5) Remember that metoclopramide (Reglan) blocks dopamine receptors and can cause this side effect in patients with cancer or diabetes.
b. Treatment.
(1) Lower the antipsychotic dose (if possible).
(2) Give low-dose β-blockers (such as propranolol 5 to 30 mg tid).
(3) Give low-dose diazepam (2 to 5 mg tid).
(4) Anticholinergics (benztropine 2 mg bid) are often not as effective.
6. Tardive dyskinesia is a hyperkinetic abnormal involuntary movement disorder caused by sustained exposure to antipsychotic medication.

Table 12-10 **Antiparkinson Medications**

Drug	Formulation	Daily dose (mg)	Half-life (h)	Receptor		
				Dopamine	Histamine	Acetylcholine
Amantadine (Symmetrel)	Tab: 100 mg	50-150 bid	24	3+ agonist	None	
Benztropine (Cogentin)	Tab: 0.5, 1, 2 mg Amp: 1 mg/mL	1-6 bid (q30min until acute symptom relief)	24	2+ agonist		3+ antagonist
Biperiden (Akineton)	Tab: 2 mg Amp: 5 mg/mL	2-8 qd-tid (q30min until acute symptom relief)				2+ antagonis
Diphenhydramine (Benadryl)	Tab: 25, 50 mg Amp: 10, 50 mg/mL	50-200/day divided bid-qid	3-5	None	Strong antagonist	1+ antagonist
Trihexyphenidyl (Artane)	Tab: 2, 5 mg Elixir: 2 mg/mL Sequels: 5 mg (sustained release)	2-30 qd	10-12	1+ agonist		4+ antagonist

amp, ampule; tab, tablet.
Level of effect: 1+, minimal; 2+, moderate; 3+, high; 4+, very high.

TD can affect neuromuscular function in any body region but is most commonly seen in the oral–facial region.

a. Incidence.

   (1) A patient needs exposure of at least 3 to 6 months to be at risk for developing TD.

   (2) The annual incidence is about 4% to 8% in patients taking typical neuroleptic agents for 2 years. About half of those cases are irreversible.

   (3) Incidence may be as high as 25% in high-risk groups such as the elderly.

   (4) Because of the potential risk:

      (a) Examine all patients for movement disorder before starting treatment.

      (b) Monitor for EPS weekly during acute treatment.

      (c) Examine for TD every 6 months on typical agents and every year on atypicals. High-risk patients such as the elderly should be examined more often with consent.

   (5) Informed consent is the common law standard in the United States.

      (a) The APA recommends informing patients about TD when they are being treated with a conventional antipsychotic medication.

      (b) One study found that disclosing information about antipsychotic medication did not have an adverse effect on patients' medication compliance and readmission rate.

   (6) The atypical antipsychotics have significantly lower (but not zero) incidence of TD potential.

b. Identification.

   (1) TD can look like a regular dyskinesia, but it responds to opposite treatment. Interventions that improve a regular dyskinesia (lowering the antipsychotic dose, adding an anticholinergic or dopamine agonist) make TD worse.

   (2) TD typically involves oral, buccal, and lingual muscles, but it can involve limbs or trunk.

c. Differential diagnosis. Other neurologic diagnoses can appear as TD (Box 12-6).

d. Monitoring.

   (1) Examine for abnormal movements before prescribing neuroleptic agents, and reexamine at regular 6-month intervals.

   (2) Consider using the Abnormal Involuntary Movement Scale (AIMS) (Box 12-7).

e. Prevention is key because of lack of effective treatment. Use the lowest neuroleptic dose for the shortest period.

f. Treatment.

   (1) There is no consistently successful treatment for TD.

   (2) Lowering the dose (or discontinuing the neuroleptic agent) if possible may remove the TD symptoms, usually after a period of weeks of exacerbation.

BOX 12-6 Differential Diagnosis of Tardive Dyskinesia

Neurologic Disorders

Brain neoplasms
Fahr's syndrome
Huntington's disease
Idiopathic dystonias (tics, blepharospasm, aging)
Ill-fitting dentures
Meige's syndrome (spontaneous oral dyskinesia)
Postanoxic extrapyramidal syndrome
Postencephalitic extrapyramidal syndrome
Torsion dystonia
Wilson's disease

Drugs

Amphetamines	Levodopa
Anticholinergics	Lithium
Antidepressants	Magnesium
Heavy metals	Phenytoin

---

(3) Drugs that may be tried (TD can reemerge after stopping the drug).
  (a) Clozapine 300 to 500 mg/day (strongest supportive evidence).
  (b) Olanzapine 5 to 20 mg/day has been shown to significantly reduce TD in a prospective clinical trial.
  (c) Branched-chain amino acids (phenylalanine) 220 mg/kg tid have been shown to improve TD in a randomized, double blind, placebo-controlled clinical trial.
  (d) Quetiapine 400 mg/day was shown to improve TD in a few studies.
  (e) Vitamin E (1200 to 1600 IU/day) showed modest positive effect in some trials. Longer multicenter placebo-controlled, randomized trials, however, showed no significant benefit.
  (f) Anticholinergics have not been helpful with TD, but they can reduce symptoms of tardive dystonia (trihexyphenidyl in doses of about 20 mg/day).
  (g) Cholinesterase inhibitors such as donepezil (Aricept) have been recently tried in open-label studies with some success. This is based on the theory that TD is caused by the damage or destruction of striatal cholinergic neurons.
  (h) Benzodiazepines, calcium channel blockers, naltrexone, γ-aminobutyric acid (GABA), baclofen, clonidine, reserpine, buspirone, essential fatty acids, insulin, and electroconvulsive therapy (ECT) have all been tried with no significant benefit.

> ## BOX 12-7   Abnormal Involuntary Movement Scale (AIMS)
>
> ### Preparation
>
> Use a firm chair, without arms.
> Remove anything (gum, candy) from the patient's mouth.
> Inquire about dentures and their condition.
> Ask if patient notices any movements and if they bother or interfere with activities.
> At some point, observe the patient unobtrusively.
>
> ### Rating Scale
>
> Rate the patient's response to the procedure with this scale:
>
> 0   None
> 1   Minimal
> 2   Mild
> 3   Moderate
> 4   Severe
>
> ### Procedure
>
> 1. Have the patient sit in chair with hands on knees, legs slightly apart, and feet flat on floor. Look at entire body for movements in this position.
> 2. Ask the patient to sit with hands hanging unsupported. If the patient is wearing trousers, hands should hang between the legs. If the patient is wearing a dress (or other unbifurcated garment), hands should hang over the knees. Observe hands and other body areas.
> 3. Ask the patient to open the mouth. Observe tongue at rest within the mouth. Do this twice.
> 4. Ask patient to protrude the tongue. Observe abnormalities of tongue movement. Do this twice.
> 5. Ask the patient to tap the thumb with each finger as rapidly as possible for 10 to 15 seconds, first with the right hand, then with the left hand. Observe facial and leg movements.
> 6. Flex and extend the patient's left and right arms one at a time.
> 7. Ask the patient to stand up. Observe in profile. Observe all body areas again, hips included.
> 8. Ask the patient to extend both arms in front with palms down. Observe trunk, legs, mouth.*
> 9. Have the patient walk a few paces, turn, and walk back to chair. Observe hands and gait. Do this twice.*

*Activated movements.

(4) Patients with severe TD are best referred to a specialty program.
(5) Tardive dystonia is a severe variant of TD, which is characterized by spastic muscle contractions in contrast to choreoathetoid movements. Tardive dystonia is often associated with great distress and physical discomfort.

BOX 12-8 Differential Diagnosis of Neuroleptic Malignant Syndrome Symptoms

Fever

Agranulocytosis
Anticholinergic syndrome
Dehydration
Heat stroke
Infection
Serotonin syndrome

Muscle Rigidity

Extrapyramidal symptoms
Lethal catatonia

Benign Elevation of Creatine Phosphokinase

Intramuscular injection
Physical restraints or other physical trauma
Severe muscle exertion

Neuroleptic Malignant Syndrome

Neuroleptic malignant syndrome (NMS) is potentially life-threatening.

1. Incidence (in some form) may be as high as 2%, though life-threatening cases are rarer; mortality is 5% to 30%. Although it is uncommon with the atypical agents, NMS can occur with them.
2. Identification. NMS is often misdiagnosed and should be considered in any patient taking antipsychotics who appears to be getting worse rather than getting better. Clinical features include the following (Box 12-8):
   a. Hyperthermia.
   b. Extreme muscle rigidity unrelieved by anticholinergics.
   c. Autonomic instability.
   d. Delirium.
   e. Elevated creatine phosphokinase (CPK). In some patients CPK can be elevated to 800 mg/dL by having intramuscular injections and physical restraints. However, elevations over this level are a result of some other pathologic process.
3. Course and treatment.
   a. Mild NMS can resolve spontaneously with discontinuation of antipsychotic agents, which should always be the first step. Supportive care and adequate hydration are also indicated.
   b. Amantadine (100 mg bid) is often used in milder cases.
   c. Daily CPK should be followed in patients with suspected NMS.
   d. More serious cases can result in death from shock, renal failure (with myoglobinuria), respiratory failure, or disseminated intravascular coagulation (DIC). Patients might need medical intensive care monitoring with supportive treatment. Pharmacologic

treatments that are often used include dopamine agonists such as bromocriptine or dantrolene, which directly reduces muscle rigidity.
  e. In resistant cases, ECT is reported to improve symptoms.
  f. When antipsychotic treatment is resumed, a drug other than the precipitating agent (preferably an atypical) should be used in lower doses with slow careful titration.

Other Adverse Neurologic Effects

1. Sedation.
    a. Sedation, which is associated with antihistaminic effects, may be helpful in the agitated patient, but it can be a liability affecting compliance and performance.
    b. Treatment.
        (1) Lower the dose if possible.
        (2) Give the dose at bedtime.
        (3) Switch to a less-sedating drug.
2. Cognitive side effects.
    a. Confusion, disturbed concentration, memory impairment, and delirium.
    b. Mediated through anticholinergic and antihistaminergic effects of antipsychotics.
    c. More common with low-potency typical antipsychotics.
    d. Treatment.
        (1) Lower the dose if possible.
        (2) Switch to a drug with less effect on cholinergic and histaminergic receptors.
3. Anticholinergic activity.
    a. Anticholinergic activity varies inversely with the tendency to cause EPS. It can impair cognition and lead to medical complications (e.g., urinary retention), especially in the elderly and medically ill.
    b. Treatment.
        (1) Switch to an agent with lower anticholinergic effects.
        (2) Sugarless mints or gum can help dry mouth.
        (3) Bulk agents or stool softeners.
        (4) For urinary retention, bethanechol may be helpful (for details, see Chapter 7).
4. Lowering seizure threshold. All antipsychotics lower the seizure threshold to some degree.
    a. This is not a reason to avoid using antipsychotics in an epileptic patient as long as the patient is taking adequate anticonvulsants.
    b. Clozapine has a clinically relevant dose-related seizure risk. Doses of less than 300 mg/day are associated with a seizure rate of 1%, doses between 300 and 600 mg/day are associated with a seizure rate of 2.7%, and doses greater than 600 mg/day are associated with a rate of 4.4%.

Cardiovascular

1. Orthostatic hypotension (associated with (α_1-adrenergic antagonism).
    a. As with the tricyclic antidepressants, orthostasis can be a problem for some patients.

      (1) Patients with intravascular volume depletion.
      (2) Patients who have been on bedrest.
      (3) The elderly, who can fall and become injured.
   b. Document lying and standing blood pressure and pulse with associated symptoms.
   c. Treatment.
      (1) Make sure the patient is hydrated.
      (2) Support stockings might help.
      (3) Switch to another medication.
2. QT prolongation is associated with development of torsades de pointes.
   a. The average QT interval in adults is about 400 msec, and the risk of torsades de pointes increases as the interval lengthens. A QTc (QT interval corrected for heart rate) interval of longer than 500 msec is considered a substantial risk for torsades de pointes.
   b. A number of medications prolong QT interval, including antipsychotics (notably thioridazine and pimozide) and some tricyclic antidepressants.
      (1) Ziprasidone prolongs the QT interval somewhat longer than the other atypicals (mean increases for ziprasidone are 20.3 msec; risperidone, 11.6 msec; olanzapine, 6.8 msec; quetiapine, 14.5 msec; thioridazine, 35.6 msec; haloperidol, 4.7 msec). Further, these prolongations were not affected by P450 inhibitors.
      (2) In the absence of increased risk factors for QT prolongation or cardiac arrhythmias, no special cardiac monitoring is indicated.
      (3) In the presence of known heart disease, history of syncope, family history of sudden death before age 40 years, or congenital long QT syndrome, a baseline electrocardiogram (ECG) is indicated for patients starting on ziprasidone, thioridazine, mesoridazine, or pimozide.
      (4) Drugs that inhibit CYP 3A4 (see Table 12-6), deplete potassium or magnesium (diuretics, cyclosporine, aminoglycosides), or prolong QTc (amiodarone, quinidine, thioridazine, pimozide, gatifloxacin, and tacrolimus) increase the risk of QTc prolongation if they are used concomitantly with ziprasidone.
3. Cerebrovascular adverse events and excess mortality in elderly dementia patients. There have been reports of increased risk for transient ischemic attack (TIA), stroke, and mortality with the atypical antipsychotics. Recent metaanalytic data seems to confirm that there is a small added risk of these complications compared to placebo. The risk also seems to be present for the conventional antipsychotics. This risk does not contraindicate the use of these agents, but it underscores the need to use them for serious and necessary clinical indications while maximizing the concurrent use of psychosocial interventions.

Endocrine and Metabolic

1. Prolactin is increased because the prolactin-inhibiting factor is dopamine.
   a. Can cause galactorrhea, breast swelling, discharge, menstrual irregularities, and impaired sexual function, as well as reduced testosterone production.

b. Symptoms usually resolve over weeks to months after lowering or stopping the drug.

c. The atypical antipsychotics (with the exception of risperidone) tend to cause less prolactin increase than the typical agents.

d. Patients on antipsychotics known to increase prolactin should be screened for symptoms of hyperprolactinemia at each visit until stable, and then yearly.

e. Prolactin level should be checked and monitored in symptomatic and in high-risk patients and in those with preexisting osteopenia or osteoporosis and women with breast cancer. Using an antipsychotic with less effect on prolactin level is indicated in these cases, if possible.

2. Weight gain.

a. Schizophrenics are more likely to be overweight. Using a body mass index (BMI) of ≥30 or higher as a definition of obesity, about 25% of the general population and 42% of schizophrenics are obese.

b. Antipsychotics have a continuum of weight gain liability: Ziprasidone and aripiprazole have low risk; risperidone and quetiapine have medium risk; olanzapine and clozapine have the highest risk. Weight gain is a potentially serious liability of antipsychotic treatment that needs to be monitored and managed.

c. Waist size larger than 35 inches for women and 40 inches for men is associated with increased health risks.

d. Focus on preventing weight gain (which seems to be associated with increased appetite) can be an issue for both typical and atypical antipsychotics.
   (1) Appetite suppressants should not be used.
   (2) Calorie restriction and weight management counseling are appropriate.

3. Diabetes.

a. Schizophrenics have a higher risk for developing diabetes.

b. All patients starting on antipsychotics should have a baseline fasting blood glucose.

c. Monitor for diabetes symptoms: weight change, polyuria, polydipsia.

4. Hyperlipidemia.

a. Schizophrenics are vulnerable to developing the metabolic syndrome (which includes abdominal obesity, elevated fasting glucose, elevated triglycerides, low high-density lipoprotein [HDL] cholesterol, and hypertension).

b. Clozapine and olanzapine appear to be associated with the greatest risk of dyslipidemia. Quetiapine and risperidone have intermediate effects, and ziprasidone and aripiprazole are associated with few or no effects.

5. Consensus guidelines (summarized in Table 12-11) have been developed conjointly by the American Diabetes Association, APA, American Association of Clinical Endocrinologists, and North America Association for the Study of Obesity.

a. Patients taking SGA should receive appropriate baseline screening and ongoing monitoring.

Table 12-11   Monitoring Protocol for Patients on Atypical (Second-Generation) Antipsychotics*

Clinical Parameter	Baseline	4 weeks	8 weeks	12 weeks	Quarterly	Annually	Every 5 years
Personal or family history of DM, obesity, dyslipidemia, CV disease, HTN	×					×	
Weight (BMI)	×	×	×	×	×		
Waist circumference	×			×		×	
Blood pressure	×			×		×	
Fasting plasma glucose	×			×		×	
Fasting lipid profile	×			×			×

BMI, body mass index; CV, cardiovascular; DM, diabetes mellitus; HTN, hypertension.
*More frequent assessment may be warranted based on clinical status.

245

  b. Baseline screening should include:
    (1) Personal and family history to identify preexisting risk factors, smoking, hypertension, hyperlipidemia, diabetes, obesity, sedentary lifestyle, ischemic heart disease, and family history of diabetes or cardiovascular disease.
    (2) Weight and height (to calculate BMI).
    (3) Waist circumference at the level of the umbilicus.
    (4) Blood pressure.
    (5) Fasting plasma glucose and lipid profile.
  c. Nutrition and physical activity counseling should be provided to all patients who are overweight (BMI 25.0 to 29.9) or obese (BMI > 30.0).
  d. Patients and their families should be aware of the signs and symptoms associated with diabetes, especially diabetic ketoacidosis.
  e. Follow-up monitoring.
    (1) Weight at 4, 8, and 12 weeks and quarterly thereafter. If the patient gains more than 5% of his or her weight, consider cross-titrating to a safer SGA.
    (2) Blood work should be reassessed 3 months after starting the antipsychotic and annually thereafter, or as clinically indicated.
    (3) Fasting plasma glucose level 126 mg/dL or higher, random plasma glucose 200 mg/dL, or hemoglobin A1c higher than 6.1% suggests the possibility of diabetes and should lead to consultation.

Sexual Dysfunction

Sexual dysfunction is common with antipsychotic use (up to 50% to 60% with typical antipsychotiics) and contribute to poor compliance on treatment. Patients are often embarrassed to talk about their sex life; less than 10% of patients mention sexual dysfunction, and physicians should ask direct questions.

1. Decreased desire (libido).
   a. May actually be due to the illness itself (negative symptoms, depression).
   b. Possible mechanisms include increased prolactin, sedation, and central dopamine blockade.
2. Decreased arousal (impotence in men).
   a. Possible mechanisms include anticholinergic effect, central dopamine blockade, or hypogonadism due to hyperprolactinemia.
   b. Thioridazine, chlorpromazine, and drugs increasing prolactin (typicals, risperidone) can cause this type of sexual dysfunction.
3. Orgasmic disorders include anorgasmia and premature, dry, and retrograde ejaculation.
   a. Possible mechanisms include α-adrenergic blockade, anticholinergic effects, and hyperprolactinemia.
   b. More common with low-potency typical drugs.
4. Treatment.
   a. Modification of other risk factors (other drugs, medical condition, depression).
   b. Lower the antipsychotic dose if possible.

   c. Switch to an atypical with little prolactin-elevation effect.

   d. Bromocriptine can help but might exacerbate psychosis.

   e. Amantadine may be beneficial.

   f. Might need referral to endocrinology or genitourinary specialist.

Other Adverse Effects of Individual Antipsychotics

1. Jaundice of a cholestatic hypersensitivity type is an uncommon side effect mostly associated with the phenothiazines within the first few months of treatment.

   a. Patients may be switched to another class of antipsychotic.

   b. More commonly, transient mild-to-moderate transaminase enzyme elevations with the phenothiazines are seen in the first few weeks of treatment, with a gradual return to normal.

2. Retinitis pigmentosa is a potential complication seen in patients taking daily doses of 800 mg or more of thioridazine.

3. Special issues with clozapine.

   a. Contraindications.

     (1) Myeloproliferative disorder.

     (2) Uncontrolled epilepsy.

     (3) History of clozapine-induced agranulocytosis or severe granulocytopenia.

   b. Unusual side effects of clozapine.

     (1) Sialorrhea and drooling occur relatively frequently and are most likely due to decreased saliva clearance related to impaired swallowing mechanism.

     (2) Agranulocytosis (defined as an absolute neutrophil count of less than $500/mm^3$) occurs at a cumulative incidence of approximately 1.3% at 1 year. It is a rare side effect with clozapine and usually occurs early in treatment. Monitoring guidelines must be followed.

       (a) The risk is highest in the first 6 months of treatment, and therefore weekly white blood cell (WBC) and neutrophil monitoring is required.

       (b) After 6 months, monitoring may be done every 2 weeks, because the risk of agranulocytosis appears to diminish considerably (an estimated rate of three cases per 1000 patients).

       (c) WBC counts must remain above $3000/mm^3$ during clozapine treatment, and absolute neutrophil counts must remain above $1500/mm^3$.

       (d) Reports of chills, fever, or sore throat should raise suspicion of this problem.

       (e) A WBC count less than $2000/mm^3$ or absolute neutrophil count (ANC) less than $1000/mm^3$ indicates impending or actual agranulocytosis. Stop clozapine immediately, check WBC and differential counts daily, monitor for infection, and consider bone marrow aspiration and protective isolation if indicated.

       (f) WBC count of 2000 to $3000/mm^3$ or ANC of 1000 to $1500/mm^3$ indicates high risk of agranulocytosis. Again, stop clozapine immediately, check WBC and differential daily, and monitor for infection. Clozapine may be resumed if no infection is present, the WBC count rises to greater than 3000, and the ANC is higher than 1500 (resume checking WBC count twice a week until it is higher than 3500).

(g) If the WBC count is 3000 to 3500/mm^3, and it falls to 3000/mm^3 over 1 to 3 weeks, or if immature WBC forms are present, repeat the WBC count with a differential. If a subsequent WBC count is 3000 to 3500/mm^3 and the ANC is higher than 1500/mm^3, repeat the WBC count with a differential count twice a week until the WBC count is higher than 3500/mm^3.

(3) Eosinophilia develops in 1% of patients. Therapy should be interrupted if levels rise above 4000/mm^3.

(4) Fever. Transient elevations above 100.4° F can occur, especially within the first month of use. Fever is usually benign and self-limited but raises the possibility of underlying infection or NMS.

(5) Myocarditis.
   (a) Symptoms include unexplained fatigue, dyspnea, tachypnea, fever, chest pain, palpitations, and other signs of heart failure.
   (b) Eighty percent of cases occur within the first 6 weeks of treatment.
   (c) Lab abnormalities include increased WBC count, eosinophilia, increased erythrocyte sedimentation rate, and ST and T wave abnormalities.
   (d) Clozapine should be stopped immediately and the patient should not be rechallenged.

OVERDOSE OF ANTIPSYCHOTICS

1. Patients can survive extremely high doses of antipsychotic agents.
2. Problems encountered with overdose (depending on the drug's side effects) could include the following:
   a. Seizures.
   b. Anticholinergic syndrome.
   c. EPS.
   d. NMS.
   e. Hypotension.
   f. Cardiac arrhythmias.
   g. Coma.
3. None of the antipsychotics can be removed by dialysis. Treatment usually includes activated charcoal and symptom-directed supportive care.

SWITCHING ANTIPSYCHOTICS

1. There are no established evidence-based methods for switching from one antipsychotic to the other. Three common methods are used.
   a. Immediately discontinuing drug A while starting drug B at full dosage.

   b. Slowly tapering drug A while starting drug B at full dosage.
   c. Slowly tapering drug A while slowly increasing drug B to full dosage (cross-titration).
2. Cross-titration is the most widely recommended method. There is no clear evidence indicating how quickly to make the transition. The general recommendation is 3 to 7 days for inpatients and 1 to 3 weeks for outpatients. If clozapine is being replaced, tapering can even take longer, because incidence of acute psychosis is higher with quick discontinuation.

USE OF ANTIPSYCHOTICS IN PREGNANCY

1. All antipsychotics are classified as pregnancy category C except clozapine, which is a category B drug.
2. No specific teratogenic deformity is associated with the typical antipsychotic agents; however, they should be used only if absolutely necessary during pregnancy, especially during the first trimester.
3. If the baby is exposed to typical antipsychotics during the last trimester, he or she can manifest EPS during the first weeks of life.
4. Chlorpromazine has been associated with neonatal jaundice.
5. Clozapine and olanzapine apparently do not increase the teratogenic risk. Data on use of other atypical agents are limited. However, there have been reports that women who have schizophrenia and who are taking atypical antipsychotics have a higher risk of neural tube defects in their infants because of the associated low intake of folate and obesity, although weight gain is not uniform with all atypicals.
6. It is not yet known whether quetiapine, ziprasidone, and aripiprazole are excreted in breast milk. All other antipsychotic agents are secreted in breast milk. The general recommendation is that women should not breast-feed while on antipsychotics.

OTHER INDICATIONS FOR ANTIPSYCHOTICS

1. Delirium.
   a. Although antipsychotics are widely and frequently used for delirium, none of the antipsychotics have FDA indication for treatment of delirium.
   b. Low-dose antipsychotics are generally helpful in decreasing the agitation, disorganization, and perceptual dysfunction in delirious patients.
      (1) Medical patients with confusion, but without significant physical agitation, can benefit from the temporary use of haloperidol 0.5 mg bid or risperidone 0.5 mg bid.
      (2) The cognitive and behavioral effects of delirium can continue for many days after the underlying medical etiology is corrected.
   c. Sundowning in elderly or medically ill patients might respond to antipsychotics, but the actual etiology for sundowning is not known.
      (1) Low-dose antipsychotics can effectively decrease agitation and confusion associated with sundowning.

(2) Such an approach might become a standing order in nursing home patients, but the drug should be tapered or reduced after several weeks to see if it is still necessary (see Chapter 5 for OBRA regulations).

(3) In general, delirium is better managed with standing orders of low-dose antipsychotic agents than with prn orders.

d. Delirium with significant physical agitation can require larger doses of antipsychotics (see Chapter 14), along with 1 to 2 mg of lorazepam every few hours.

2. Psychotic depression and bipolar disorder.

   a. Combination treatment with an antipsychotic and an antidepressant is the treatment of choice for major depression with psychotic features, although ECT may be more effective. Because of potential for side effects, these drugs are not indicated for maintenance treatment and should be discontinued once remission is achieved.

   b. Of the atypicals, olanzapine and quetiapine are currently approved for acute and maintenance treatment of bipolar mania. Ziprasidone and risperidone are only approved for acute bipolar mania.

3. Dementia.

   a. Alzheimer's disease has a psychotic component in 20% to 40% of Alzheimer's patients, and many of these patients warrant judicious use of antipsychotics (see Chapter 5).

   b. The atypical agents used in low doses appear to be better tolerated in this population.

   c. Agitated dementia patients can benefit from doses as low as risperidone 0.25 mg bid.

4. Nausea, emesis, and hiccups.

   a. Low-potency typical antipsychotics exert potent antiemetic effect via H_1 antagonism

   b. Chlorpromazine is also approved as oral, IM, or IV treatment of intractable hiccup, depending on severity.

5. Tourette's syndrome. Pimozide is the only atypical approved for this disorder.

6. For psychotic patients who do not respond to antipsychotics, consider the following:

   a. Is the diagnosis correct? Could there be, for example, an underlying sedative withdrawal syndrome that is not responsive to antipsychotics, requiring benzodiazepines?

   b. Has the patient developed akathisia, with increased restlessness and agitation, requiring dose reduction or the use of β-blockers or benzodiazepines?

   c. Has the patient developed NMS, with increased delirium, requiring immediate discontinuation of the antipsychotic and close medical observation?

   d. Has the patient been taking an adequate dose (and actually taking the medication) for long enough?

   e. Is the patient taking the medication?

12.5 Alternatives to Antipsychotics for Psychotic Symptoms of Schizophrenia

1. Electroconvulsive therapy (ECT) is generally not effective in schizophrenia, but it is occasionally tried to treat nonresponsive patients who have severe symptoms. ECT is effective, however, in catatonia.
2. Mood stabilizers. Of all the mood stabilizers, only valproic acid and lamotrigine have been shown to have benefit when combined with antipsychotics.
3. Adjunctive use of antidepressants can help accompanying depressive symptoms.
4. Adjunctive benzodiazepines are occasionally helpful in controlling agitated behavior.

12.6 Nonpharmacologic Aspects of Treating Schizophrenia

Nonpharmacologic treatment is important to rehabilitation and recovery.

1. A number of psychosocial treatments have demonstrated effectiveness during the stable phase. They are often best coordinated by a case manager, especially for patients with chronic illness.
   a. Family intervention.
   b. Supported employment.
   c. Assertive community treatment.
   d. Social skills training.
   e. Cognitive behavior therapy (focusing on residual positive symptoms using belief modification, using focusing and reattribution, and normalizing the psychotic experience).
2. The chronic schizophrenic patient cannot usually be adequately treated unless these multidimensional, community-based methods are individually tailored for each patient in an integrated program.

SUGGESTED READINGS

Adams CE, Fenton MK, Quraishi S, David AS: Systematic meta-review of depot antipsychotic drugs for people with schizophrenia. Br J Psychiatry 179:290-299, 2001.

Altamura AC, Sassella F, Santini A, et al: Intramuscular preparations of antipsychotics: Uses and relevance in clinical practice. Drugs 63(5):493-512, 2003.

Arnold LM, Strakowski SM, Schwiers ML, et al: Sex, ethnicity, and antipsychotic medication use in patients with psychosis. Schizophr Res 66(2-3):169-175, 2004.

Bressan RA, Jones HM, Pilowsky LS: Atypical antipsychotic drugs and tardive dyskinesia: Relevance of D_2 receptor affinity. J Psychopharmacol 18(1):124-127, 2004.

Gentile S: Clinical utilization of atypical antipsychotics in pregnancy and lactation. Ann Pharmacother 38(7-8):1265-1271, 2004.

Green AI, Canuso CM, Brenner MJ, Wojcik JD: Detection and management of comorbidity in patients with schizophrenia. Psychiatr Clin North Am 26(1):115-139, 2003.

Holt RI, Peveler RC, Byrne CD: Schizophrenia, the metabolic syndrome and diabetes. Diabet Med 21(6):515-523, 2004.

Jeste DV, Gladsjo JA, Lindamer LA, Lacro JP: Medical comorbidity in schizophrenia. *Schizophr Bull* 22(3):413-430, 1996.

Kane JM, Aguglia E, Altamura AC, et al: Guidelines for depot antipsychotic treatment in schizophrenia. European Neuropsychopharmacology Consensus Conference in Siena, Italy. *Eur Neuropsychopharmacol* 8(1):55-66, 1998.

Kane JM, Davis JM, Schooler N, et al: A multidose study of haloperidol decanoate in the maintenance treatment of schizophrenia. *Am J Psychiatry* 159(4):554-560, 2002.

Knegtering H, van der Moolen AE, Castelein S, et al: What are the effects of antipsychotics on sexual dysfunctions and endocrine functioning? *Psychoneuroendocrinology* 28(Suppl 2):109-123, 2003.

Koren G, Cohn T, Chitayat D, et al: Use of atypical antipsychotics during pregnancy and the risk of neural tube defects in infants. *Am J Psychiatry* 159(1):136-137, 2002.

Kroeze WK, Hufeisen SJ, Popadak BA, et al: H_1-histamine receptor affinity predicts short-term weight gain for typical and atypical antipsychotic drugs. *Neuropsychopharmacology* 28(3):519-526, 2003.

Lehman AF, Kreyenbuhl J, Buchanan RW, et al: The Schizophrenia Patient Outcomes Research Team (PORT): Updated treatment recommendations 2003. *Schizophr Bull* 30(2):193-217, 2004.

Lehman AF, Lieberman JA, Dixon LB, et al: Practice guideline for the treatment of patients with schizophrenia, second edition. *Am J Psychiatry* 161(2 Suppl):1-56, 2004.

Littrell KH, Johnson CG, Peabody CD, Hilligoss N: Antipsychotics during pregnancy. *Am J Psychiatry* 157(8):1342, 2000.

Prior TI, Baker GB: Interactions between the cytochrome P450 system and the second-generation antipsychotics. *J Psychiatry Neurosci* 28(2):99-112, 2003.

Sacchetti E, Valsecchi P: Quetiapine, clozapine, and olanzapine in the treatment of tardive dyskinesia induced by first-generation antipsychotics: A 124-week case report. *Int Clin Psychopharmacol* 18(6):357-359, 2003.

Schachter DC, Kleinman I: Psychiatrists' attitudes about and informed consent practices for antipsychotics and tardive dyskinesia. *Psychiatr Serv* 55(6):714-717, 2004.

Tauscher J, Hussain T, Agid O, et al: Equivalent occupancy of dopamine D_1 and D_2 receptors with clozapine: Differentiation from other atypical antipsychotics. *Am J Psychiatry* 161(9):1620-1625, 2004.

Somatoform Disorders

13

Colin J. Harrington

13.1 Overview

1. The somatoform disorders are defined as a group of disorders in which:
   a. Physical symptoms suggest a medical disorder for which there is no demonstrable pathology or inadequate evidence of an underlying physical basis, and
   b. There is a strong presumption that the symptoms are linked to psychological factors.
2. The *process of somatization* is common to all somatoform disorders and is marked by:
   a. The manifestation of psychological stress in somatic symptoms.
   b. Abnormal *illness behavior* notable for a mismatch between perceived illness and documented disease.
   c. Amplification is the process by which physical sensation and symptoms lead to anxiety about their significance, then anxiety and its associated autonomic activation lead to a focus on and exacerbation of symptoms.
   d. Significant patient distress and repeat medical visits.
   e. Not all somatizing patients have frank somatoform disorders. Some degree of association between psychological stress and physical symptoms is normal.
3. The somatoform disorders include the following:
   a. Somatization disorder.
   b. Undifferentiated somatoform disorder.
   c. Conversion disorder.
   d. Pain disorder (associated with psychological factors or with both psychological factors and a general medical condition).
   e. Hypochondriasis.
   f. Body dysmorphic disorder (BDD).
   g. Somatoform disorder not otherwise specified (NOS).
4. Although not classified in the *Diagnostic and Statistical Manual of Mental Disorders*, fourth edition (DSM-IV), as "somatoform disorders," the following will also be addressed in this chapter:
   a. Acute somatized symptoms.
   b. Factitious disorder (classified as a distinct category or diagnosis).
   c. Malingering (listed under "other conditions that may be a focus of clinical attention").

13.2 Somatization Disorder

DEFINITION AND IDENTIFICATION

1. Somatization *disorder* represents an extreme form of somatization in which multiple unexplained symptoms are experienced across numerous organ systems.
2. Some chronic forms of somatization might not meet the full diagnostic criteria for somatization disorder and are classified as undifferentiated somatoform disorders as discussed later.
3. Somatization disorder is marked by:
   a. A history of many physical complaints (or the belief that one is sick) beginning before 30 years of age, lasting for several years, and resulting in either medical seeking behavior or significant impairment.
   b. A combination of the following unexplained symptoms:
      (1) Four pain symptoms (involving at least four different sites or functions, including head and neck, abdomen, back, joints, extremities, chest, rectum, during menstruation, during sexual intercourse, during urination).
      (2) Two gastrointestinal symptoms other than pain (including nausea, bloating, vomiting, diarrhea, or food intolerance).
      (3) One sexual symptom (e.g., sexual indifference, sexual dysfunction, irregular menses, excessive menstrual bleeding, vomiting during pregnancy).
      (4) One pseudoneurologic symptom not limited to pain (including balance difficulties, weakness, difficulty swallowing, aphonia, urinary retention, hallucinations, loss of sensation, double vision, blindness, deafness, seizures, dissociation, loss of consciousness other than fainting).
   c. These symptoms are not the result of an identified medical condition, or if a medical condition does exist, the symptoms and their effects on the patient exceed what would be expected for this condition.
   d. The symptoms are not consciously feigned or intentionally produced.

PREVALENCE

1. Lifetime prevalence for somatization disorder is less than 2% and is higher in female patients.
2. More common are patients who have unexplained somatic symptoms but do not meet full criteria for somatization disorder. Most primary care practitioners recognize chronic somatization as a common problem.
3. Patients with a history of somatization who do not meet full (specific symptom number and site) criteria for somatization disorder are classified as having "undifferentiated somatoform disorder" (a residual diagnostic category), which is marked by:
   a. One or more physical complaints not limited to pain (typically fatigue, loss of appetite, or gastrointestinal or urinary symptoms).
   b. Symptoms are not a result of a known medical condition, or if a medical condition is present, the symptoms and their effects on the patient are in excess of what would be expected.

   c. Symptoms are not consciously feigned or intentionally produced.

   d. Duration of symptoms is 6 months or longer.

   e. Symptoms are not the result of another mental disorder associated with physical complaints (such as depression).

4. There is a potential association between sexual abuse and somatization, with high rates of abuse noted in patients with chronic pelvic pain syndromes and functional gastrointestinal disorders.

DIFFERENTIAL DIAGNOSIS

1. Medical disorders that manifest with multiple, vague, and unexplained chronic somatic symptoms can be misdiagnosed as somatization. Occult cancers, chronic infections, and endocrine, rheumatologic, and neurologic disorders must be carefully considered before arriving at a diagnosis of somatization. Medical evaluation of polysomatic complaints might reveal the following diagnoses:

   a. Thyroid and parathyroid disease.

   b. Adrenal disease.

   c. Porphyria.

   d. Multiple sclerosis.

   e. Systemic lupus erythematosus and other vasculitides.

   f. Myasthenia gravis.

   g. Endometriosis.

   h. Fibromyalgia.

   i. Early stages of occult malignancy.

   j. Syphilis.

   k. Lyme disease.

   l. Human immunodeficiency virus (HIV) infection.

   m. Temporomandibular joint syndrome.

   n. Irritable bowel disease and frank inflammatory bowel disease.

   o. Chronic fatigue syndrome.

2. Psychiatric disorders that are often associated with somatic symptoms must also be considered in the primary differential diagnosis or as co-occurring diagnoses. Relevant psychiatric diagnoses include:

   a. Schizophrenia with multiple somatic delusions and delusional disorder (somatic type).

     (1) In schizophrenia, somatic complaints are usually more bizarre, and frank psychotic signs and symptoms such as hallucinations and thought disorder are noted (see Chapter 12)

     (2) In delusional disorder (somatic type), specific somatic preoccupation of delusional proportions exists in isolation (without associated signs and symptoms of schizophrenia), beliefs about somatic symptoms are less bizarre (and possibly plausible), and thought disorder is absent.

   b. Panic disorder, in which the physical symptoms are episodic and occur only during a panic attack.

   c. Malingering, in which symptoms are consciously produced for the purpose of clearly definable secondary gain such as acquisition of medication or for avoidance of financial, legal, family, or work obligations. The presence of an unresolved lawsuit or disability claim can make assessment complicated.

   d. Factitious disorder, in which the person fabricates symptoms or misrepresents history for no clear secondary gain, presumably for the purpose of playing the sick role. Factitious disorder patients are thought not to be fully aware of the motivations for their behavior.
   e. Chronic depression, in which the patient might present with physical symptoms as a component of the affective illness.
   f. Generalized anxiety, with multiple somatic manifestations (see Box 9-1).
   g. Substance abuse, which can account for many confusing symptoms, especially if it is surreptitious.

PROGNOSIS

1. Somatization disorder tends to be chronic and fluctuating in its course. Complete remission is rare.
2. With proper management (see next section) somatization disorder can be contained, but it is usually not cured.

TREATMENT

1. Realistic expectations of treatment must be established in approaching the somatization disorder patient. The focus of clinical attention should be on management rather than cure.
2. The following clinical points help to guide a generally accepted treatment strategy that is based on assumptions about the underlying psychological needs of these patients:
   a. Patients do not necessarily desire relief but may seek a relationship with and understanding from the practitioner.
   b. Patients want and require the physician to acknowledge they are sick.
   c. Titrate reassurance carefully. Patients are often resistant to reassurance that nothing is physically, identifiably wrong with them and are sensitive to the suggestion that symptoms are psychologically based.
   d. Treatment should emphasize "care not cure" because a medical diagnosis will not fully resolve symptoms.
   e. Avoid dichotomous "mind—body" approaches to symptom interpretation.
   f. Acknowledge patient distress and that a problem exists, and show a willingness to help.
   g. Little is gained by a premature explanation that symptoms are based on emotions or psychological factors.
      (1) Avoid engaging in early discussion of primary versus secondary relationships between physical and psychological symptoms.
      (2) When such an explanation is eventually offered, it should be done gradually and in a way that makes the patient feel understood and taken seriously. Avoid any suggestion that symptoms are "all in their head" because these patients are sensitive to the perception of being dismissed.
   h. The emphasis should be on optimization of function.
      (1) Try to understand the patient's stresses and coping resources and set targets for more adaptive health-related behavior.

(2) Reinforce nonillness behavior and communication. Whenever possible, discuss and address things other than physical symptoms.
(3) Educate about the intimate relationship between symptoms of body, brain, and mind using examples from everyday life (e.g., flushing when embarrassed, dry mouth when speaking in public, headache when chronically stressed, chest tightness and racing heart when acutely anxious).

  i. Schedule regular appointments to eliminate the need for the patient to manifest symptoms to seek help.
  j. Limit diagnostic tests and unnecessary medications. Some focused physical examination and occasional laboratory tests may be helpful (for both physician and patient), with more reliance on signs than symptoms.
  k. Group therapy with a cognitive behavior focus may be helpful as well.
3. Psychiatric input can lower costs of managing somatizing patients. Low-cost educational interventions can have a significant impact on the medical care costs and functional level of some somatizing patients (Smith, 1995).

13.3 Acute Somatized Symptoms

DEFINITION
Acute somatized symptoms are defined as abrupt-onset somatic symptoms occurring in the setting of and associated with marked psychological stress. Most people experience transient physical manifestations of stress. Acutely somatized distress is a common reason for medical visits.

PREVALENCE
Acute somatized symptoms are ubiquitous and are likely to account for a high percentage of symptoms in primary care.

DIFFERENTIAL DIAGNOSIS
1. Medical disorders. In addition to the chronic, recurrent medical disorders needing diagnostic consideration in the patient with somatization disorder, acute medical problems can be associated with novel, difficult emotional situations.
   a. Patients under intense stress can develop myocardial ischemia or infarction, stroke, or asthma exacerbation. DSM-IV refers to this as a stress-related physiologic response.
   b. No matter what the emotional context, acute somatic symptoms must always be medically evaluated.
2. Psychiatric disorders. The psychiatric differential diagnosis is the same as that for chronic somatization, with possible extra emphasis on panic disorder (see Box 9-4).

PROGNOSIS
Acute somatized symptoms generally respond to brief interventions including education, psychosocial support, and limited pharmacologic treatment (e.g., short-term benzodiazepine use).

TREATMENT

1. Identify the relevant psychosocial issues by a thorough psychiatric assessment (see "Psychosocial Review of Systems" in Chapter 2).
2. Do a physical evaluation and examination to assure the patient (and physician) that appropriate medical diagnoses are being considered.
3. Explain that the acute physical symptom is linked to the underlying distress. For example, you might explain that "when people get very stressed, they often experience chest tightness."
4. Reassure the patient that there is no acute, life-threatening illness that requires urgent medical treatment.
5. Follow up with treatment or referral that addresses the underlying psychosocial distress (e.g., office counseling or brief therapy).

13.4 Conversion Disorder

DEFINITION AND IDENTIFICATION

1. *Conversion disorder* is defined as the loss of physical or neurologic function that suggests a physical disorder but that cannot be accounted for by examination, laboratory, or imaging findings. The diagnostic name suggests that unconscious psychic conflict is *converted* into somatic symptoms, with associated reduction in anxiety, symbolic resolution of conflict, and prevention of conflict from reaching conscious awareness. These functions are referred to as *primary gain* to differentiate them from the *secondary gain* of malingering.
2. Criteria for conversion disorder.
   a. Loss of or alteration in voluntary motor or sensory functioning that suggests a neurologic or other medical disorder (e.g., paralysis, anesthesia, paresthesia, ataxia, blindness, convulsions).
   b. Symptoms do not conform to known anatomic patterns or physiologic mechanisms (sometimes referred to as *pseudoneurologic*).
   c. Psychological factors are judged to be associated with symptom onset or exacerbation. Current criteria, however, do not require the demonstration of a specific symbolic relationship between physical symptoms and a psychological stressor, as in earlier psychodynamic theory.
   d. Symptoms are not consciously produced.
   e. Symptoms are not the result of a medical condition, substance use, or culturally sanctioned behavior.
   f. The symptom causes distress or impairment in functioning.
   g. Symptoms are not limited to pain or sexual dysfunction. When psychological factors are thought to play a significant role in the onset, severity, exacerbation, or maintenance of pain as the primary complaint, the disorder is classified as *pain disorder*.
   h. Symptoms are not better accounted for by some other mental disorder.

PREVALENCE

1. There are limited data on the prevalence of conversion disorders. Estimates of the prevalence of conversion disorder in outpatient medical practice range from 1% to 3% of visits.
2. Conversion disorder is significantly more common in women.
3. Conversion disorder is more prevalent in rural populations, developing countries, and settings of lower socioeconomic status and medical knowledge.
4. Classic pseudoneurologic symptoms, such as loss of function of a limb, are unusual but are still seen.
5. Less dramatic conversion symptoms, such as chest pain developing after the death of a loved one by heart attack, remain quite common.
6. Psychogenic nonepileptic seizures (pseudoseizures) are considered by many to be a common presentation of conversion disorder.

DIFFERENTIAL DIAGNOSIS

1. Medical disorders.
    a. A similar list of medical disorders presented in the section on somatization should be considered before making a diagnosis of conversion disorder.
    b. In earlier follow-up studies of conversion disorder, a substantial fraction of cases were eventually identified as medical problems, such as multiple sclerosis. More recent studies suggest less frequent mislabeling of conversion disorder, perhaps due to the use of more sensitive diagnostic laboratory and imaging tools.
2. Psychiatric disorders. Refer to the list of diagnoses in the section on somatization disorders.

PROGNOSIS

1. Conversion disorder symptoms are generally of short duration, with or without intervention. Symptoms typically resolve in 2 weeks or less.
2. Conversion symptom recurrence is common, with up to 25% of patients re-experiencing symptoms within a year of the initial presentation.
3. Some patients experience chronic symptoms.
4. Good prognostic features include acute onset of symptoms, identifiable precipitating stressors, short duration of symptoms, higher level of intelligence, symptoms of paralysis, and symptoms of blindness. Symptoms of seizure or tremor suggest a poorer prognosis.

TREATMENT

Before initiating treatment, keep the following in mind:

1. Conversion symptoms exist for the theoretical purpose of protecting the patient from some intolerable psychological situation.
2. Removal of this defense (e.g., by use of hypnosis) can leave the patient feeling overwhelmed and vulnerable.
3. Treatments must include a component that addresses the underlying psychological distress as well as the specific physical symptom.

Nonpharmacologic Treatment

Strong suggestion and empathic education and reassurance are the mainstays of treatment for conversion symptoms. As in the case of somatization, explanations about the intimate relationship among mind, brain, and physical symptoms should be explained. The physician is advised to speak realistically and humbly about the understanding of these symptoms and to speak confidently about their typically prompt resolution.

Interviewing under Amobarbital or Hypnosis

When suggestion and education are unsuccessful, hypnosis and amobarbital (Amytal) interviewing can be considered.

1. Use of these methods requires special training and experience.
2. These methods can facilitate uncovering of a suspected underlying psychological conflict.
3. Under the altered state induced by hypnosis or amobarbital, the symptom can temporarily or permanently disappear:
   a. For many physical complaints, the nonspecific effects of relaxation can account for symptom improvement (such as decreased pain, tremors, or autonomic symptoms).
   b. The "reversal" of a major symptom, such as limb paralysis, is a strong indicator of a psychological basis for the symptom.
   c. Because amobarbital is a barbiturate with anticonvulsant effects, it can ameliorate symptoms caused by a real seizure disorder.
4. Sequential clinical interviews may be required.
5. It is not clear that amobarbital or hypnosis results in faster resolution of conversion symptoms than sequential clinical interviews.

Indications

Hypnosis and amobarbital interviews are indicated as an aid in the differential diagnosis and treatment of the following conditions:

1. Recovery of function of conversion pseudoneurologic symptoms.
2. Differentiation between conversion and malingering.
3. Abreaction of posttraumatic stress disorder.
4. Recovery of memory in psychogenic fugue and amnesia.

Contraindications and Risks

1. Medical contraindications to amobarbital interviewing.
   a. Absolute contraindications.
      (1) Barbiturate allergy.
      (2) History of porphyria.
   b. Relative contraindications.
      (1) Respiratory infection or inflammation compromising airway function.
      (2) Severe cardiac impairment, including congestive heart failure (CHF), and hepatic, renal, or pulmonary impairment.
      (3) Barbiturate addiction.
      (4) Hypotension or significant hypertension, if more than 500 mg is to be used.
      (5) It is necessary to wait at least 12 hours after the last drink if alcohol intoxication is suspected.

2. Psychiatric contraindications to hypnosis and amobarbital interviewing.
   a. Paranoia. For example, the patient might feel that "the doctor is attempting to read my mind" or may be concerned of ideas of "thought control" or manipulation.
   b. Patient refusal of the procedure.
   c. Unrealistic expectations or expectations of a magical cure.
3. Risks of amobarbital interviewing.
   a. Primary risk is respiratory, usually associated with too-rapid administration of the amobarbital solution (> 50 mg/min) or too much total drug (> 500 mg), leading to excessive sedation, apnea, or airway closure.
   b. Vasomotor collapse and laryngospasm are rare complications and are also typically associated with excessive sedation and deeper levels of anesthesia.
   c. Psychotic regression.
   d. Prolonged abreactive states mimicking a psychotic break.

Method

Amobarbital interviewing procedure.

1. The purpose of the procedure should be explained fully and the patient should be reassured. Patients should be invited to ask any questions they have.
2. The patient (or an appropriate surrogate decision maker) should give formal consent.
3. It should be emphasized that amobarbital is not a "truth serum."
4. Patients should be told that any remarks made and information learned are confidential.
5. A relative or trusted friend should be available to accompany the patient home if the procedure is done on an outpatient basis and to remain in attendance during the procedure if the patient wishes.
6. Additional hospital personnel should be available if restraint is required for an untoward abreaction.
7. A quiet room should be used.
8. Resuscitation equipment and staff knowledgeable in its use must be available.
9. Vital signs must be regularly monitored.
10. Patients should recline and be told that the medication will make them relax and feel like talking.
11. Insert a 21-gauge intravenous needle.
12. Infuse a 5% solution of amobarbital (500 mg of amobarbital dissolved in 10 mL of sterile water) at a rate of no faster than 1 mL/min (50 mg/min) to prevent respiratory depression or apnea. If using a 10% solution, do not exceed 1 mL/min.
13. Engage the patient.
    a. Begin with neutral topics.
    b. If the patient is mute, suggest to the patient that he or she will soon feel like talking.
    c. Prompt the patient with known facts about his or her life.

14. The infusion should be continued until one of the following occurs:
    a. Drowsiness, slurring of speech, or sustained lateral nystagmus.
    b. The patient begins making mistakes while counting backwards from 100.
    c. Sedation threshold is usually between 150 mg and 350 mg (3 to 7 mL). However, elderly or cognitively impaired patients might respond to as little as 75 mg (1.5 mL).
15. Proceed gradually with questions aiming at more affect-laden topics.
16. If the patient is mute or verbally inhibited, do not press too hard on potentially frightening topics so as to prevent undue anxiety during the interview.
17. Continue to infuse amobarbital at a rate of 0.5 to 1.0 mL approximately every 5 minutes with the 5% solution to maintain an adequate level of narcosis.
18. The interview may last from 15 minutes to 1 hour; the average interview length is 30 minutes.
19. The interview may be concluded by returning to neutral topics and/or by making generally supportive statements.
20. The patient should remain supine for a minimum of 15 minutes until he or she is able to walk without assistance. Some advise 2 to 5 hours of in-bed supervision.

13.5 Pain Disorder

DEFINITION
1. Pain is the predominant focus of clinical attention (acute or chronic).
2. Psychological factors are considered to play a role in the patient's experience of pain and treatment-seeking behavior.
3. Pain symptoms are not feigned or intentionally misreported or produced.
4. Two subtypes.
    a. Pain disorder associated with psychological factors, where identifiable medical disorders are thought to play little or no role in the onset, severity, or persistence of pain.
    b. Pain disorder associated with both psychological factors and a general medical condition, where medical and psychological factors are operative in the patient's experience of pain, and pain is out of proportion to or in excess of what would be expected from the medical condition alone.

PREVALENCE
1. Pain complaints and disorders are extremely common in general medical and psychiatric practice.
2. Pain complaints and disorders are often associated with iatrogenic opioid and benzodiazepine dependence.
3. Chronic pain is often associated with depressive symptoms.

DIFFERENTIAL DIAGNOSIS
1. Acute or chronic pain complaints that are fully explained by an identifiable medical disorder are coded in Axis III as *medical*

pain disorders. Thus, a full medical evaluation of pain complaints is necessary before arriving at a diagnosis of psychologically based pain disorder.

2. Somatization disorder is marked by pain complaints, but patients also experience pseudoneurologic and other unexplained nonpain symptoms across numerous organ systems that are specific to a diagnosis of somatization disorder.

3. Conversion disorder is marked by loss of function (pseudoneurologic) rather than by pain symptoms.

4. Hypochondriasis can involve the experience of pain, but it is the misinterpretation of and worry about the diagnostic significance of pain or nonpain symptoms that defines hypochondriasis.

5. Pain complaints may be a part of factitious and malingering disorders, but unlike pain disorder, these patients intentionally misrepresent their symptoms and misreport their history of alleged underlying medical conditions. Secondary gain, including the acquisition of narcotic analgesic medications, can often be identified in cases of malingering.

TREATMENT

1. Identify and treat any identifiable medical contributors to pain symptoms.

2. Like somatization and hypochondriasis, the goal of treatment is *management* rather than frank *cure.*

3. Chronic pain clinics with a multidisciplinary approach are often helpful and demonstrate to the patient that their symptoms are being taken seriously.

4. Behavioral approaches that emphasize acceptance of a certain degree of pain and the goal of optimization of function despite residual pain are most successful.

5. Treatment contracts that carefully outline the prescription and use of opiates and benzodiazepines can help to minimize problems of iatrogenic dependence.

13.6 Hypochondriasis

DEFINITION

1. Preoccupation with or fear that one has a disease despite a negative diagnostic evaluation.

2. Fears are based upon misinterpretation and misattribution of normal somatic sensation and findings (e.g., headache, abdominal distention, chest tightness, rapid heart rate, cough, musculoskeletal pains, skin changes).

3. The fear or preoccupation persists despite medical reassurance.

4. The duration of symptoms and preoccupation is 6 months or longer.

PREVALENCE

Estimates of prevalence in outpatient general medical practice range from 4% to 9%.

DIFFERENTIAL DIAGNOSIS

1. Medical disorders. Refer to the list of differential diagnostic considerations in somatization disorder patients.
   a. Rheumatologic, endocrinologic, neurologic, chronic infectious, and occult malignant conditions must be *ruled out before* arriving at a diagnosis of hypochondriasis.
   b. Fibromyalgia, irritable bowel syndrome, chronic fatigue syndrome, and temporomandibular joint syndrome are common *comorbid* diagnoses in patients considered to be hypochondriacal.
2. Psychiatric disorders. Refer to the list for somatization disorder.
   a. Preoccupation with illness and physical symptoms may be a form of obsessive–compulsive disorder (OCD). These two disorders can be difficult to distinguish.
   b. Somatic concerns are a common aspect of affective illness and anxiety diagnoses (e.g., major depression and generalized anxiety disorder) but resolve with effective treatment of these disorders.
   c. Somatic concerns can emerge in the early stages of dementing illness. Cognitive dysfunction is a primary finding in these cases.
   d. Schizophrenic patients sometimes focus on a delusional belief of a physical disorder, but other psychotic-spectrum signs and symptoms predominate.
   e. Isolated somatic preoccupation of delusional proportions can qualify as "delusional disorder, somatic type" when other signs and symptoms of frank schizophrenia are absent (e.g., hallucinations, thought disorder, bizarre delusions, flat affect).
   f. Somatic preoccupation restricted to a concern about personal appearance may be categorized as BDD (see later).
   g. If there is clear evidence of secondary gain, the presentation may be better explained by a diagnosis of malingering.
   h. Hypochondriacal patients often have depression, anxiety, or some other somatoform disorder.

PROGNOSIS

Hypochondriasis tends to be chronic, with periods of remission and exacerbation associated with stress.

TREATMENT

1. Patience and reassurance are crucial because hypochondriacal patients are high utilizers of medical resources and physician time.
2. Psychotherapy.
   a. Psychoanalytic psychotherapy is generally not helpful.
   b. Supportive therapy may be helpful when it consists of the following:
      (1) Accurate information about symptoms.
      (2) Education about misperception and misinterpretation of symptoms and somatic sensation.
      (3) Regular brief visits and physical examinations.
      (4) Reassurance.
      (5) Brief use of anxiolytic medications during periods of high stress.

   c. Cognitive behavior therapy (CBT) has become the treatment of choice when available and consists of:
      (1) Methods aimed to educate about and alter the patient's automatic dysfunctional thought pattern and misinterpretation of internal stimuli.
      (2) Behavioral methods of exposure to the feared situations and somatic cues that trigger anxiety and its escalation in the face of associated autonomic activation.
3. Pharmacotherapy.
   a. Antidepressants often reduce the hypochondria symptoms in somatically preoccupied depressed patients.
   b. Selective serotonin reuptake inhibitors (SSRIs) and serotoninergic tricyclic agents (clomipramine) may be helpful for patients whose somatic preoccupation is part of an OCD syndrome.
   c. Antipanic agents may be helpful for patients with comorbid panic disorder and hypochondriasis (e.g., SSRIs, benzodiazepines).
   d. For hypochondriacal patients without comorbid psychiatric diagnoses, there is some evidence that SSRIs alone may be helpful, usually in higher doses than those used for depression (e.g., fluoxetine or paroxetine in doses up to 60 mg/day or sertraline in doses of at least 150 mg/day).
   e. Antipsychotic agents are indicated when hypochondriacal preoccupation is part of a psychotic disorder such as schizophrenia or delusional disorder, somatic type.

13.7 Body Dysmorphic Disorder

DEFINITION

1. Body dysmorphic disorder (BDD) is marked by preoccupation with imagined defects in or exaggeration of real features of physical appearance.
2. The disorder typically begins between adolescence and midlife and consists of a pervasive feeling that some body part is ugly, distorted, or defective:
   a. Patients can usually acknowledge some degree of exaggeration of their concern, but they still feel that the problem is significant.
   b. When insight into the abnormal nature of BDD symptoms is lost, these patients can appear frankly delusional.
3. BDD patients often consult dermatologists, primary physicians, and plastic surgeons and often undergo unnecessary surgery and other cosmetic procedures.

DIFFERENTIAL DIAGNOSIS

1. Depression. Somatic preoccupation resolves with treatment of the mood disorder.
2. BDD is phenomenologically (and possibly neurobiologically) related to OCD and may be difficult to distinguish. BDD patients often spend hours thinking about their appearance and engage in repetitive mirror checking.

3. Anorexia nervosa. Preoccupation is with body weight, size, and shape and is associated with compensatory behavior such as diet restriction, diuretic and/or cathartic use, and excessive exercise (see Chapter 18).
4. Transsexualism. Somatic preoccupation is limited to gender-related physical characteristics.
5. Schizophrenia with somatic delusions. Patients have associated psychotic signs and symptoms.
6. Delusional disorder, somatic type. Schizophrenia-spectrum symptoms other than delusions are absent and the somatic delusion is not restricted to concern of body appearance.

TREATMENT

1. There is little evidence to support the effectiveness of performing requested surgery to repair the perceived defect. Indeed, surgery should be assiduously avoided when a diagnosis of BDD is suspected.
2. Among psychotherapy options, cognitive behavior treatments appear to be most effective.
3. Medications used to treat OCD (SSRIs and clomipramine) can offer some relief to patients with BDD.
4. Antipsychotic agents may be indicated if insight into preoccupation with bodily appearance is lost and/or symptoms are of psychotic proportions.
5. BDD is often comorbid with depression, and antidepressants are indicated in this case.

13.8 Factitious Disorder

DEFINITION

1. Factitious disorder is marked by the intentional production or feigning of physical or psychological signs or symptoms.
2. Patients often misreport their medical histories in dramatic fashion.
3. The motivation for the behavior is unclear and is presumed to be for the purpose of assuming the sick role. While the patient is aware of the voluntary production of symptoms, he or she is thought to be unaware of any conscious motivations for the behavior.
4. In contrast to malingering, external incentives and secondary gain such as financial compensation or avoidance of work, social, legal, or military obligations cannot be easily identified.

MUNCHAUSEN SYNDROME

1. *Munchausen syndrome* is a term that has been used to describe a severe form of factitious disorder characterized by:
   a. Pathologic lying and dramatic accounts of medical history (pseudologica fantastica).
   b. Extensive travel across multiple medical settings and institutions for the purpose of seeking medical care (and presumably to avoid detection).

CLINICAL PRESENTATION

1. Patients with factitious disorder are often:
   a. Young women employed in the health professions.

    b. Men of lower socioeconomic class with a lifelong pattern of social maladjustment.
2. Common accompanying features include:
    a. Personality disorders, typically cluster B (borderline and antisocial types).
    b. Higher than expected knowledge of medicine.
    c. Willingness to undergo uncomfortable and invasive procedures.
    d. History of multiple hospitalizations.
    e. Multiple surgical scars.

DIFFERENTIAL DIAGNOSIS

1. Diagnosis of factitious disorder requires a high index of suspicion. Factitious disorder should be considered when there are notable inconsistencies in examination findings and history.
2. Differential diagnosis includes:
    a. Conversion disorder. Symptoms are pseudoneurologic, associated with an identifiable stressor, and not intentionally produced.
    b. Malingering. Symptoms are intentionally produced, and identifiable secondary gain can be identified (as noted earlier).
    c. Mixed presentations are common, and features of each of these diagnoses can be seen in patients *within* and *across* different presentations. Differentiation between factitious disorder and malingering can be particularly difficult when administration of psychotropic medications (e.g., opiate narcotics and benzodiazepines) is part of the treatment. In some cases, both diagnoses are appropriate.

TREATMENT

1. General approaches used with somatizing patients (see earlier) can be helpful.
2. Performance of unnecessary invasive procedures should be carefully avoided.
3. Treatment of coexisting psychiatric conditions (e.g., depression, anxiety, psychotic symptoms) may be helpful.
4. Confrontation is typically met with denial and anger, and factitious disorder patients often sign out of the hospital against medical advice.
5. Patients with factitious disorder should be approached forthrightly and empathically in an attempt to clarify the diagnosis and enlist them into treatment.
6. Physicians must avoid acting negatively, angrily, or accusingly.
7. A description of the diagnosis and characteristics of factitious disorder, an explanation of the risks associated with factitious behavior, a genuine expression of interest in achieving accurate diagnosis, and an offer of treatment may succeed in gaining the patient's trust and an honest report of their history.
8. Any decision to search the patient, their room, or their belongings should be thoroughly discussed with both the patient and risk management and should be carefully documented.

13.9 Malingering

DEFINITION

1. The intentional production of signs or symptoms and/or misrepresentation of history.
2. The behavior is associated with and driven by clearly identifiable secondary gain (e.g., financial compensation, acquisition of psychotropic medication, or avoidance of work, social, legal, or military obligations).

CLINICAL CHARACTERISTICS

1. Malingering patients are more often male.
2. Malingering is often comorbid with cluster B personality disorders, typically borderline and antisocial types.

DIFFERENTIAL DIAGNOSIS

1. Conversion and factitious disorders must be considered before arriving at a sole diagnosis of malingering (as noted in factitious disorder discussion).
2. Mixed presentations with conversion and factitious features can occur both within and across patients and admissions.

TREATMENT

1. Like factitious disorder, malingering patients often react angrily to the suggestion that they may be intentionally producing their symptoms and leave the hospital against medical advice.
2. Malingering patients should be given the benefit of the doubt diagnostically (short of having unequivocal evidence of their behavior) and treated respectfully and compassionately with the goal of clarifying diagnosis and targeting safe treatment as described in the section on factitious disorders.
3. Any decision to search the patient, their room, or their belongings should be thoroughly discussed with both the patient and risk management and should be carefully documented.

13.10 Somatoform Disorder Not Otherwise Specified

This is a residual diagnostic category reserved for unexplained somatic presentations that do not meet criteria for any of the specific DSM-IV somatoform disorders described in this chapter.

SUGGESTED READINGS

Abbey SE: Somatization and somatoform disorders. In Levenson JL (ed): *Textbook of Psychosomatic Medicine*. Washington, DC, American Psychiatric Publishing, 2004, pp 271-296.

Abramowitz JS, Schwartz SA, Whiteside SP: A contemporary conceptual model of hypochondriasis. *Mayo Clin Proc* 77:1323-1330, 2002.

Allen LA, Escobar JI, Lehrer PM, et al: Psychosocial treatments for multiple unexplained physical symptoms: A review of the literature. *Psychosom Med* 64:939-950, 2002.

American Psychiatric Association: *Diagnostic and Statistical Manual of Mental Disorders*, 4th ed. Washington, DC, American Psychiatric Association, 1994.

Barsky AJ: The patient with hypochondriasis. N Engl J Med 345:1395-1399, 2001.

Barsky AJ, Ahern DK: Cognitive behavior therapy for hypochondriasis: A randomized controlled trial. JAMA 292:1464-1470, 2004.

Barsky AJ, Borus JF: Somatization and medicalization in the era of managed care. JAMA 274:1931-1934, 1995.

Barsky AJ, Klerman GL: Overview: hypochondriasis, bodily complaints, and somatic styles. Am J Psychiatry 140(3):273-283, 1983.

Brown FW, Golding JM, Smith GR: Psychiatric comorbidity in primary care somatization disorder. Psychosom Med 52:445-451, 1990.

deGruy F, Columbia L, Dickinson P: Somatization disorder in a family practice. J Fam Pract 25(1):45-51, 1987.

Epstein RM, Quill TE, McWhinney IR: Somatization reconsidered: Incorporating the patient's experience of illness. Arch Intern Med 159:215-222, 1999.

Fallon BA, Klein BW, Liebowitz MR: Hypochondriasis: Treatment strategies. Psychiatric Annals 23(7):374-381, 1993.

Folks DG, Feldman MD, Ford CV: Somatoform disorders, factitious disorders, and malingering. In Stoudemire A, Fogel BS, Greenberg DB (eds): Psychiatric Care of the Medical Patient. New York, Oxford University Press, 2000, pp 459-476.

Ford CV: Deception syndromes: Factitious disorders and malingering. In Levenson JL (ed): Textbook of Psychosomatic Medicine. Washington, DC, American Psychiatric Publishing, 2004, pp 297-310.

Goldberg RJ, Novack DH, Gask L: The recognition and management of somatization: What is needed in primary care training. Psychosomatics 33(1):55-61, 1992.

Heruti RJ, Reznik J, Adunski A, et al: Conversion motor paralysis disorder: Analysis of 34 consecutive referrals. Spinal Cord 40:335-340, 2002.

Hiller W, Fichter MM, Rief W: A controlled treatment study of somatoform disorders including analysis of healthcare utilization and cost-effectiveness. J Psychosom Res 54:369-380, 2003.

Kanner AM: More controversies on the treatment of psychogenic pseudoseizures: An addendum. Epilepsy Behav 4:360-364, 2003.

Kaplan C, Lipkin M, Gordon GH: Somatization in primary care: Patients with unexplained and vexing medical complaints. J Gen Int Med 3:177-190, 1988.

Kellner R: Functional somatic symptoms and hypochondriasis: A survey of empirical studies. Arch Gen Psychiatry 42:821-833, 1985.

Kirmayer LJ, Robbins JM (eds): Current Concepts of Somatization: Research and Clinical Perspectives. Washington, DC, American Psychiatric Publishing, 1991.

Kroenke K, Swindle R: Cognitive-behavioral therapy for somatization and symptom syndromes: A critical review of controlled clinical trials. Psychother Psychosom 69:205-215, 2000.

Lidbeck J: Group therapy for somatization disorders in primary care: Maintenance of treatment goals of short cognitive-behavioral treatment one-and-a-half-year follow-up. Acta Psychiatr Scand 107:449-456, 2003.

Looper KJ, Kirmayer LJ: Behavioral medicine approaches to somatoform disorders. J Consult Clin Psychol 70:810-827, 2002.

Mayou R, Levenson J, Sharpe M: Somatoform disorders in DSM-V. Psychosomatics 44:449-451, 2003.

Moene FC, Landberg EH, Hoogduin KAL: Organic syndromes diagnosed as conversion disorder: Identification and frequency in a study of 85 patients. J Psychosom Res 46:7-12, 2002.

Noyes R, Kathol RG, Fisher MM, et al: The validity of DSM-III-R hypochondriasis. Arch Gen Psychiatry 50:961-970, 1993.

Phillips KA, Grant J, Siniscalchi J, et al: Surgical and nonpsychiatric medical treatment of patients with body dysmorphic disorder. Psychosomatics 42:504-510, 2001.

Roelofs K, Keijsers GP, Hoogduin KA, et al: Childhood abuse in patients with conversion disorder. Am J Psychiatry 159:1908-1913, 2002.

Sharpe M, Carson A: "Unexplained" somatic symptoms, functional syndromes, and somatization: Do we need a paradigm shift? Ann Intern Med 134:926-930, 2001.

Smith GR, Monson RA, Ray DC: Patients with multiple unexplained symptoms: Their characteristics, functional health, and health care utilization. Arch Intern Med 146:69-72, 1986.

Smith GR, Monson RA, Ray DC: Psychiatric consultation in somatization disorder: A randomized controlled study. N Engl J Med 314(22):1407-1413, 1986.

Smith GR, Rost K, Kashner M: A trial of the effect of a standardized psychiatric consultation on health outcomes and costs in somatizing patients. Arch Gen Psychiatry 52:238-243, 1995.

Spiro HR: Chronic factitious illness. Arch Gen Psychiatry 18:569-579, 1968.

Toomey TC, Hernandez JT, Gittelman DF, Hulka JF: Relationship of sexual and physical abuse to pain and psychological assessment variables in chronic pelvic pain patients. Pain 53:105-109, 1993.

Walker EA, Roy-Byrne PP, Katon WJ, Jemelka R: An open trial of nortriptyline in women with chronic pelvic pain. Int J Psychiatry Med 21:245-252, 1991.

Warwick HMC, Salkovskis P: Hypochondriasis. Behav Res Ther 28(2):105-117, 1990.

Behavioral Emergencies and Forensic Issues

14

Ali Kazim

14.1 Behavioral Emergencies

A behavioral emergency is defined as any agitated (or potentially threatening) physical behavior toward self or others.

HANDLING THE SITUATION

1. Step one: Create a safe environment. The first priority is to create a safe environment for the patient, staff, and other patients.
   a. Do not put yourself in danger where a patient could trap or assault you.
   b. Assess the patient in a room with no breakable or dangerous objects.
   c. Separate patients from overstimulating situations.
   d. Consider the use of security guards to perform the following functions:
      (1) Stand nearby if needed.
      (2) Stay in the room to indicate that acting out will not be tolerated.
      (3) Assist in applying physical restraints if trained to do so.
      (4) Search for (or remove) weapons.
2. Step two: Avoid escalating the situation. Skillful interviewing can prevent escalation of the behavior. Such techniques generally consist of:
   a. Practicing nonthreatening behavior.
   b. Avoiding physical proximity.
   c. Avoiding threatening behavior (e.g., clenching fists).
   d. Remaining calm in voice and manner.
   e. Using clear and simple communication that does not create ambiguity or stimulate paranoia.
   f. Helpful listening; be empathic.
   g. Provide support.
   h. Be aware of your own feelings about the patient and how that might influence care.
3. Step three: Brief initial assessment.
   a. Should be done in the first 5 minutes.
   b. Items from a brief history, physical examination, and mental status examination provide data for initial diagnostic decisions (Box 14-1). Use collateral data sources including chart, family, referral sources.

BOX 14-1   Data Summary Sheet for Behavioral
Emergencies

Target Symptoms

☐ Agitation   ☐ Hallucinations   ☐ Suicidal
☐ Bizarre behavior   ☐ Homicidal   ☐ Violence
☐ Delirium   ☐ Incoherent   ☐ Other: _____
☐ Delusions   ☐ Mute

History

☐ Alcohol   ☐ Headache   ☐ Sedatives
☐ Cocaine   ☐ Head injury   ☐ Seizures
☐ Hallucinogens   ☐ Narcotics
☐ Medical diagnoses: _____
☐ Psychiatric diagnoses: _____
☐ Surgery: _____

Physical Examination

☐ Cranial nerve abnormality   ☐ Meningeal signs
☐ Head trauma   ☐ Motor abnormality
☐ Temp _____
☐ BP _____
☐ Heart rate _____
☐ Resp rate _____

Preliminary Diagnosis

☐ Delirium   ☐ Mania   ☐ Schizophrenia
☐ Delirium tremens   ☐ Paranoia
☐ Depression   ☐ Personality disorder

Management

☐ Constant observation   ☐ Security   ☐ Transfer
☐ Restraints   ☐ Medication: _____

  c. Differential diagnosis.
    (1) A behavioral emergency can have a wide range of etiologies.
        The medical history and sociodemographics influence the
        probability of which disorders are most likely.
      (a) Substance use and intoxication are extremely common
          issues.
    (2) Delirium. Agitated behavior resulting from some underlying
        medical cause (see Boxes 3-2 and 3-3). Because of the preva-
        lence of substance abuse and alcoholism, withdrawal delirium is
        a common cause of agitated behavior.
    (3) Manic disorder. Inquire about history of mood swings and
        previous manic episodes.

(4) Schizophrenia. Relapse often occurs when medication is stopped.

(5) Personality disorder. Some antisocial or borderline personalities have aggressive—destructive behavior tendencies, especially if the patient is depressed or using drugs.

d. History.

  (1) Onset.

    (a) Acute onset usually implies delirium.

    (b) Mania can have a sudden onset, but it usually builds up over time and often follows a depressive episode with treatment noncompliance.

    (c) Schizophrenic decompensation often follows increasing withdrawal, paranoia, or other psychotic symptoms with treatment noncompliance.

  (2) Past psychiatric history.

    (a) Mania, schizophrenic agitation, or antisocial or borderline behavior all have high rates of recurrence.

    (b) A thorough assessment is always needed because of frequent medical comorbidity (and substance abuse) in psychiatric patients.

  (3) Medical problem list. The longer the list of medical problems, the more likely is delirium (see Box 3-2).

  (4) Drugs and medication.

    (a) Common cause of behavioral emergencies (see Box 3-1).

    (b) Establish a complete drug list.

    (c) Obtain additional history from people who are with the patient.

    (d) Obtain a toxicology screen.

  (5) History of head injury. Patients, especially the elderly, might forget or overlook a minor head injury that can result in a subdural hematoma.

e. Mental status.

  (1) Delirium is characterized by the following:

    (a) Disorientation.

    (b) Impaired (or fluctuating) level of consciousness.

    (c) Visual hallucinations or sensory illusions.

    (d) Impaired attention.

  (2) However, those with acute mania and schizophrenia also may be disoriented and might have disorganized attention.

f. Physical examination.

  (1) Vital signs should be obtained as soon as possible.

    (a) Elevated temperature with altered mental status or behavior should raise suspicion of central nervous system (CNS) infection, especially in patients with acquired immunodeficiency syndrome (AIDS), cancer, or diabetes and those taking immunosuppressive drugs and steroids.

    (b) Elevated blood pressure, if extreme, can indicate intracranial bleeding or stroke.

(c) Rapid respiratory rate can indicate pulmonary embolism, salicylate intoxication, or acid–base abnormalities.

(d) Pulse irregularities, tachyarrhythmias, and bradyarrhythmias can indicate myocardial infarction or other cardiac disorders.

(2) Head injury. Always examine the patient for signs of head injury, because alcoholics or schizophrenics are at high risk for accidents and assaults.

(3) Screening neurologic examination. Minimal observations should include the following:

(a) Movement of extremities.

(b) Extraocular movements.

(c) Pupillary function.

(d) Facial asymmetry.

TREATMENT

Medication Strategies

1. Prevention.

   a. With the escalating or mildly agitated patient, offer some oral medication with the following suggestion, "You might find this medication will help you feel calmer." Giving the patient a choice of taking the medication intramuscularly (IM) or orally (PO) may convey some sense of control.

   b. Once medicated, the patient may feel in enough control to decrease further confrontation.

2. Rapid medication use in emergencies.

   a. Benzodiazepines and antipsychotics can be rapidly administered to decrease behavioral agitation. No medication rapidly cures schizophrenia.

   b. Once the patient is physically calm, a more thorough physical examination and interview can take place.

   c. Benzodiazepines versus antipsychotic agents (Table 14-1).

      (1) For agitation resulting from sedative withdrawal, benzodiazepines are more effective. Antipsychotics do not cover sedative withdrawal.

      (2) Benzodiazepines (unlike antipsychotics) do not create any risk for dyskinesia.

      (3) There are not sufficient studies to determine which medication is preferable in behavioral emergencies other than sedative withdrawal.

      (4) Benzodiazepines and antipsychotics are often used in combination.

3. Dosing medication in emergencies.

   a. Start with a single dose, such as:

      (1) Lorazepam 0.5 to 2 mg IM or PO (lorazepam is the only benzodiazepine that is absorbed well from IM sites and also does not cause potential hepatic complications).

      (2) Lorazepam may also be added to the following antipsychotics:

         (a) Haloperidol 2 to 5 mg IM or PO elixir.

         (b) Risperidone 0.5 to 2 mg PO elixir.

Table 14-1   **Psychotropic Medication in Physically Agitated Patients**

Drug	NMS	EPS	Hypotension	Anticholinergic	Respiration Depression	Cardiac Conduction Impairment
Haloperidol	Possible	+++	+	0	0	Rare
Lorazepam	0	0	0	0	Possible	0
Olanzapine	Possible	‡‡	+	+	0	Rare
Risperidone	Possible	+	‡‡	0	0	Rare
Ziprasidone	Possible	+	‡‡	0	0	Rare

EPS, extrapyramidal symptoms; NMS, neuroleptic malignant syndrome.

(c) Olanzapine 5 to 10 mg IM or zyprexa (Zydis rapidly dissolving oral formulation).

(d) Ziprasidone 20 mg IM q4h or 10 mg IM q2h.

b. If sufficient calming response is not obtained within 30 to 120 minutes, the initial dose may be repeated (assuming no change in diagnostic assessment).

c. Most patients respond (i.e., become physically calm) with a few doses.

d. Oral elixir is usually well absorbed and can produce a response in about 10 to 20 minutes, which is about the same for IM injections.

e. Haloperidol is sometimes used intravenously (IV) in the general hospital (not a Food and Drug Administration [FDA]-approved route).

f. A subset of delirious patients appear to require very high doses. Psychiatric consultation should be sought if a patient does not respond to the usual standard of two or three doses.

g. Once the patient is calmed, the total amount of psychotropic medication used can be added up and prescribed in divided doses over each of the following several days to avoid relapse.

Side Effects

Table 14-1 lists relative importance of potential complications resulting from anticholinergic, hypotensive, or cardiac side effects or from extrapyramidal side effects (EPS).

1. Respiratory depression is a risk with benzodiazepines for CO_2 retainers and those taking other respiratory depressants such as narcotics.

2. Antipsychotics can rarely lead to prolonged QTc interval, resulting in torsades de pointes.

3. Antipsychotics rarely lead to clinically relevant orthostatic hypotension, which is more likely in patients who are volume depleted or autonomically impaired.

4. Neuroleptic malignant syndrome (NMS) (see Chapter 12) is extremely rare with antipsychotics but should be considered if the patient seems to get worse instead of better. Watch for fever, rigidity, increasing confusion.

5. Akathisia (see Chapter 12), resulting in increased agitation, can occur in 10% to 40% of patients receiving continued doses of antipsychotics.

6. Acute dystonia can occur with antipsychotics (though mostly with the potent D_2 antagonists). With haloperidol, the incidence is as high as 40% in young muscular male patients. Acute dystonia is rare with the atypical antipsychotics.

   a. Cogentin 2 mg can be added to the first dose of haloperidol to prevent dystonia (see Chapter 12); or it can be ordered prn if dystonia occurs.

   b. In patients with cervical traction or spinal instability, a dystonia can be life-threatening. Antipsychotics are best avoided in such patients.

7. Issues with benzodiazepine use (also see Chapter 10).

   a. Potential respiratory depression.

b. Psychomotor impairment can lead to falls if the patient is not monitored.

c. Excessive sedation. Patients do not like to be put to sleep.

d. Some personality disorders may become disinhibited and require haloperidol.

8. Do not give psychotropics to a patient who might have an evolving intracranial process, such as subarachnoid hemorrhage, intracranial bleeding, or swelling following trauma.

a. Level of consciousness is important in determining the need for neurosurgical intervention.

b. Medication may be given in conjunction with the attending trauma surgeon.

Other Medication Options

1. Narcotics.

a. Morphine is used to control agitation in postsurgical, trauma, or acute myocardial infarction patients.

b. In general, the calming effect is only temporary and the patient might require larger and more frequent doses.

2. β-Blockers and buspirone.

a. Not useful in acute situations.

b. Can decrease episodic aggression after head injury or other brain damage. See Chapter 5 for additional details.

3. Rapid loading with divalproex (Depakote) can be successful in calming acute bipolar mania (see Chapter 8 for specifics). It should not be used in patients with abnormal liver function tests.

a. Start 20 mg/kg/day until a blood level is available; or

b. Start 30 mg/kg for 2 days, followed by 20 mg/kg starting on day 3.

14.2 Suicide Evaluation

1. Suicide is completed by more than 30,000 Americans each year and is the eighth leading overall cause of death (second among youth).

2. Evaluation and documentation of suicidal ideation are core components of any psychiatric assessment (see Box 6-4 for mental status questions regarding suicide).

3. A high percentage of patients who commit suicide visit a primary care provider in the prior few months.

4. Risk factors provide a general context for an evaluation. The individual patient requires individual assessment, not just a "score" on a risk factors scale.

a. Chronic medical illness.

(1) Suicide risk is almost twice as high among patients with cancer and is significantly elevated among patients with AIDS.

(2) Hemodialysis patients have a higher than expected suicide rate (as high as 5%); it is as high as in patients with chronic schizophrenia.

(3) Other medical patients with higher than expected risk include those with delirium tremens and respiratory diseases.

b. Old age. White elderly men have a rapidly increasing incidence of completed suicide, four times higher than the national rate.

c. Male sex. (Women attempt more often; men succeed more often.)

d. Recent major mental illness accounts for a high percentage of suicides.
   (1) Major depression (50%).
   (2) Chronic alcoholism (20%).
   (3) Schizophrenia (10%).
   (4) Borderline personality (5% to 15%).

e. Previous suicide attempts (present in 30% to 40%).

f. Suicidal ideation (communicated in 60%).

g. Panic attacks (20% of those with panic disorder have a lifetime history of suicide attempts).

h. Poor sleep.

i. Unemployment.

j. Unmarried status.

k. Recent discharge from hospital.

5. Clinical questions to evaluate suicide potential (Table 14-2).

   a. The clinician is not expected to read the patient's mind or force the patient into a confession.

   b. However, the clinician is expected to ask questions and document answers that allow a judgment about suicide risk. Box 6-4 provides an escalating series of questions leading up to direct questions about suicidal ideation and planning.

   c. Every suicide evaluation should record (at least) the following:
      (1) Suicidal ideation and plan.
         (a) Patients with definite ideas or a plan should be considered at high risk no matter what else is going on.
         (b) The presence of suicidal ideation or planning does not mean the patient must be hospitalized; however, alternate plans must be carefully worked out.
      (2) What would keep you from taking your life at this point?
         (a) Lack of a reason to live or lack of any future planning implies higher risk.
         (b) Reasons to live (e.g., children, religion, or insurance money) or signs of future plans (not wanting to miss too much work) mitigate risk.
      (3) Presence or absence of significant cognitive impairment.
         (a) Delirium or other cognitive impairment make the interview less reliable.
         (b) Suicide risk evaluation should be deferred until the patient is clear from a drug-altered state or other delirium.
      (4) Presence or absence of psychosis.
         (a) Command hallucinations for suicide are ominous.
         (b) Any psychotic symptoms increase suicide risk.
      (5) Presence of a depressive prodrome. Major depression with intensifying suicidal thoughts is a significant risk.
      (6) What the patient says it makes sense to do.
         (a) One of the best questions for clinical assessment of suicide risk is, "What do you think it makes sense to do now?"

TABLE 14-2 Mental Status Component of Suicide, Homicide, and Violence Evaluation

Component	Ideas			Plans		
	No	Indefinite	Definite	No	Indefinite	Definite
Suicide						
Homicide						
Violence						
What inhibits:				Reason to live:		

       (b) Patients at high suicide risk often give answers like, "It really doesn't matter what happens to me anymore" or "I don't think anything can help."

       (c) Signs of future orientation can indicate that the suicidal planning is not imminent; for example, if a patient shows concern about going back to work, being around for a child's birthday, or keeping an appointment with a therapist.

    (7) Confirmation by a third party.

       (a) When a story seems unclear, more information is often helpful. As described in Chapter 2, talking to another person can be extremely important, as long as the patient gives consent.

       (b) In an emergency, it may be possible to bypass the patient's permission to talk to someone else.

6. The chronically suicidal patient.

  a. Chronically suicidal patients may have borderline personality disorders (see Chapter 17).

    (1) These patients are often angry and manipulative, making management decisions difficult.

    (2) These patients have a high risk of eventual suicide, perhaps as high as 25%.

  b. Unfortunately, many borderline patients are not helped by hospitalization.

    (1) In fact, hospitalization may reinforce regressive behaviors.

    (2) A decision not to hospitalize such a patient must be accompanied by an alternative outpatient treatment plan and documentation of why hospitalization is not considered the best therapeutic approach.

  c. A number of psychotropic drugs have been tried with borderline patients with varying degrees of success (see Chapter 17).

  d. Consider concurrent diagnoses in the patient with personality disorder. For example, concurrent major depression, acute grief, or drug-induced delirium are treatable conditions, which might warrant a brief hospitalization.

7. What to do if the patient is suicidal.

  a. If you believe the patient is at significant suicidal risk, the patient should not be allowed to leave the interview setting without an appropriate treatment plan.

  b. Alternative plans.

    (1) Referral and direct transport to a more experienced psychiatric clinician or emergency psychiatry setting.

    (2) Hospitalization, voluntary if possible or by commitment if necessary.

    (3) If commitment is necessary, tell patients that you feel there is significant suicide risk and that you must make decisions that will protect them at this time. (See commitment section later in this chapter.)

    (4) An outpatient alternative if supervision can be arranged that is responsible and reliable.

    (5) Establishing a contract for safety with the patient may be appropriate for some patients with lower levels of suicidal ideation.

14.3 Evaluation of the Violent or Homicidal Patient

1. Because violence and murder are so prevalent, violent behavior is important to consider in the mental status assessment.
2. Risk factors for violence.
    a. Previous history of violence.
    b. Antisocial personality traits.
    c. Substance abuse.
    d. Brain impairment associated with disinhibition and episodic impulsiveness.
    e. Signs of extreme anger or irritability.
    f. Age. Violence peaks in late teens and early 20s.
    g. Sex. Violence is more common in men than women. Among those with mental disorders, base rates are more equivalent.
    h. Violent behavior is inversely related to IQ.
3. Psychiatric disorders associated with violence.
    a. Agitated schizophrenic patients can cause injury during attempts to control their behavior.
    b. Patients with paranoia disorders, including schizophrenia, have an increased risk of violent behavior as a response to the delusions.
    c. Patients who have mania with irritability can be provoked to violent behavior.
    d. Patients with severe personality disorders including borderline, narcissistic, and antisocial can be provoked to violence when they do not get what they want.
    e. Dementia or delirium (especially with delusions).
4. Medical disorders associated with violence.
    a. Drug use.
        (1) Phencyclidine (PCP).
        (2) Alcohol intoxication.
        (3) Stimulant abuse (cocaine, amphetamines).
        (4) Sedative withdrawal.
    b. Epilepsy.
        (1) Prodromal irritability can lead to aggression.
        (2) Ictal aggression is rare and generally not goal directed
        (3) Periictal aggression can result from the following:
            (a) Postictal automatisms.
            (b) Postictal confusion or disinhibition.
5. Violence assessment.
    a. History (the best predictor of future behavior is past behavior).
        (1) Past episodes (number of episodes and means of violence).
        (2) Nature and number of arrests.
        (3) Presence of premeditation or impulsiveness.

    (4) Precipitants of violence.

    (5) Access to weapons.

b. Mental status (see Box 14-1).

    (1) As with the suicide evaluation, use a series of questions such as the following.

        (a) "Have you been having thoughts of hurting anyone?"

        (b) "Have you gone so far as to have plans to harm someone?"

        (c) "You mentioned how angry you were with that guy. Have you been thinking about what you might do to get back at him?"

    (2) As with suicidal ideation and planning, it is possible to have a spectrum of responses.

        (a) Indefinite (e.g., "I'm so mad I could kill someone.")

        (b) Definite (e.g., "When I get home, I'm really going to let her have it.")

    (3) Define the degree of planning and the access to the means to carry out any plan. For example, if a patient threatens to shoot someone, does he own or have access to a gun?

    (4) Delirium or dementia can impair impulse control or judgment.

    (5) Command hallucinations to harm someone are dangerous symptoms.

    (6) Paranoia creates risk if there is a strong patient delusion focused on some individual.

    (7) Irritability raises risk of violent behavior.

c. Physical examination.

    (1) Issues relevant to violence potential include signs associated with drug intoxication or withdrawal (see Chapter 15).

    (2) Signs include ataxia, dysarthria, nystagmus, dilated pupils, sweating, tachycardia, and increased blood pressure.

d. The Overt Aggression Scale (Box 14-2) is used to evaluate signs of aggression.

e. Management of homicidal ideation.

    (1) If a patient appears to pose a serious risk of harm to a specific person, the physician must do something appropriate.

    (2) Although laws differ regionally, physicians are generally expected to do the following:

        (a) Inform the intended victim of the risk and inform the police.

        (b) Detain the patient under mental health commitment (if necessary) and arrange for hospitalization.

        (c) Most states require an actual threat made against a clearly identifiable person before a duty to warn or to protect arises.

        (d) When in doubt, obtain some guidance from a specialist in psychiatry or law.

BOX 14-2   Overt Aggression Scale

Verbal Aggression

- ☐ Makes loud noises, shouts angrily.
- ☐ Yells mild personal insults (e.g., "You're stupid!").
- ☐ Curses viciously, uses foul language in anger, makes moderate threats to others or self.
- ☐ Makes clear threats of violence toward others or self ("I'm going to kill you") or requests help to control self.

Physical Aggression against Objects

- ☐ Slams doors, scatters clothing, makes a mess.
- ☐ Throws objects down, kicks furniture without breaking it, marks the wall.
- ☐ Breaks objects, smashes windows.
- ☐ Sets fires, throws objects dangerously.

Physical Aggression against Self

- ☐ Picks or scratches skin, hits self, pulls hair (with no or minor injury only).
- ☐ Bangs head, hits fist into objects, throws self onto floor or into objects (hurts self without serious injury).
- ☐ Small cuts or bruises, minor burns.
- ☐ Mutilates self, causes deep cuts, bites that bleed, internal injury, fracture, loss of consciousness, or loss of teeth.

Physical Aggression against Other People

- ☐ Makes threatening gestures, swings at people, grabs at clothes.
- ☐ Strikes, kicks, pushes, pulls hair (without injury to others).
- ☐ Attacks others, causing mild to moderate physical injury (bruises, sprain, welts).
- ☐ Attacks others, causing severe physical injury (broken bones, deep lacerations, internal injury).

From Yudofsky S, Stevens L, Silver J: *Am J Psychiatry* 141:114-115, 1984.

14.4 Use of Physical Restraints

1. The use of physical restraints may be indicated for the following patients:
   a. Patients whose safety would otherwise be impaired or who might harm others.
   b. Intensely agitated patients (who often calm down when placed in restraints).
2. Patients placed in restraints usually have underlying diagnoses.
   a. Agitated delirium.
   b. Schizophrenic agitation.
   c. Manic agitation.

    d. Patients with intense suicidal or homicidal behavior who cannot control their impulses.

    e. Agitated drug intoxication or withdrawal.

3. Restraints should never be used as punishment or as a substitute for adequate staffing.

4. Restraints should be used only if there is no less-restrictive alternative.

5. The use of restraints should be managed as follows (specific rules are prescribed by the Joint Commission for Accreditation of Hospitals):

    a. The specific indication should be clearly documented.

    b. There must be a signed physician's order (even if the procedure was initiated by some other staff member).

    c. The order should specify a time limit.

    d. Anyone impaired enough to require restraints should have continuous staff observation.

    e. Restraints should be properly designed. Do not use bed sheets tied into a knot.

    f. Restraints should be applied by experienced staff.

        (1) Five staff members are necessary to restrain a resistant patient.

        (2) Security should be called to assist.

        (3) Nursing and security staff should receive training in this procedure.

    g. During the procedure, the patient should be told in calm, simple terms what is happening.

        (1) Patients may be confused or psychotic and misperceive the situation.

        (2) Say something like, "You are in a hospital. These people are nurses and security staff. No one is going to hurt you; we are trying to help make things safe for you."

    h. The need for restraints must be reevaluated (at least every shift), with documentation supporting continued use.

    i. When to remove restraints.

        (1) As soon as the patient has demonstrated a reasonable period of behavioral stability.

        (2) The patient's promise that there will be no dangerous behavior might not be enough to warrant removal.

14.5 Commitment under Mental Health Statutes

1. Strictly speaking, commitment is a judicial rather than a medical procedure.

2. Physicians generally are involved in filling out papers that allow a period of detention before a formal commitment proceeding.

3. In a formal commitment hearing, the patient is represented by an attorney or mental health advocate.

4. Laws vary in different states; therefore, when in doubt, check with a psychiatrist or legal consultant regarding criteria and procedures for commitment. However, most states share features of criteria for commitment.

a. Immediate dangerousness to self or others by virtue of a mental disorder and need of immediate care and treatment.

b. Incapability of caring for self in terms of food, clothing, and shelter.

5. In many states, a psychiatrist's signature is not necessary on a commitment paper. Often other physicians (or allied health professionals) may sign.

6. Qualifying for commitment does not mean that a patient is incompetent to make decisions about treatment.

a. A committed patient is considered competent to refuse psychotropic medication or medical procedures.

b. Medication may be used against the patient's wishes in emergency situations only.

7. In most states, commitment allows a short period of detention (usually several days) for an assessment before a formal legal proceeding to evaluate the need to commit the patient to a longer period of care.

8. How does commitment under mental health statutes apply to medical patients who want to leave the hospital against medical advice or refuse treatment?

a. If the patient is judged to be in immediate danger as a result of a mental disorder and can be treated in a setting under the jurisdiction of their mental health statutes, the patient could be committed under the mental health statutes.

b. Patients in need of medical treatment who are delirious and show impaired judgment are generally not committed on the basis of the mental health statutes. Instead, they are detained on the basis of implied consent associated with their incompetence to make a decision about the need for immediate treatment.

c. When in doubt about what to do, base the decision on clinical judgment for the patient's health and safety, and then seek legal advice. Maintaining the safety and health of the patient should always be the guiding principle.

14.6 Competence Evaluations

1. Psychiatrists are commonly asked to help decide if a patient is competent.

2. Technically, competence is a judicial decision, not a medical one. However, judges often rely on the opinions of psychiatrists, who are considered experts in obtaining and evaluating interview information.

3. Questions of competence should refer to some specific aspect of competence, for example:

a. Competence to refuse a medical procedure.

b. Competence to manage finances.

c. Competence to be at home without supervision.

4. The competence evaluation should focus on the specific aspect of competence in question. To be considered competent, a patient

must be able to demonstrate an understanding of the issues in question. For example:

   a. To be competent to manage finances, patients need to show that they know their assets, income, expenses, how to process financial transactions, and the consequences of not paying a bill.

   b. To be competent to refuse a medical treatment, patients have to demonstrate that they know and understand their medical condition and the treatment being suggested, can process the information provided, and understand the consequences of refusing the treatment, the alternatives, and the risks and benefits of the treatment.

5. Refusal of treatment does not always mean the patient is not competent. Reasons patients refuse treatment include the following:

   a. Lack of information necessary to decide what to do.

   b. Anger at the medical system because of delays, disappointments, or perceived oversights, which should be identified and addressed.

   c. Disagreements within the family about what to do.

   d. Confusion or delirium, inability to retain or process information.

   e. Depression with undue pessimism. Because "nothing could help anyway," why agree to treatment?

6. Questions about a patient's wishes for treatment can involve such documents as living wills or durable powers of attorney. When in doubt, consult with a hospital risk manager.

SUGGESTED READINGS

Adamek ME, Kaplan MS: Firearm suicide among older men. *Psychiatric Serv* 47: 304-305, 1996.

American Psychiatric Association. Practice guidelines for the assessment and treatment of patients with suicidal behaviors. *Am J Psychiatry* 160(11 Suppl):1-60, 2003.

Bongar B: *The Suicidal Patient: Clinical and Legal Standards of Care*, 2nd ed. Washington, DC, American Psychological Association, 2001.

Cornelius JR, Salloum IM, Mezzich J, et al: Disproportionate suicidality in patients with comorbid major depression and alcoholism. *Am J Psychiatry* 152:358-364, 1995.

Hughes DH: Implications of recent court rulings for crisis and psychiatric emergency services. *Psychiatric Serv* 47:1332-1333, 1996.

Jacobs D, Brewer M: APA practice guideline provides recommendations for assessing and treating patients with suicidal behaviors. *Psychiatr Ann* 34(5):373-384, 2004.

Simon RI, Gutheil TG: A recurrent pattern of suicide risk factors observed in litigated cases: Lessons in risk management. *Psychiatr Ann* 32(7):384-387, 2002.

VandeCreek L, Knapp S: Tarasoff and Beyond: Legal and Clinical Considerations in the Treatment of Life-Endangering Patients, 3rd ed. Sarasota, Fla, Professional Resource Press, 2001.

Yudofsky SC, Silver JM, Jackson W, et al: The Overt Aggression Scale for the objective rating of verbal and physical aggression. *Am J Psychiatry* 143:35-39, 1986.

Alcohol and Substance Abuse

15

Michael D. Stein

15.1 Alcohol Abuse

1. Definition. The American Medical Association (AMA) defines alcoholism as an illness characterized by significant impairment (physiologic, psychological, or social) directly associated with persistent and excessive use of alcohol.
2. Prevalence.
   a. Estimated prevalence in the United States is 7% to 10%.
   b. Prevalence in medically hospitalized patients is 20% to 40%.
3. Morbidity and mortality.
   a. Alcohol is involved in about 30% of suicides and 60% of homicides. The lifetime suicide risk in alcoholics is 2% to 3.5% (60 to 120 times the level of risk in the normal population)
   b. Alcohol is a major factor in accidents and domestic violence.
   c. Alcohol use is associated with the following:
      (1) Intoxication.
      (2) Withdrawal.
      (3) Wernicke–Korsakoff syndrome.
      (4) Cerebral cortical atrophy (dementia).
      (5) Cerebellar degeneration.
      (6) Polyneuropathy.
      (7) Myopathy.
      (8) Pellagra.
      (9) Gastrointestinal disorders and bleeding (e.g., esophagitis, gastritis, hepatitis, pancreatitis, cirrhosis, and gastrointestinal cancers).
         (a) Seventy-five percent of patients with chronic pancreatitis have alcoholism.
         (b) Elevated serum glutamic-oxaloacetic transaminase (SGOT), serum glutamic-pyruvic transaminase (SGPT), and lactate dehydrogenase (LDH) levels are common.
         (c) Elevated serum γ-glutamyl transpeptidase (SGGT) is particularly sensitive.
      (10) Cardiovascular disorders include hypertension and cardiomyopathy.
      (11) Hematologic disorders include thrombocytopenia, anemia, and leukopenia (elevated mean corpuscular volume (MCV) is common).
      (12) Infections.

BOX 15-1   CAGE Questionnaire

Have you ever felt the need to **C**ut down on drinking?
Have you ever felt **A**nnoyed by criticisms of drinking?
Have you ever had **G**uilty feelings about drinking?
Have you ever needed a morning **E**ye-opener?

---

(13) Dehydration.
(14) Trauma. Each year more than 25,000 persons die and 150,000 are permanently disabled because of alcohol-related traffic accidents.
(15) Seizures.
(16) Decreased albumin, vitamin B_{12}, folate.
(17) Increased uric acid, elevated amylase, prolonged prothrombin times (with cirrhosis).

4. Recognition.
   a. Alcoholism is poorly recognized. Casual interviewing of a patient is not sufficient.
   b. Several brief screening questionnaires can be useful.
      (1) The CAGE questionnaire (Box 15-1) is a simple four-item test with high sensitivity. An affirmative answer to more than one question is considered a basis for suspicion of alcoholism.
      (2) The Michigan Alcohol Screening Test (short version) is a 10-item form (Box 15-2).

5. Treatment. Alcoholism is a chronic medical illness.
   a. Detoxification is the first step in treatment.
   b. Maintenance of sobriety requires a maintenance program consisting of the following:
      (1) A support program such as Alcoholics Anonymous.
      (2) Treatment of psychiatric comorbidities such as depression or anxiety.
      (3) Family treatment to address enabling behavior and support adaptive behavior.
      (4) Consideration of medication options.

15.2 Alcohol Dependence

A number of medications assist in preventing relapse in alcohol-dependent patients. Optimal dosage, duration, and patient profile remain unclear. Adherence is a major factor in effectiveness. Medications should be used as part of a psychosocial treatment plan.

1. Medications that modify intoxication.
   a. Naltrexone.
      (1) Used daily, it can reduce relapse to heavy drinking, and it has a modest effect on abstinence.
      (2) It works best with a relapse-prevention approach that includes coping skills training or cognitive behavior therapy.

BOX 15-2   **Michigan Alcohol Screening Test***

Do you feel you are a normal drinker?
Do friends or relatives think you are a normal drinker?
Have you ever attended a meeting of Alcoholics Anonymous?
Have you ever lost friends or girlfriends/boyfriends because of drinking?
Have you ever gotten in trouble at work because of drinking?
Have you ever neglected your obligations, your family, or your work for 2 or more days in a row because of your drinking?
Have you ever had DTs, severe shaking, heard voices, or seen things that were not there after heavy drinking?
Have you ever gone to anyone for help about your drinking?
Have you ever been in a hospital because of your drinking?
Have you ever been arrested for drunk driving or driving after drinking?
Scoring: Answering "yes" to three or more questions indicates alcoholism.

*Brief version.
From Pokorny AD, Miller BA, Kaplan HB: *Am J Psychiatry* 129:342-345, 1972.

      (3) Common side effects include insomnia, nausea, headache, and fatigue.
  b. Disulfiram.
      (1) It inhibits acetaldehyde dehydrogenase, which increases the unpleasant actions of alcohol such as nausea, vomiting, and flushing.
      (2) It may be effective with supervised daily ingestion in motivated persons, but it is generally out of favor.
2. Medications that reduce craving or urge to drink.
  a. Ondansetron.
      (1) Ondansetron is a serotonin-3 receptor antagonist that might alter alcohol's acute reinforcing effects.
      (2) Its use may be limited to early-onset alcoholism.
      (3) It is not yet Food and Drug Administration (FDA)-approved for alcoholism treatment.
  b. Acamprosate.
      (1) The main effect is on glutamate receptors, with lesser effect on γ-aminobutyric acid (GABA) receptors.
      (2) It has modest effects in reducing relapse to drinking and maintaining more abstinent days.
      (3) Side effects include headache and diarrhea.
3. Medications that modulate the behavioral effects of alcohol.
  a. Selective serotonin reuptake inhibitors (SSRIs) have had inconsistent success with alcohol-dependent patients.
  b. The best outcomes with SSRIs are seen in early-onset and antisocial alcoholics.

15.3 Alcohol Intoxication

1. Intoxication is the most common problem associated with alcohol use.
2. Intoxication is associated with serious potential for dangerous behavior and violence directed toward self or others.
3. When dealing with the intoxicated patient, the following principles may be helpful.
   a. Security. If there is potential for aggressive behavior or if the patient could be armed, call security or police.
   b. Minimize threatening behavior. Some principles in managing the aggressive patient are presented in Chapter 14. It is important to avoid making the patient feel more paranoid or threatened (e.g., challenging or yelling back at the patient).
   c. Create a sociable environment. For example, offering food or coffee helps channel behavior into a social context.
4. Consider the need for transfer to a detoxification site for patients with a history of continuous ingestion of large amounts of alcohol.
5. Medical differential diagnosis of the intoxicated patient.
   a. Hepatic encephalopathy.
   b. Hypoglycemia.
   c. Postictal state.
   d. Head trauma.
   e. Central nervous system (CNS) infection.
   f. Intoxication by other drugs.
   g. Confusion from Wernicke–Korsakoff syndrome.
6. Laboratory tests that can help in diagnosis.
   a. Blood alcohol level (BAL) (see later).
   b. Glucose level (can reveal alcohol-related hypoglycemia).
   c. Electrolytes and blood urea nitrogen (BUN) (can reveal alcoholic ketoacidosis as well as dehydration).
   d. Toxicology screen (can reveal other substances).
   e. Complete blood count (CBC) (can reveal blood loss or infection).
   f. In a patient with hemorrhage or symptomatic liver disease, a prothrombin time (PT), partial thromboplastin time (PTT), and platelet count should be checked.
7. Treatment.
   a. Protect the patient and others from physical harm.
   b. Thiamine 100 mg intramuscular (IM), then orally tid for 2 weeks.
   c. Multivitamins given daily.
   d. For agitation, lorazepam 1 to 2 mg by mouth (PO) or intravenous (IV), with repeated doses if needed.
   e. Treat alcohol-related medical problems.
   f. Constantly re-evaluate for other problems.

15.4 Alcoholic Paranoia

1. Patients become intensely jealous, hostile, and paranoid while under the influence of alcohol.

BOX 15-3   COMA: Symptoms of Wernicke–Korsakoff Syndrome

Confusion
Ophthalmoplegia
Memory impairment
Ataxia

---

2. This disorder is very difficult to treat.
   a. Try small amounts of antipsychotic agents (which usually do not help very much).
   b. Refer to an alcohol program that can help with abstinence.
3. Potential for violence is increased during this state (often with a history of aggressive behavior).

15.5 Pathologic Intoxication

1. Intoxication with small amounts of alcohol (often only 2 to 4 ounces).
2. The intoxicated state can consist of aggressive, impulsive behavior with paranoia, which the patient does not remember afterward.
3. Managed with medication as described in Chapter 14.
4. Personality disorders often coexist.

15.6 Wernicke–Korsakoff Syndrome (Alcohol Amnestic Syndrome)

The full syndrome can be described with the mnemonic COMA (Box 15-3).
1. Patients might not show the complete syndrome.
2. Confabulation is not typical and is a consequence of the memory impairment.
3. Treatment is a medical emergency. When suspected, give thiamine 100 mg and folate 1 mg IV followed by thiamine 100 mg daily for several weeks.

15.7 Alcoholic Hallucinosis

1. Vivid auditory hallucinations without other cognitive impairment.
2. Other sensory hallucinations can also occur.
3. The patient remains oriented and may be aware that the voices are hallucinations.
   a. Voices are often accusatory and threatening. Because of the nature of the hallucinations, these patients are at some risk for harming themselves or others.
   b. Hallucinations can occur while drinking, during withdrawal, or between episodes.

4. Hallucinations are less common than delirium tremens (DTs) and not associated with delirium, tremor, disorientation, and agitation.
5. Hallucinations may be difficult to differentiate from intoxication in paranoid schizophrenia.
6. Treatment.
   a. If warranted, detain the patient in a protected setting.
   b. If the behavior creates immediate danger, treat as a behavioral emergency (see Chapter 14).
   c. The hallucinations generally clear within 30 days after cessation of drinking.

15.8 Alcoholic Dementia

1. Cognitive testing is abnormal in a high percentage of sober alcoholics.
2. Among the causes of impaired cognition in alcoholics are the following:
   a. Direct ethanol neurotoxicity.
   b. Premorbid intellectual deficits.
   c. Thiamine deficiency (dementia in alcoholics is usually nutritional).
   d. Recurrent head trauma.
   e. Hepatocerebral degeneration.
   f. Marchiafava–Bignami disease (necrosis of corpus callosum).

15.9 Hepatic Encephalopathy

1. Hepatic encephalopathy is usually of rapid onset, with delirium progressing to stupor and coma.
2. Asterixis or tremor is present.
3. It occurs in about 5% of patients with cirrhosis.
4. Benzodiazepine antagonists are being tested as a treatment.

15.10 Fetal Alcohol Syndrome

1. About 4 to 12 ounces of 100-proof alcohol must be consumed daily during pregnancy to produce this disorder.
2. Defects in child's CNS include:
   a. Mental retardation.
   b. Poor coordination.
   c. Hyperactivity.
   d. Growth deficiencies.
   e. Facial abnormalities.

15.11 Alcohol Comorbidities

1. Depression. Approximately 33% of alcoholics have a comorbid affective disorder.
   a. Depressive symptoms may be secondary to alcohol, or alcohol use may be a result of underlying depression.
      (1) History might reveal which came first.
      (2) Patient might need to go through detoxification and remain alcohol free for at least 6 weeks to sort out the diagnosis.

b. Antidepressants may be helpful in treating depression and prevent-ing relapse of drinking.

c. It is difficult to successfully treat a mood disorder while a patient is actively drinking. In such cases, regard the alcohol use as the pri-mary problem and reassess and treat the mood disorder once the patient is free of alcohol.

2. Anxiety.

a. Approximately 25% of alcoholics have a comorbid anxiety disorder. Anxiety may be secondary to alcohol withdrawal, or alcohol use may be a result of underlying anxiety.

b. Generalized anxiety is a common comorbidity, and if identified and treated, it can decrease some of the patient's need to drink.

(1) Buspirone 10 mg tid may be useful (especially in the context of ongoing psychosocial treatment) because it is not addicting and does not augment the sedative properties of alcohol.

(2) There are no published controlled trials of SSRI efficacy for alcoholism.

c. It is difficult to successfully treat an anxiety disorder while a patient is actively drinking. Regard the alcohol use as the primary problem and reassess once the patient is free of alcohol.

d. Benzodiazepines have potential for misuse in persons with more severe alcoholism, a history of misuse of other drugs, and comorbid antisocial personality disorder.

3. Chronic mental illness. At least 25% of the chronically mentally ill have some complicating alcohol use.

4. Borderline personality disorder. Substance abuse is a common comor-bidity and adds significantly to suicide risk.

15.12 Alcohol and Sedative Withdrawal

OVERVIEW

1. The severity of alcohol or other sedative withdrawal ranges from mild discomfort requiring no treatment (minor abstinence) to life-threaten-ing symptoms requiring acute hospitalization (DTs) (Box 15-4). Patients who discontinue alcohol or other sedatives too quickly are at risk for withdrawal.

2. Prevalence. In a general medical hospital, about 40% of patients have been using alcohol or other sedatives. When a medical patient sud-denly becomes agitated, confused, or psychotic, DTs should be first in the differential diagnosis.

3. Significance. If untreated, DTs have a 10% mortality rate; the mortal-ity rate can increase to 25% with other acute medical disorders. With treatment, alcohol withdrawal delirium mortality is 0% to 1%.

ALCOHOL WITHDRAWAL

1. Symptoms (see Box 15-4) can appear within 8 hours of the last drink and peak between 24 and 36 hours.

a. Morning hangover.

b. Morning shakiness.

BOX 15-4   **Abstinence Signs in Alcohol Withdrawal**

Minor Withdrawal

Appears within a few hours after alcohol discontinuance and generally disappears within 48 hours.
- Symptoms include:
- Hyperreflexia
- Irritability
- Nausea
- Sleeplessness
- Sweating
- Tremor
- Weakness

Major Withdrawal

Usually appears from 48 to 72 hours after discontinuance (or lowering of dose).
Symptoms include:
- Confusion
- Fever
- Hallucinations
- Hypertension
- Seizures
- Tachycardia
- Tachypnea
- Tremulousness
- Weakness

   c. Craving for alcohol.
   d. Insomnia, vivid dreams.
   e. Anxiety, irritability.
   f. Nausea, vomiting.
   g. Sweating, weakness, myalgias.
   h. Tachycardia, hypertension.
   i. Coarse tremor of hands and tongue.
   j. Transient visual, tactile, or auditory hallucinations or illusions.
   k. Grand mal seizures.
2. Repeated episodes of minor withdrawal can appear to be a chronic anxiety disorder.
3. Minor withdrawal can be managed effectively in an outpatient setting, often with no medication. Outpatient management can be performed using chlordiazepoxide, diazepam, or lorazepam, with decreasing doses as symptoms resolve, and daily outpatient visits to monitor abstinence and provide referral for long-term treatment or self-help meetings.

MAJOR ABSTINENCE SYNDROME: ALCOHOL WITHDRAWAL DELIRIUM

1. Risk factors for alcohol withdrawal delirium (AWD) or DTs.
   a. Long, intense history of alcohol exposure.
   b. Recent binge followed by abrupt cessation.
   c. Previous history of AWD or DTs.
   d. Infection, head trauma, pancreatitis, gastrointestinal hemorrhage, myocardial infarction, poor nutrition.
2. Timing. Onset and severity of withdrawal symptoms are determined by the half-life of the substance.
   a. Sedatives other than alcohol.
      (1) Major abstinence is unlikely to follow use of long-acting sedatives such as diazepam or chlordiazepoxide, whose active metabolites have a half-life of about 100 hours (see Chapter 10).
      (2) Short-acting sedatives (such as butalbital or triazolam) have a rapid onset of severe withdrawal symptoms often within 24 hours.
   b. Alcohol.
      (1) Symptoms typically develop 2 to 3 days after cessation or reduction in drinking.
      (2) Symptom onset may be delayed as long as 7 days, especially if there has been use of some cross-tolerant sedative.
3. Symptoms (see Box 15-4).
   a. Symptoms may be obscured by concurrent medications or medical conditions. For example,
      (1) β-Blockers can mask tachycardia.
      (2) Narcotics can mask mydriasis.
      (3) Antipyretics can mask fever.
   b. Symptoms may be rated using the Clinical Institute Withdrawal Assessment for Alcohol (CIWA-A) Scale (Box 15-5).
4. Treatment.
   a. Sedative withdrawal syndromes can be managed with cross-tolerant sedatives (Table 15-1).
      (1) Alcohol is cross-tolerant but has a short half-life, causes gastric irritation and excessive sedation, and provides a confusing message for the patient.
      (2) Antihistamines, chloral hydrate, and buspirone are not cross-tolerant.
      (3) β-Blockers can decrease autonomic symptoms, but they do not prevent or treat DTs and should not be given to persons with alcohol withdrawal delirium.
      (4) Antipsychotic agents are not cross-tolerant sedatives.
      (5) Carbamazepine has been shown to reduce withdrawal symptoms and can reduce rebound drinking, particularly for persons who have experienced multiple previous detoxifications.
      (6) Chloral hydrate is no longer considered a standard treatment approach.

BOX 15-5   Clinical Institute Withdrawal Assessment for Alcohol (CIWA-A)

Within this test, the maximum possible score is 67. Facilities generally have ranges for which they give certain amounts of detox medication. The usual cutoff below which medication is deemed unnecessary is a score of 10. A separate assessment, the CIWA-B, is available for benzodiazepine withdrawal.

Nausea and vomiting (0-7)

Ask the patient, "Do you feel sick to your stomach? Have you vomited?" Observe.

0   No nausea and no vomiting
1   Mild nausea with no vomiting
2
3
4   Intermittent nausea with dry heaves
5
6
7

Tremor (0-7)

Ask the patient to stand with arms extended and fingers spread apart. Observe.

0   No tremor
1   Not visible but can be felt fingertip to fingertip
2
3
4   Moderate tremor
5
6
7   Severe, even with arms not extended

Paroxysmal Sweats (0-7)

Observe.

0   No sweat visible
1   Barely perceptible sweating with moist palms
2
3
4   Beads of sweat obvious on forehead
5
6
7   Drenching sweats

Box continued on following page

BOX 15-5   **Clinical Institute Withdrawal Assessment for Alcohol (CIWA-Ar)** *(Continued)*

Anxiety (0-7)

Ask, "Do you feel nervous?" Observe.

0   No anxiety; at ease
1   Mildly anxious
2
3
4   Moderately anxious, or guarded with anxiety implied
5
6
7   Acute panic state as seen in severe delirium or acute schizophrenic presentations

Agitation (0-7)

Observe.

0   Normal activity
1   Somewhat more than normal activity
2
3
4   Moderately fidgety and restless
5
6
7   Pacing back and forth or constantly thrashing about

Tactile Disturbances (0-7)

Ask, "Have you any itching, pins and needles, burning, or numbness? Do you feel bugs crawling on or under your skin?" Observe.

0   None
1   Very mild itching, pins and needles, burning or numbness
    Mild itching, pins and needles, burning or numbness
3   Moderate itching, pins and needles, burning or numbness
4   Moderately severe hallucinations
5   Severe hallucinations
6   Extremely severe hallucinations
7   Continuous hallucinations

Auditory Disturbances (0-7)

Ask, "Are you more aware of sounds around you? Are they harsh? Do they frighten you? Are you hearing anything that is disturbing to you? Are you hearing things you know aren't there?" Observe.

0   Not present
1   Very mild harshness or ability to frighten
2   Mild harshness or ability to frighten
3   Moderate harshness or ability to frighten
4   Moderately severe hallucinations

Box continued on following page

> BOX 15-5   **Clinical Institute Withdrawal Assessment for Alcohol (CIWA-Ar)** *(Continued)*
>
> 5   Severe hallucinations
> 6   Extremely severe hallucinations
> 7   Continuous hallucinations
>
> **Visual Disturbances (0-7)**
>
> Ask, "Does the light appear to be too bright? Is the color different? Does it hurt your eyes? Are you seeing anything that is disturbing to you? Are you seeing things you know aren't there?" Observe.
>
> 0   Not present
> 1   Very mild sensitivity
> 2   Mild sensitivity
> 3   Moderate sensitivity
> 4   Moderately severe hallucinations
> 5   Severe hallucinations
> 6   Extremely severe hallucinations
> 7   Continuous hallucinations
>
> **Headache, Fullness in Head (0-7)**
>
> Ask, "Does your head feel different? Does it feel like there is a band around your head?" Do not rate dizziness or lightheadedness. Otherwise, rate severity.
>
> 0   Not present
> 1   Very mild
> 2   Mild
> 3   Moderate
> 4   Moderately severe
> 5   Severe
> 6   Very severe
> 7   Extremely severe
>
> **Orientation and Clouding of Sensorium (0-4)**
>
> Ask, "What day is this? Where are you? Who am I?"
>
> 0   Oriented; can do serial additions
> 1   Cannot do serial additions or is uncertain about date
> 2   Disoriented for date by no more than 2 calendar days
> 3   Disoriented for date by more than 2 calendar days
> 4   Disoriented for place and/or person

    b. DTs require medical management capabilities.
       (1) Patients at risk for DTs should be closely monitored for changes in pulse, respiration, temperature, and heart rate.
       (2) Increased autonomic discharge occurs first, followed by the delirium, hallucinations, and physical agitation. Occasionally, behavioral symptoms precede.

Table 15-1   **Dose Conversions for Sedative–Hypnotic Drugs**

Drug	Dose (mg)
Benzodiazepines	
Alprazolam	1
Chlordiazepoxide	25
Clonazepam	0.5-1
Clorazepate	15
Diazepam	10
Estazolam	1
Flurazepam	15
Halazepam	40
Lorazepam	2
Oxazepam	30
Prazepam	80
Temazepam	15
Triazolam	0.25
Zolpidem	10
Barbiturates	
Amobarbital	100
Butabarbital	100
Pentobarbital	100
Phenobarbital	30
Secobarbital	100

c. Modal treatment involves the use of a benzodiazepine, which reduces mortality and duration of symptoms. Do not write 24-hour orders. It is important to observe the patient on a regular basis (e.g., every 3 hours) to adjust the dose according to response. Drug options include the following:

(1) Long-acting benzodiazepines.

(a) Once the patient is loaded with a long-acting benzodiazepine for 24 hours and there are no withdrawal symptoms, the medication can be stopped (based on long half-life) or at least decreased by 25% to 50% each subsequent day to avoid oversedation.

(b) Chlordiazepoxide 25 to 100 mg PO every 3 to 6 hours on the first day. Decrease the dose by 20% (of the original dose) per day over 5 days or discontinue after 24 hours.

(c) Diazepam 2 to 20 mg PO (or IV) every 3 to 6 hours on first day. Decrease the dose by 20% (of the original dose) per day over 5 days.

(2) Short-acting benzodiazepines.

(a) Lorazepam 2 mg PO or IM every 3 to 6 hours for the first 24 hours (based on symptoms), then taper.

(b) Because of the shorter half-life and lack of age-related hepatic metabolism, lorazepam is preferable in the elderly and in those with liver impairment.

(3) Pentobarbital or propofol can be used if the patient demonstrates agitation uncontrolled by large doses of benzodiazepines.

(4) See Box 15-5 for the CIWA protocol.

 d. Thiamine. Treat alcoholics with 100 mg IV thiamine immediately and then orally for at least 3 more days. Should be given before administration of fluids containing glucose.
 e. Magnesium. Hypomagnesemia is common in chronic alcoholics.
   (1) Magnesium sulfate 1 g IM or IV every 6 to 12 hours for 48 hours.
   (2) Magnesium oxide 250 to 500 mg PO four times a day for 48 hours (diarrhea is the most common side effect).
 f. Neuroleptic agents are not recommended because they are associated with higher mortality, longer duration of delirium, and more complications than sedative–hypnotics. They can play an adjunctive role in reducing severe psychotic symptoms.

ALCOHOL WITHDRAWAL SEIZURES

1. Withdrawal seizures can occur in one fourth to one third of continuous heavy drinkers, more commonly in those with a history of epilepsy.
2. Seizures usually occur within 8 to 38 hours after cessation of drinking, with a peak incidence at about 24 hours (and therefore almost always precede AWD). One third of patients with withdrawal seizures go on to develop AWD.
3. Check for and correct low magnesium.
4. Anticonvulsants are not helpful prophylactically and should be reserved for use in patients with a history of non–alcohol-related seizures. For patients with non–alcohol-related seizure history, phenytoin can be given in a loading dose of 15 mg/kg dissolved in 250 to 500 mL of D$_5$W over 4 hours, followed by 100 mg PO every 8 hours for 3 to 4 days or chronically if the electroencephalogram (EEG) is abnormal.
5. An etiology other than an alcohol withdrawal seizure should be sought in the following seizures:
 a. Occurring after the onset of delirium.
 b. Focal or multiple.
 c. Accompanied by elevated temperature.
 d. Occurring in the context of head trauma.

15.13 Blood Alcohol Level

1. Blood alcohol levels (BALs; Table 15-2) are fairly reliable indicators of ethanol in the blood and a reflection of brain ethanol levels.
2. BAL is reported as percent or mg% (to obtain mg%, multiply percent by 1000).
3. BAL is influenced by a person's weight, rapidity of drinking, time elapsed since the last drink, ability to metabolize alcohol, and presence of food.
4. On average, a person can decrease their BAL by 15 mg% an hour; a person with a history of drinking and activated enzymes can metabolize 30 mg% an hour.
 a. A heavy drinker with a BAL of 300 will have a BAL of 0 in about 10 hours.
5. On average:
 a. One drink gives a BAL of 30 mg%.
 b. Two drinks give a BAL of 50 to 60 mg% with mild coordination problems.

Table 15-2 **Blood Alcohol Levels**		
Blood Alcohol Level		
%	**mg/dL**	**Clinical Findings (In Nontolerant Patients)***
0.05	50	Inattention, unsteadiness
0.10	100	Impaired memory, abnormal Romberg (eyes closed)
0.15	150	Slurred speech, abnormal Romberg (eyes open)
0.20	200	Stupor
0.25	250	Anesthesia
0.35	>350	Respiratory arrest

*Patients with significant alcohol consumption develop tolerance and can have minimal findings even with a blood alcohol level of 250 mg/dL.

    c. Four or five drinks in an hour give a BAL of 100 mg%, with some psychomotor impairment and ataxia.
    d. BALs between 150 and 300 are associated with staggering gait, passing out, blacking out (a period of amnesia following drinking), and irrational behavior.
6. A patient showing no symptoms at a high BAL has a high tolerance from chronic, significant alcohol use.
    a. A BAL of 150 mg% with no symptoms of intoxication indicates alcoholism.
    b. A BAL of 350 to 400 mg% is considered the LD_{50} (a lethal dose for 50% of the population).
7. The first-pass metabolism is lower in women, leading to increased alcohol levels and lower thresholds for intoxication in women.

15.14 Abuse of Cocaine and Other Stimulants

1. Prevalence. After alcohol, cocaine is the most frequently abused drug with significant medical consequences.
2. Symptoms (Table 15-3).
    a. Typical intranasal dose onset takes only minutes. Inhaled (smoked) cocaine (crack) has faster onset and more intense autonomic and psychic effect, along with increased addicting reinforcement.
    b. Common acute medical effects.
        (1) Anorexia.
        (2) Insomnia.
        (3) Hyperactivity.
        (4) Pressured speech.
        (5) Rapid thoughts.
        (6) Hyperreflexia.
        (7) Tachycardia.
        (8) Diaphoresis.
    c. Less common serious consequences.
        (1) Hyperpyrexia.
        (2) Hypertension.
        (3) Seizures.

Table 15-3 Stimulant and Hallucinogen Symptoms and Treatments

Drug	Behavioral Effects	Physical Effects	Laboratory Findings	Treatment
Amphetamine and other sympathomimetics (including cocaine) and amphetamine-like substances.	Alertness, loquaciousness, euphoria, hyperactivity, irritability, aggressiveness, agitation, paranoid trends, impotence, visual and tactile hallucinations	Mydriasis, tremor, halitosis, dry mouth, tachycardia, hypertension, weight loss, arrhythmias, fever, convulsions, perforated nasal septum (with snorting)	Detected in blood and urine	For agitation: diazepam IM or PO 5-10 mg q3h; for tachyarrhythmias: propranolol (Inderal) 10-20 mg PO q4h, vitamin C 0.5 g qid PO can increase urinary excretion by acidifying urine
Hallucinogens: LSD, psilocybin (mushrooms), mescaline (peyote), DET, DMT, DOM or STP, MDA	Duration of 8-12 h with flashback after abstinence, visual hallucinations, paranoid ideation, false sense of achievement and strength, suicidal or homicidal tendencies, depersonalization, derealization	Mydriasis, ataxia, hyperemic conjunctiva, tachycardia, hypertension	None	Emotional support (talking down) For mild agitation: diazepam 10 mg IM or PO q2h for 4 doses For severe agitation: haloperidol 1-5 mg IM and repeat q6h prn. May have to continue haloperidol 1-2 mg/d PO for weeks to prevent flashback syndrome.

PCP and phencyclidine-like substances (including ketamine, TCP)	Duration of 8-12 h (about 2 h for ketamine), hallucinations, paranoid ideations, labile mood, loose associations (can mimic schizophrenia), catatonia, violent behavior, convulsions	Nystagmus, mydriasis, ataxia, tachycardia, hypertension	Detected in urine up to 5 days after ingestion	Phenothiazines may be used only with LSD. *Caution:* Phenothiazines can produce *fatal* results if used with other hallucinogens (e.g., DET, DMT), especially if they are adulterated with strychnine or belladonna alkaloids. Phenothiazines contraindicated for first week after ingestion. For violent delusions: haloperidol 1-4 mg IM or PO q12-4h until patient is calm
Volatile hydrocarbons and petroleum derivatives: glue, benzene, gasoline, varnish thinner, lighter fluid, aerosols	Euphoria, clouded sensorium, slurred speech, ataxia, hallucinations in 50% of cases, psychoses, permanent brain damage if used daily over 6 mo	Odor on breath, tachycardia with possible ventricular fibrillation, possible damage of brain, liver, kidneys, myocardium	Relevant to determine tissue damage (aspartate aminotransferase)	For agitation: haloperidol 1-5 mg q6h until calm; avoid epinephrine because of myocardial sensitization
Other inhalants: nitrous oxide	Euphoria, drowsiness, ataxia, confusion			

DET, diethyltryptamine; DMT, dimethyltryptamine; DOM, 4-methyl-2,5-dimethoxyamphetamine; LSD, lysergic acid diethylamide; MDA, 3,4-methylene-dioxyamphetamine; PCP, phencyclidine; STP, serenity, tranquility, peace (nickname for DOM); TCP, 1-[1-(2-thienyl)-cyclohexyl]-piperidine.

      (4) Myocardial infarction.

      (5) Brain hemorrhage.

  d. Acute psychiatric effects.

      (1) Similar to a panic attack, including palpitations and hyperventilation; however, unlike the fear and dysphoria of a panic attack, cocaine often produces euphoria.

      (2) Chronic effects.

         (a) Auditory and visual hallucinations.

         (b) Paranoid delusions.

         (c) Tendency to violent behavior.

         (d) Tactile hallucinations.

         (e) Autonomous panic attacks.

3. Recognition.

  a. Patients may be reluctant to admit their habit and instead report related symptoms such as panic attacks or chest pain.

  b. Patients need to be asked directly, and when in doubt, a toxicology urine screen may be helpful.

      (1) Although the plasma half-life elimination of cocaine is brief (hours), cocaine's metabolite, benzoyl ecgonine, may be detected in the urine for up to several days.

  c. Physical symptoms of cocaine use.

      (1) Frequent intranasal use can cause abnormal nasal septum, rhinitis, and sinusitis.

      (2) Freebase inhalers can develop bronchitis.

      (3) Seizures.

      (4) Snowlights (flashes of light in the periphery of the visual fields).

      (5) Overdoses are associated with stroke, ventricular fibrillation, or cardiac arrest.

4. Selected medical treatment aspects of cocaine abuse.

  a. The cocaine habit is powerful. Rats given an opportunity to self-inject with cocaine sometimes continue until they die of hyperthermia, seizures, or cardiac arrhythmias.

  b. Extreme autonomic hyperactivity can be counteracted to some extent with β-blockers.

  c. Neuroleptic agents help associated psychosis.

  d. Chronic cocaine can kindle abnormal brain activity, leading to seizures and panic attacks even after stopping cocaine.

  e. Withdrawal can lead to profound depression with increased suicide risk.

  f. Treatment must address both behavioral and physical habits. In general, a physician working alone will not be successful in treating cocaine (or other substance) addiction because a comprehensive behavioral program, including peer feedback and support, is usually necessary.

  g. Medications to treat cocaine abuse. Studies of disulfiram, dopamine-selective antagonists, citicoline, anticonvulsants, and a cocaine-specific vaccine are early but promising. β-Blockers and amantadine are promising in reducing cocaine withdrawal symptoms.

  h. Treatment of associated psychiatric comorbidity is important. There is no evidence supporting the use of antidepressants in the treatment of cocaine dependence. Given the high rate of treatment attrition, psychotherapeutic support to keep patients in treatment may be helpful.

15.15 Hallucinogens

1. Lysergic acid diethylamide (LSD), mescaline, psilocybin, dimethyltryptamine (DMT), methylenedioxymethamphetamine (MDMA, "ecstasy"), and phencyclidine (PCP) all can produce hallucinations, delusions, and intense affective symptoms.
2. PCP use is associated with violence.
   a. Physical symptoms of PCP intoxication include nystagmus, myoclonus, and ataxia.
3. Treatment.
   a. Create a safe setting.
   b. Decrease sensory stimulation.
   c. Use verbal reassurance.
   d. Autonomic symptoms can be lessened with β-blockers.
   e. Benzodiazepines or neuroleptic agents may be helpful for agitation or psychosis.
   f. Avoid use of drugs with anticholinergic side effects, which could increase the confusion.

15.16 Issues in Narcotics Use

1. Respiratory depression is the major medical concern with acute use of narcotics. In general, this is a problem for the following patients:
   a. Those who have not had time to develop tolerance to this effect.
   b. Patients taking large intravenous doses.
   c. Those taking other sedatives (such as benzodiazepines) that depress respiratory function.
2. Common problems in pain management.
   a. The major reason for continued pain in medical and surgical patients is underuse of narcotic analgesics. Inadequate pain relief can take the form of:
      (1) Inadequate amount of narcotic per dose.
      (2) Excessive time duration between doses.
   b. One method to establish the problem in pain control is to ask the patient to rate pain on a scale from 0 to 10 in which 0 is "no pain" and 10 is "the worst pain the patient has experienced."
      (1) The first rating should be done about one half hour after the narcotic dose to see if the dose amount is adequate. If the rating is high at that point, a larger dose should be given.
      (2) The patient should be rated again just before the next dose is given. If that rating is high, the duration between doses might be too long.
   c. Scheduled versus as needed (prn) dosages.
      (1) In general, a schedule is better.
      (2) Pain can often be managed with lower overall doses if it is kept from reemerging.

        (3) Drawbacks of prn schedule.

           (a) Low numbers of nursing staff can result in delays.

           (b) It rewards the patient for reporting pain.

        (4) A "reverse prn" schedule gives the patient the option, on a schedule, of refusing a dose.

3. Patient-controlled analgesia (PCA).

   a. Patients control the release of small amounts of parenteral narcotics as they feel they need them.

   b. A lock-out period keeps the patient from using too much too quickly.

   c. Overall, studies of PCA in the context of acute (usually postoperative) pain indicate better pain control using less narcotic.

4. Constipation.

   a. Constipation occurs acutely and remains a serious problem during narcotic use. It can progress to paralytic ileus and obstruction.

   b. Patients requiring continuous narcotics should be put on a prophylactic bowel regimen, such as daily docusate sodium (Colace) or fiber-containing stool softeners.

   c. Constipation is made worse by concurrent anticholinergic drugs.

5. Psychiatric effects of narcotics.

   a. Many narcotics users seek narcotics to self-medicate underlying psychiatric disorders.

   b. Psychiatric disorders often reemerge after chronic users discontinue narcotics.

6. Dose conversion.

   a. It is helpful to be able to interconvert doses of narcotics when:

        (1) Simplifying drug orders.

        (2) Detoxing a patient.

        (3) Converting any narcotic.

        (4) Converting from one narcotic to another.

   b. Box 15-6 lists a formula for interconverting narcotics.

7. Tolerance, dependence, and addiction.

   a. *Tolerance* refers to nervous system adaptation to continued exposure.

        (1) Over a few weeks, tolerance develops to the respiratory depressant effects, analgesic effects, and some psychotropic effects.

        (2) After about 3 weeks, patients might require a higher dose to achieve the same pain relief.

        (3) This dose escalation does not mean the patient is an addict or is abusing the medication.

   b. *Dependence* refers to a state resulting in the emergence of withdrawal symptoms if the drug is stopped.

        (1) Every patient who has continued exposure to narcotics for a few weeks and then stops will experience typical withdrawal symptoms (Box 15-7).

        (2) The time of onset and symptom severity are proportional to drug half-life (Table 15-4).

        (3) This physiologic dependence is related to but not equivalent to the psychological or behavioral dependence that patients also can develop.

BOX 15-6   Narcotic Dose Conversions*

Oral Dose Conversion

To convert an oral dose of any narcotic to an equivalent oral dose of morphine, multiply by:
0.33 for codeine
8 for hydromorphone
0.2 for meperidine
3 for methadone
2 for oxycodone
0.5 for pentazocine
0.15 for propoxyphene

Intramuscular Dose Conversion

To convert an intramuscular dose of any narcotic to an equivalent oral dose of morphine, multiply by:
30 for butorphanol
40 for hydromorphone
0.8 for meperidine
6.0 for methadone
3.0 for morphine
1.5 for pentazocine

Intranasal Butorphanol

Another alternative for acute pain is intranasal butorphanol (Stadol NS). A 2-mg dose is equivalent to 75 mg IM meperidine. Because this drug is a mixed agonist–antagonist it should not be used in a patient already taking narcotic agonists, because withdrawal could be precipitated.

*Equivalent doses are approximate and may need to be adjusted, especially in early treatment.

    c. *Addiction* refers to a state of tolerance and dependence, with a behavioral component consisting of a preoccupation with obtaining and using the drug in question.
      (1) Patients with chronic malignant pain (e.g., from cancer) who are maintained with morphine are not addicts.
      (2) Paradoxically, physicians who withhold narcotics from patients who legitimately need them can create addicts by forcing a preoccupation with obtaining the drugs they need.
8. Narcotics withdrawal.
    a. Onset and duration.
      (1) Proportional to duration of action (see Table 15-4).
      (2) Starts within a half day for short-acting narcotics, such as heroin, and usually ends after several days.
      (3) Starts after a few days for longer-acting drugs, such as methadone, and continues in some drawn-out form for a number of weeks.

BOX 15-7   Clinical Institute Narcotic Assessment (CINA)

Nausea and Vomiting (0-6)

Ask the patient, "Do you feel sick to your stomach? Have you vomited?" Observe.

0   No nausea and no vomiting
1
2   Mild nausea with no vomiting
3
4   Intermittent nausea with dry heaves
5
6   Constant nausea, frequent dry heaves, and/or vomiting

Tremor (0-3)

Ask the patient to stand with arms extended and fingers spread apart. Observe.

0   No tremor
1   Not visible, but can be felt fingertip to fingertip
2   Moderate, with patient's arms extended
3   Severe, even if arms are not extended

Sweating (0-3)

Observe.

0   No sweat visible
1   Barely perceptible sweating with moist palms
2   Beads of sweat obvious on forehead
3   Drenching sweat over face and chest

Restlessness (0-3)

Observe.

0   Normal activity
1   Somewhat more than normal activity (might move legs up and down and shift position occasionally)
2   Moderately fidgety and restless, shifting position frequently
3   Gross movements most of the time or constantly thrashes about

Goose Flesh (0-3)

Observe.

0   No goose flesh visible
1   Occasional goose flesh but not elicited by touch, not prominent
2   Prominent goose flesh in waves and elicited by touch
3   Constant goose flesh over chest and arms

Lacrimation (0-2)

Observe.

0   None
1   Eyes watering, tears at corners of eyes
2   Profuse tearing from eyes over face

BOX 15-7   Clinical Institute Narcotic Assessment (CINA) (*Continued*)

Nasal Congestion (0-2)

Observe.
0   No nasal congestion, sniffling
1   Frequent sniffling
2   Constant sniffling with watery discharge

Yawning (0-2)

Observe.
0   None
1   Frequent
2   Constant, uncontrolled yawning

Abdominal Changes (0-2)

Ask, "Do you have any pains in your lower abdomen?"
0   No complaints, normal bowel sounds
1   Reports waves of abdominal crampy pain, active bowel sounds
2   Reports crampy abdominal pain, diarrheal movements, active
      bowel sounds

Changes in Temperature (0-2)

Ask, "Do you feel hot or cold?"
0   No report of temperature change
1   Reports feeling cold, hands cold and clammy to touch
2   Uncontrollable shivering

Muscle Aches (0-2)

Ask, "Do you have any muscle aches?"
0   No muscle aching reported, e.g., arm and neck muscles soft at
      rest
1   Mild muscle pains
2   Reports severe muscle pains; muscles of legs, arms, and neck in
      constant state of contraction

Heart Rate

$(X - 80)/10 = $ _____

Systolic Blood Pressure

$(X - 130)/10 = $ _____

    b. Severity and multiple drug abuse issues.
       (1) Patients rarely die from narcotics withdrawal.
       (2) Sedative withdrawal, with seizures and autonomic dysfunction,
           is much more dangerous.
       (3) In cases of multiple addictions, withdraw the patient from one
           drug at a time.

Table 15-4 **Substance Half-Lives**	
Agent	**Duration of Action (h)**
Codeine	4-7
Heroin	3-4
Hydromorphone	4-6
Levomethadyl acetate	48-96
Meperidine	2-4
Methadone	12-24
Morphine	2.5-7
Oxycodone	3-5
Pentazocine	2-3
Propoxyphene	6-8

      (4) Because of physiologic stress, maintain narcotics until other medical problems are stabilized.

   c. Recognition and treatment. See Box 15-7 for the Clinical Institute Narcotics Assessment (CINA) protocol.

      (1) Should be based on observation of symptoms rather than on history.

         (a) Some addicts make up their dose to obtain a supply from a naive physician.

         (b) The composition and identity of street drugs are uncertain.

      (2) The principle is to achieve a narcotic level comparable to habitual level of use and then decrease the daily dose in increments that balance withdrawal symptoms with time.

         (a) The taper can be 10% to 33% a day.

         (b) There is no way to eliminate all withdrawal symptoms.

         (c) For most street addicts, 10 to 20 mg of methadone PO is usually sufficient to control withdrawal symptoms, with rapid taper (5 to 10 mg per day) if hospitalized. Patients must be tapered off methadone because it cannot be prescribed for outpatient use other than through licensed treatment programs. For opiate-dependent persons enrolled in a methadone maintenance program, confirmation from the treatment program is essential. If the program cannot be reached immediately, using half the patient-stated dose should be adequate to prevent discomfort.

      (3) Whatever dose is selected, observe and adjust on the basis of toxicity or withdrawal.

      (4) Clonidine as an alternative or adjunct.

         (a) An α-adrenergic agonist, which blocks autonomic discharge, can be used alone or with a narcotic taper to reduce withdrawal symptoms.

         (b) About one third of patients do not tolerate clonidine because of hypotension.

      (5) Treatment of heroin overdose.

         (a) Naloxone is a specific opiate antagonist with no agonist properties or euphoriant potential. It is nonscheduled and

inexpensive. It reverses the respiratory depression and sedation caused by opiates.
   (b) The initial intramuscular or subcutaneous dose is 0.4 mg of naloxone, followed by 1 to 2 mg if no response in 3 to 5 minutes.
   (c) Complications. Low rate of seizures, arrhythmia, severe agitation. The half-life is short and there is concern that sedation and respiratory depression will recur after 20 to 30 minutes.
9. Methadone maintenance.
   a. Methadone maintenance programs provide treatment for narcotics addicts unable to succeed at abstinence. It is the most effective narcotics addiction treatment in reducing drug use, street crime, incarceration, and human immunodeficiency virus (HIV) infection. Programs typically include daily dosing, individual and group counseling, and urine toxicology monitoring.
   b. Physicians outside of hospitals or methadone programs may not provide methadone for the treatment of opiate addiction.
   c. If a methadone maintenance patient is admitted to the hospital, call the program to confirm the methadone dose and maintain the patient with that dose during the admission.
   d. Methadone is dosed once daily by most programs, and average doses are 100 mg. Higher doses are used for persons with continued craving, for rapid metabolizers, or for those on concomitant medications that affect metabolism.
   e. Methadone side effects include insomnia and constipation. There is no liver toxicity related to methadone; if liver function tests are abnormal, other reasons should be sought.
10. Buprenorphine.
   a. Buprenorphine offers an outpatient opioid addiction treatment that may be prescribed by qualified physicians in the medical office outside the methadone clinic system.
   b. Buprenorphine is a partial agonist: It activates the opioid receptor (although not to the same degree as methadone), creating a ceiling dose effect, but blocking effects of full agonist.
   c. Buprenorphine treatment is not recommended for patients:
      (1) On high doses of benzodiazepines, alcohol, or other CNS depressants.
      (2) With significant untreated psychiatric morbidity.
      (3) With previous drug abuse treatments.
   d. Buprenorphine abuse is possible, but the current formulation containing buprenorphine in combination with naloxone decreases potential for injection use.
   e. Buprenorphine plus naloxone can be used for medically supervised detoxification or maintenance treatment.
   f. Maintenance treatment involves three phases.
      (1) Induction to find the minimum dose of buprenorphine at which the patient discontinues use of other opioids.
      (2) Stabilization, when withdrawal symptoms abate, treatment side effects are minimal, and cravings are reduced.

(3) Maintenance, when attention to psychosocial and family issues predominate.
11. What to do when the narcotic addict requires analgesics.
    a. Narcotics addicts should not be deprived of adequate analgesia.
    b. Remember that the patient will have tolerance. Therefore addicts often need somewhat higher doses to achieve the expected effects.
    c. When treating pain in a methadone maintained patient, it is usually helpful to continue the methadone and to use another narcotic for pain control. This keeps the two issues separate.
12. Chronic malignant pain.
    a. Pain secondary to a malignancy (or other "malignant" medical condition) should be treated without prejudice about potential addiction.
        (1) There is an imperative to provide terminal patients with adequate analgesia.
        (2) Oral morphine is the standard for chronic malignant pain. It does not require injections, and it can be titrated easily.
            (a) Oral morphine elixir is used on an every-3-hours basis.
            (b) Oral morphine can provide relief equivalent to parenteral doses.
            (c) Box 15-6 shows the interconversions of different narcotics to the oral morphine equivalent.
            (d) Once a daily dose has been established, it can be converted to a sustained-release form (such as controlled-release morphine sulfate [MS Contin]) that is more convenient for the patient.
        (3) Give half the daily oral morphine elixir dose every 12 hours in the controlled-release formulation or one third every 8 hours.
        (4) Oral or parenteral morphine can be used prn for breakthrough pain.
        (5) Fentanyl patches are another alternative for chronic malignant (and postsurgical) pain.
            (a) Once the patient's narcotics requirement has been established, convert to the equivalent patch dose (Table 15-5).
            (b) Oral (or parenteral) narcotics doses can be used to supplement breakthrough pain if necessary.
        (6) Butorphanol nasal spray is available as an alternative to the IM route, with comparable acute pain relief. Dose is usually 1 mg (1 spray) in each nostril, with a repeat if needed. Because butorphanol is a mixed agonist–antagonist, it cannot be used in patients already taking narcotics because it can precipitate withdrawal.
13. Nonmalignant chronic pain (such as chronic low back pain or chronic headache) creates significant treatment dilemmas and problems.

Table 15-5 **Converting Narcotics to Fentanyl Patch**	
Oral 24-Hour Morphine Dose (mg)	**Fentanyl Patch Dose (μg/h)**
45-134	25
135-224	50
225-314	75
315-404	100
405-494	125
495-584	150
585-674	175
675-764	200
765-854	225
855-944	250
945-1034	275
1035-1124	300

a. Some patients with chronic pain seem to be able to maintain fairly low, consistent doses of narcotic.
b. Many chronic pain patients show addictive behavior that contributes to management problems.
   (1) Using multiple providers to prescribe analgesics.
   (2) Using multiple medications.
   (3) Running out of prescriptions early.
   (4) "Losing" their supply of medication.
   (5) Using the emergency department for refill.
c. The correct medication is rarely the cure for chronic pain, even though these patients feel some medical treatment will cure them. Chronic pain represents a complex behavioral problem rather than a limited medical symptom.
d. Treatment.
   (1) Convert the patient from the acute to the chronic pain paradigm.
      (a) In the acute paradigm, pain is seen as a symptom of an underlying treatable medical problem. Therefore acute pain is evaluated aggressively, treated with surgery when possible, or treated with medication if needed.
      (b) The acute paradigm does not apply very well to chronic pain.
      (c) In the chronic pain paradigm, there is no simple surgical cure, and narcotics do not solve the problem. Treatment involves a program combining the following:
         (i) Behavioral elements (stressing adaptive functions and positive behavior).
         (ii) Physical therapy and exercise components.
         (iii) Attention to underlying psychosocial stresses and psychiatric comorbidity.

15.17 Psychotropic Medications as Analgesic Augmenters

1. Nonnarcotic analgesics such as the nonsteroidal antiinflammatory drugs (NSAIDs).
   a. Work by different mechanisms and can significantly augment pain relief for patients already taking narcotics.
   b. Antiinflammatory properties may be effective in inflammatory conditions in which narcotics are more nonspecific.
2. Antidepressants.
   a. Most patients with chronic pain should have a trial of some antidepressant because of the prevalence of coexisting depression, leading to amplification of symptoms.
   b. Antidepressants have some analgesic augmenting properties demonstrated in:
      (1) Diabetic neuropathy.
      (2) Postherpetic neuralgia.
      (3) Tension and migraine headache.
      (4) Myofascial pain.
   c. Amitriptyline or imipramine is used in starting doses of 25 to 50 mg/day, increasing every 4 to 7 days by 25-mg increments.
   d. Duloxetine has a recent FDA indication for diabetic neuropathic pain.
   e. Pain conditions are heterogeneous, and some may be helped by noradrenergic rather than serotoninergic augmentation.
   f. Nefazodone potentiates morphine analgesia.
3. Antihistamines.
   a. Hydroxyzine (Vistaril) is often used as a coanalgesic. Its mechanism of analgesic action is unknown. Hydroxyzine 25 mg given alone appears to have the analgesic potency of about 2 mg of IM morphine.
4. Stimulants. Dextroamphetamine in oral doses of 5 to 10 mg has been demonstrated to augment narcotic analgesia.
5. Cocaine. Despite its use in Brompton's mixture, no study has ever documented the analgesic potency of cocaine.
6. Steroids are important in a number of pain conditions including metastatic bone disease, epidural cord compression, headache resulting from increased intracranial pressure, and tumor infiltration of nerves.
7. Antipsychotic agents generally do not have significant analgesic properties and are more often used for their anxiolytic and antiemetic properties.
8. Anticonvulsants can act as membrane stabilizers that help exert some analgesic effect. Low doses of carbamazepine (e.g., 50 mg tid) and phenytoin have been used in neuropathic pain syndromes, though there are few controlled data.
9. Neurontin has been used for neuropathic pain syndromes at doses up to 2700 mg per day (tid dosing). Neurontin has soporific effects as well, and it helps with insomnia related to pain.

15.18 Marijuana Abuse

1. Definition.
   a. Problems in controlling use despite experiencing adverse personal consequences.
   b. Complaints of loss of control over use and of cognitive and motivational impairments.
2. Prevalence.
   a. Cannabis (including hashish, marijuana, blunts, and other forms of tetrahydrocannabinol) is the most prevalent psychoactive substance used in the United States.
   b. Approximately 7% of 18-year-olds meet criteria for dependence.
   c. Past year use in the general population was 9%, and 32% reported lifetime use.
   d. The leading substance found in adolescent arrests, emergency department admissions, and autopsies.
3. Morbidity and mortality.
   a. Physiologic changes produced within minutes of inhalation include tachycardia, feelings of euphoria, sedation, and analgesia. Occasionally, apprehension, depression, and anger are intensified.
   b. Dose—response relationships are difficult to establish because cannabis does not come in standard doses. Tetrahydrocannabinol (THC) amounts have increased from 0.5% two decades ago to nearer 5%.
   c. Acute marijuana intoxication affects motor performance, complex reaction time, and recall and comprehension of written information.
      (1) Performance effects can last up to 24 hours.
      (2) Alcohol and marijuana have additive detrimental effects.
   d. Cardiopulmonary harm.
      (1) Most cannabis smokers also smoke tobacco, making epidemiologic data difficult to dissect. There are indications that cannabis has effects similar to those of tobacco.
      (2) Risk of chronic bronchitis, emphysema, and lung cancer are increased.
      (3) Myocardial infarction is four times more likely to occur within an hour of smoking.
      (4) The relationship to coronary artery disease is unclear.
   e. Injuries include increased rates of motor vehicle accidents, assaults, and self-inflicted injuries resulting in hospitalization. Concurrent use of alcohol and other illegal drugs can confound findings.
   f. Psychological harm.
      (1) Regular use has been associated with an increased incidence of depression.
      (2) Can exacerbate symptoms of schizophrenia.
      (3) High-risk behavior, including sexual risk taking.
4. Marijuana withdrawal in heavy, chronic users.
   a. Anxiety.
   b. Insomnia.
   c. Appetite disturbance.

5. Treatment.
   a. Cognitive behavior therapy alone and in combination with motivational interviewing.
   b. Group psychoeducational approaches.
   c. Twelve-step therapies.
   d. Family therapy.

SUGGESTED READINGS

Abbott PJ, Quinn D, Knox L: Ambulatory medical detoxification for alcohol. *Am J Drug Alc Abuse* 21:549-563, 1995.

Anton RF, Swift RM: Current pharmacotherapies of alcoholism: A US perspective. *Am J Addictions* 12:S53-S68, 2003.

Ewing JA: Detecting alcoholism: The CAGE questionnaire. *JAMA* 252:1905-1907, 1984.

Fiellin DA, O'Connor PG: Office based treatment of opioid dependence. *N Engl J Med* 347:817-823, 2002.

Fudala PJ, Bridge TP, Herbert S, et al: Office-based treatment of opiate addiction with a sublingual tablet formulation of buprenorphine and naloxone. *N Engl J Med* 349:949-958, 2003.

Holder HD, Blose JO: The reduction of health care costs associated with alcoholism treatment: A 14-year longitudinal study. *J Stud Alcohol* 53(4):293-302, 1992.

Hoskin PJ, Hanks GW: Opioid agonist—antagonist drugs in acute and chronic pain states. *Drugs* 41(3):326-344, 1991.

Max MB, Lynch SA, Muir J, et al: Effects of desipramine, amitriptyline, and fluoxetine on pain in diabetic neuropathy. *N Engl J Med* 326:1250-1256, 1992.

Mayo-Smith MF, Beecher LH, Fischer TL, et al: Management of alcohol withdrawal delirium: An evidence-based practice guideline. *Arch Intern Med* 164:1405-1412, 2004.

O'Connor PG, Fiellin DA: Pharmacologic treatment of heroin-dependent patients. *Ann Intern Med* 133:40-54, 2000.

Selzer ML: The Michigan Alcoholism Screening Test: The quest for a new diagnostic instrument. *Am J Psychiatry* 127:89-94, 1971.

Electroconvulsive Therapy

16

David A. Solomon

16.1 Overview

1. Electroconvulsive therapy (ECT) is often neglected as a treatment option by nonpsychiatrists because of the lack of knowledge of its modern applications and technology and because of ongoing stigma.
2. ECT is a medical procedure in which a brief electrical stimulus is used to induce a seizure under controlled conditions to treat certain major mental disorders.
3. The psychobiologic mechanisms responsible for the therapeutic effects of ECT remain unknown.

16.2 Indications

1. ECT is generally not a first-line treatment. ECT should be considered when the following has occurred:
   a. A patient has failed trials of medication.
   b. A patient cannot tolerate the risks or side effects of medication.
   c. There is a need for an immediate response, because of potential for the following:
      (1) Suicidal behavior.
      (2) Malnutrition.
      (3) Severe psychosis with agitation.
      (4) Prolonged catatonia.
2. ECT should be considered for the following disorders:
   a. Unipolar major depressive episode.
   b. Bipolar disorder, major depressive episode.
   c. Bipolar disorder, manic or mixed episode.
   d. Schizoaffective disorder, manic or major depressive episode.
   e. Unremitting psychosis.
      (1) Schizophrenia.
      (2) Schizoaffective disorder.
3. ECT may also be effective in the following disorders:
   a. Some severe psychoses secondary to a general medical condition.
   b. Delirium.
   c. Refractory epilepsy.
   d. Neuroleptic malignant syndrome.
   e. Parkinson's disease.

16.3 Contraindications

1. There are no absolute contraindications and few relative contraindications for ECT. Pregnancy is *not* a contraindication, and ECT may be used in all trimesters in consultation with the obstetrician.
2. Certain situations have a substantially increased risk associated with ECT.
   a. Space-occupying intracranial lesions or other conditions associated with increased intracranial pressure.
   b. Recent myocardial infarction (MI). The standard practice is to wait at least 3 months after an MI to give ECT.
   c. Recent intracerebral hemorrhage.
   d. Bleeding or unstable vascular aneurysm or malformation.
   e. Retinal detachment.
   f. Pheochromocytoma.
   g. Anesthetic risk rated at American Society of Anesthesiologists (ASA) level 4 or 5.
   h. Ventricular arrhythmias.
3. Certain medical conditions require special consideration in technique to avoid complications.
   a. Chronic obstructive pulmonary disease (COPD) or other significant pulmonary disease.
   b. Asthma.
   c. Hypertension.
   d. Cardiac arrhythmia.
   e. History of cerebrovascular accident (CVA).
   f. Coronary artery disease.
   g. Significant osteoporosis or major bone fractures.
   h. Extreme obesity.

16.4 Adverse Effects

OVERALL MORTALITY

1. Contemporary ECT, including preoxygenation, brief anesthesia, muscle relaxation, and careful physiologic and cardiac monitoring, is associated with a low rate of morbidity and mortality.
   a. Significant medical complications are reported in the range of 0.3% to 0.4% of patients treated.
      (1) The most common complications involve cardiac arrhythmias and myocardial ischemia.
      (2) Transient benign arrhythmias occur in 10% to 40% of patients with cardiac disorders.
      (3) Infrequent but serious complications.
         (a) MI.
         (b) Congestive heart failure.
         (c) Coronary insufficiency.
         (d) Exacerbation of hypertension.
         (e) Prolonged seizures.
         (f) Pulmonary aspiration.

(g) Pulmonary edema.
(h) Laryngospasm.
(i) Prolonged apnea.
(4) Less serious injuries.
(a) Musculoskeletal injury.
(b) Damage to teeth.
(c) Oral lacerations.
(d) Myalgias.
b. Common complaints.
(1) Anxiety (anticipation of treatment).
(2) Headaches.
(3) Muscle aches.
(4) Memory loss. The seizure produced by ECT almost always causes a retrograde amnesia for the event.
(5) Cognitive impairment.
2. Mortality associated with ECT is comparable to (if not lower than) anesthesia mortality among surgical outpatients (about 0.9 deaths per 10,000 cases).
3. The majority of deaths are cardiorespiratory complications.

COGNITIVE EFFECTS

1. Memory impairment has been considered the principal adverse effect of ECT.
2. ECT is associated with four types of short-term memory impairment.
a. Postictal confusion immediately following treatment.
b. Retrograde amnesia for a variable period of minutes to hours before the treatment.
c. Anterograde amnesia for a variable period of minutes to hours to days.
d. Longer lasting subjective complaints of memory impairment, which are difficult to evaluate. Possible explanations include the following:
(1) A genuine neuropsychologic impairment too subtle for standard neuropsychological testing to detect.
(2) Patients use this complaint for secondary gain.
(3) Patients become more aware of memory problems that preceded treatment.
(4) Memory difficulty may be part of a residual psychopathologic condition such as major depression.
3. Acquisition and retention of new memories and long-term memory are not impaired.
4. The incidence and severity of cognitive effects depend to some extent on technical variables. The following variables are associated with increased chance of cognitive impairment.
a. Bilateral electrode placement.
b. Higher stimulus intensity.
c. Sine wave stimulation (should not be used).
d. More frequent treatments (i.e., less time between treatments).
e. Concomitant psychotropic use.
f. Higher anesthesia dose.

5. For most young, healthy patients, post-treatment confusion is generally limited to a few hours. For the elderly or those with other risk factors for confusion, post-treatment confusion can last all day, several days, or in unusual cases, up to a few weeks.
   a. If a patient does not recover cognitive function sufficiently, additional treatments may have to be delayed.
   b. Recording cognitive mental status before treatments is important to assess changes from baseline.
6. If severe cognitive dysfunction develops during ECT:
   a. Decrease stimulus dose.
   b. Decrease frequency of treatments.
   c. Switch from bilateral to unilateral.
   d. Review concurrent medications.

CARDIOVASCULAR EFFECTS

1. The majority of deaths attributed to ECT are a result of cardiac complications. Cardiac complications occur in about 10% of patients, although the majority are transient.
2. ECT is associated with several significant physiologic events that contribute to cardiovascular risk.
   a. Increased parasympathetic tone within the first 15 seconds, with potential for bradycardia or asystole, as well as various arrhythmias.
   b. Immediate sympathetic discharge with marked increase in circulating catecholamines (plasma epinephrine is released mainly from the adrenal medulla), creating potential for tachyarrhythmias and hypertension.
      (1) Associated increased myocardial oxygen consumption can cause myocardial ischemia in susceptible patients.
      (2) Patients within 6 months of myocardial infarction should be treated cautiously if at all.
3. Attenuation of autonomic changes can decrease cardiovascular complications. Patients with preexisting hypertension or hypertensive responses to ECT should be premedicated using labetalol 5 to 10 mg IV about 90 seconds before induction of seizures.

PULMONARY EFFECTS

1. General anesthesia creates a risk for patients with pulmonary disease.
2. Mild hypoxia, hypercapnia, and respiratory acidosis are not uncommon.

CEREBROVASCULAR EFFECTS

There is a brief but marked increase in intracranial pressure associated with increased cerebral blood flow following the electrical stimulus.

INTRAOCULAR EFFECTS

Increases in intraocular pressure may be relevant for patients with poorly controlled glaucoma.

INTRAGASTRIC EFFECTS

Increases in intragastric pressure can lead to regurgitation or pulmonary aspiration, especially for patients with hiatal hernia.

OTHER COMPLICATIONS

Estimated rate of complications is about 1 per 1400 treatments. These complications include the following:

1. Laryngospasm.
2. Prolonged apnea.
3. Prolonged seizures and status epilepticus. Many ECT devices now allow monitoring of seizure duration.
4. Tooth damage.
5. Laceration of lip or tongue.
6. Fractures or dislocations. Risks are quite minor with proper use of muscle relaxants.
7. Post-treatment nausea, headache, and muscle soreness are not uncommon but usually respond to symptomatic treatments.

16.5 Drug Interactions

1. Reserpine and chlorpromazine are contraindicated because of reports of cardiovascular collapse and respiratory depression.
2. Lithium can prolong neuromuscular blockade of succinylcholine, and it can contribute to severe post-treatment delirium. In general, lithium should be discontinued before ECT.
3. There is no specific evidence for contraindications to giving ECT to a patient taking monoamine oxidase inhibitors (MAOIs) or tricyclic antidepressants.
4. Patients taking warfarin (Coumadin) may continue taking that medication, but they should have prothrombin time maintained at less than two times control.
5. Acetylcholinesterase inhibitors (e.g., donepezil, rivastigmine, galantamine) can prolong the duration of succinylcholine effects. These medications are generally best discontinued prior to ECT. The clinical relevance of this interaction is debated; however, the anesthesiologist should know if a patient continues on an acetylcholinesterase inhibitor.

16.6 Procedure

CONSENT

1. Patients must provide signed informed consent.
2. If the patient is not considered competent to provide consent, it may be possible to proceed with consent provided by a spouse or family member. When in doubt about the legality of a substituted decision maker, consult a risk manager.

PRE–ELECTROCONVULSIVE THERAPY ASSESSMENT

1. The minimal assessment before ECT should include the following:
   a. Psychiatric assessment to document appropriate diagnosis and history.
   b. Mental status examination.
   c. Physical and neurologic examination to establish presence of any risk factors.

    d. Laboratory studies.
      (1) Complete blood count (CBC).
      (2) Electrolytes (especially for patients receiving diuretics or digitalis).
      (3) Renal function (blood urea nitrogen [BUN], creatinine).
      (4) Electrocardiogram (ECG).
    e. Consultation from specialists (including pre-ECT anesthesiology consultation) should be obtained if there is concern about cardiac, pulmonary, or other special medical risk factors.
    f. Studies such as neuroimaging, electroencephalography (EEG), or chest x-ray depend on the clinical condition.
2. Most consultants recommend tapering and discontinuing psychotropic medication before ECT (because no additive benefit has been demonstrated).
    a. It is important to discontinue lithium because of reports of associated delirium.
    b. Although it is possible to do ECT on patients who are taking MAOIs, because of the potential for drug interactions, MAOIs should be stopped 2 weeks before treatment whenever possible.
    c. Reserpine should be discontinued 2 weeks before ECT in order to avoid risk of apnea, hypotension, and cardiac dysrhythmia.
3. Other potential medical interactions.
    a. Prolonged seizures secondary to theophylline.
    b. Increased seizure threshold with anticonvulsants and benzodiazepines.

PRE–ELECTROCONVULSIVE THERAPY ORDERS

1. Nothing by mouth (NPO) for 8 hours before treatment.
    a. Cardiac drugs or medication for gastric reflux may be given if necessary with sips of water about 2 hours before ECT.
    b. Diuretics may be withheld, because being NPO lowers fluid levels.
    c. Rauwolfia alkaloids should be discontinued several weeks before ECT to prevent apnea, hypotension, and cardiac dysrhythmias.
2. Diabetic patients treated with insulin in the morning are typically given half the dose of insulin in the morning before each ECT treatment and the other half after the ECT treatment.
3. To dry secretions and provide anticholinergic blockade of the vagal bradycardias or asystole:
    a. Glycopyrrolate 0.2 to 0.4 mg IV (which does not cross the blood-brain barrier) is often the first line of treatment.
    b. Atropine (0.4 to 1 mg IV) 30 to 40 minutes before ECT.

ELECTROCONVULSIVE THERAPY TECHNIQUE

1. Patients are given a short-acting anesthetic agent such as methohexital or ketamine. Other agents include etomidate (expensive); propofol (highly anticonvulsant); and thiopental (anticonvulsant and associated with cardiac arrhythmias).
2. Once asleep, patients receive a muscle relaxant (usually IV succinylcholine 0.5 to 1 mg/kg) to minimize muscle response to the seizure.

a. A blood pressure cuff may be inflated on an ankle before giving succinylcholine in order to observe motor activity associated with the seizure.

b. Neuromuscular blockade generally takes about 100 seconds.

3. The anesthetist ventilates the patient with a bag-valve-mask with 100% oxygen and monitors vital signs (pulse, blood pressure, respiration) along with pulse oximetry and cardiac rhythm. A bite block is inserted in the mouth to prevent oral injury.

4. Electrodes are applied by the psychiatrist (unilateral or bilateral placement), and an electrical stimulus is administered to induce a seizure.

a. Parameters involved in stimulus dosing involve waveform, stimulus duration, and intensity.

b. Electrode placement.

(1) Bilateral placement is generally more effective, but it is also associated with more cognitive impairment. High-dose right unilateral ECT may be as efficacious as bilateral with less morbidity.

(a) Bilateral placement should be used on patients with severe illness (e.g., suicidal or psychotic).

(b) The electrode site is prepared by cleansing the site and applying electrode jelly.

(2) If a patient has not improved with four to six unilateral nondominant placement treatments, the placement should be changed to bilateral.

(3) If severe cognitive impairment develops with bilateral placement, the placement should be changed to unilateral.

c. Stimulus dosing is calculated by one of several methods.

(1) Based on age. Age in years equals the percentage of intensity (e.g., a patient 65 years old is treated at 65% maximum intensity).

(2) High fixed dose to all patients (contributes to cognitive impairment).

(3) Dose titration (the preferred approach). Each successive dose is increased during the first treatment until a seizure is produced.

(a) For Mecta Spectrum 5000Q, use 12, 20, 40, 80 J.

(b) For Thymatron DGX, use 10%, 20%, 40%, 80% energy.

(c) Stimulus threshold is then estimated as the midpoint between the stimulus producing the seizure and the previous stimulus that did not produce a seizure.

(d) On the second treatment, stimulus provided should be slightly above the seizure threshold when using bilateral ECT and two and a half times the threshold when using unilateral ECT.

(e) On subsequent treatments, increase the stimulus dose by about 5 J. in order to remain above the threshold.

5. Missed seizures.

a. If a seizure is not induced, a higher intensity stimulus is applied (up to a total of four attempts) after a 20- to 40-second delay.

b. Causes.

(1) Excessively high dose of anesthesia.

(2) Concomitant use of anticonvulsants (including benzo-diazepines).

(3) Inadequate oxygenation.

(4) Inadequate hydration.

c. Seizure threshold can be reduced with caffeine sodium benzoate 500 to 2000 mg IV over 1 minute, given 2 to 3 minutes before anesthesia induction. Other options include:

(1) Hyperventilate the patient immediately before ECT.

(2) Increase the stimulus charge.

(3) Give 200 mg, 300 mg, or 400 mg of sustained-release theophylline the night before ECT.

(4) Use an anesthetic that is not an anticonvulsant.

6. Prolonged seizures (greater than 180 seconds) should be terminated pharmacologically, using one of the following:

a. IV diazepam 5 to 15 mg.

b. IV midazolam 1 to 3 mg.

7. Seizure duration. The seizure itself generally lasts 20 seconds (considered a minimum effective seizure duration) to 90 seconds.

8. Treatment conclusion.

a. The patient begins to wake up within a minute and is monitored until fully alert.

b. Many patients are able to resume normal activities within 1 or 2 hours. ECT can be done as an outpatient procedure in patients without medical complications.

9. Number of treatments.

a. A full course of ECT is generally 6 to 9 treatments.

(1) Because treatments are usually given three times per week on alternate days, a full course can take 3 weeks.

(2) A trial of ECT can consist of 2 to 20 ECT treatments, depending upon the clinical response.

b. Relapse is an important clinical problem.

(1) Antidepressant medication (re)started after successful ECT can help prevent relapse.

(2) Some patients require episodic continued ECT to maintain remission (maintenance ECT).

16.7 Considerations with Specific Medical Diseases

1. Physiologic effects of ECT.

a. Cardiovascular effects.

(1) Immediate. Parasympathetic stimulation can lead to bradycardia, hypotension, and asystole.

(2) After 1 minute.

(a) Sympathetic stimulation leads to tachycardia, hypertension, and dysrhythmias, with increased cardiac output and myocardial oxygen consumption.

(b) Cerebral effects.

(i) Increased oxygen consumption.

         (ii) Increased cerebral blood flow.

         (iii) Increased intracranial pressure.

      (c) Other effects include increased intragastric pressure.

   b. Increased intraocular pressure.

2. Cardiovascular disease.

   a. Myocardial infarction and ischemic heart disease are the most common causes of ECT-associated death.

   b. Wait, if possible, at least 6 months to give ECT after myocardial infarction or cerebrovascular hemorrhage.

     (1) Use of nitrates and intravenous (IV) β-blockers and careful attention to oxygenation can minimize cardiovascular risk.

      (a) Labetalol (5 to 20 mg IV) or esmolol (5 to 60 mg IV) can reduce risk in patients with hypertension or tachycardia.

      (b) Nitroglycerin paste or sublingual aerosol can diminish risk in patients with coronary artery disease.

      (c) Regularly prescribed cardiac medications should be given with a small sip of water before ECT.

     (2) Arrhythmias.

      (a) Those at risk for bradyarrhythmias (or asystole) should be given glycopyrrolate or atropine before treatment.

      (b) Those at risk for tachyarrhythmias should be given IV β-blockers.

      (c) When in doubt, consult cardiology before treatment course.

     (3) Cardiac pacemakers and defibrillators.

      (a) Because the ECT electrical stimulation does not reach the heart, there is little risk of interfering with pacemaker or defibrillator function.

      (b) Typically, pacemakers and defibrillators are turned off before treatment and then turned back on afterward.

3. Parkinson's disease.

   a. ECT may be helpful in depression associated with Parkinson's disease, although this is not well accepted.

   b. ECT also diminishes motor symptoms of Parkinson's disease (although the effect is temporary).

4. CVA.

   a. There are no specific guidelines on how long ECT should be deferred after CVA (months). Waiting is especially important following hemorrhagic stroke because of risk of recurrent bleeding.

   b. Curare may be preferable to succinylcholine in patients with spastic paralysis following stroke.

5. COPD.

   a. Be sure inhalant bronchodilators are used before treatment.

   b. Keep theophylline levels at 15 µg/mL or less to prevent prolonged seizures.

6. Neuroleptic malignant syndrome. ECT can be effective treatment, with a response rate comparable to pharmacologic treatment.

7. Delirium.

   a. ECT has been reported to be of benefit for alcohol withdrawal delirium as well as several other etiologies of delirium.

   b. However, use of ECT for delirium is rare, given that ECT can cause delirium.
8. Central nervous system space-occupying lesions.
   a. ECT causes a transient increase in intracerebral pressure (ICP). However, modifications in ECT technique can allow ECT treatment even for these patients. Modifications include the following:
      (1) Antihypertensives.
      (2) Steroids.
      (3) Osmotic diuretics.
      (4) Hyperventilation.
   b. Small meningiomas probably pose little risk.
   c. Subdural hematomas should be evacuated before ECT.
9. Epilepsy.
   a. ECT increases seizure threshold; therefore ECT can reduce the number of seizures in this disorder.
   b. Patients with epilepsy should continue anticonvulsants during ECT, although higher stimulus settings are therefore necessary to produce adequate seizures.
10. Pregnancy.
ECT may be used during all trimesters of pregnancy (and the postpartum period).

a. In the English literature up to 1992, two fetal deaths and three birth defects have been reported among the 69 reported cases of ECT during pregnancy. The role of ECT in these complications is difficult to assess.
b. Anesthetics, anticholinergics, and neuromuscular blocking agents have not been thoroughly studied in pregnant women. They have been used safely but with limited documentation in the first trimester. Effects of numerous and prolonged use have not been determined.
   (1) Monitoring of fetal heart rate should be done before and after each ECT treatment when the gestational age is more than 14 to 16 weeks.
   (2) An obstetric consultant should be part of the planning and treatment process.

SUGGESTED READINGS

American Psychiatric Association: The Practice of Electroconvulsive Therapy: Recommendations for Treatment, Training, and Privileging, 2nd ed. Washington, DC, American Psychiatric Association, 2001.
Casey DA, Davis MH: ECT in the very old. Gen Hosp Psychiatry 18:436-439, 1996.
Coffey CE: The Clinical Science of Electroconvulsive Therapy. Washington, DC, American Psychiatric Association, 1993.
Coffey CE, Weiner RD, Djang WT, et al: Brain anatomic effects of electroconvulsive therapy: A prospective magnetic resonance imaging study. Arch Gen Psychiatry 48:1013-1021, 1991.
Cohen D, Taieb O, Flament M, et al: Absence of cognitive impairment at long-term follow-up in adolescents treated with ECT for severe mood disorder. Am J Psychiatry 157:460-462, 2000.
Dwork AJ, Arango V, Underwood M, et al: Absence of histological lesions in primate models of ECT and magnetic seizure therapy. Am J Psychiatry 161:576-578, 2004.

Ferrill MJ, Kehoe WA, Jacisin JJ: ECT during pregnancy: Physiologic and pharmacologic considerations. *Convulsive Ther* 8:186-200, 1992.

Gagne GG Jr, Furman MJ, Carpenter LL, Price LH: Efficacy of continuation ECT and antidepressant drugs compared to long-term antidepressants alone in depressed patients. *Am J Psychiatry* 157:1960-1965, 2000.

Husain MM, Rush AJ, Fink M, et al: Speed of response and remission in major depressive disorder with acute electroconvulsive therapy (ECT): A consortium for research in ECT (CORE) report. *J Clin Psychiatry* 65:485-491, 2004.

Lisanby SH, Maddox JH, Prudic J, et al: The effects of electroconvulsive therapy on memory of autobiographical and public events. *Arch Gen Psychiatry* 57:581-590, 2000.

McCall WV, Reboussin DM, Weiner RD, Sackheim HA: Titrated moderately suprathreshold vs fixed high-dose right unilateral electroconvulsive therapy: Acute antidepressant and cognitive effects. *Arch Gen Psychiatry* 57:438-444, 2000.

Petrides G, Fink M: The "half-age" stimulation strategy for ECT dosing. *Convulsive Ther* 12:138-146, 1996.

Sackheim HA, Prudic J, Devenand DP, et al: A prospective, randomized, double-blind comparison of bilateral and right unilateral electroconvulsive therapy at different stimulus intensities. *Arch Gen Psychiatry* 57:425-434, 2000.

UK ECT Review Group: Efficacy and safety of electroconvulsive therapy in depressive disorders: A systematic review and meta-analysis. *Lancet* 361:799-808, 2003.

Personality Disorders

17

Daniela A. Boerescu

17.1 Overview

PREVALENCE

1. Overall, about 10% of the population has a personality disorder.
2. The prevalence appears to be higher in medical and psychiatric populations, increasing to about one third of psychiatric patients seen in general hospital psychiatry and outpatient psychiatry, and to about one half of alcohol and substance-abuse patients.
3. Personality disorders tend to become exacerbated following significant stresses or losses and during the course of disorders such as dementia associated with disinhibition.

COMORBIDITY

1. Both major depression and anxiety disorders (generalized anxiety disorder, panic disorder, social phobia, post-traumatic stress disorder) have a high rate of comorbidity of personality disorder, estimated to occur in about 40% to 70% of patients.
2. Comorbid personality disorder is likely to be found in patients who have somatization, eating disorder, and chronic pain, and in those who recurrently attempt suicide.
3. Personality disorder is often overlooked as a diagnosis in the elderly, in whom it often coexists with a dementia or depression diagnosis.

DEFINITION

1. Personality traits are enduring patterns of perceiving the world and oneself and relating to others.
   a. Traits are not pathologic, nor are they mental disorder diagnoses.
   b. Recognition of traits can be helpful in understanding reaction to stresses, including illness.
2. Personality disorders are made up of personality traits that show a maladaptive persistence and inflexibility. They are defined by the *Diagnostic and Statistical Manual of Mental Disorders*, fourth edition, text revision (DSM-IV-TR) using the following criteria:
   a. An enduring pattern of inner experience and behavior that deviates from cultural expectations. This pattern is manifested in two or more of the following areas.
      (1) Cognition (ways of perceiving self, others, or events).
      (2) Affect (range, intensity, lability, and appropriateness of emotional responses).

      (3) Interpersonal functioning.

      (4) Impulse control.

  b. The pattern is inflexible and pervasive.

  c. The pattern leads to significant distress or impairment in important areas of functioning.

  d. The pattern is stable and can be traced back to adolescence or early adulthood.

  e. The pattern is not better accounted for by another mental disorder, substance use, or a general medical condition.

3. Personality disorders and traits are recorded on Axis II of the DSM-IV-TR multiaxial diagnostic system.

RECOGNITION

1. The purpose of recognizing personality disorder is to understand a patient's behavior and how it might influence the presentation of his or her medical or psychiatric illnesses.

  a. For example, substance abuse cannot be treated in most cases without understanding accompanying personality features.

  b. Personality disorders often complicate the doctor–patient relationship.

2. Personality disorders are often overlooked, especially in the elderly.

3. Problem behavior in medical patients is often labeled personality disorder when actually the patient's problem is delirium.

4. Both personality traits and disorders tend to become exaggerated and more fixed during the course of dementia.

5. Becausee personality tends to be enduring, a change in personality often indicates some underlying brain disorder. Frontal lobe disease, for example, often manifests with a "change in personality."

6. Recognition of a personality disorder is not easy except when the patient has an exaggerated form of behavior. Information helpful in describing personality may be obtained from the following:

  a. Observation of dress and interview participation. Is the patient meticulous, disorganized, sociable, or guarded?

  b. Listening to how patients express their needs. Is the presentation overly dramatic or excessively complaining? Does the patient try to convey self-importance?

  c. Ask some specific questions.

    (1) How has the person interacted with significant people?

    (2) Does the patient feel close to or confide in anyone? You could ask, "How is your current problem affecting your closest relationship?" Listen for evidence of manipulation or overdependence.

    (3) What illness behavior has the patient shown in the past? You may inquire, "When you were in the hospital (or sick) before, what was that like for you?" Listen for feelings of helplessness or a pattern of conflict with caretakers. Ask about what was helpful or problematic with previous physicians.

    (4) "What sort of interests do you have and what do you enjoy doing?" This question can reveal many personality features

including range of affect, level of social involvement, and degree of maturity.

(5) If possible ask friends, family, and staff about what type of person the patient is. You may hear, for example, "Father never really trusts anyone," or "Mother has always been a complainer like this, no matter what anyone does for her."

7. Use of testing. A wide range of instruments is available for investigating personality disorder:

a. (Semi-)structured interviews like the Diagnostic Interview for Personality Disorders (DIPD-IV) or the Structured Interview for DSM Personality IV (SIPD-IV) are mostly used in research.

b. Self-report instruments, like the Minnesota Multiphasic Personality Inventory (MMPI). This test is self-administered, takes a few hours to complete, and for a small fee can be rapidly scored by computer. The MMPI can be useful when one is puzzled by a patient with possible factitious illness or chronic pain. However, its use should be limited to situations in which the personality information can be critical to the diagnosis or management and cannot be reasonably obtained otherwise.

SPECIFIC PERSONALITY DISORDERS AND THEIR MANAGEMENT

Personality types in medical management and appropriate interventions are listed in Table 17-1.

17.2 Paranoid Personality Disorder

1. Definition. Paranoid personalities exhibit the following characteristics:
   a. Have a pervasive mistrust and are suspicious of others' motives.
   b. Are preoccupied with doubts of loyalty of friends or associates.
   c. Have trouble confiding because of fear of betrayal.
   d. Read threats into benign remarks or events.
   e. Persistently bear grudges.
   f. Misperceive attacks on character and are quick to counterattack.
   g. Distrust fidelity of spouse or sexual partner.
2. Impact on medical care. Paranoid patients feel especially vulnerable in a weakened or ill condition because they have an excessive need for autonomy.
   a. Often blame other people for their illness.
   b. Have a litigious strain and easily take offense.
   c. Continually question whether there are hidden reasons for events.
   d. Are sensitive to the intrusions of history taking and the ambiguities of the diagnostic process.
   e. Might suddenly flee (sign out against medical advice) because of suspicion and fear.
   f. In response to stress they can experience very brief psychotic episodes (lasting minutes to hours).
3. Intervention.
   a. To counteract fear, provide straightforward explanations of tests and procedures, including history taking.

Table 17-1 Personality Types in Medical Management

Personality	Meaning	Type of Illness Response	Intervention
Antisocial	A potential opportunity	Looks for an advantage	Set limits
Avoidant	Invisible	Avoids interaction	Be supportive, not critical
Borderline	More anxiety	Increased disorganization	Set limits
Dependent	Expects limitless care and interest	Demanding or withdrawn	Satisfy needs with limit setting
Depressive	Love and care = suffering	Complaining, rejecting	Acknowledge difficulties
Histrionic	Defect, punishment	Seductive	Reassure; avoid collusion
Narcissistic	Threatens grandiosity	Grandiosity; disparaging	Confidence, professionalism
Obsessive–compulsive	Threatens control	Obstinate, uncooperative	Information; give control
Paranoid	Confirms weakness; expects assault	Blames others; hostility	Clear plans, keep distance
Passive–aggressive	Another frustration	Complains, blames	Avoid angry response
Schizoid	Anxiety with forced contact	Reclusive, uncooperative	Accept distance

b. Warn about possible side effects; explain changes in treatment, and offer reasons for delays. A written treatment plan can help enlist cooperation.
c. Appealing for tolerance may be helpful.
d. Avoid unexpected changes in scheduling of events without providing the reasons.
e. Be careful about calling the patient's family or asking any others for information without explicit consent. Short-term low-dose antipsychotic treatment is helpful for psychotic paranoid ideation, but it is usually difficult to convince these patients of the need for this medication.

17.3 Schizoid and Schizotypal Personality Disorders

1. Definition. Schizoid personalities are detached from social relationships and show a limited range of emotional expression. Schizoid patients exhibit the following characteristics:
   a. Neither desire nor enjoy close relationships. They are "loners."
   b. Choose solitary activities, including their occupation.
   c. Have little interest in sexual relationship.
   d. Do not take pleasure in activities.
   e. Lack close friends. The schizoid patient does not seem to care about social contacts. If the social isolation is a result of fear of rejection, with an underlying desire for acceptance, the patient may be an avoidant personality.
   f. Appear indifferent to praise or criticism.
   g. Show emotional detachment.
   h. If, in addition to social isolation, there are additional eccentricities in communication or behavior, the patient may be classified as having a schizotypal personality disorder. Such eccentricities can include the following:
      (1) Ideas of reference ("everything going on pertains to me").
      (2) Odd beliefs or magical thinking (telepathy or clairvoyance).
      (3) Unusual perceptual experiences.
      (4) Odd thinking or communication (wandering or metaphorical speech).
      (5) Suspiciousness or paranoid thinking.
      (6) Inappropriate or constricted affect.
      (7) Odd or eccentric appearance.
      (8) Excessive social anxiety.
2. Impact on medical care. Schizoid and schizotypal personalities:
   a. Are uncomfortable with forced contact with medical providers.
   b. Deal with anxiety by withdrawing; therefore emotional or physical disorders can go unreported.
   c. Might prompt well-meaning providers to draw them out. However, such attempts at engagement only increase their distress.
   d. Can become acutely psychotic for short periods, particularly while under stress (e.g., the stress of hospitalization).

3. Intervention.
   a. Do not try to resocialize these patients. Accept their need to remain uninvolved.
   b. Rely on diagnostic thoroughness to avoid overlooking disorders that the patient is reluctant to volunteer.
   c. The treatment of choice is individual (supportive) psychotherapy. Antipsychotic medication can be used short term for transient psychotic states. Long-term use is not recommended.

17.4 Antisocial Personality Disorder

1. Definition. Antisocial personalities (previously classified as "sociopaths" or "psychopaths") have a pervasive disregard for the rights of others.
   a. Extended history of multiple kinds of antisocial behavior beginning in childhood and continuing into adulthood. However, the diagnosis should not be made before the age of 18. Antisocial behavior before age 15 constitutes a conduct disorder. Before the age of 15 years, these personalities show several of the following: truancy, expulsion from school, delinquency, running away from home, persistent lying, vandalism, early sexual behavior, or substance abuse.
   b. Repeated acts that are grounds for arrest.
   c. Lying.
   d. Impulsiveness and failure to plan ahead.
   e. Irritability or aggressiveness.
   f. Reckless disregard for the safety of self or others.
   g. Consistent irresponsibility.
   h. Lack of remorse.
2. Impact on medical care. The antisocial personality is incompatible with the culture of medical care. They often are involved with medical care because of their drug use and trauma. Once in the medical system, they act in the following ways:
   a. Lie about their history.
   b. Try to manipulate prescriptions.
   c. Might attempt to steal drugs or supplies.
   d. Make persistent, inappropriate demands.
   e. Might have visitors who cause these problems if unsupervised.
3. Intervention.
   a. To avoid being manipulated, document objective physical signs in managing clinical problems. This is important when dealing with drug withdrawal, for example.
   b. Provide straightforward confrontation with a reasonable treatment plan. Provide clear boundaries and consequences.
   c. Be aware that these patients try to make the physician feel guilty for not providing what they want.
   d. Treatment of substance abuse is best handled by well-organized treatment systems, not by individual clinicians.
   e. Very few treatment modalities have proven success. Group treatment appears to be most effective, with all group members having the same disorder and in a confined setting (e.g., in prison).

17.5 Borderline Personality Disorder

1. Definition. Borderline personalities have a pervasive pattern of instability of interpersonal relationships, self-image, and affects. There is also marked impulsivity beginning in early adulthood. Other features include the following:

   a. Frantic efforts to avoid real or imagined abandonment.
   b. Unstable and intense relationships characterized by alternating idealization and devaluation.
   c. Unstable self-image.
   d. Behavior that is impulsive and self-damaging involving areas such as substance abuse, eating, spending, or driving.
   e. Recurrent suicidal or self-mutilating behaviors, gestures, or threats.
   f. Affective instability with intense episodic moods usually lasting hours to days.
   g. Chronic feelings of emptiness (often misdiagnosed as depression).
   h. Inappropriate intense anger.
   i. Brief psychotic episodes consisting of transient paranoia or dissociation.

2. Interaction with the medical system.

   a. Relationships with physicians or other providers are unstable and intense, alternating between intense dependence and rejection.
   b. "Splitting," that is, a positive relation with one member of the treatment team and a negative relation with another, is common. When team members find themselves fighting with each other, suspect the patient has a borderline personality disorder.
   c. In early meetings, the borderline patient appears attractive and hopeful. It is not unusual to hear "You are the best doctor I have ever had." However, some real or imagined disappointment leads to anger and rejection.
   d. Evaluation and disposition of suicide attempts is complex because of the need to assess chronic suicidal behavior (see Chapter 14). The self-destructive behavior is usually precipitated by a real or perceived abandonment, and self-mutilation brings relief that reinforces the behavior.
   e. Treatment is complicated by the use of medical conditions (such as diabetes) as a way of carrying out self-destructive tendencies.
   f. These personalities do everything they can to destroy the professional relationship, but then they intensify pathologic behavior at any suggestion of termination.

3. Intervention.

   a. Maintain balanced, realistic expectations. Do not collude in unrealistic expectations.
   b. Do not use "borderline" as a pejorative term.
   c. Understanding that there is a stable pattern of instability may put a more long-term perspective on a frustrating situation.
   d. Be realistic about what is possible.
   e. Provide clear and consistent boundaries and limits.
   f. Communication should be simple and straightforward.

g. A single clinician should be in charge of all phases of therapy to prevent splitting. It is important to have periodic meetings of the treatment team members to discuss the case. This will help to prevent splitting and offer education and support to the treatment providers.

h. Avoid being manipulated by the patient's implicit or stated demands. Instead, reassure the patient that the best possible treatment will be provided.

i. When behavioral problems emerge, calmly review the therapeutic goals and boundaries of treatment. Such limit setting is definitely necessary, but in the short run it can lead to new complaints, noncompliance, outright hostility, a suicide attempt, or termination of treatment.

j. Do not underestimate the significance of going on vacation or transferring the patient to another doctor. Prepare the patient for referral early on and be prepared for reactions that may be interpreted and contained.

k. Therapy is very important for the prognosis of these patients. Several forms of individual and group therapy have been developed and researched. Dialectical behavior therapy (a form of cognitive behavior therapy) has the most evidence to support its effectiveness.

l. Role of psychotropics.
  (1) Antipsychotics are the best-studied medications in borderline personality disorder. Acute treatment in crisis situations can be effective in reducing symptom severity, psychotic symptoms, and irritability. The evidence for maintenance therapy is debatable.
  (2) Antidepressants are recommended for managing affective symptoms. Tricyclics should be avoided because of danger in overdose. Monoamine oxidase inhibitors (MAOIs) are problematic due to dietary noncompliance. First-line treatments are selective serotonin reuptake inhibitors (SSRIs) or serotonin and norepinephrine reuptake inhibitors (SNRIs).
  (3) Anticonvulsants (carbamazepine and possibly valproic acid) can be helpful in borderline patients with an affective presentation and behavioral dyscontrol.
  (4) Lithium may be useful for treatment of irritability, anger, and aggression.
  (5) Antianxiety agents. Benzodiazepines often lead to dependence and occasionally to disinhibition. Buspirone may be an alternative for chronic anxiety.

17.6 Histrionic Personality Disorder

1. Definition. The histrionic personality is described as follows:
   a. Needs to be the center of attention.
   b. Often is inappropriately seductive, provocative, or self-dramatizing.
   c. Shows rapidly shifting or shallow emotional expression.
   d. Uses physical appearance to draw attention.
   e. Uses impressionistic and vague speech.

f. Is suggestible.
g. Considers relationships to be more intimate than they actually are.
h. Acts very emotionally when little things go wrong.
i. Has poor frustration tolerance and need for immediate gratification.
2. Impact on medical care. The histrionic patient is characterized by the following actions:
   a. Creates problems not so much from the disorders they present as from the way they present their disorders. They run the risk of being labeled "hysterical" even when presenting bona fide symptoms. However, they are more likely to present with somatization disorder and conversion disorder.
   b. Provides vague, nonfactual histories. They pay more attention to impressions and feelings than to logic and detail. History taking can be frustrating.
   c. Often have a certain seductive appeal and might tempt the provider into an inappropriate personal relationship.
   d. Experiences illness as a threat to attractiveness, leading to efforts to be desirable and be taken care of.
3. Intervention.
   a. Appreciate the threat that illness poses to a person to whom attractiveness is so important.
   b. Understand seductive behavior as a response to distress. Reassure the patient of an interest in taking care of the illness.
   c. Maintain a professional stance despite any temptation to collude with the patient in a flirtatious and misleading way.
   d. If the patient's behavior is especially seductive, tell the patient that such behavior makes treatment more difficult and that a "special" relationship is not necessary (and will not be allowed) for the best medical treatment.
   e. Low-dose benzodiazepines are useful for short-term management of extreme emotional states. Another option (without the risk of abuse or dependency) is small doses of antipsychotics. Long-term pharmacotherapy is indicated only for associated Axis I disorders (i.e., major depressive disorder).

17.7 Narcissistic Personality Disorder

1. Definition. There is a pervasive pattern of grandiosity, need for admiration, and lack of empathy. Narcissistic personalities have the following characteristics:
   a. A grandiose sense of self-importance.
   b. Preoccupation with fantasies of unlimited success. They often talk about their accomplishments or claimed accomplishments.
   c. Belief they are special and should relate only to other special people.
   d. Need for special admiration. They are sensitive to criticism, which can provoke rage, humiliation, or both.
   e. A sense of entitlement.
   f. A tendency to take advantage of others.
   g. Lack of empathy.

  h. Envy of others and feeling that others are envious of them.
  i. Arrogance.
2. Impact on medical care. The narcissistic patient:
  a. Experiences a damaged sense of superiority in accepting the sick role, because this involves being placed in an inferior position.
  b. Makes disparaging remarks about providers as a defense.
  c. Astutely notices professional weakness, and disqualifies providers as not "good enough."
  d. Often demands referral to a specialist.
  e. Can provoke an argument or power struggle. The doctor–patient relationship is characterized either by disruption (because of inability to accept criticism) or control.
3. Intervention.
  a. Treating the narcissistic patient involves maintaining a balance between two positions.
    (1) If the physician appears too controlling or powerful, the patient cannot tolerate the relative inferiority and weakness.
    (2) If the patient feels the physician is not special, they feel devalued and worry about getting special treatment.
  b. Convey unassuming self-confidence.
  c. The treatment of choice for narcissistic personality disorder is individual psychodynamic psychotherapy. Pharmacotherapy is needed when an Axis I disorder is present (comorbidity with dysthymia and major depressive disorder).

17.8 Avoidant Personality Disorder

1. Definition. The avoidant personality is characterized by the following:
  a. Avoids relationships (despite desiring them) due to fear of criticism, disapproval, and rejection.
  b. Is unwilling to get involved with people unless certain of being liked.
  c. Suffers from very low self-esteem and feelings of inadequacy.
  d. Does not take personal risks for fear of embarrassment.
2. Impact on medical care. These patients tend to be "invisible" and their medical conditions remain undiagnosed and/or undertreated because of the following characteristics:
  a. Need of strong assurance of uncritical acceptance and safety before they can engage in a doctor–patient relationship.
  b. Excessive guilt and shame if their lifestyle has contributed to their illness (e.g., smoking, alcohol abuse).
  c. Tendency to feel very hurt if the provider is being slightly disapproving.
  d. Uncomfortable in medical settings where they have to interact often with new staff or multiple providers.
3. Intervention.
  a. Avoid being critical.
  b. Be supportive, especially at the beginning of treatment, in order to engage the patient.

    c. Be aware that they need encouragement in order to contact you for emergencies or new symptoms. Educate them when it is appropriate for them to seek care.

    d. Recommend cognitive behavior therapy. Group therapy can be particularly helpful.

    e. Anxiolytics are helpful for short-term management of situational anxiety. Antidepressants (SSRIs, SNRIs, or MAOIs) are indicated for comorbid major depression or anxiety disorders.

17.9 Dependent Personality Disorder

1. Definition. The dependent personality can be described as follows:
   a. Has difficulty making everyday decisions without excessive input and reassurance.
   b. Needs others to assume responsibility.
   c. Has difficulty expressing disagreement because of fear of loss of support or approval.
   d. Feels helpless when alone due to exaggerated fear of being unable to care for self.
   e. Does not initiate projects on their own due to lack of self-confidence.
   f. Goes to extreme lengths to obtain support and maintain a relationship, no matter how abusive it might be; seeks another relationship as soon as one ends.
2. Impact on medical care. These patients often cause problems because they demand too much of their providers, who then become frustrated and rejecting.
   a. The dependent patient often exhibits the following characteristics:
      (1) Often has a strong attachment and involvement with one or a series of medical providers.
      (2) Is uncomfortable when separated from the provider and feels helpless.
      (3) Has difficulty making medical decisions without turning to others for advice or reassurance.
   b. As a result of these characteristics, dependent personalities:
      (1) Make frequent, often unnecessary, office visits or phone calls or unwarranted requests for special attention.
      (2) Insist on having everything done for them.
      (3) Might withdraw from treatment if they feel too deprived and find another provider.
3. Intervention. Dependent personalities are among the most common personality problems encountered in medical care. This is not surprising because medical symptoms are a stress on these persons and bring out their underlying fears and concerns.
   a. Avoid the tendency to become annoyed with their excessive demands, which would only lead to rejection and an escalating cycle of dependency.
      (1) Instead, inquire about and help address current stresses.
      (2) Say, "I know your recent illness (symptom) has you very worried, and that accounts for your many attempts to call.

Let's set up some regular times to talk. Of course, you can call me any time if you feel there is a real emergency."

b. Drawing boundaries must be done in a way the patient does not experience as punishment or withdrawal.

c. Try to patiently describe what you feel you can and should do for the patient and what is reasonable for the patient to do.

d. Recommend individual or group therapy focused on cognitive change, assertive training, and social skills.

17.10 Obsessive–Compulsive Personality Disorder

1. Definition. The obsessive–compulsive (OC) personality disorder is described as follows:
   a. Preoccupied with rules, order, details to the extent that the major point of the activity is lost.
   b. Perfectionistic to the extreme that interferes with task completion.
   c. Work-oriented to the exclusion of leisure activities.
   d. Inflexible and rigid about matters of morality, ethics, values.
   e. Has a need to be in control and cannot delegate responsibility.
   f. Can be miserly and stingy, or unable to discard worn-out or worthless objects, even when they have no sentimental value.

2. Impact on medical care.
   a. OC patients exhibit the following characteristics that can affect medical care:
      (1) When established procedure does not dictate the correct answer and they are faced with different options, making decisions is time consuming and painful.
      (2) They can become upset or angry in situations in which they are not able to maintain control (e.g., when they are faced with the diagnosis of an illness).
      (3) They are particularly conscious about their relative status in relationships, including those with medical providers, and may display excessive deference to an authority they respect and excessive resistance to authority they do not respect.
      (4) They can be intolerant of affective behavior in others and usually express emotions in a highly controlled manner.
      (5) They demonstrate rigidity about things being done the one "correct" way (their way).
      (6) Miserliness about spending that might affect their medical care (refusing care due to copayments).
   b. As a result of these features, OC personalities can be:
      (1) Frustrated because of trying to get more and more medical opinions, and dissatisfied with care that does not match their rigid values.
      (2) Noncompliant as a way of keeping control.
      (3) Unsure about instructions.

3. Intervention. These patients typically cause problems when they refuse to follow medical advice as a result of needing to be in control.

a. These patients are not comfortable simply being told what to do.
b. Appropriate amounts of information (enough but not too much detail) must be provided to allow participation in management decisions. Ways to return some control can include asking patients to monitor their own blood pressure or to initiate an exercise program.
c. Be responsive to concerns and complaints, but do not get embroiled in detailed descriptions of insignificant side effects.
d. The use of benzodiazepines is controversial (it could decrease the anxiety associated with their behavior, but sedative effects may be perceived as a further interference with autonomy).
e. Group therapy may be helpful because the other group members can point out bothersome behavior and call for a change.

17.11 Depressive Personality Disorder

1. Definition. Although included in the DSM system in the category of personality disorder not otherwise specified, the depressive personality disorder warrants consideration, because it often presents clinical problems. It is characterized by:
   a. Depressive thinking and behavior with gloomy mood, unhappiness, and pessimism.
   b. Poor self-esteem and self-criticism.
   c. Prone to feeling worried and/or guilty.
   d. Judgmental toward others.
   e. Have been called "manipulative help rejecters," and have features of the "pain-prone patient."
   f. Regards sacrifice as the necessary burden of life, and little is done for personal pleasure. Very often, those who are supposed to "benefit" from their sacrifices feel guilty and frustrated.
2. Interaction with the medical system. The depressive personality might never acknowledge anything positive about what is done for them.
3. Intervention.
   a. There may be no way to alter this self-pitying behavior.
   b. Recognize the problem as a lifelong style.
   c. It may be worthwhile to confront the patient in a nonrejecting way by pointing out the negative behavior.
   d. It might help to suggest that recovery is another burden. This allows continued complaining while behaving more positively. One might say, "It seems that in a life of trials, you have one more burden to take on."
   e. Suggest that the patient work on recovery for the sake of someone else (e.g., the children).

17.12 Passive–Aggressive (Negativistic) Personality Disorder

1. Definition. Although included in DSM IV-TR's "personality disorder not otherwise specified" category, this type of

patient is also commonly encountered and is characterized by the following:

   a. Passive resistance (angry reluctance, procrastination, forgetfulness, or intentional inefficiency when they have to do things).

   b. Complaints of being misunderstood and unappreciated.

   c. Complaints of personal misfortune.

   d. A pervasive sense of underlying resentment.

   e. Disguised hostility.

   f. Moodiness and argumentativeness.

2. Impact on medical care. In interaction with medical providers, the passive–aggressive personality patient is characterized by the following:

   a. Has a need to gain attention and is angry at the lack of attention. The tendency to resist authorities can be dangerous when it is directed against a medical provider.

   b. Ends up in a chronic state of dissatisfaction, frustration, and angry resentment about medical care.

   c. Holds a conviction of being treated poorly, which is reinforced when the doctor loses patience with the constant sense of dissatisfaction.

   d. Might seek litigation and complain to administration and directors about care.

3. Intervention.

   a. Accept that the complaining and dissatisfaction will not change.

   b. Provide and document a solid standard of clinical care.

   c. Guard against doing too little ("digging in your heels" to a dissatisfied customer) or going too far as a defensive measure.

SUGGESTED READINGS

American Psychiatric Association: *Diagnostic and Statistical Manual of Mental Disorders*, 4th ed., text revision. Washington, DC, American Psychiatric Press, 2000.

Bender S, Dolan T, Skodol E, et al: Treatment utilization by patients with personality disorder. *Am J Psychiatry* 158(2):295-302, 2001.

Casey PR, Tryer P: Personality disorder and psychiatric illness in general practice. *Br J Psychiatry* 156:261-265, 1990.

Coccaro EF, Kavoussi RJ: Biological and pharmacological aspects of borderline personality disorder. *Hosp Community Psychiatry* 42(10):1029-1033, 1991.

Elliot RL: The masochistic patient in consultation-liaison psychiatry. *Gen Hosp Psychiatry* 9:241-250, 1987.

Groves JE: Taking care of the hateful patient. *N Engl J Med* 298:883-887, 1978.

Kunik ME, Mulsant BH, Rifai AH: Diagnostic rate of comorbid personality disorder in elderly psychiatric inpatients. *Am J Psychiatry* 151:603-605, 1994.

Linehan MM: *Cognitive Behavioral Treatment of Borderline Personality Disorder*. New York, Guilford Press, 1993.

Livesley WJ: *Handbook of Personality Disorders*. New York, Guilford Press, 2001.

Shea MT, Pilkonis PA, Beckham E, et al: Personality disorders and treatment outcome in the NIMH Treatment of Depression Collaborative Research Program. *Am J Psychiatry* 147:711-718, 1990.

Soloff PH: Psychopharmacology of borderline personality disorder. *The Psychiatr Clin North Am* 23(1):169-190, 2000.

Stoudemire A, Thompson T: The borderline personality in the medical setting. *Ann Intern Med* 96:76-79, 1982.

Ursano RJ, Epstein RS, Lazar SG: Behavioral responses to illness: Personality and personality disorders. In Rundell JR, Wise MG (eds): *Textbook of Consultation Liaison Psychiatry*. Washington, DC: American Psychiatric Press, 2002, pp 107-125.

Zimmerman M: Diagnosing personality disorders. *Arch Gen Psychiatry* 51:225-245, 1994.

Zimmerman M, Rothschild L, Chelminski I: The prevalence of DSM-IV personality disorders in psychiatric outpatients. Submitted to *Am J Psychiatry* 162(10):1911-1918, 2005.

Eating Disorders, Obesity, and Nicotine Dependence

18

Mark B. Elliot

18.1 Anorexia Nervosa

DEFINITION

1. Refusal to maintain minimal normal body weight (less than 85% of expected weight).
2. Intense fear of gaining weight or becoming fat, even though the patient is underweight.
3. Disturbance in self-perception of weight, body size, or shape.
4. In female patients, absence of at least three consecutive menstrual cycles (associated with low follicle-stimulating hormone [FSH] and luteinizing hormone [LH] levels).

EPIDEMIOLOGY

1. Ninety-five percent of patients are women.
2. Most cases develop during adolescence.
3. Estimated lifetime prevalence is 0.5% to 3.7%.
   a. Eighty-five percent of patients have clinical onset between the ages of 13 and 20 years.

ETIOLOGY

1. Genetic contributions. Monozygotic twin concordance is greater than dizygotic twin concordance.
2. Psychodynamic theories. Patients have symptoms indicating difficulty with separation and autonomy (i.e., parental enmeshment), poor affect regulation, and difficulty negotiating psychosexual development.
3. There are many theories but no known single etiology.

RECOGNITION

1. There are two subtypes of anorexia based upon methods patients use to control weight.
   a. In the restricting subtype, patients use low-calorie intake and exercise.
   b. In the binge-eating and purging subtype, patients alternate bingeing and starvation along with purging and laxative or diuretic abuse. Purging can occur in up to 70%.
   c. Many patients, particularly in younger age groups, have symptoms that evade categorization into either. In this case, the technical diagnosis is "eating disorder not otherwise specified."
2. Symptoms.
   a. Extreme fear of gaining weight.

BOX 18-1   Screening Laboratory Evaluation of Eating Disorder Patients

Amylase	Glucose
Bone density	Liver function
Blood urea nitrogen (BUN), creatinine	Magnesium
	Phosphate
Calcium	Serum osmolality
Complete blood count	Thyroid function
Electrocardiogram	Urinalysis (with electrolytes)
Electrolytes	

---

   b. Obsessive—compulsive behavior is common.

   c. Patients have poor social adjustment but often with some areas of high functioning (e.g., intellectual).

   d. Patients have odd food habits (hoarding, hiding).

   e. Hyperactivity is common, and patients have compulsive, extreme training programs.

   f. Mood and sleep disturbances are not uncommon.

3. Physical signs.

   a. Emaciated physical appearance.

   b. Dry yellowish skin and some hair loss.

   c. Loss of tooth enamel and scarring of the back of the hand from inducing vomiting.

   d. Neuropathies and seizures may be an outcome.

   e. Cardiomyopathy (especially with concurrent use of ipecac, showing creatine phosphokinase (CPK) abnormalities along with non-specific electrocardiographic (ECG) changes.

4. Laboratory abnormalities (Box 18-1).

5. Medical disorders (Box 18-2).

DIFFERENTIAL DIAGNOSIS

1. Normal thinness. Anorexia nervosa is a distinct disorder and is not simply the low end of the normal weight distribution.

2. Medical disorders.

   a. Endocrine disorders.

      (1) Hypothalamic disease (growth hormone deficiency can result in diminished appetite).

      (2) Diabetes mellitus (there seems to be an increased statistical association).

      (3) Addison's disease (cortisol insufficiency may be associated with early satiety).

      (4) Hyperthyroidism.

   b. Gastrointestinal disorders.

      (1) Malabsorption.

      (2) Inflammatory bowel disease.

BOX 18-2   Medical Disorders in Patients with Eating Disorders

Cardiovascular

Arrhythmias: supraventricular beats and ventricular tachycardia, rare QT prolongation.
Nonspecific ECG changes: T wave inversions, ST depressions (electrolyte abnormalities)
Sinus bradycardia from malnutrition
Use of ipecac can lead to irreversible myocardial damage and diffuse myositis

Endocrine

Abnormal LH and FSH levels
Euthyroid sick syndrome
Hypothalamic amenorrhea
Osteopenia

Gastrointestinal

Chronic vomiting can lead to esophageal damage, including Mallory–Weiss tears
Hypercholesterolemia (abnormal lipoprotein metabolism)
Nonspecific LFT changes
Pancreatitis
Steatohepatitis

Hematologic

Anemia (low iron, vitamin B_{12}, folate)
Coagulopathies
Leukopenia
Thrombocytopenia

Neurologic

Cortical atrophy of both white and gray matter. Structural studies indicate that although white matter loss may be reversible with weight gain, loss of gray matter might not be.
Seizures

Renal and Electrolytes

Azotemia
Diabetes insipidus
Hypochloremic alkalosis
Hypokalemia
Hyponatremia
Laxative use can induce metabolic acidosis due to loss of potassium bicarbonate
Metabolic alkalosis
Increased risk of nephrolithiasis

ECG, electrocardiogram; FSH, follicle-stimulating hormone; LFT, liver function test; LH, luteinizing hormone.

       (3) Superior mesenteric artery syndrome (with postprandial vomit-
ing secondary to intermittent gastric outlet obstruction).

       (4) Celiac disease.

  c. Genetic disorders.

       (1) Turner's syndrome.

       (2) Gaucher's disease.

  d. Other medical disorders.

       (1) Occult malignancies, such as central nervous system (CNS)
tumors.

       (2) Acquired immunodeficiency syndrome (AIDS).

3. Psychiatric disorders.

  a. Major depression with poor appetite.

  b. Obsessive–compulsive disorder with focus on food.

  c. Psychotic disorder such as schizophrenia or paranoid disorder in
which food is feared as part of a delusion.

  d. Phobic disorders in which food is avoided.

       (1) Swallowing phobia occurring after a choking episode.

       (2) Food fears after oral surgery.

       (3) Fear of vomiting in public (as a component of an agoraphobia
disorder).

  e. Tourette's disease (may have accompanying anorexia).

TREATMENT

Hospitalization

Hospitalization is one of the most important decisions a clinician has to
make, especially because the consequences of this disease can be fatal.
Although the decision to hospitalize should be based on comprehensive
consideration of the whole person, specific criteria for hospitalization
include the following:

1. Rapid or persistent decline in oral intake.
2. Behavior that is dangerous to the person's health, is out of control,
   and cannot be managed on an outpatient basis (e.g., suicidal behavior, severe depression, psychotic decompensation, or bingeing and
   purging out of control).
3. Continued decline despite maximally intensive outpatient treatment
   or partial hospitalization.
4. Degree of patient's denial and resistance prohibits less-intensive treatment options.
5. Weight loss of more than 30% over 6 months or body mass index
   (BMI) lower than 75% of ideal or knowledge of weight at which
   instability previously occurred.
6. Hypokalemia of less than 3 mEq/L or other electrolyte disturbance
   not corrected by oral supplementation.
7. ECG changes (especially arrhythmias).
8. Heart rate (HR) less than 40 or greater than 110.
9. Systolic blood pressure (BP) less than 90.
10. Marked orthostatic hypotension (including HR > 20 beats above
    normal or decreased pressure > 20 mm Hg below normal).
11. Hypothermia (temperature < 97°F [36°C]) or dehydration.

BOX 18-3   Example of Refeeding Protocol

1. Contract with patient for a weight goal. Goal should not exceed 1 to 2 pounds in the first week and 3 to 5 pounds afterward.
2. Begin 30-40 kcal/kg/day (approx. 1000 to 1600 kcal) in frequent small meals to avoid bloating sensation.
3. Increase calories to as high as 70-100 kcal/kg/day, depending on height and age (consult with nutrition service).
4. Add, as necessary, vitamin and mineral supplements (monitor electrolytes closely).

In severe cases, nasogastric feeding or total parenteral nutrition must be used starting at 800 to 1200 kcal/day.

12. Laxative or diuretic abuse that cannot be controlled with outpatient treatment.

Interventions in the Hospital

1. Identification and management of medical problems. Monitor vital signs, ECG, hydration, and electrolytes (pay particular attention to potassium imbalance in the context of vomiting).
2. Bedrest with supervised feedings using constant observation.
3. Refeeding protocol (Box 18-3).
4. Complications of refeeding.
   a. Edema (use support stockings, leg elevation, and salt restriction). Need to monitor serum electrolytes and perform frequent physical examinations.
   b. Abdominal distention and bloating. Use reassurance. May also try metoclopramide 5 mg PO bid.
   c. Congestive heart failure. Patient might require diuretics and careful medical management.
5. Setting weight goals and patient involvement in a program with positive behavior reinforcements.
6. Forced feeding should be used in patients with medically serious status.
7. Medications.
   a. Cyproheptadine might stimulate appetite (initial doses of 8 mg/day PO may be increased to 32 mg/day).
   b. Antidepressants should be used if there are depressive symptoms. Selective serotonin reuptake inhibitors (SSRIs) are unlikely to be helpful before successful weight gain, but there is some evidence that fluoxetine may improve weight maintenance.
   c. Antipsychotics in low doses may be tried for patients whose preoccupations seem to be of psychotic proportions, though no controlled studies support this practice.
   d. Short-term anxiolytics might help some very anxious patients if given before mealtime.
   e. There have been some case reports of the use of naltrexone (50 to 150 mg/day) to assist in weight gain.

8. Psychotherapy.
   a. There are very few studies addressing the efficacy of therapy in the acute phase of treatment.
   b. There has been some concern that group therapy might worsen prognosis by increasing competition between patients to remain thin.
   c. Family intervention is almost always necessary because of the pathologic family dynamics that usually develop around the eating problems.
   d. Cognitive behavior therapy and interpersonal therapy are often preferred initially to correct cognitive distortions, improve coping mechanisms, and improve eating behavior.
   e. Following weight restoration, individual and group psychodynamic treatment may be employed to address any persistent personality disorders.

PROGNOSIS

1. This disease might have a mortality rate of 5% to 20%.
2. Most patients improve with treatment, although the illness may be relapsing (approximately two thirds have an enduring morbid food and weight preoccupation).
3. Favorable prognostic indicators.
   a. Earlier age at onset.
   b. Return of menses.
   c. Good premorbid school or work history.
4. Negative prognostic indicators.
   a. Lower minimum weight.
   b. Vomiting.
   c. Failure to respond to prior treatments.
   d. Disturbed family relationships before onset of the eating disorder.
   e. Being married.
   f. Hospitalizations.
   g. Being male.
   h. Having a comorbid psychopathologic condition.

18.2 Bulimia Nervosa

DEFINITION

1. Recurrent episodes of binge eating (several episodes a week for several months). A binge is defined as the following:
   a. Eating more in some discrete period of time than most people would eat.
   b. A lack of control over eating during the episode.
2. Regular episodes of self-induced vomiting, use of laxatives or diuretics, fasting, or vigorous exercise to prevent weight gain.
3. Binge eating and inappropriate compensatory behavior both occur at least twice a week, on average, for 3 months.
4. Persistent overconcern with body shape and weight.

5. Two subtypes exist.
   a. Purging. Regularly engages in self-induced vomiting or use of laxatives or diuretics.
   b. Nonpurging. Uses other compensatory behavior such as fasting and excessive exercising.

EPIDEMIOLOGY

1. Some binge eating is extremely common in adolescents (about 90% are girls).
2. Some bulimic features are present in 5% to 25% of the young adult population.
3. Lifetime prevalence is about 1.1% to 4.2% (male-to-female ratio about 1:10).
4. No known etiology.
   a. Family and twin studies demonstrate a significant genetic contribution.
   b. Psychodynamic theories include bingeing as behavioral dysregulation due to dearth of maternal involvement and dissociated self states with angry attacks on one's own body due to masochistic or sadistic needs.

RECOGNITION

1. Uncontrollable bingeing episodes. Foods consumed are usually high in carbohydrates and fats and can exceed 5000 kcal per episode.
2. Food buying and bingeing are often done in secret and can occur at any time.
3. Bingeing usually alternates with purging, terminating a bingeing episode with forced vomiting. Urine screens for laxative and diuretics may be helpful. Diuretics generally also increase urine electrolytes.
4. Comorbid emotional difficulties are common.
   a. Feelings of guilt.
   b. Concurrent depression (in up to 75%).
   c. Other impulse control problems can co-occur, including substance abuse (involving 30% to 37%).
   d. Sexual dysfunction is also common.
   e. Obsessive–compulsive symptoms in up to 25% of patients.
   f. Panic disorder in up to 20%.
   g. Sexual abuse has been reported in 20% to 50% of patients.
   h. Increased prevalence of cluster B and C personality disorders.
5. Medical complications (seen in up to 40% of patients).
   a. Electrolyte imbalances.
   b. Metabolic acidosis.
   c. Increased blood urea nitrogen (BUN).
   d. Esophageal tears.
   e. Decalcification of teeth.
   f. Parotid swelling, with increased amylase (usually elevated in binge–purge patients and not in restrictive anorexic patients). Serial amylase level can help detect covert purging.
   g. Altered thyroid and cortisol function.

DIFFERENTIAL DIAGNOSIS
1. Anorexia nervosa (see last section).
2. Major depression.
3. Bipolar affective disorder.
4. Adjustment disorder (bulimia as a reaction to a stress).
5. Kleine–Levin syndrome (hypersomnia and hyperphagia).
6. Klüver–Bucy syndrome (visual agnosia, hypersexuality, hyperphagia).
7. Compulsive hyperphagia has been reported in patients with seasonal affective disorder.

MEDICAL EVALUATION
1. Electrolytes.
2. Glucose.
3. Thyroid function tests.
4. Neuroimaging of pituitary.
5. Complete blood count (CBC).
6. ECG.
7. Serum amylase level.

TREATMENT
1. Medical stabilization is the first priority.
2. Behavior therapy (and nutrition education) with scheduling and positive reward mechanisms.
3. Group therapy with other bulimic patients may be helpful; meta-analysis of 40 group treatment studies suggested moderate efficacy.
4. Family therapy is usually needed to assist the family in how best to interact with the patient, though systematic studies are not available.
5. Individual psychotherapy.
   a. Cognitive behavior therapy is the individual therapy modality with the most evidence for efficacy; however, only a minority of patients achieve full abstinence from bingeing and purging behavior.
   b. Interpersonal psychotherapy modality and dialectical behavior therapy also have demonstrated efficacy.
6. Medication.
   a. Antidepressants are clearly superior to placebo in the short-term treatment of bulimia and probably have an additive effect when used in conjunction with cognitive behavior therapy.
      (1) Binge frequency can decline by 50% to 75%.
      (2) Improvement often occurs in the first few weeks, unrelated to effects on depressive symptoms.
      (3) SSRIs are first-line medication. Fluoxetine is the only agent with Food and Drug Administration (FDA) approval; doses are often in the range of 60 mg/day.
      (4) Tricyclic antidepressants (after correction of underlying electrolyte and ECG abnormalities) can help to treat comorbid affective symptoms, but they also have been reported helpful even in patients without identifiable depressive symptoms.
      (5) Monoamine oxidase inhibitors (MAOIs) show evidence of efficacy, but diet restraints complicate use.

     (6) Buproprion should not be used due to risk of seizures in context of bingeing and purging.

     (7) Long-term effects on binge frequency and depression are not as good.

  b. A trial of anticonvulsants (phenytoin or carbamazepine in the usual anticonvulsant doses) can help a subgroup of patients with abnormal electroencephalograms (EEGs) even without a formal seizure disorder. Plasma levels should be monitored carefully.

  c. Some preliminary studies indicate possible beneficial effects of naltrexone, topiramate, and ondansetron in reduced bingeing and purging.

PROGNOSIS

1. Overall short-term success with treatment is 50% to 70%.
2. Relapse rates in 6 months to 6 years are between 30% and 50%.
3. Mortality may be 1% to 15%.
4. Treatment of psychiatric comorbidity is important to outcome.

18.3 Obesity

DEFINITION

1. Characterized by accumulation of excess adipose tissue and associated with increased risk of mortality and morbidity.
2. *Obesity* is often defined as BMI > 30 (BMI is weight in kilograms divided by height in meters squared). BMI > 25 defines *overweight*.

EPIDEMIOLOGY

1. In 2000, about 65% of the adult population in the United States had a BMI > 25 (up 40% from the 1980 rate of 46%).
2. In 2000, about 30% of the adult population had a BMI > 30 (up 200% from the 1980 rate of 15%).
3. More than 10% of children 2 to 5 years old and 15% of children 6 to 19 years old are overweight.
4. Obesity is more common in women and overweight is more common in men.
5. Obesity is especially common in African Americans, some Latin American populations, and Native Americans.

ETIOLOGY

1. Genetic.
  a. Family, twin, and adoption studies have indicated that genetics influences 40% to 75% of variation in BMI.
  b. With the exception of rare single gene mutations that result in severe obesity (e.g., loss of leptin production), numerous genes contribute modestly to predisposition.
2. Behavioral. About 60% of the U.S. population does not participate in regular physical activity, and 25% are almost entirely sedentary.
3. Environmental.
  a. Television viewing is associated with greater weight in children and adults.
  b. Physical exertion for work and daily living has decreased.

4. Psychodynamic.
   a. Food consumption may be used to fill unmet dependency needs.
   b. The complex demands of sexuality may be mitigated by becoming unattractive.
5. Psychiatric comorbidity.
   a. Children and adolescents with depression may be at increased risk for overweight.
   b. Patients with bipolar disorder might have elevated rates of overweight, obesity, and abdominal obesity.
   c. Obese persons seeking weight-loss treatment might have elevated rates of mood disorders, although most overweight persons in the community do not have mood disorders.

DIFFERENTIAL DIAGNOSIS (i.e., SECONDARY CAUSES)

1. Cushing's syndrome. Signs are buffalo hump and central obesity; look for supraclavicular fat, proportionally thin extremities, and easy bruising.
2. Hypothalamic tumor such as craniopharyngioma often manifests with headache and papilledema.
3. Head trauma with hypothalamic injury of appetite center (imaging does not rule out injury).
4. Hypothyroidism.
   a. Mild hypothyroidism (thyroid-stimulating hormone [TSH] 4-9 IU/mL) can promote 2- to 6-lb weight gain per year.
   b. Often associated with fatigue.
5. Rare genetic disorders (e.g., Prader—Willi syndrome manifests with mental retardation and morbid obesity since childhood).
6. Medication side effects.
   a. Weight gain is a potential side effect of many medications.
   b. Examples include antipsychotic drugs, tricyclic and heterocyclic antidepressants, MAOIs, lithium, and glucocorticoids.

COURSE AND PROGNOSIS

1. About 300,000 deaths each year in the United States may be attributed to obesity.
2. Obesity is the second leading cause of preventable death in the United States (behind smoking).
3. Morbidity increases in a fairly linear fashion with BMI, beginning at the upper end of the normal range.
4. In the United States, association between excess body weight and mortality may be weaker for African Americans than for whites.
5. Cardiovascular disorders.
   a. Risk is strongest for cardiovascular disorders.
      (1) Patients with BMI > 25 are two to three times more likely to have cardiovascular disease and are more likely to die from it.
      (2) Women with BMI > 25 are three times more likely to have high blood pressure and women with BMI > 30 are six times more likely to have high blood pressure.

6. Diabetes.
   a. Up to 80% of cases of type 2 diabetes may be attributed to the combined effect of inactivity and obesity.
   b. Patients with a BMI > 30 have 10 times the risk of developing diabetes.
7. Cancer.
   a. Breast, colon, uterine, renal, esophageal, and ovarian cancer incidence all increase with BMI.
   b. Overweight and obesity can account for 14% of cancer deaths in men and 20% of cancer deaths in women.
8. Gallstones. Overweight women have twice the risk of gallstones, and obese women have 2.5 to 3 times the risk.
9. Osteoarthritis.
   a. Overweight adults are more than twice as likely to develop arthritis in the hip.
   b. Overweight and obesity are associated with an increased risk of hip replacement.

TREATMENT

1. Diet, exercise, and behavior interventions.
   a. Counseling typically aims to promote change in diet and/or exercise; behavior interventions help patients acquire the skills, motivation, and support to change diet and exercise patterns.
   b. Behavior interventions typically include self-monitoring, stimulus control, exercise programs, and cognitive restructuring.
   c. Behavior approach has been summarized in several publications (e.g., *The LEARN Program for Weight Management 2000*).
   d. A National Institutes of Health (NIH) review of 29 trials with at least a 1-year follow-up indicates that those treated with diet, exercise (and sometimes behavior) interventions lost between 1.9 kg and 8.8 kg (mean, 3.3 kg) when corrected for change in controls.
   e. Although very-low-calorie diets did produce greater initial weight loss than low-calorie diets, results were similar beyond 1 year.
2. Pharmacology.
   a. Consider in patients with BMI > 27 when conservative measures have been unsuccessful.
   b. Realistic goal is loss of 5% to 10% of initial body weight over 6 to 12 months, followed by long-term maintenance of this loss.
   c. NIH guidelines recommend that if a chosen medication does not result in loss of 2 kg in the first month, the dose should be adjusted or the medicine discontinued.
   d. The FDA has approved only two drugs for long-term use and one for short-term use.
      (1) Sibutramine.
         (a) Inhibits norepinephrine and serotonin reuptake.
         (b) Ineffective as antidepressant (for which it was designed) but found to reduce body weight and appetite and to increase satiety.

(c) More than 10 prospective randomized clinical trials supported its efficacy.

(d) Three trials of at least 1 year's duration demonstrate that patients on sibutramine lost 4.3 kg, or 4.6% more weight than those on placebo.

(e) Common side effects are dry mouth, constipation, and insomnia.

(f) Although safety has been shown in patients with controlled hypertension, patients experience average increased systolic blood pressure (SBP) of 4 mm Hg, increased diastolic blood pressure (DBP) of 2 to 4 mm Hg, and increased heart rate of 4 beats/min so that regular pulse and blood pressure monitoring are recommended.

(g) Contraindicated in patients with poorly controlled hypertension, cardiovascular disease, and patients taking either MAOIs or SSRIs.

(2) Orlistat.

(a) Inhibits pancreatic and gastrointestinal lipases.

(b) Prevents absorption of approximately 30% of dietary fat.

(c) Results of 11 prospective randomized, controlled trials together indicate 2.7 kg or 2.9% greater weight reduction for treated patients compared with placebo at 1-year follow-up.

(d) Also decreases low-density lipoprotein (LDL) and cholesterol independent of weight change.

(e) Decreases progression to diabetic state and leads to better glycemic control in patients with diabetes.

(f) Side effects include oily spotting, liquid stools, fecal urgency or incontinence, flatulence, and abdominal cramping.

(g) Recommend taking a multivitamin 2 hours before or after medication because medication can impair absorption of fat-soluble vitamins.

(3) Phentermine.

(a) Noradrenergic agent.

(b) Approved for use of up to 3 months due to lack of long-term studies.

(c) Studies demonstrate a 2- to 10-kg greater weight loss in treated patients than in those receiving placebo.

(d) Side effects include insomnia, dry mouth, constipation, restlessness, euphoria, nervousness, increased pulse rate, and blood pressure.

(e) Contraindicated in patients with cardiovascular disease, hypertension, or a history of drug abuse and in those taking MAOIs.

e. Medications with positive trials but not yet FDA approved.

(1) Rimonabant. CB_1 cannabinoid-receptor antagonist that is in phase III trials.

(2) Topiramate. Antiepileptic medication with phase III trials held due to adverse events while the extended-release formulation is developed.

      (3) Zonisamide. Antiepileptic medication with a single randomized, double-blind, placebo-controlled study indicating efficacy.

      (4) Buproprion. Dopamine and norepinephrine reuptake inhibitor with an 8-week positive study.

3. Surgery.
  a. Limited to patients with BMI > 40 or BMI > 35 plus associated health complications who have not responded to more conservative measures.
  b. Procedures.
    (1) Bariatric surgery. Restrictive or malabsorptive; the current technique is primarily restrictive.
    (2) Gastric bypass. Complete gastric partitioning with anastomosis of the proximal gastric segment to the jejunal loop.
    (3) Adjustable gastric banding. Inflatable band around the stomach that can be adjusted to different diameters.
    (4) Vertical banded gastroplasty. Partial gastric partitioning at the proximal gastric segment with placement of gastric outlet stoma of a fixed diameter.
  c. Practical and ethical concerns limit ability to perform true randomized, blinded, placebo-controlled trials.
  d. NIH reviewed five trials and found 10- to 159-kg surgical weight loss over 12 to 48 months in patients who received surgery.

18.4 Nicotine Dependence

PREVALENCE AND SIGNIFICANCE

1. Cigarette smoking remains the most important preventable contributor to death, disability, and unnecessary health expenditures in the United States.
2. More than 48 million American adults still smoke (24%).

NICOTINE PHARMACOLOGY

1. Nicotine from tobacco smoke is rapidly absorbed and achieves maximum brain concentrations within 1 minute.
  a. Cigarettes usually contain 6 to 11 mg of nicotine, of which 1 to 3 mg is absorbed. Therefore a one-pack-a-day smoker absorbs about 40 mg of nicotine each day, achieving plasma concentrations of 25 to 35 ng/mL by the afternoon.
  b. The plasma half-life of nicotine is about 2 hours.
2. Because tolerance develops, people have to smoke more to obtain the desired effects of nicotine.
3. Effects of nicotine.
  a. Relaxes skeletal muscles.
  b. Activates the brain, with increases in serotonin, endogenous opioids, catecholamines, and vasopressin.
  c. Stimulates the brain's "reward center" through effects on dopamine pathways in the mesolimbic system.
  d. Increases attention, memory, and learning.
  e. Decreases anxiety.
  f. Decreases negative affect.

> ### BOX 18-4   Drugs Whose Metabolism Is Accelerated by Nicotine
>
> | | | |
> |---|---|---|
> | Acetaminophen | Imipramine | Tacrine |
> | Amitriptyline | Mexiletine | Theophylline |
> | Caffeine | Naproxen | Tizanidine |
> | Clomipramine | Olanzapine | Verapamil |
> | Clozapine | Ondansetron | Warfarin |
> | Cyclobenzaprine | Phenacetin | Zileuton |
> | Estradiol | Propranolol | Zolmitriptan |
> | Fluvoxamine | Riluzole | |
> | Haloperidol | Ropivacaine | |

    g. High doses can produce cocaine-like stimulation.
    h. Suppresses appetite.
4. Addictive properties of nicotine.
    a. Nicotine produces physiologic changes that account for tolerance, physical dependence, and withdrawal.
    b. Nicotine withdrawal syndrome.
        (1) Timing. Appears within 2 hours of cessation of smoking and peaks within 24 to 48 hours. The syndrome can last days to weeks, with great individual variation.
        (2) Symptoms.
            (a) Nicotine craving.
            (b) Irritability, anger.
            (c) Anxiety.
            (d) Difficulty concentrating.
            (e) Restlessness.
            (f) Decreased heart rate.
            (g) Increased appetite and weight gain (smoking cessation is associated with an average weight gain of about 6 pounds).
            (h) Depression.
5. Drug interactions.
    a. Nicotine accelerates the metabolism of many drugs, including many (but not all) of the tricyclic antidepressants, benzodiazepines, and some antipsychotic agents (Box 18-4).
    b. Smoking increases activity of the P450 1A2 isoenzyme (see Chapter 20).

SMOKING AND PSYCHIATRIC DISORDERS

1. Psychiatric patients are more likely than the general population to smoke.
2. Smokers have higher levels of depression.
3. Patients with depression who smoke are less likely to quit.

4. Depression may be a strong predictor of relapse in people who try to quit smoking.
5. Substance abusers have a high rate of smoking.
6. Alcohol use is associated with more difficulty in trying to quit smoking.
7. There appears to be a unique association between nicotine use and schizophrenia.
   a. From 80% to 90% of those with schizophrenia smoke compared with 25% to 30% of the general population.
   b. Some studies have indicated that use of tobacco transiently restores the cognitive and sensory deficits associated with schizophrenia.
   c. Smoking cessation appears to exacerbate the symptoms of schizophrenia.
   d. There is suggestion that schizophrenic patients have aberrant nicotine receptors in various cerebral areas (specifically α_7, α_4, and β_2 subunits).

TREATMENT OF NICOTINE DEPENDENCE
Overview

1. Tobacco dependence is a chronic condition that often requires repeated intervention. However, there are effective treatments that can produce long-term or even permanent abstinence.
2. Because effective tobacco dependence treatments are available, every patient who uses tobacco should be offered at least one of these treatments.
   a. Patients *willing* to try to quit tobacco use should be provided treatments identified as effective in this guideline.
   b. Patients *unwilling* to try to quit tobacco use should be provided a brief intervention designed to increase their motivation to quit.
3. It is essential that clinicians and health care delivery systems (including administrators, insurers, and purchasers) institutionalize the consistent identification, documentation, and treatment of every tobacco user seen in a health care setting.
4. Brief tobacco dependence treatment is effective, and every patient who uses tobacco should be offered at least brief treatment.
5. There is a strong dose–response relation between the intensity of tobacco dependence counseling and its effectiveness. Treatments involving person-to-person contact (via individual, group, or proactive telephone counseling) are consistently effective, and their effectiveness increases with treatment intensity (e.g., minutes of contact).
6. The best treatment programs combine pharmacologic with cognitive behavior and social therapies.
7. Tobacco dependence treatments are both clinically effective and cost-effective relative to other medical and disease prevention interventions. Therefore, insurers and purchasers should ensure that:
   a. All insurance plans include as a reimbursed benefit the counseling and pharmacotherapeutic treatments identified as effective.
   b. Clinicians are reimbursed for providing tobacco dependence treatment just as they are reimbursed for treating other chronic conditions.

Pharmacologic Approaches to Nicotine Dependence

The U.S. Public Health Service recommends that all patients who are trying to quit smoking be given pharmacotherapy, unless it is contraindicated. First-line treatments that reliably increase long-term smoking abstinence rates include nicotine replacement and buproprion.

Nicotine Replacement

Comparative trials of the various types of nicotine replacement do not indicate significantly different rates of abstinence. Most studies indicate a 15% to 25% abstinence rate with treatment after 1 year, nearly twice the rate for those treated with placebo.

1. Nicotine resin complex (nicotine gum [Nicorette]).
   a. Most frequent side effects are hiccups, nausea, anorexia, oral or jaw soreness, and gastrointestinal distress.
   b. Instructions for use.
      (1) Do not use with cigarettes.
      (2) Use as a substitute for smoking.
      (3) Chew slowly and park the gum to titrate release of nicotine to simulate smoking.
      (4) One piece substitutes for about two cigarettes.
      (5) Establish a maintenance level for 2 to 3 months, then slowly decrease.
      (6) Avoid acidic drinks (coffee, juice) before and during gum chewing.
2. Nicotine transdermal patches.
   a. Has the advantage of once-a-day application.
   b. Can be used with patients who would have trouble following the instructions for chewing nicotine gum.
   c. Disadvantage is that some patients are helped by more of a direct substitute (the patch is abstract).
   d. Side effects.
      (1) Skin irritation (causes discontinuance in up to 5%).
      (2) Insomnia and disturbing dreams.
      (3) Cardiac arrhythmias if combined with smoking in susceptible patients with coronary disease.
   e. Habitrol, Nicoderm, Nicotrol.
      (1) Various forms between 30 to 40 $\mu g/cm^2/h$.
      (2) Nicotine content varies by size of patch.
      (3) Dosage ranges from about 5 to about 20 mg over 24 hours depending on size of patch.
   f. Usual treatment involves 4 to 6 weeks at the 21-mg level, followed by 2 to 4 weeks at 14-mg and then 7-mg levels.
   g. Use a lower starting dose in patients with coronary disease, those who weigh less than 100 pounds, or those who smoke less than half a pack a day.
   h. Some patients benefit from combined therapy: Nicotine gum is used to supplement the patch for momentary needs.

    i. Transdermal nicotine does not appear to cause a significant increase in cardiovascular events in outpatients with cardiac disease.

    j. Nicotine patches can cause some short-term improvements in depression in patients with depressive symptoms.

    k. Conversely, some patients are at risk for developing major depression after smoking cessation.

3. Nicotine nasal spray.

    a. Each 0.05-mL spray delivers 0.5 mg of nicotine.

    b. Recommended dose is 1 to 2 sprays every hour for 6 to 8 weeks, with a maximum dose of 40 mg/day.

    c. Minimum recommended treatment is 8 doses per day for 3 to 6 months.

    d. Recommend tapering over subsequent 4- to 6-week period to prevent withdrawal.

    e. Common adverse effects include nasal irritation, rhinorrhea, sneezing, throat irritation, and coughing.

4. Nicotine inhaler.

    a. Consists of mouthpiece and plastic cartridge containing 4 mg of nicotine.

    b. About 80 inhalations are necessary to obtain nicotine typically found in a single cigarette.

    c. Recommended use of 6 to 16 cartridges per day for 6 to 12 weeks followed by tapering over a 3-month period.

    d. Common adverse effects include throat irritation and coughing.

5. Nicotine lozenges.

    a. Those who smoke less than 30 minutes after waking should start with 4-mg lozenges; those who smoke after more than 30 minutes should start with a 2-mg lozenge.

    b. Do not eat or drink anything 15 minutes before or while using the lozenge because nicotine is absorbed only through the mouth. Allow the lozenge to slowly dissolve over 20 to 30 minutes, occasionally shifting from one side of the mouth to the other.

    c. Use 2 to 4 mg up to 10 times daily for 6 weeks, then slowly taper over the next 6 weeks.

Buproprion SR

1. Bupropion sustained-release tablets (Zyban) have FDA approval for use in smoking cessation.

2. Begin medication 1 week before the planned date of smoking cessation.

3. Begin with 150 mg qAM for 3 days, then increase the dose to 150 bid for the duration of the treatment.

4. In addition to its dopamine and norepinephrine reuptake inhibition, buproprion might also act as a nicotine receptor antagonist.

5. Failure to obtain abstinence after 4 weeks merits termination of trial.

6. Side effects include:

    a. Headache.

    b. Jitteriness.

    c. Dry mouth.

    d. Initial insomnia.
    e. Gastrointestinal symptoms.
7. Bupropion is contraindicated in patients with seizures or eating disorders.

Other Medications

Second-line treatments include clonidine and nortriptyline.

1. Clonidine.
    a. Attenuates nicotine withdrawal symptoms and has been used as an adjunct to smoking cessation programs.
    b. Usually used in doses of 0.1 to 0.3 mg/day for 2 weeks, then tapered.
    c. Side effects include dizziness, lightheadedness, sedation, and dry mouth.
2. Nortriptyline.
    a. Five trials have demonstrated efficacy.
    b. Start with 25 mg/day and increase to a target dose of 75 to 100 mg/day.
3. Other antidepressants (selegiline, doxepin, fluoxetine, paroxetine, buspirone, and venlafaxine) have been studied to some extent, but strength of evidence is insufficient to make them the initial treatment of choice.

COGNITIVE BEHAVIOR TREATMENTS

1. Three types of counseling and behavioral therapy are especially effective and should be used with all patients attempting to quit smoking.
    a. Practical counseling (problem solving and skills training).
    b. Social support as part of treatment (intratreatment social support).
    c. Help in securing social support outside of treatment (extratreatment social support).
2. The cognitive behavior component is essential to any treatment program. It usually involves three stages.
    a. Preparation.
        (1) Review reasons and readiness for quitting.
        (2) Establish a target quit date.
        (3) Keep a daily diary to establish baseline levels as well as what prompts smoking.
    b. Quitting.
        (1) Self-management (stimulus control).
        (2) Identify, alter, or avoid cues that trigger smoking.
        (3) Substitute another stimulus for cues that cannot be avoided.
        (4) Aversion strategies (increase usual smoking rate to the point where it becomes distasteful) have sometimes been used.
        (5) Nicotine fading involves gradually switching brands to ones with lower nicotine content.
    c. Maintenance.
        (1) Identify high-risk relapse situations.
        (2) Rehearse how to deal with those situations.
        (3) Avoid seeing a "slip-up" as a total failure.
        (4) Get involved in other rewarding activities.

NICOTINE VACCINE

1. Immunologic approaches target the drug itself rather than the brain.
2. Phase I clinical trials have not produced any serious adverse events in humans and have produced dose-dependent increases in serum antibody levels.
3. Although preliminary data from small trials suggest vaccination can facilitate abstinence, more advanced trials are needed.

SUGGESTED READINGS

American Academy of Pediatrics, Committee on Adolescence: Identifying and treating eating disorders. *Pediatrics* 111(1):204-211, 2003.

American Psychiatric Association: Treatment of patients with eating disorders, third edition. American Psychiatric Association. *Am J Psychiatry* 163(7 Suppl):4-54, 2006.

Borrelli B, Niaura R, Keuthen NJ, et al: Development of major depressive disorder during smoking-cessation treatment. *J Clin Psychiatry* 57:534-538, 1996.

Brownell KD: *The LEARN Program for Weight Management 2000.* Dallas, Tex: American Health Publishing, 2000.

Ciraulo DA, Piechniczek-Buczek J, Iscan EN: Outcome predictors in substance abuse disorders. *Psychiatr Clin North Am* 26(2):381-409, 2003.

Damcott C, Sack P, Shuldiner A: The genetics of obesity. *Endocrinol Metab Clin North Am* 32(4):761-786, 2003.

Fisher M: The course and outcome of eating disorders in adults and adolescents: A review. *Adolesc Med* 14(1):149-158, 2003.

Hughes JR: Antidepressants for smoking cessation. *Cochrane Database Syst Rev* (2):CD000031, 2003.

Indiana University School of Medicine: Drug interactions: Defining genetic influences on pharmacologic responses. Available at http://medicine.iupui.edu/flockhart/ (accessed October 14, 2006).

Joseph AM, Norman SM, Ferry LH, et al: The safety of transdermal nicotine as an aid to smoking cessation in patients with cardiac disease. *N Engl J Med* 335:1792-1798, 1996.

Karnath B: Smoking cessation. *Am J Med* 112(5):399-405, 2002.

Kerem NC, Katzman DK: Brain structure and function in adolescents with anorexia nervosa. *Adolesc Med* 14(1):109-118, 2003.

Klump K, Kaye W, Strober M: The evolving genetic foundations of eating disorders. *Psychiatr Clin North Am* 24(2):215-225, 2001.

Korner J, Arrone LJ: Pharmacologic approaches to weight reduction: Therapeutic targets. *J Clin Endocrinol Metab* 89(6):2616-2621, 2004.

LeSage MG, Keyler DE, Pentel PR: Current status of immunologic approaches to treating tobacco dependence: Vaccines and nicotine-specific antibodies. *AAPS J* 8(1):E65-E75, 2006.

Marlow SP: Smoking cessation. *Respir Care* 48(12):1238-1254, 2003.

McTigue K, Harris R, Hemphill B, et al: Screening and interventions for obesity in adults: Summary of the evidence for the U.S. Preventive Services Task Force. *Ann Intern Med* 139(11):933-949, 2003.

Quigley EMM, Hasler WL, Parkman HP: AGA technical review on nausea and vomiting. *Gastroenterology* 120(1): 263-286, 2001.

Ripoll N: Nicotine receptors and schizophrenia. *Curr Med Res Opin* 20(7):1057-1074, 2004.

Schneider M: Bulimia nervosa and binge-eating disorder in adolescents. *Adoles Med* 14(1):119-131, 2003.

Stein C, Colditz G: The epidemic of obesity. *J Clin Endocrinol Metab* 89(6):2522-2525, 2004.

Talwar A, Jain M, Vijayan VK: Pharmacotherapy of tobacco dependence. *Med Clin North Am* 88:1517-1534, 2004.

United States Department of Health and Human Services: Tobacco cessation—You can quit smoking now! Clinician materials. Available at http://www.surgeongeneral.gov/tobacco/(accessed October 15, 2006).

Wadden T, Butryn M: Behavioral treatment of obesity. *Endocrinol Metab Clin North Am* 32(4):981-1003, 2003.

Yager J: Implementing the Revised American Psychiatric Association practice guideline for the treatment of patients with eating disorder. *Psychiatr Clin North Am* 24(2):185-199, 2001.

Yager J, Andersen A, Devlin M, et al: American Psychiatric Association practice guidelines for eating disorders. *Am J Psychiatry* 150:207-228, 1993.

Sexual Disorders

19

John P. Wincze

19.1 Phases of Sexual Function

Sexual dysfunction involves a disturbance in one of the following phases of sexual activity.

1. Desire involves fantasies and interest in sexual activity.
2. Excitement includes subjective pleasure as well as physiologic arousal.
   a. Male changes include penile tumescence and erection.
   b. Female changes include pelvic vasocongestion, vaginal lubrication and expansion, and swelling of the external genitalia.
3. Orgasm consists of the peak of sexual pleasure, with release of sexual tension and rhythmic contraction of perineal muscles and reproductive organs.
   a. With ejaculation of semen in men.
   b. With contractions of the outer third of the vagina in women.
   c. Rhythmic anal sphincter contraction in both sexes.
4. Resolution phase involves muscle relaxation in both sexes and a physiologic refractory period for erection and orgasm in men.

19.2 Sexual History

1. Aspects to include in the sexual history.
   a. Substance abuse history.
   b. History of physical abuse.
   c. History of sexually transmitted diseases.
   d. Past and present relationships.
   e. Satisfaction with current sexual relationship.
   f. Level of sexual activity.
   g. Sexual practices and preferences (includes primary partner and sexual outlets besides primary partner).
   h. Gender preferences (of a sexual partner).
   i. History of childhood sexual abuse or assault.
   j. Contraceptive choice.
   k. Past and present problem areas.
   l. Mental health history.
2. How to obtain the history.
   a. Normalize inquiry by stating, "It is very common for many of my patients to report problems related to sexual matters. What has been your experience in this area?"

    b. Be prepared to explain why the questions are relevant and important.

    c. Avoid appearances of being anxious or judgmental.

    d. At times, a simple open-ended invitation, such as "Tell me about any problems in your sex life" may be effective.

3. Patient obstacles to obtaining a history.

    a. Religious or familial prohibitions.

    b. Fear of appearing deviant or abnormal.

    c. Prior traumatic experiences.

    d. Fear of appearing inadequate.

    e. Fear of lack of confidentiality.

    f. Discomfort with the subject.

4. Clinician obstacles to obtaining a history.

    a. Lack of time.

    b. Religious or familial prohibitions.

    c. Concerns about what to do if a problem is presented.

    d. Discomfort with the subject.

5. System obstacles to obtaining a history.

    a. Social attitudes.

    b. Time.

    c. Lack of resources to manage problems once they are discovered.

    d. Lack of confidentiality of medical records.

6. Ruling out medical factors is the first diagnostic task with all sexual problems.

    a. Medications (Table 19-1).

    b. Street drugs.

    c. Depression.

    d. Menopause.

    e. Medical illness or chronic pain.

19.3 Sexual Dysfunction

All the following dysfunctions can be lifelong, acquired, generalized, or situational. Criteria from the *Diagnostic and Statistical Manual of Mental Disorders*, fourth edition (DSM-IV), are followed for making a diagnosis.

DISORDERS OF SEXUAL DESIRE

1. Hypoactive sexual desire disorder.

    a. Deficiency or absence of sexual fantasies or desire for sexual activity.

    b. The patient is distressed or is involved in interpersonal difficulty as a result.

    c. Dysfunction is not a result of another psychiatric or medical cause or drug (see following section).

    d. Consider major depression, obsessive–compulsive disorder (OCD), and posttraumatic stress disorder (PTSD).

2. Sexual aversion disorder.

    a. Persistent or recurrent aversion to, or avoidance of, genital sexual contact with a sexual partner.

    b. The disturbance causes distress or interpersonal difficulty.

Table 19-1 Medications and Substances Causing Sexual Dysfunction

Drug	Loss or Decrease of Libido	Loss or Decrease of Potency	Inhibition of Orgasm	Delayed or No Ejaculation	Priapism	Increased Libido	Painful Ejaculation	Dyspareunia	Spontaneous Orgasm	Penile Anesthesia	Retrograde Ejaculation
Anticholinergics or Antihistamines											
Atropine		×									
Benztropine		×									
Diphenhydramine		×									
Hydroxyzine		×									
Propantheline		×									
Trihexyphenidyl		×									
Anticonvulsants											
Carbamazepine		×									
Phenytoin	×	×			×						
Primidone	×	×									
Antidepressants											
Amitriptyline	×	×	×	×							
Amoxapine		×	×	×							
Clomipramine		×	×	×			×				
Desipramine		×	×	×							
Doxepin	×			×							
Fluoxetine	×		×	×					×		
Fluvoxamine	×		×	×							
Imipramine	×		×	×			×				
Isocarboxazid	×		×	×						×	
Nortriptyline	×	×	×	×							
Paroxetine	×										

Table continued on following page.

Table 19-1 **Medications and Substances Causing Sexual Dysfunction** (Continued)

Drug	Loss or Decrease of Libido	Loss or Decrease of Potency	Inhibition of Orgasm	Delayed or No Ejaculation	Priapism	Increased Libido	Painful Ejaculation	Dyspareunia	Spontaneous Orgasm	Penile Anesthesia	Retrograde Ejaculation
Protriptyline	×						×				
Sertraline			×	×	×						
Trazodone	×		×	×	×	×					
Trimipramine	×		×	×							
Venlafaxine	×		×	×							
Cancer											
Chemotherapeutics											
Busulfan		×									
Chlorambucil		×									
Clofibrate	×	×									
Cyclophosphamide		×									
Cytosine arabinoside		×									
Interferon	×	×						×			
Methotrexate	×	×									
Tamoxifen					×						
Vinblastine	×	×						×			
Cardiovascular Agents											
Amiloride		×									
Amiodarone	×	×									
Atenolol		×									
Captopril		×									
Chlorthiazide	×	×		×							
Clonidine	×	×		×							×
Digoxin	×	×									
Etretinate		×									

Drug							
Famotidine		×					×
Guanethidine	×	×		×			
Labetalol	×	×		×	×		
Methyldopa	×	×		×			
Mexiletine	×	×					
Nadolol	×	×		×	×		
Nifedipine		×					
Phentolamine		×			×		
Pindolol		×					
Prazosin		×					
Propranolol		×					
Spironolactone	×	×					
Thiazide diuretics	×	×					
Verapamil	×						
Dopaminergics							
Bromocriptine		×		×			
Carbidopa–levodopa	×	×					
Pimozide				×	×	×	
Selegiline			×				×
Drugs of Abuse							
Alcohol		×		×			
Amphetamines (chronic use)		×					
Amyl nitrate	×	×					
Cannabis	×				×		
Cocaine						×	
Heroin	×			×		×	
LSD	×			×		×	
Phencyclidine	×	×		×			
H₂ Blockers							
Cimetidine	×	×					

Table continued on following page.

Table 19-1 **Medications and Substances Causing Sexual Dysfunction** (Continued)

Drug	Loss or Decrease of Libido	Loss or Decrease of Potency	Inhibition of Orgasm	Delayed or No Ejaculation	Priapism	Increased Libido	Painful Ejaculation	Dyspareunia	Spontaneous Orgasm	Penile Anesthesia	Retrograde Ejaculation
Hormones											
Estrogen	×					×					
Leuprolide		×									
Progestins		×									
Steroids	×					×					
Testosterone					×						
Narcotics											
Methadone	×	×	×	×							
Morphine	×	×									
Neuroleptic Agents											
Chlorpromazine	×	×		×	×						
Chlorprothixene				×	×						
Clozapine					×						
Fluphenazine	×	×		×	×						
Haloperidol		×		×	×		×				
Mesoridazine		×		×	×						
Metoclopramide	×				×						
Molindone					×						
Perphenazine				×							

Risperidone	×		×							
Sertindole		×								
Thioridazine	×	×	×							×
Thiothixene			×						×	
Trifluoperazine										×
Sedative–Hypnotics										
Benzodiazepines	×		×		×					
Barbiturates	×			×						
Other Drugs										
Baclofen	×									
Danazol	×									
Fenfluramine	×			×					×	
Indomethacin	×							×		
Ketoconazole	×							×		
Lithium	×									
Naltrexone	×		×		×		×			
Naproxen						×				
Omeprazole						×				
Papaverine									×	
Propofol										

    c. The dysfunction is not accounted for by some other disorder.

    d. Consider major depression, OCD, PTSD, and phobia.

DISORDERS OF SEXUAL AROUSAL

1. Female sexual arousal disorder.

    a. Persistent or recurrent inability to attain, or maintain until completion of sexual activity, an adequate lubrication—swelling response of sexual excitement.

    b. The disturbance causes distress or interpersonal difficulty.

    c. The dysfunction is not accounted for by some other disorder.

    d. Medical issues to consider.

      (1) Menopausal reductions in estrogen levels.

      (2) Atrophic vaginitis.

      (3) Diabetes mellitus.

      (4) Pelvic radiation therapy.

      (5) Reduced lubrication is associated with the following:

        (a) Lactation.

        (b) Antihypertensives.

        (c) Antihistamines.

      (6) Medications (see Table 19-1), especially tricyclic antidepressants or selective serotonin reuptake inhibitors (SSRIs). The estimated prevalence of sexual impairments associated with these antidepressants is between 20% and 60%. There is a lower prevalence (5%) with bupropion, nefazodone, and mirtazapine. See Chapter 7.

      (7) Psychiatric disorders.

        (a) Major depression.

        (b) OCD.

        (c) PTSD.

2. Male erectile disorder.

    a. Persistent or recurrent inability to attain or maintain an adequate erection until completion of sexual activity.

    b. The disturbance causes distress or interpersonal difficulty.

    c. The dysfunction is not accounted for by some other disorder.

    d. Medical issues to consider.

      (1) Diabetes mellitus.

      (2) Multiple sclerosis.

      (3) Autonomic injury as a result of surgery or radiation.

      (4) Peripheral neuropathy.

      (5) Renal failure.

      (6) Peripheral vascular disease.

      (7) Medications (see Table 19-1).

        (a) Antihypertensives.

        (b) Antidepressants.

        (c) Neuroleptic agents.

        (d) Substances of abuse.

    e. Medical diagnostic tests such as nocturnal penile tumescence studies, ultrasound, or angiography can assess physiologic erectile functions.

f. Treatments (available or under Food and Drug Administration [FDA] review):
   (1) Oral medications.
      (a) Sildenafil (Viagra), tadalafil (Cialis), and verdenafil (Levitra) act as a smooth muscle relaxant and increase blood flow into the corpus cavernosum.
      (b) Apomorphine, which apparently affects brain center involved in triggering erections.
      (c) Phentolamine relaxes smooth muscles and dilates arteries.
   (2) Penile suppository. Alprostadil.
   (3) Injection into base of penis. Alprostadil (Caverject) relaxes smooth muscles.
   (4) Surgery.
      (a) Useful when problem results from a medical etiology.
      (b) Implants can be reliable, but they destroy erectile tissue and are a last-resort treatment.

ORGASMIC DISORDERS

1. Female or male orgasmic disorder.
   a. Persistent or recurrent delay in or absence of orgasm following a normal sexual excitement phase.
   b. The disturbance causes marked distress or interpersonal difficulty.
   c. The problem is not better accounted for by another psychiatric or medical disorder.
   d. Common medications inhibiting orgasm.
      (1) Tricyclic or SSRI antidepressants.
      (2) Benzodiazepines.
      (3) Neuroleptic agents.
      (4) Antihypertensives.
      (5) Narcotics.
   e. The common psychiatric disorder accounting for this problem is major depression.
2. Premature ejaculation.
   a. Persistent or recurrent ejaculation with minimal sexual stimulation before or shortly after penetration and before the person wishes it.
   b. The disturbance causes marked distress or interpersonal difficulty.
   c. The problem is not a result of medications, medical conditions, or other psychiatric problems.
   d. Treatment.
      (1) Often focused on providing accurate information about male sexual functioning.
      (2) Often involves reducing conflict between partners.
      (3) SSRIs, associated with delayed ejaculation, can be used therapeutically for premature ejaculation. Typical starting dose is sertraline 25 mg qd or paroxetine 10 mg qd.

SEXUAL PAIN DISORDERS

1. Dyspareunia.
   a. Genital pain associated with penetration or genital manipulation.
   b. Can occur in men and women.

   c. Causes marked distress or interpersonal difficulty.
   d. Is not a result of other medical problems, such as:
    (1) Vaginismus.
    (2) Lack of vaginal lubrication.
    (3) Pelvic or urinary tract infections.
    (4) Vaginal or penile scar tissue.
    (5) Endometriosis.
    (6) Abdominal adhesions.
    (7) Postmenopausal vaginal atrophy.
    (8) Temporary estrogen depletion during lactation.
    (9) Gastrointestinal disorders.
    (10) Medications (see Table 19-1).
     (a) Fluphenazine.
     (b) Thioridazine.
     (c) Amoxapine.
   e. Not a result of another psychiatric disorder.
    (1) Somatization disorder.
    (2) PTSD.
    (3) Major depression.
  2. Vaginismus.
   a. Recurrent or persistent involuntary contraction of the perineal muscles surrounding the outer third of the vagina when vaginal penetration is attempted.
   b. The disturbance causes distress or interpersonal problems.
   c. The disturbance is not better accounted for by a medical or psychiatric problem.
   d. Evaluate history for psychiatric problems.
    (1) Sexual abuse or trauma.
    (2) Somatization disorder.
   e. Medical issues to consider.
    (1) Endometriosis.
    (2) Vaginal infection.

SEXUAL DYSFUNCTION ASSOCIATED WITH MEDICAL CONDITIONS

There are a wide variety of physical and psychological issues involving sexual dysfunction accompanying medical illness. The clinician has the obligation to inquire about concerns regarding sexual activity with patients (and partners).

 1. Patients with cardiac disease are often fearful of resuming sexual activity after a myocardial infarction, angioplasty, or coronary artery bypass. Resuming sexual activity postinfarction does not increase morbidity.
  a. Changes in heart rate, blood pressure, and oxygen uptake during conventional sexual activity with an established partner are similar to those experienced during light to moderate short-term exercise.
  b. The greatest physiologic stress is brief, occurring during orgasm, and quickly returns to baseline.

2. Cancer and its treatment creates a wide variety of physical problems that can interfere with sexuality.
   a. Disfigurement.
   b. Distortions in body image.
   c. Loss of physiologic functions.
   d. Pain.
   e. Loss of sexual desire.
   f. Infertility.
3. Diabetes mellitus. Although physical factors (e.g., neuropathy) play a significant role in sexual dysfunction, psychological factors also contribute to loss of interest, arousal, and orgasmic potential.
4. Renal failure.
   a. Male erectile dysfunction in 20% to 80% of patients.
      (1) Male dysfunction is associated with the following:
         (a) Decreased testosterone.
         (b) Increased estradiol.
         (c) Autonomic dysfunction.
         (d) Vascular insufficiency.
         (e) Zinc deficiency and anemia.
      (2) Dialysis does not generally improve sexual function.
   b. More than half of uremic women are amenorrheic before menopause. A similar number complain of loss of sexual interest.
   c. Successful kidney transplant is usually associated with improved sexual function.
5. Human immunodeficiency virus (HIV) and acquired immune deficiency syndrome (AIDS).
   a. Decrease in sexual desire and activity is extremely common in both men and women with early-stage HIV disease.
   b. Relationship problems can be expected.
6. Spinal cord injury.
   a. Cervical or thoracic injuries can impair psychogenic arousal and orgasm without impairing responses to direct mechanical stimulation (although the patient cannot feel the stimulation).
   b. Lumbar–sacral injuries impair the genital–spinal reflex, so direct stimulation is not effective for arousal. If the autonomic system is spared, psychogenic arousal is still possible.
   c. Bowel and bladder incontinence also interferes with sexual function.
   d. Neurogenic erectile dysfunction in paraplegic or quadriplegic men can be addressed with the following:
      (1) Intracavernosal pharmacotherapy.
         (a) Combinations of phentolamine mesylate and papaverine HCl injected into the lateral base of the penis.
         (b) Other medications include vitamin E and prostaglandin E_1.
      (2) Penile prostheses.
      (3) Topical nitroglycerin.
      (4) Vacuum pressure devices.
7. Stroke.
   a. Impairs all phases of sexual response.

    b. In women, left hemisphere lesions are associated with more sexual dysfunction.

    c. In men, left hemisphere lesions are associated with less sexual dysfunction.

    d. Fear of a repeated cerebrovascular accident (CVA) is a common cause of sexual dysfunction. Other causes include the following:

      (1) Diminished self-esteem.

      (2) Anxiety about performance.

      (3) Fear of rejection.

      (4) Medication effects.

8. Dementia is associated with numerous sexual problems.

    a. Disinhibition leading to public masturbation, genital exposure, fondling of others, or inadvertent self-harm from self-stimulation.

    b. More than 60% of patients with Huntington's disease, for example, are reported to have exhibitionism, sexual aggression, voyeurism, or hypersexuality.

    c. Antiandrogen treatment is sometimes used in hypersexual demented men. Medroxyprogesterone acetate 300 mg IM given weekly has been used successfully in some patients.

9. Multiple sclerosis and spinal cord lesions.

    a. Have a high incidence of sexual dysfunction.

    b. Erectile dysfunction is the most common effect in men, and 90% of diagnoses are neurogenic.

    c. Anorgasmia and impaired desire are the most common effects in women.

    d. Pelvic sensory deficits and loss of energy also contribute.

    e. Incontinence jeopardizes intimacy.

10. Temporal lobe disorders.

11. Other endocrine conditions.

    a. Hypothyroidism.

    b. Hypoadrenocorticism and hyperadrenocorticism.

    c. Hyperprolactinemia.

    d. Hypogonadal conditions.

    e. Pituitary dysfunction.

    f. Genitourinary disorders.

      (1) Testicular disease.

      (2) Peyronie's disease.

      (3) Urethral infections.

      (4) Prostatectomy complications.

      (5) Genital injury or infection.

      (6) Atrophic vaginitis.

      (7) Infections of vagina or external genitalia.

      (8) Episiotomy scars.

      (9) Cystitis.

    g. Endometriosis.

    h. Prolapsed uterus.

    i. Pelvic neoplasms.

MEDICATIONS THAT IMPAIR SEXUAL FUNCTIONING

See Table 19-1.

19.4 Paraphilias

DEFINITION

The essential features of paraphilias are recurrent, intense, sexually arousing fantasies, sexual urges, or behavior involving nonhuman objects, suffering or humiliation of oneself or others, or children or other nonconsenting partners. The fantasies or behavior are essential or preferred for sexual arousal to occur and cause distress to oneself or others.

1. Exhibitionism is recurrent, intense, sexually arousing fantasies, urges, or behavior involving exposure of genitals to unsuspecting strangers.
2. Fetishism is recurrent, intense, sexually arousing fantasies, urges, or behaviors involving the use of nonliving objects (such as female lingerie).
3. Frotteurism is recurrent, intense, sexually arousing fantasies, urges, or behavior involving touching and rubbing against a nonconsenting person.
4. Pedophilia is recurrent, intense, sexually arousing fantasies, urges, or behavior involving sexual activity with a prepubescent child or children. DSM-IV specifies that the patient be at least 16 years of age and at least 5 years older than the victim.
5. Sexual masochism. Recurrent, intense, sexually arousing fantasies, urges, or behavior involving the act (real, not simulated) of being humiliated, beaten, bound, or otherwise made to suffer. A particularly dangerous form of this disorder, which results in accidental deaths, involves hypoxyphilia, in which oxygen deprivation is used to enhance sexual arousal. Deprivation can be produced by chest compression, noose, plastic bag, or a volatile nitrite (producing temporary decrease in brain oxygenation by producing peripheral vasodilation).
6. Sexual sadism is recurrent, intense, sexually arousing fantasies, urges, or behavior involving acts (not simulated) in which the psychological or physical suffering (including humiliation) of the victim is sexually exciting to the person. There are few examples of reported treatments and no long-term outcome studies.
7. Transvestic fetishism is generally described as cross-dressing in heterosexual men for the purpose of sexual arousal. This is distinguished from other conditions in which a man cross-dresses, as in transsexualism and effeminate homosexuality.
8. Voyeurism. Recurrent, intense, sexually arousing fantasies, urges, or behavior involving the act of observing an unsuspecting person who is naked, disrobing, or engaging in sexual activity.

TREATMENT

Antiandrogens have been used to decrease aberrant sexual tendencies in male patients when the behavior is a danger to others, as in rape and pedophilia.

1. Intramuscular antiandrogens combined with psychotherapy and relapse prevention programs have been successful.
2. Long-term use of antiandrogens is associated with the following:
   a. Increased systolic blood pressure.
   b. Gallstone formation.
   c. Infertility.
   d. Changes in glucose tolerance.
   e. Depression.
   f. Weight gain.
3. Leuprolide (a synthetic gonadotropin-releasing hormone analogue approved for the treatment of prostate cancer) decreases testosterone to the castrate level.
   a. The most common side effect is hot flushes.
   b. There may be initial worsening of symptoms and transient testosterone increase.
   c. Monthly depot preparations are available.
4. Orally administered estrogen (such as ethinyl estradiol 0.10 mg/day) has been used but with lower success than antiandrogen drugs.

19.5 Gender Identity Disorder

1. Two criteria must be met for diagnosis.
   a. A strong and persistent cross-gender identification with the desire to be, or insistence that one is, the opposite gender.
      (1) Psychological testing may be helpful in confirming the sexual preferences.
      (2) Onset is usually ages 2 to 4 years.
      (3) The patient might present in medical settings with genital self-mutilation.
      (4) Differential diagnosis.
         (a) Opposite sex impersonator.
         (b) Malingering.
         (c) Borderline personality disorder.
         (d) Schizophrenia.
         (e) Transvestic fetishism.
         (f) Primary or secondary transsexualism.
   b. Persistent discomfort with one's assigned gender.
2. This condition cannot be diagnosed if there is a medical condition resulting in sexual ambiguity (intersex conditions), such as the following:
   a. Androgen insensitivity syndrome.
   b. Congenital adrenal hyperplasia.
   c. Ambiguous genitalia with hypogonadism.
3. There must be significant distress or functional impairment.
4. Medical and surgical treatments used by patients with gender identity disorders.
   a. For men.
      (1) Estrogen treatments (lifelong).
      (2) Electrolysis.
      (3) Laryngeal cartilage shaving.

        (4) Vocal cord shortening.
        (5) Jaw reconfiguration.
        (6) Penectomy.
        (7) Augmentation mammoplasty.
        (8) Liposuction.
        (9) Neovaginal construction.
    b. For women.
        (1) Testosterone treatment.
        (2) Facial plastic surgery.
        (3) Hysterectomy.
        (4) Oophorectomy.
        (5) Mastectomy.
        (6) Chest wall contouring.
        (7) Genitoplasty.
        (8) Testicular implants.
        (9) Neophallus construction.

SUGGESTED READINGS

Bancroft J: Biological factors in human sexuality. *J Sex Res* 39:15-21, 2002.

Cain V, Johannes C, Avis N, et al: Sexual functioning and practices in a multi-ethnic study of midlife women: Baseline results from SWAN. *J Sex Res* 40:266-276, 2003.

Carroll R: Assessment and treatment of gender dysphoria. In Leiblum S, Rosen R (eds): *Principles and Practice of Sex Therapy*, 3rd ed. New York, Guilford Press, 2000, pp 368-397.

Carson CC, Kirby RS, Goldstein I (eds): *Textbook of Erectile Dysfunction*. Oxford, Isis Medical Media, 1999.

Charlton RS (ed): *Treating Sexual Disorders*. San Francisco, Jossey–Bass, 1997.

DeLamater J, Freidrich W: Human sexual development. *J Sex Res* 39:10-14, 2002.

Heiman J: Sexual dysfunction: Overview of prevalence, etiological factors, and treatment. *J Sex Res* 39:73-78, 2002.

Johnson S, Phelps D, Cottler L: The association of sexual dysfunction and substance use among a community epidemiological sample. *Arch Sex Behav* 33:55-63, 2004.

Laws DR, O'Donohue W: *Sexual Deviance: Theory, Assessment, Treatment*. New York, Guilford, 1997.

Meyer W, Bockting W, Cohen-Kettenis P, et al: The standards of care for gender identity disorders, sixth version. *J Psychol Hum Sex* 13:1-30, 2001.

Schover L: Sexual problems in chronic illness. In Leiblum S, Rosen R (eds): *Principles and Practice of Sex Therapy*, 3rd ed. New York, Guilford Press, 2000, pp 398-422.

Wincze J, Carey M: *Sexual Dysfunction: A Guide for Assessment and Treatment*, 2nd ed. New York, Guilford, 2001.

The P450 System: Drug Interactions

20

Richard J. Goldberg

20.1 Definition

1. The cytochrome P450 enzyme system is a collection of more than 40 different isoenzymes that are responsible for the oxidative metabolism of many endogenous and exogenous compounds.
2. P450 system activity is inhibited by several widely used selective serotonin reuptake inhibitors (SSRIs).
3. The relevance of the P450 system, however, extends beyond the SSRIs to include a multiplicity of commonly prescribed medications.
4. P450 inhibition. The clearance of many drugs involves several P450 families as well as other systems. Therefore, finding a potential drug interaction listed in Boxes 20-1 and 20-2 does not necessarily mean that the combination will always result in a significant interaction.
   a. Nevertheless, caution should guide coprescribing when interactions are possible.
   b. When interactions are possible, it would be judicious to start with lower doses and increase doses gradually.
5. Substrate competition. Plasma elevations can occur from substrate competition as well as from inhibition.
   a. Caution is in order when coprescribing two substrates of the same enzyme system.
   b. For example, substrate competition might explain the interaction reported between alprazolam and desipramine.
6. Onset and termination of inhibition.
   a. Enzyme inhibition might begin immediately (or, more often, within the first week), increase over time until a drug reaches a steady state, and persist for as long as the drug is circulating (e.g., for weeks after terminating long-acting drugs such as fluoxetine).
   b. Enzyme inhibition will last for as long as an enzyme is saturated. Inhibition can disappear quite rapidly with shorter-acting drugs.

20.2 P450 System Terminology

The P450 system enzymes are classified into families based on amino acid sequences.

1. The members of this system are referred to as *isoenzymes* because they share significant homologies in their peptide chains.

BOX 20-1 Inhibitors of P450 Enzymes

1A2

Amiodarone
Fluoroquinolone antibiotics: Ciprofloxacin, enoxacin, norfloxacin,
   lomefloxacin
SSRIs: Fluvoxamine
Ticlopidine (Ticlid)
Other: Flutamide, mexiletine, propafenone

2C9

Amiodarone
Fluconazole (Diflucan)
Fluvastatin (Lescol)
SSRIs: Fluoxetine, fluvoxamine, paroxetine, sertraline
Sulfamethoxazole (e.g., Bactrim, Septra)
Zafirlukast (Accolate)

2C19

Esomeprazole
Lansoprazole (Prevacid)
Omeprazole (Prilosec)
SSRIs: Fluoxetine, fluvoxamine, norfluoxetine, paroxetine
Ticlopidine (Ticlid)
Topiramate (Topamax)

2D6

Amiodarone
Chlorpromazine (Thorazine)
Cimetidine (Tagamet)
Metoclopramide (Reglan)
Quinidine
SSRIs: Fluoxetine, norfluoxetine, paroxetine, sertraline
Terbinafine (Lamisil)
Other: Bupropion

3A4

Amiodarone
Antidepressants: Norfluoxetine, nefazodone
Antibiotics: Ciprofloxacin, norfloxacin, macrolides
Antifungals: Itraconazole, ketoconazole
Antivirals: Indinavir, ritonavir
Cimetidine
Diltiazem
Grapefruit juice
Verapamil (Calan, Covera, Isoptin)

SSRI, selective serotonin reuptake inhibitor.

BOX 20-2   Substrates of P450 Enzymes

1A2

ANTIDEPRESSANTS
Tricyclics: Amitriptyline, clomipramine, fluvoxamine, imipramine
Other: Mirtazapine

ANTIPSYCHOTICS
Atypical: Olanzapine, ziprasidone
Conventional: Chlorpromazine, fluphenazine, haloperidol,
 mesoridazine, perphenazine, thioridazine, thiothixene,
 trifluoperazine

NEUROLEPTIC AGENTS
Clozapine
Haloperidol

XANTHINES
Caffeine
Theophylline

OTHER

Exogenous steroids	Phenacetin
Melatonin	Propranolol
Methadone	Tacrine

2C9

ANTIDEPRESSANTS
Fluoxetine
Sertraline

SULFONYLUREA HYPOGLYCEMICS

Glipizide	Tolbutamide
Glyburide	

OTHERS

NSAIDs	Tamoxifen
Phenytoin	S-Warfarin

2C19

ANTIDEPRESSANTS
Tricyclics: Amitriptyline, clomipramine, imipramine, trimipramine
SSRIs: Citalopram, fluoxetine, sertraline
Other: Venlafaxine

OTHER
Diazepam
Propranolol
Proton pump inhibitors: Omeprazole

BOX 20-2   Substrates of P450 Enzymes (*Continued*)

2D6

ANALGESICS

Codeine*	Methadone
Hydrocodone	Oxycodone
Lidocaine	Tramadol*

ANTIDEPRESSANTS

SSRIs: Fluoxetine, fluvoxamine, paroxetine, sertraline
Tricyclics: All
Other: Mirtazapine, nefazodone, trazodone, venlafaxine

ANTIPSYCHOTICS

Conventional: Chlorpromazine, fluphenazine, haloperidol,
   thioridazine
Atypicals: Clozapine, quetiapine, risperidone, aripiprazole

CARDIOVASCULAR MEDICATIONS

Diltiazem	Nifedipine
Encainide	Propafenone
Flecainide	Propranolol
Mexiletine	Timolol

OTHER

Amphetamine	Donepezil
Chlorpheniramine	Galantamine
Dextromethorphan	Loratadine

3A4

ANALGESICS

Buprenorphine	Meperidine
Codeine	Propoxyphene
Fentanyl	Tramadol

ANTIARRHYTHMICS

Amiodarone	Propafenone
Lidocaine	Quinidine
Mexiletine	

ANTIDEPRESSANTS

SSRIs: Citalopram, fluoxetine, paroxetine, sertraline
Tricyclics: Most
Other: Mirtazapine, venlafaxine

ANTIPSYCHOTICS

Atypical: Aripiprazole, clozapine, pimozide, quetiapine, risperidone,
   ziprasidone
Conventional: Chlorpromazine, haloperidol, perphenazine

Box continued on following page

BOX 20-2   **Substrates of P450 Enzymes** (*Continued*)

SEDATIVES

Benzodiazepines: Clonazepam, diazepam
Triazolobenzodiazepines: Alprazolam, estazolam, midazolam, triazolam
Others: Buspirone, donepezil, galantamine, zaleplon, zolpidem

---

*Prodrug conversion issue.
SSRI, selective serotonin reuptake inhibitor.

2. Each of the families is referenced by a number that follows the root term P450 (or "CYP450," used interchangeably).
   a. The family number may be followed by a subfamily letter, which in turn may be followed by the number for an individual enzyme form.
   b. For example, P450 2D6 is also referred to as CYP2D6, where 2 refers to the family, *D* to the subfamily, and 6 to the individual form.
3. New information on P450 interactions and characterization is being reported continuously.

20.3 Genetic Polymorphism

Each of the isoenzymes of the P450 system is under genetic control and each has activity for different classes of drugs.

1. Because of genetic polymorphism, different people have different levels of activity of different CYP450 isoenzymes.
2. People with genetically determined low levels of activity are referred to as "poor" metabolizers.
   a. For 2D6, approximately 5% to 14% of white North Americans are poor metabolizers. The percentage of poor metabolizers among Asians, Africans, and African Americans is higher. Poor metabolizers can be identified through genotype testing or drug challenge tests using dextromethorphan.
   b. For 2C19, 2% to 6% percent of whites, 15% to 20% of Japanese, and 10% to 20% of Africans are poor metabolizers. Poor metabolizers can be identified through a drug challenge test using S-mephenytoin.
   c. For 2C9, 10% of whites are poor metabolizers. Tolbutamide has been used as a probe of 2C9 activity.
   d. For 1A2, 12% of the population are slow metabolizers, and about 40% are fast metabolizers. Slow metabolizers may be at higher risk of nonfatal myocardial infarction (MI) associated with higher caffeine levels. Poor metabolizers can be identified through a drug challenge test using caffeine.
   e. For 3A4 there is 10- to 30-fold interindividual genetic variation, although there is some question of how this translates into clinical drug metabolism.

f. There are no clinical parameters useful in predicting the metabolizing status of a particular patient.

20.4 Age Effects

1. 2D6 activity does not appear to change with age. However, age-related changes in hepatic and/or renal function can influence metabolic activity.
2. Activity of the 3A4 system does not appear to decline with age, but it is higher on average in women and lower in obese persons.
3. 2C19 activity does seems to show age-related decreases in activity.

20.5 P450 Inhibitors

P450 inhibitors are listed in Box 20-1.

1. Some medications inhibit, that is, interfere with or compete for, the activity of one or more isoenzymes, resulting in elevated drug levels of coprescribed medications metabolized by those isoenzymes.
2. Inhibitors of 2D6.
   a. Among the SSRIs.
      (1) Paroxetine is the most potent inhibitor.
      (2) Fluoxetine is a relatively strong inhibitor.
      (3) Sertraline is a relatively weak inhibitor, though there appears to be increased inhibition with increasing dose.
      (4) Citalopram and escitalopram show the lowest inhibition activity (and therefore have the lowest potential for 2D6 interactions).
   b. Other antidepressants.
      (1) Bupropion appears to have some potentially relevant 2D6 inhibition.
      (2) Venlafaxine, nefazodone, and mirtazapine inhibition of this system is probably not clinically relevant.
      (3) Duloxetine is a moderate inhibitor of 2D6.
   c. Other potent 2D6 inhibitors include cimetidine, quinidine, ritonavir, terbinafine, and ticlopidine.
3. Inhibitors of 3A4.
   a. Psychotropics (norfluoxetine, nefazodone).
   b. Other potent inhibitors.
      (1) Azole antifungals, diltiazem, macrolide antibiotics, ciprofloxacin, indinavir, ritonavir.
      (2) Grapefruit juice.
4. Inhibitors of 1A2.
   a. Psychotropics (fluvoxamine).
   b. Other potent inhibitors include ciprofloxacin, mexiletine, and propafenone.
5. Inhibitors of 2C9.
   a. Psychotropics (fluvoxamine, modafinil).
   b. Other potent inhibitors include ritonavir, fluconazole, and amiodarone.
6. Inhibitors of 2C19.

a. Psychotropics (fluvoxamine, fluoxetine, paroxetine).
b. Other potent inhibitors include ticlopidine, omeprazole, ritonavir.

20.6 P450 Substrates

Cytochrome P450 substrates are shown in Box 20-2.

1. Medications that are metabolized by the P450 system (i.e., substrates) are at risk for elevations of plasma levels if they are coprescribed with an inhibitor. All substrates have the potential also to be inhibitors; however, not all inhibitors are substrates.
2. 2D6 substrates.
   a. Antidepressants.
      (1) Two SSRIs: paroxetine and fluoxetine. This accounts for their nonlinear pharmacokinetics, because they inhibit their own metabolism.
      (2) Imipramine, amitriptyline, and nortriptyline.
      (3) Venlafaxine is converted to its active metabolite by the 2D6 system; however, there does not appear to be much clinical significance to interference with this conversion.
      (4) A metabolite of both trazodone and nefazodone (m-CPP) is a 2D6 substrate that can act as an anxiogenic agent if it accumulates. Normally, trazodone, nefazodone, and this metabolite are cleared without significant clinical effects. However, if a patient is taking a 2D6 inhibitor, high levels of this common metabolite, m-CPP, can become relevant, leading to increased anxiety.
      (5) Duloxetine is a 2D6 substrate.
   b. Antipsychotic agents.
      (1) The metabolism of many antipsychotic agents involves the 2D6 system.
         (a) Haloperidol.
         (b) Perphenazine.
         (c) Thioridazine.
         (d) Risperidone.
         (e) Clozapine.
      (2) An unexpected increase in neuroleptic levels may be associated with increased extrapyramidal side effects or akathisia (or any other potential antipsychotic side effect), resulting in clinical impairment.
   c. Other medical drugs.
      (1) Type IC cardiac antiarrhythmics such as encainide, mexiletine, and propafenone.
      (2) Beta-blockers, including metoprolol.
      (3) Codeine, oxycodone, and tramadol.
         (a) These are metabolized by this system to produce active forms.
      (4) Pentazocine.
      (5) Dextromethorphan (at high levels, dextromethorphan can produce psychotic symptoms).

(6) Phentermine, a sympathomimetic used in weight-loss programs, at high doses can lead to anxiety and excessive sympathetic autonomic activity.
(7) Benztropine.
d. Illicit drugs. 3,4-Methylenedioxymethamphetamine (MDMA, "ecstasy").
3. 3A4 substrates.
a. Secondary amine tricyclics such as desipramine and nortriptyline.
b. Calcium channel blockers such as nifedipine and diltiazem.
c. Other drugs.
(1) Lidocaine.
(2) Quinidine.
(3) Tamoxifen.
(4) Carbamazepine.
(5) Cyclosporine.
(6) Testosterone.
(7) Cortisol.
(8) Dexamethasone.
(9) Lovastatin.
d. Benzodiazepines. Increased benzodiazepine levels can lead to unexpected psychomotor impairment or other toxicity.
(1) Triazolam.
(2) Midazolam.
(3) Estazolam.
(4) Alprazolam.
(5) Diazepam.
e. Nonbenzodiazepine hypnotics (zolpidem and zaleplon).
f. Buspirone.
4. 1A2 substrates.
a. Benzodiazepines.
(1) Alprazolam.
(2) Diazepam.
b. Neuroleptic agents.
(1) Clozapine.
(2) Haloperidol.
c. Antidepressants
(1) Imipramine (and probably amitriptyline and clomipramine).
(2) Mirtazapine.
d. Tacrine.
e. Phenacetin.
f. Caffeine and theophylline.
g. Propranolol.
h. Warfarin.
i. Methadone.
j. Endogenous steroids.
5. 2C9 substrates.
a. S-warfarin.
b. Phenytoin.
c. Oral hypoglycemics (thiazolidinediones).

6. 2C19 substrates.
   a. Mephenytoin.
   b. Diazepam and desmethyldiazepam.
   c. Imipramine, clomipramine, and amitriptyline.
   d. Propranolol.
   e. Tolbutamide.
   f. Phenytoin.

20.7 P450 Inducers

Cytochrome P450 inducers are shown in Box 20-3.

1. The activity of P450 microsomal enzymes can be increased by several hundred compounds. It is unclear whether 2D6 is inducible.
2. Nonspecific inducers.
   a. Alcohol (long-term use).
   b. Barbiturates.
   c. Carbamazepine.
   d. Meprobamate.
   e. Phenytoin.
3. Specific inducers of the 1A2 system.
   a. Cigarette smoke. When a patient stops smoking, drug toxicity can occur for 1A2 substrates several weeks later (e.g., with theophylline, clozapine, and olanzapine).
   b. Cabbage.
   c. Brussels sprouts.
4. Inducers of the 3A4 system.
   a. Dexamethasone and other glucocorticoids.
   b. Rifampicin.
   c. Carbamazepine and oxcarbazepine.
   d. Reverse transcriptase inhibitors: nivirapine and efavirenz.
   e. Modafinil.
   f. St. John's wort.
   g. Ritonavir. Note, for example, that if meperidine metabolism is increased by an induced 3A4 system, the amount of its neurotoxic metabolite, normeperidine, can increase.
5. Inducers of 2C9 and 2C19: Rifampin.
6. Because induction requires protein synthesis, maximum effects of induction take several weeks to develop (unlike inhibition, which can occur within several days).

20.8 Therapeutic Implications

The significance of an elevated plasma level of a particular drug is determined largely by whether serious adverse effects increase as the level of the drug increases. Examples are as follows:

1. Paroxetine.
   a. Added to nortriptyline can lead to tricyclic toxicity.
   b. Added to a schizophrenic patient who is on haloperidol and benztropine can lead to anticholinergic delirium.

BOX 20-3   Inducers of P450 Enzymes

1A2

Caffeine
Carbamazepine
Chronic smoking
Modafinil
Nafcillin
Omeprazole
Rifampin
Ritonavir

2C9

Carbamazepine
Ethanol
Phenobarbital
Phenytoin
Rifampin
Ritonavir

2C19

Carbamazepine
Phenobarbital
Phenytoin
Prednisone
Rifampin
Ritonavir

3A4

Carbamazepine
Phenobarbital
Phenytoin
Rifabutin
Rifampin
Ritonavir

---

2. Carbamazepine is a paninducer and can reduce the levels of many coadministered drugs. Carbamazepine added to oral contraceptives can lead to contraceptive failure.
3. If cimetidine and nortriptyline are taken together, and cimetidine is stopped, nortriptyline levels can become subtherapeutic.
4. If a chronic smoker on clozapine stops smoking, clozapine levels can become toxic.
5. Fluoxetine.
   a. Can reduce analgesic effects of tramadol.
   b. Can exaggerate hypnotic effects of estazolam.
   c. Can increase levels of risperidone.
6. Sertraline can slightly increase the maximum concentration of diazepam and pimozide. Concomitant use of sertraline and pimozide is considered contraindicated.
7. Depressed acquired immunodeficiency syndrome (AIDS) patients who are taking a tricyclic antidepressant and then start taking ritonavir can develop toxic levels of the antidepressant.
8. Patients taking fluvoxamine can experience pronounced caffeine effects.
9. Modafinil can prolong S-warfarin effects.
10. Omeprazole can increase diazepam effects.
11. Sertraline inhibits glucuronidation and can lead to toxic interactions with lamotrigine.

SUGGESTED READINGS

Azaz-Livshits TL, Danenberg HD: Tachycardia, orthostatic hypotension and profound weakness due to concomitant use of fluoxetine and nifedipine. *Pharmacopsychiatry* 30:274-275, 1997.

Carrillo JA, Benitez J: Clinically significant pharmacokinetic interactions between dietary caffeine and medications. *Clin Pharmacokinet* 39:127-153, 2000.

Centorrino F, Baldessarini RJ, Frankenburg FR, et al: Serum levels of clozapine and norclozapine in patients treated with selective serotonin reuptake inhibitors. *Am J Psychiatry* 153:820-822, 1996.

Cornelis MC, El-Sohemy A, Kabagambe EK, Campos H: Coffee, CYP1A2 genotype, and risk of myocardial infarction. *JAMA* 295:1135-1141, 2006.

DeLeon J, Armstrong SC, Cozza KL: Clinical guidelines for psychiatrists for the use of pharmacogenetic testing for CYP450 2D6 and CYP450 2C19. *Psychosomatics* 47:75-85, 2006.

DeVane CL, Nemeroff CB: 2002 guide to psychotropic drug interactions. *Prim Psychiatry* 9:28-57, 2002.

Fischer V, Vogels B, Maurer G, Tynes RE: The antipsychotic clozapine is metabolized by the polymorphic human microsomal cytochrome P450 2D6. *J Pharmacol Exp Ther* 260(3):1355-1360, 1992.

Fuhr U: Drug interactions with grapefruit juice. Extent, probable mechanism and clinical relevance. *Drug Saf* 18:251-272, 1998.

Fuhr U, Anders E, Mahr G: Inhibitory potency of quinolone antibacterial agents against cytochrome P4501A2 activity in vivo and in vitro. *Antimicrob Agents Chemother* 36:942-948, 1992.

Grimsley S, Jann M, Carter J: Increased carbamazepine plasma concentrations after fluoxetine coadministration. *Clin Pharmacol Ther* 50:10-15, 1991.

Honig P, Wortham D, Zamani K: Terfenadine—ketoconazole interaction: Pharmacokinetic and electrocardiographic consequences. *JAMA* 269: 1513-1518, 1993.

Honig P, Wortham D, Zamani K, et al: Comparison of the effect of the macrolide antibiotics erythromycin, clarithromycin, and azithromycin on terfenadine steady-state pharmacokinetics and electrocardiographic parameters. *Drug Invest* 7(3):148-156, 1994.

Karnik NS, Maldonardo JR: Antidepressants and statin interactions: A review and case report of simvastatin and nefazodone-induced rhabdomyolyis and transaminitis. *Psychosomatics* 46:565-568, 2005.

Maurer PM, Bartkowski RB: Drug interactions of clinical significance with opioid analgesics. *Drug Saf* 8(1):30-48, 1993.

Owen JR, Nemeroff CB: New antidepressants and the cytochrome P450 system: Focus on venlafaxine, nefazodone and mirtazapine. *Depress Anxiety* 7(suppl 1):24-32, 1998.

Schadel M, Wu D, Otton S, et al: Pharmacokinetics of dextromethorphan and metabolites in humans: Influence of the CYP2D6 phenotype and quinidine inhibition. *J Clin Psychopharmacol* 15:263-269, 1995.

Schillevoort I, de Boer A, van der Weide J, et al: Antipsychotic-induced extrapyramidal syndromes and cytochrome P450 2D6 genotype: A case controlled study. *Pharmacogenetics* 12:235-240, 2002.

Varhe A, Olkkola K, Neuvonen P: Oral triazolam is potentially hazardous to patients receiving systemic antimycotics ketoconazole or itraconazole. *Clin Pharmacol Ther* 56:6:601-607, 1992.

Zevin S, Benowitz NL: Drug interactions with tobacco smoking: An update. *Clin Pharmacokinet* 36:425-438, 1999.

Child and Adolescent Psychiatry

21

Joseph V. Penn

21.1 General Principles

OVERVIEW

1. Psychiatric conditions in childhood and adolescence are associated with substantial morbidity and, if untreated, can become chronic and recurrent disorders.
2. Comorbid psychiatric conditions are common in children and adolescents.
3. To diagnose a disorder, there must be clear evidence of significant impairment in social or academic functioning.
4. Appreciation of the familial, social, and neurodevelopmental context is essential.
5. Knowledge regarding psychopharmacologic treatments is expanding but limited.
6. Multidisciplinary assessment and treatment planning are usually needed.
7. Anecdotally, the prescribing of multiple psychotropic medications (combined treatment or polypharmacy) in the pediatric population seems on the increase. Few data exist to support advantageous efficacy for drug combinations, which are used primarily to treat comorbid conditions. The current clinical state of the art supports judicious use of combined medications, keeping such use to clearly justifiable circumstances. Medication management requires the informed consent of the parents or legal guardians and must address benefits versus risks, side effects, and the potential for drug interactions.

COMPLETE DIAGNOSTIC ASSESSMENT

1. Interview the youth and parents, both separately and together; other important adults or siblings might also be useful sources of information.
2. Clarify the onset, development, and context of current symptoms.
3. Obtain information from schools, counselors, past and current health care providers, and others.
4. Review the developmental, medical, school, social, and family psychiatric history.
5. Mental status examination, assessment of school functioning, and degree of involvement with peer group and social competence are important. Assess the larger context of the child's personality, functioning, and developmental adaptation to family, school, and social environment.

389

6. Assess the family for possible problems such as familial stressors, losses, conflicts, marital difficulties, inappropriate roles or boundaries, domestic violence, and emotional, sexual, or physical abuse.
7. Rule out general medical or neurologic conditions or disorders resulting from the direct physiologic effects of a substance or medication.
8. Have a high index of suspicion for substance abuse (e.g., alcohol, cannabis, nicotine, other illicit substances) in adolescents and youths engaging in high-risk behavior.

21.2 Anxiety Disorders

SEPARATION ANXIETY DISORDER
Definition and Identification
1. Separation anxiety disorder is the developmentally inappropriate and excessive anxiety precipitated by separation from attachment figures (parents or others), home, or other familiar surroundings.
2. The child excessively worries that harm might come to either a parent (or attachment figure) or the child, which would result in their separation.
3. This disorder can manifest as refusal to go to school, nightmares about separation, fears and distress on separation, or multiple somatic complaints (e.g., stomachaches, headaches).

Epidemiology
1. Estimated prevalence is 3% to 4% of all school-age children and 1% of all adolescents.
2. Incidence is equal in boys and girls.
3. It is more common in young children than in adolescents and most common between ages 7 and 8 years.

Differential Diagnosis
1. Nonpathologic anxiety or developmentally appropriate separation anxiety.
2. Social phobia.
3. Generalized anxiety disorder (GAD).
4. Specific phobia occurs in about one third of all referred separation anxiety cases.
5. Pervasive developmental disorders.
6. Schizophrenia.
7. Depressive disorders.
8. Panic disorders with agoraphobia.
9. Conduct disorder.

Course and Prognosis
Course and prognosis are variable and related to age at onset, duration of symptoms, and development of comorbid anxiety or depressive disorders.

Treatment
1. Feedback and education to the parents and child.
2. School refusal should be regarded as a problem needing urgent and specific intervention, in particular, a plan for separation from the

attachment figure (e.g., return to school or day care center) as soon as possible. Additional consultation with school personnel is critical.
3. A multimodal treatment approach (e.g., individual and family therapy). Specific cognitive behavior therapy (CBT) and other behavior strategies.
4. Studies of medications (Tables 21-1 and 21-2) are limited.

SPECIFIC PHOBIA

Definition and Identification

1. Specific phobia (formerly known as simple phobia) is the excessive and unreasonable fear or dread of circumscribed objects or situations (phobic stimuli), such as fear of animals, blood, heights, closed spaces, or flying, that provokes immediate anxiety.
2. Avoidance, anxiety, or distress related to the fear is associated with functional impairment or significant distress.
3. Children might not realize that their fears are marked or unreasonable.
4. Phobic children report somatic symptoms and avoidance or fearful anticipation when confronted with the phobic stimulus, and they might exhibit crying, tantrums, freezing, or clinging.

Epidemiology

1. Phobias are the most common mental disorders in the United States.
2. The natural environmental type (e.g., heights, storms, and water) and the blood, injection, and injury types are most common in children under 10 years old.
3. Specific phobia tends to run in families, particularly the blood, injection, and injury types.

Differential Diagnosis

1. Developmentally appropriate fear or normal anxiety.
2. Social phobia.
3. GAD.
4. Panic disorders with agoraphobia.
5. Obsessive–compulsive disorder (OCD).
6. Schizophrenia.

Course and Prognosis

1. Not a great deal is known. Need to assess level of impairment and amenability to treatment.
2. Specific phobias may be associated with more morbidity than previously recognized, such as development of substance-related disorders.
3. Phobias can affect school performance and socialization.

Treatment

1. Transitory, developmentally appropriate fears do not require treatment, whereas specific phobias might.
2. Present treatment options and plan, enlisting the parents' and child's involvement. Include information regarding how progress will be evaluated.
3. Behavior therapy and CBT may be helpful.
4. More complicated cases might require more intensive individual and family psychotherapy.

Table 21-1 Antianxiety Drugs: High-Potency Benzodiazepines

Drug (Brand)	Preparations	Duration of Action	Main Uses	Daily Dose	Adverse Effects	Comments
Alprazolam (Xanax)	Tabs: 0.25, 0.5, 1, 2 mg ER tabs: 0.5, 1, 2, 3 mg Soln: 1 mg/1 mL concentrate	Peak plasma levels 1-3 h after ingestion; half-life 6-20 h	Anxiety disorders; adjunct treatment in refractory psychosis; adjunct in mania; severe agitation; Tourette's; severe insomnia; MDD and anxiety; akathisia	Initial dosing: 7-16 y: 0.005 mg/kg/dose or 0.125 mg tid Max: 0.02-0.06 mg/kg/day	Same as other benzodiazepines Higher risk for rebound and withdrawal reactions	
Buspirone (BuSpar)	Tabs: 5, 7.5, 10, 15, 30 mg	Variable Best taken between meals to increase rate of absorption	Anxiety disorders (GAD); adjunct treatment in refractory OCD; aggressive behavior in children with developmental disorders	Start with 2.5-5 mg bid; ↑ weekly by 5 mg to 30 mg/day max (adult max, 60 mg/day)	Drowsiness, disinhibition No cross-tolerance with benzodiazepines	
Clonazepam (Klonopin)	Tabs: 0.5, 1, 2 mg Wafers: 0.125, 0.25, 0.5, 1, 2 mg	Peak plasma levels 1-3 h after ingestion; half-life 20-40 h	Same as alprazolam	Not studied in psych disorders for youth <18 y Consult PDR for dosage requirements for seizure disorders	Drowsiness, disinhibition, agitation, confusion, depression, withdrawal reactions, potential risk for abuse and	Avoid benzodiazepines if possible due to high risk of abuse, dependence, and diversion Taper slowly to

Lorazepam (Ativan)	Tabs: 0.5, 1, 2 mg Injectable Soln: 2 mg/1 mL	Peak plasma levels 1-3 h after ingestion; half-life 10-20 h	Same as other high-potency benzodiazepines Temporary use in severe adjustment disorder with anxious mood	0.02 mg/kg/day; usual 0.05 mg/kg/dose Max dose: 2 mg/dose Range: 0.02-0.1 mg/kg	Same as other benzodiazepines Higher risk for withdrawal and rebound reactions

dependence, less risk for rebound and withdrawal reactions
Withdrawal effects and rebound; tics, headache, dizziness, irritability; abdominal discomfort, lethargy, fatigue.
Cognitive dulling or irritability 1-2 h after dose can indicate excessive dose

avoid withdrawal reactions

Note: Consult the *Physicians' Desk Reference* for complete listing of adverse effects.
ER, extended release; GAD, generalized anxiety disorder; max, maximum; MDD, major depressive disorder; OCD, obsessive–compulsive disorder; soln, solution; tab, tablet.

Table 21-2 Antianxiety Drugs: Noradrenergic Agents

Drug (Brand)	Preparations	Main Uses	Typical Starting Dose	Max Dose/Day	Adverse Effects	Comments
Clonidine (nonspecific) (Catapres)	Tabs: 0.1, 0.2, 0.3 mg Patches: 0.1, 0.2, 0.3 mg/24 h	Sleep disturbances, tics; alternative for ADHD*	< 100 lb: 0.05 mg hs, titrate in 0.05-mg increments bid, tid, qid > 100 lb: 0.1-mg qhs, titrate in 0.1-mg increments bid, tid, qid	60-90 lb: 0.2 mg 90-100 lb: 0.3 mg > 100 lb: 0.4 mg	Sedation (very frequent), hypotension (rare), dry mouth, confusion (with high dose), depression, rebound hypertension with abrupt withdrawal (taper to avoid), localized irritation with patch	Avoid coadministering clonidine and β-blockers Use caution with methylphenidate (sudden death has been reported in a few cases) Blood pressure and ECG monitoring are recommended at baseline and regular intervals throughout treatment
Guanfacine (selective α₂ agonist) (Tenex)	Tabs: 1, 2 mg	Sleep disturbances, tics; alternative for ADHD*	< 100 lb: 0.5 mg hs, titrate in 0.5-mg increments bid, tid, qid > 100 lb: 1 mg hs, titrate in 1-mg increments bid, tid, qid	60-90 lb: 2 mg 90-100 lb: 3 mg > 100 lb: 4 mg	Same as clonidine; less sedation, hypotension Higher risk for bradycardia and hypotension (dose dependent) and rebound hypertension	Blood pressure and ECG monitoring are recommended at baseline; follow-up at regular intervals throughout treatment

Propranolol (β-blocker) (Inderal)	Tabs: 20, 40, 60, 80 mg; 60, 80, 120, 160 mg long-acting	Aggresion and self-abuse in children with developmental disorders, including mental retardation and pervasive developmental disorders Severe agitation, akathisia.	Young child: initial starting target dose range of 20 mg may be set, e.g., 5 mg qid Older child, adolescent: 10 mg tid; no clearly defined target dose ranges	Younger child might require lower doses Consider qid dosing for 7 days, then ↑ to 10 mg qid for 6-8 wk. Consider ↑ to 15 mg qid for 4-6 wk	Bronchospasm (contraindicated in asthmatics) Rebound abrupt withdrawal with hypertension (taper to avoid) Nausea, vomiting, depression, allergic reactions Higher risk of bradycardia and hypotension (dose dependent) and rebound hypertension Bronchospasm (contraindicated in asthmatics) Nausea, vomiting, depression, allergic reactions Can interact with many drugs Gradually taper to discontinue (to avoid rebound tachycardia)	Blood pressure and ECG monitoring recommended at baseline and follow-up at regular intervals Avoid in patients with distinct medical contraindications

* No FDA approval for this indication.

5. There are few pharmacologic studies to date in children and adolescents.

SELECTIVE MUTISM
Definition and Identification

1. Recently conceptualized as a type of social phobia.
2. The hallmark of this disorder is when a child who is fluent with language consistently fails to speak in specific social situations, such as school, but speaks fluently in other situations, such as at home and in certain familiar settings.
3. Most children are silent in their mute situations, but some whisper or use single-syllable words.
4. Selective mutism can develop gradually or suddenly after a disturbing or traumatic experience.
5. History of delayed onset of speech or speech abnormalities may be contributory.

Epidemiology

1. Selective mutism is uncommon, and prevalence is estimated at 3 to 8 children per 10,000.
2. Young children are more vulnerable. Selective mutism usually occurs in children 4 to 8 years old.
3. It is more common in girls.
4. Children with selective mutism are often abnormally shy in preschool years.

Differential Diagnosis

1. Shy children exhibiting transient muteness in new, anxiety-provoking situation.
2. Mental retardation.
3. Pervasive developmental disorders.
4. Expressive language disorder.
5. Separation anxiety.
6. Social phobia.
7. Conversion disorder.
8. Depressive disorders.
9. Oppositional defiant disorder.

Course and Prognosis

1. Most cases last only a few weeks or months, but some persist for years.
2. Children who do not improve by the age of 10 years have a worse prognosis.

Treatment

1. Consultation with school personnel is essential.
2. Multimodal approach across settings. Provide positive reinforcement for speech and lack of reinforcement for mutism.
3. The preschool child might benefit from a therapeutic nursery, and parents might benefit from counseling.
4. Individual psychotherapy and/or behavioral therapy may be helpful, as well as group therapy with speaking peers to promote social skills, peer involvement, and age-appropriate assertiveness.

5. Consider adjunctive selective serotonin reuptake inhibitors (SSRIs) (see Table 21-5) (efficacy data are limited).

PANIC DISORDER AND AGORAPHOBIA
Definition and Identification
1. Panic disorder and agoraphobia are recurrent, unexpected panic attacks. A panic attack is a discrete period of intense fear or discomfort that develops abruptly and reaches a peak rapidly. It is accompanied by specific somatic symptoms, fear, and worry. Other common symptoms include palpitations, chest pain, faintness, and trembling or shaking.
2. Panic disorder can occur with or without agoraphobia, which is anxiety about being in places or situations from which escape might be difficult (or embarrassing) or in which help may not be available in the event of having a panic attack or panic-like symptoms.
3. Panic disorder with or without agoraphobia most often begins in adolescence or early adult life but can develop at any age.

Epidemiology
1. Prevalence in persons aged 14 to 17 years is less than 1%.
2. The incidence is much higher than panic disorder without agoraphobia and increases greatly with the onset of puberty.

Differential Diagnosis
Panic attacks are the hallmark of panic disorder, but they can be associated with other anxiety disorders.
1. Specific phobia.
2. Social phobia.
3. OCD.
4. Posttraumatic stress disorder (PTSD).
5. Agoraphobia can occur without a history of panic disorder.
6. Separation anxiety (may be a comorbid condition).
7. Depressive disorders.
8. Attention-deficit/hyperactivity disorder (ADHD).
9. Substance abuse.

Course and Prognosis
The long-term outcome is unknown, but adult studies indicate that panic disorder can become chronic.

Treatment
1. Educate patient, family, and school (if appropriate).
2. Consult with primary care, mental health providers, and school personnel when appropriate.
3. CBT appears to be effective for panic symptoms.
4. Individual, group, or family therapy are useful for issues complicating recovery.
5. Pharmacotherapy should not be the sole intervention. To date there are no randomized trials for children or adolescents.
6. SSRIs may be promising (see Table 21-5). Responses reported are similar to those in adults.

7. Because of the risks of diversion, abuse, tolerance, dependence, withdrawal, and behavioral disinhibition with benzodiazepines, their risk-to-benefit ratio should be considered carefully.

SOCIAL PHOBIA

Definition and Identification

1. Social phobia is a persistent fear of one or more social situations (e.g., speaking in front of others, attending social gatherings, speaking to strangers) in which the exposure provokes marked anxiety.
2. The anxiety results in interference with functioning or marked distress about experiencing the fear. The child might avoid participating in classroom activities, presentations, or physical education.
3. Adults recognize that the fear is excessive or unreasonable, but children might not.
4. Young children might cry, have a tantrum, or cling or hide behind parents when confronted with a feared social situation, and they might refuse to attend school.
5. Adolescents might avoid classes or drop out of school. They might have difficulty interviewing for jobs or in social interactions or with dating or relationships.

Epidemiology

1. Occurs in approximately 1% of children and adolescents, but this number may be underestimated.
2. Early age at onset, with a mean of 15 years, with peaks before the age of 5 years and at about 13 years.
3. Similar numbers of boys and girls.

Differential Diagnosis

1. Comorbidity with other anxiety and depressive disorders is common.
2. Panic attacks, panic disorder, or agoraphobia.
3. Substance abuse, especially alcohol.
4. Specific phobia.
5. OCD.
6. PTSD.
7. Separation anxiety.
8. Depressive disorders.
9. ADHD.

Course and Prognosis

Long-term outcome is unknown, but adult studies indicate that social phobia is often chronic.

Treatments

1. Present options and plan to patient, enlisting parents' involvement. Include information regarding how progress will be evaluated.
2. Provide CBT to promote successful experience in social interactions.
3. Individual or group psychotherapy for developing a sense of self, addressing internal conflicts, and promoting social skills, peer involvement, and age-appropriate assertiveness.
4. Additional family intervention.
5. SSRIs may be considered (see Table 21-5).

GENERALIZED ANXIETY DISORDER

Definition and Identification

1. Generalized anxiety disorder (including overanxious disorder of childhood) is excessive anxiety and worry (apprehensive expectation) about a number of events or activities (such as future events, social acceptability, competence and performance in school and athletics, or meeting others' expectations) that the child finds difficult to control.
2. Feelings of restlessness, fatigability, difficulty concentrating, irritability, muscle tension, or sleep disturbance are present for 6 months. Only one of these symptoms is required in children.
3. This worry is pervasive and persistent, occurs without precipitant, and causes impairment in social or other important areas of functioning.

Epidemiology

Generalized anxiety disorder is not well researched in children and adolescents.

Differential Diagnosis

1. Normal anxiety.
2. Depressive disorders.
3. Panic attacks and panic disorder (anxiety or worry about having a panic attack).
4. Social phobia (being embarrassed in public).
5. OCD (being contaminated).
6. Separation anxiety (being away from home or close relatives).
7. Anorexia nervosa (gaining weight).
8. Somatization disorder (having multiple physical complaints).
9. Hypochondriasis (having a serious illness).
10. PTSD.

Course and Prognosis

Untreated anxiety disorder can have a chronic course and a low remission rate.

Treatment

1. Treatment combines education, consultation with schools and primary care providers, psychotherapies, and pharmacotherapy (see Table 21-5). Additional family intervention is recommended.
2. Although there are limited data, if severity warrants, consider SSRIs (see Table 21-5).
3. Buspirone (see Table 21-1) has been used in open studies in adolescents and shown decreases in anxiety.

POSTTRAUMATIC STRESS DISORDER

Definition and Identification

1. Posttraumatic stress disorder (PTSD) is the direct, witnessed, or verbal exposure to an event characterized by threat to life, potential for physical injury, or violence to a family member. A wide variety of stressors can lead to PTSD.

2. The youth's response involves fear, surprise, helplessness, horror, and disorganized or agitated behavior.
3. To meet criteria for PTSD, the response must include a specific number of symptoms from each of three broad categories: reexperiencing the event, consequent avoidance of stimuli or numbing of general responsiveness, and persistent increased arousal.
4. Specific PTSD symptoms vary by developmental stage of the child and the nature of the stressor.
5. Children might have fearful or traumatic dreams. They might exhibit traumatic play (e.g., repetitive dramatization in play of the event) or reenactment behavior (replication of some of the experience).
6. There may be a loss of previously acquired skills, causing a child to be less verbal and to exhibit regressed behavior, such as thumb sucking or enuresis, or to fail to acquire new skills.
7. There may be physiologic reactivity including hypervigilance, an exaggerated startle response, somatic symptoms, sleep disturbance, sleepwalking, and nightmares.
8. Adolescents might seek out opportunities to engage in reenactment behavior or dangerous thrill seeking.
9. Self-mutilation, sexual or aggressive play, and suicidal behavior warrant further evaluation for sexual or physical abuse.
10. There are important role differences between clinical and forensic evaluations and evaluators. These roles should remain separate.
11. Assessment of PTSD relies primarily on the clinical interview of the youth and parents or guardian and information from collateral historians and records whenever possible.

Epidemiology

Incidence and prevalence are unclear in children and adolescents, but they are clearly higher in children exposed to life-threatening events.

Differential Diagnosis

1. Acute stress disorder.
2. Adjustment disorders.
3. Panic disorder.
4. GAD.
5. Depressive disorders.
6. ADHD.
7. Substance use disorders.
8. Dissociative disorders.
9. Conduct disorder.
10. Borderline personality traits or other emerging personality disorder.
11. Schizophrenia or other psychotic disorder.
12. Malingering or secondary gain issues if the youth or family presents for medicolegal or disability evaluation.
13. Factitious disorder.

Course and Prognosis

The course and prognosis are highly variable and depend on circumstantial factors (the stressor), child intrinsic factors, coping and resiliency, and extrinsic influences over the recovery environment. Although most studies indicate that some youth have a spontaneous recovery, PTSD can persist for many years.

Treatment

1. The prevention–intervention model incorporates prompt triage for children exposed to stressors, support, and strengthening of coping skills for anticipated grief and trauma responses, treatment of other disorders that can develop or be exacerbated in the context of PTSD, and treatment of acute PTSD symptoms.
2. Psychological education for child, parents, teachers, and/or significant others about the symptoms, clinical course, treatment options, and prognosis.
3. Careful decision making before beginning direct exploration of the trauma, use of specific stress-management techniques, exploration and correction of inaccurate attributions regarding the trauma, and inclusion of parents in treatment.
4. Few controlled drug studies exist. Children might have pharmacologic response similar to that of adults.
5. Antidepressants (see Table 21-5) may be useful for concurrent major depressive or panic disorder symptoms.
6. Psychostimulants or α-adrenergic agonists (e.g., clonidine or guanfacine) may be useful for concurrent ADHD symptoms (see Table 21-3).
7. Antianxiety medications (benzodiazepines, propranolol) generally have not been useful.
8. Outpatient psychotherapy is the preferred initial treatment, with psychotropics used adjunctively for prominent depressive or panic symptoms.
9. The clinical efficacy of eye movement desensitization and reprocessing (EMDR) and hypnosis in child and adolescent populations remains unclear.

OBSESSIVE–COMPULSIVE DISORDER
Definition and Identification

1. OCD is the occurrence of recurrent obsessions and compulsions that cause marked distress or impairment.
2. Obsessions are persistent thoughts, ideas, or images that intrude into awareness, for example, germs, contamination, harm or danger, worries about right and wrong, or having a tune in the head.
3. Compulsions are urges or impulses for repetitive intentional behavior, rituals, or mental acts to attempt to reduce anxiety or in response to an obsession and can include excessive cleaning, repeating, checking, counting, symmetry, ordering and arranging, touching, or hoarding.
4. Adults recognize that the fear is senseless, excessive, or unreasonable, but children might not.
5. Children often initially disguise their rituals, and symptoms can change over time.
6. It is important to distinguish OCD from the broad range of mild rituals and obsessions that occur as common experiences throughout the life span and as developmental phenomena in youths.

Table 21-3 **Attention-Deficit/Hyperactivity Disorder Medications**

Drug (Brand)	Preparations	Duration of Action	Typical Starting Dose	Adverse Effects	Comments
Stimulants *Dextroamphetamine* Dextroamphetamine (Dexedrine, DextroStat)	Tabs: 5, 10 mg	4-5 h	3-5 y: 2.5 mg q$_{AM}$ > 6 y: 5 mg q$_{AM}$ or bid	Insomnia, decreased appetite, weight loss, depression, psychosis, tachycardia, hypertension? Reduction in growth velocity with long-term use Withdrawal effects and rebound; motor tics, headache, dizziness, irritability; abdominal discomfort, lethargy, fatigue Cognitive dulling or irritability 1-2 hours after dose can indicate excessive dose Can lower seizure threshold	D-Amphetamine tablet FDA max/day: 40 mg

Drug	Formulation	Duration	Dosing	Comments
Dextroamphetamine SR (Dexedrine spansules)	Caps: 5, 10, 15 mg	6-8 h	5 mg qAM Some benefit from 2.5-10 mg regular D-amphetamine in afternoon	Same as for other stimulants
Dextroamphetamine mixed salts (Adderall)	Tabs: 5, 7.5, 10, 12.5, 15, 20, 30 mg (crushable)	4-6 h	3-5 y: 2.5 mg qAM > 6 y: 5 mg qAM-bid	Same as for other stimulants	Tab of D,L-amphetamine isomers (75% D- and 25% L-) FDA warning of sudden death Suggest cardiology consult for those with cardiac abnormalities
Dextroamphetamine mixed salts ER (Adderall XR)	Caps: 5, 10, 15, 20, 25, 30 mg	10-12 h	5-10 mg qAM Some can benefit from 5-10 mg IR in afternoon	Same as for other stimulants	Bimodal delivery (50% IR and 50% DR) Can be sprinkled on soft food Recent FDA warning of sudden death; suggest cardiology consult for those with cardiac abnormalities

Table continued on following page

Table 21-3 Attention-Deficit/Hyperactivity Disorder Medications *(Continued)*

Drug (Brand)	Preparations	Duration of Action	Typical Starting Dose	Adverse Effects	Comments
Methylphenidate					
Dexmethylphenidate (Focalin)	Tabs: 2.5, 5, 10 mg	3-5 h	2.5 mg bid (doses are 1/2 MPH doses)	Same as for other stimulants	Tablet of D-threo MPH FDA max/day 20 mg
Dexmethylphenidate ER (Focalin XR)	Caps: 5, 10, 20 mg	Similar to bid dosing of IR formulation	5 mg/day	Same as for other stimulants	SODAS formulation: 50% IR beads, 50% ER beads
Methylphenidate (Ritalin)	Tabs: 5, 10, 20 mg	30-60 min (onset) 3-6 h (duration) 1-3 h (peak) SR: 1-5 h (peak)	5 mg bid (doses are 2× dexMPH doses)	Same as for other stimulants	FDA max/day: 60 mg
Methylphenidate (Methylin)	Tabs: 2.5, 5, 10 mg (chewable) Elixir: 5 mg/5 mL	3-5 h	5 mg bid	Same as for other stimulants	Tablet of 50:50 racemic D,L-threo MPH FDA max/day: 60 mg
Methylphenidate ER (Metadate ER)	Tabs: 10, 20 mg	6-8 h	Start w/short-acting; replace w/same daily dose of inter-mediate-release preparation	Same as for other stimulants	Hydroxypropyl methylcellulose base tab of 50:50 racemic D,L-threo MPH FDA max/day: 60 mg

Methylphenidate ER (Methylin ER)	Tabs: 20, 30, 40 mg	6-8 h	20 mg qAM	Same as for other stimulants	Hydroxypropyl methylcellulose base tab of 50:50 racemic D,L-threo MPH FDA max/day: 60 mg
Methylphenidate LA (Ritalin LA)	Caps: 10, 20, 30, 40 mg	6-8 h	10-20 mg qAM	Same as for other stimulants	Bimodal delivery (50% IR, 50% DR) of 50:50 racemic D,L-threo MPH FDA max/day: 60 mg
Methylphenidate (Concerta)	Tabs: 18, 27, 36, 54 mg	12 h	18 mg qAM	Same as for other stimulants	Swallow whole with liquids Nonabsorbable tab shell may be seen in stool Osmotic pressure system delivers 50:50 racemic D,L-threo MPH FDA max/day: 6-12 y, 54 mg/day; 13-17 y, 72 mg/day

Table continued on following page

Table 21-3 **Attention-Deficit/Hyperactivity Disorder Medications** (Continued)

Drug (Brand)	Preparations	Duration of Action	Typical Starting Dose	Adverse Effects	Comments
Methylphenidate CD (Metadate CD)	Caps: 10, 20, 30 mg (can be sprinkled)	8 h	20 mg qAM	Same as for other stimulants	Bimodal delivery, 30% immediate and 70% delayed, of 50:50 racemic D,L-threo MPH FDA max/day 60 mg
Methylphenidate SR (Ritalin SR)	Tabs: 20 mg	3–8 h variable	Start w/short-acting MPH and replace w/ same daily dose of intermediate-release preparation	Same as for other stimulants	FDA max/day: 60 mg
Magnesium pemoline (Cylert)	No longer on the market				
Nonstimulant Serotonin and Norepinephrine Reuptake Inhibitor					
Atomoxetine (Strattera)	Caps: 10, 18, 25, 40, 60, 80 mg (do not open cap)	5-h plasma half-life; CNS effects longer	Give qAM or divided bid; titrate slowly over weeks; do not open cap. <155 lb: 0.5 mg/kg/day × ≥3 days, then 1.2 mg/kg/day. Total daily dose should not exceed	Sedation, liver injury	Discontinue for jaundice or abnormal LFTs. Not Schedule II FDA max/day: lesser of 1.4 mg/kg or 100 mg/day. FDA warnings: Risk

of severe liver injury (2004). Black box warning: suicidal ideation (2005)

1.4 mg/kg/day or 100 mg, whichever is less.
>155 lb: 40 mg/d × ≥3 days, then 80 mg/d in 1 or 2 doses. May ↑ to 100 mg/day after additional 2-4 wk (slower titration can reduce uncomfortable side effects)

Notes: Consult the *Physicians' Desk Reference* for complete listing of adverse effects.

Consult the most recent FDA safety labeling revisions for use of stimulants for youth with preexisting structural cardiac abnormalities.

Caution is advised when administering stimulants to patients with underlying medical conditions that may be compromised by increases in blood pressure or heart rate, such as preexisting hypertension, heart failure, recent myocardial infarction, or hyperthyroidism. Stimulants should be used cautiously in patients with marked anxiety, motor tics, Tourette's disorder or family history of Tourette's, or history of substance abuse or dependence. Avoid stimulants if patient has glaucoma or is on an MAOI.

cap, capsule; CD, controlled delivery; CNS, central nervous system; DR, delayed release; ER, extended release; FDA, United States Food and Drug Administration; IR, immediate release; LA, long acting; LFT, liver function test; MAOI, monoamine oxidase inhibitor; MPH, methylphenidate; SODAS, spheroidal oral drug absorption system; SR, sustained release; tab, tablet.

7. The context and type of onset and course of symptoms should be ascertained. Assess the degree to which parents have become entangled or reinforce the child's symptoms.
8. Because of close association of tic disorders and OCD, inquire specifically about a history of motor tics (e.g., blinking; grimacing; head, neck, or jaw movements) or phonic tics (e.g., sniffing, throat clearing). In the case of some symptoms (e.g., spitting, complex tapping and touching patterns) it may be difficult to distinguish compulsive habits from complex tics.

Epidemiology

1. Prevalence rates range from 1.0% to 3.6% in the adolescent community.
2. Before puberty there is a higher male-to-female ratio; this reverses after puberty.
3. The usual age of onset can range from 3 to 18 years, but it is typically 9 to 11 years.
4. There is a higher incidence of OCD in first-degree relatives of patients with OCD.
5. Familial links have been demonstrated connecting OCD, tic disorders, and Tourette's syndrome.

Differential Diagnosis

1. Depressive disorders.
2. Anxiety disorders.
3. ADHD or disruptive behavior disorders.
4. Mental retardation, pervasive developmental disorders, and brain damage syndromes.
5. Eating disorders (anorexia and bulimia).
6. Tic disorders and Tourette's syndrome.
7. Trichotillomania
8. Childhood schizophrenia (rare).
9. Body dysmorphic disorder
10. Postinfectious conditions. Abrupt prepubertal onset of OCD and/or tic disorder after group A β-hemolytic streptococcal (GABHS) infection (autoimmune) or Sydenham's chorea. There has been recent identification of pediatric autoimmune neuropsychiatric disorders associated with streptococcal infections. A throat culture and an antistreptolysin O or antistreptoccocal DNase B titer may be considered to assist in diagnosing a GABHS infection.
11. Schizotypal personality traits or emerging disorder.

Course and Prognosis

1. Waxing and waning, with worsening related to psychosocial stressors.
2. Patients with late-onset OCD appear to have a better prognosis.

Treatments

1. CBT and SSRIs alone or in combination have been shown to reduce the core symptoms of OCD.

2. Monitor treatment response, assess symptom frequency, intensity, distress, and impairment, both at home and in school, using parent, teacher, and self-reports. Ongoing evaluation is necessary.
3. SSRIs are effective and generally well tolerated (see Table 21-5). They might require a longer trial (12 weeks) at adequate doses. In children, start with a low dose and make small increases based on clinical effect. Monitor for overactivating side effects. Treatment-resistant cases might require higher doses and other multimodal treatment interventions.
4. CBT using exposure with response prevention and individual and family therapy are also important.
5. Because OCD often occurs in the context of other psychopathology, additional individual and family, pharmacologic, and educational interventions are often necessary.

21.3 Attention-Deficit/Hyperactivity Disorder

DEFINITION AND IDENTIFICATION

1. Attention-deficit/hyperactivity disorder (ADHD) begins early in life, is persistent over time, is pervasive across different settings, and causes functional impairment.
2. Three major subtypes are designated.
   a. ADHD, combined type (inattention and hyperactivity–impulsivity).
   b. ADHD, predominantly inattentive type.
   c. ADHD, predominantly hyperactivity–impulsive type.
3. Symptoms that cause significant impairment in two or more situations, such as at school (or work) and at home, must be present.
4. Distinguish ADHD from response to acute stressors, response to inconsistent parenting and limit-setting, or sensory impairment.
5. Onset of symptoms is usually before the age of 7 years, but more severely affected children may be recognized in preschool.
6. Symptoms are present for at least 6 months.
7. Core symptoms.
   a. Inattention (difficulty sustaining attention; careless mistakes; does not seem to listen).
   b. Hyperactivity may be seen in some situations but not others. For example:
      (1) Fidgets with hands and feet or squirms in seat.
      (2) Leaves seat when remaining seated is expected.
      (3) Runs or climbs during inappropriate situations.
      (4) Difficulty playing or engaging in leisure activities quietly.
      (5) Often "on the go" or "driven by a motor."
      (6) Talks excessively.
   c. Impulsivity. Blurts out answers to questions before the questions have been completed; has difficulty awaiting turn; interrupts or intrudes on others (e.g., butts into conversations or games).
   d. Distractibility. Difficulty staying focused on task; difficulty screening out external stimuli.

8. Core symptoms and manifestations can change with development from preschool through adult life.
9. Adolescents might exhibit more impulsive risk-taking behavior.
10. Many ADHD children, adolescents, and adults have difficulty picking up on social cues, leading to difficulties in interpersonal relationships.

EPIDEMIOLOGY

1. Incidence is 3% to 5% of school-age children in the United States. Some studies report incidence of 2% to 20% in grade school.
2. ADHD is more common in boys than girls. The male-to-female ratio is 4:1 in epidemiologic samples and 9:1 in clinical samples. The hyperactive—impulsive type is especially common in boys (this may be a result of referral bias, because girls may have primarily inattention and cognition problems).
3. Prevalence declines with age, although up to 65% of hyperactive children are still symptomatic as adults. Frequency in adults is estimated to be 2% to 7%.
4. Family history can include ADHD, hyperkinesis, sociopathy, alcohol use disorders, and conversion disorder.

EVALUATION

ADHD is a clinical diagnosis. The diagnostic process must occur in a developmental context. The assessment consists of clinical interviews and standardized ratings from parents and teachers. Testing of intelligence and academic achievement usually are required. Comorbid learning disorders and other mental disorders are common.

1. Conduct a comprehensive interview with all parenting figures to specify symptoms, frequency, social and family context, and developmental factors.
2. Identify comorbid conditions.
3. Direct observation. Observe in the waiting room. Look for tics (eye blinking, nose twitching, shoulder shrugging, grunting, sniffing, facial grimacing, throat clearing).
4. Review school history and teacher reports (grades, conduct, history of detentions, suspensions, expulsions, current class size and time, teacher-to-student ratio, special educational resources, specific learning difficulties).
5. Review previous developmental, school, psychological, speech and language, or neuropsychological evaluations. Good performance on individually administered testing does not rule out ADHD.
6. Assess general cognitive and receptive—expressive language levels. Ask about child's understanding and explanation of behavioral problems. Screen for anxiety, depression, suicidal ideation, hallucinations, and unusual thinking. Perform cognitive assessment of ability and achievement.
7. Observe parent—child interaction. See how the parent redirects or manages problematic behavior.
8. Medical evaluation should include a complete medical history and examination within the past 12 months. History should include use of prescribed, over-the-counter, and illicit drugs.

9. Perform formal audiology and vision testing and speech and language evaluation if indicated.
10. Medical evaluation should screen for sensory deficits, neurologic problems, or other medical problems for symptoms (e.g., petit mal seizures, lead intoxication, obstructive sleep apnea).
11. Although some children with ADHD have impaired motor coordination, the measurement of neurologic soft signs is not useful in ADHD diagnosis. Soft signs include visual–motor–perceptual or auditory–discriminatory immaturity or impairments without overt signs of disorders of visual or auditory acuity; problems with fine and gross motor coordination, copying age-appropriate figures, rapid alternating movements, right–left discrimination problems, ambidexterity; and reflex asymmetries.
12. Rule out medication (e.g., theophylline, phenobarbital, carbamazepine) or alcohol, cannabis, or other illicit substances with behavioral effects.
13. No specific laboratory measures are pathognomonic for ADHD.
14. Consider standardized ADHD questionnaires and behavior rating scales (Child Attention Profile, Connor's Parent and Teacher Questionnaires, Achenbach's Child Behavior Checklist and Teacher Report Form).
15. If learning disabilities are suspected, recommend cognitive testing or neuropsychological assessment.
16. Neuropsychological tests are useful to evaluate specific deficits but are not sufficiently helpful to be used routinely.

DIFFERENTIAL DIAGNOSIS AND COMORBID CONDITIONS

1. As many as two thirds of elementary school-age children with ADHD who are referred for clinical evaluation have at least one other diagnosable psychiatric disorder.
2. Maintain a high index of suspicion for other disorders.
   a. Physical causes for poor attention (e.g., impaired vision or hearing, seizures, sequelae of head trauma, acute or chronic medical illness, poor nutrition, or insufficient sleep due to a sleep disorder or environment).
   b. Oppositional defiant disorder (comorbid up to 60%).
   c. Conduct disorder (up to 45% of older children).
   d. Learning disorders and language and communication disorders (reading disorder, mathematics disorder, and disorder of written expression). Prevalence is estimated in ADHD at 10% to 35%.
   e. Anxiety disorders such as OCD.
   f. Depressive disorders (may be exacerbated by school failures, trouble making friends, and poor self-esteem). Early-onset bipolar disorder may be particularly difficult to distinguish from ADHD or may be comorbid.
   g. Temperamental constellation of high activity level and short attention span.
   h. Tic disorders and Tourette's syndrome.

    i. Mental retardation, borderline intellectual functioning, and learning disabilities are commonly mislabeled ADHD, even by teachers, even though they often co-occur with ADHD.

    j. Schizophrenia or other psychotic disorder is extremely rare before puberty.

COURSE AND PROGNOSIS

1. ADHD can be successfully treated.
2. The course is highly variable. About two thirds of patients have symptoms into adolescence or adulthood.
3. Outcome may be influenced by effective treatment and family functioning.
4. Children can remain impulsive and accident-prone and have lower educational attainments.
5. Psychiatric comorbidity complicates the diagnosis, course, and prognosis.
6. Children with comorbid ADHD and conduct disorder have an increased risk of developing substance-related disorder and antisocial personality disorder as adults.

TREATMENTS

The cornerstones are support and education of parents, appropriate school placement, and pharmacologic interventions. Multimodal treatment includes a classroom management program, regular monitoring of patient and family, and close collaboration with the school.

1. Parent education and training in techniques of behavioral management are crucial.
2. Structured school and home environment with a predictable structure of reward and punishment using behavior modification such as incentives and tangible rewards, reprimands, and time-outs.
3. Pharmacotherapy (see Table 21-3).
    a. General principles.
       (1) Establishing a baseline for target symptoms is essential.
       (2) Medication treatment alone is rarely effective.
       (3) Medication is not a substitute for appropriate educational curricula, student-to-teacher ratios, or other environmental accommodations.
    b. Psychostimulants (methylphenidate or amphetamine compounds) remain first-line treatment.
       (1) All are equally effective, but response is idiosyncratic and cannot be predicted.
       (2) Usual side effects include decreased appetite, insomnia, stomachache, headache, and irritability, but most dissipate with time.
       (3) Stimulants should be used cautiously in patients with marked anxiety or history of substance abuse.
       (4) Growth suppression appears to be dose-related, if it occurs at all.

(5) Neurologic or psychiatric consultation is recommended before initiating stimulants for patients with tics or Tourette's syndrome or if new tics develop during stimulant treatment.

(6) Recent Food and Drug Administration (FDA) safety labeling revisions have been made regarding use of stimulants for youth with preexisting structural cardiac abnormalities. Caution is advised when administering stimulants to patients with underlying medical conditions that may be compromised by increases in blood pressure or heart rate, such as preexisting hypertension, heart failure, recent myocardial infarction, or hyperthyroidism.

(7) Avoid stimulant use if the patient has glaucoma or is on a monoamine oxidase inhibitor (MAOI).

c. Recent advances.

(1) New drugs and formulations include extended release methylphenidate formulations, extended release amphetamine formulations, and one norepinephrine reuptake inhibitor. A transdermal delivery system has been introduced. These new agents are all long-acting, potentially once-daily agents, reduce school-dosing difficulties, minimize stigma, and might improve medication compliance.

(2) The ability to sprinkle pill contents onto food has appeared effective in two methylphenidate compounds (Ritalin LA and Metadate CD) and one amphetamine formulation (Adderall XR). Methylin is available in liquid and chewable forms. These are potential stimulant treatment options for some younger children or youths who have problems swallowing pills.

(3) Dextro isomer formulations of stimulant medications such as D-threo-methylphenidate (Focalin) have been developed. The clinical benefit of these more specific agents remains unclear.

d. FDA-approved medications (see Table 21-3).

(1) Dextroamphetamine (Dexedrine, Dextrostat) and amphetamines (Adderall) are FDA-approved for patients 3 years and older.

(2) Methylphenidate (Ritalin) is FDA-approved for patients 6 years and older.

(3) Atomoxetine (Strattera) is a new selective norepinephrine reuptake inhibitor that is a second-line agent for ADHD. There have been some reports of elevations in liver enzymes, suggesting a need for consideration of liver enzyme monitoring and caution in youths with hepatic insufficiency.

(4) Magnesium pemoline (Cylert) is off the market as a result of past concerns over hepatotoxicity and liver failure.

e. Off-label medications.

(1) Antidepressants (desipramine, nortriptyline; see Table 21-5) require a baseline electrocardiogram (ECG) because of concerns about cardiovascular effects and sudden death. Bupropion (Wellbutrin) has positive results but needs controlled studies.

(2) α_2-Agonists (clonidine [Catapres] and guanfacine [Tenex]; see Table 21-2) have limited information regarding efficacy. Need to monitor sedation, orthostasis. Baseline ECG is recommended.

(3) Methylphenidate (see Table 21-3) transdermal delivery systems have demonstrated some initial research success.

(4) Modafinil (Provigil) is currently approved for treatment of narcolepsy and is also being studied as a potential ADHD agent.

4. School interventions.
   a. The child should be in a structured classroom and placed in the front of the room, close to the teacher.
   b. Use predictable, well-organized schedules with rules that are known and clearly reinforced.
   c. The ADHD child might need individual tutoring, resource programs, a self-contained special classroom, or a special school.
5. Individual psychotherapy.
   a. Address and treat depressed mood, low self-esteem, anxiety, or other complicating symptoms.
   b. Focus on impulse control, anger control, peer interactions, and social skills.
6. Social skills deficits might need additional specific treatment interventions.
7. Family therapy.
   a. Parent counseling and education about what ADHD is and what it is not.
   b. Address other family pathology.
8. Provide interventions and treatment for any coexisting learning disorder or comorbid condition.
9. Support groups, such as Children with Attention Deficit Disorder (CHADD) and Attention Deficit Disorder Association (ADDA), are helpful in the psychoeducational process, providing group support and knowledge and resources in the community.

21.4 Disruptive Behavior Disorders

CONDUCT DISORDER
Definition and Identification

1. Conduct disorder is a repetitive and persistent pattern of behavior in which the basic rights of others or major age-appropriate societal norms or rules are violated and that lasts at least 12 months.
2. Behavior can appear in diverse settings (i.e., home, school, or in the community) and can include fighting, aggression to people or animals, destruction of property, deceitfulness or theft, and serious violation of rules, such as truancy or running away.
3. The behavior causes impairment in social, academic, or occupational functioning.
4. It is often difficult to distinguish these acts from those classified as delinquent.

5. Clarify the onset of symptoms (before or after 10 years of age) and severity (mild, moderate, or severe). Childhood-onset conduct disorder has a different comorbidity profile than adolescent-onset conduct disorder. Childhood onset has a greater frequency of neuropsychiatric disorders, low intelligence quotient (IQ), ADHD, aggression, and family clustering of externalizing behavior.

Epidemiology

1. Estimated prevalence in children younger than 18 years is approximately 9% for boys and 2% for girls.
2. Social class variables might have an effect; for example, persons of lower socioeconomic status (SES) are processed through court and juvenile correctional systems, whereas those of higher SES are referred for clinical evaluation and treatment.
3. Boys have higher rates of delinquency and higher childhood onset of conduct disorder before age 10 years. The preponderance of boys is less prominent in adolescent-onset conduct disorder.
4. Parental conflict and family discord can result in a higher probability of becoming early legal offenders.

Diagnosis

1. Careful sequencing of contacts with authority figures (school, social service agencies, family courts, and juvenile justice system). Conduct a thorough history and direct evaluation of the patient, family, and current milieu. Evaluate for history of neglect, abuse, social problems, or gang involvement.
2. Obtain collateral information (i.e., reports from schools, juvenile probation, social service agencies) because a child or family might minimize the extent or degree of antisocial behavior or omit events that indicate disturbance.
3. Evaluate for disturbed peer relations and history of oppositional defiant disorder during early childhood.
4. Look for family history of criminality, substance abuse, somatization, parental psychopathology, and other conditions.
5. Rule out neurologic etiologies or deficits.
6. Features not required for a diagnosis of conduct disorder, but with implications for treatment and prognosis, include lack of empathy or concern for others, misperception of the intent of others in ambiguous social situations, lack of guilt or remorse, and low self-esteem.
7. High suspicion for comorbid cannabis, alcohol, nicotine abuse, and other illicit substance abuse versus dependence. The youth may have other comorbid conditions.

Differential Diagnosis

1. Substance abuse versus dependence.
2. Learning disorders.
3. ADHD.
4. Oppositional defiant disorder.
5. Adjustment disorder; may be striving to cope with a recent disruptive environment or stressor.
6. Mental retardation and pervasive developmental disorder.

7. Seizure disorders.
8. Tic disorders or Tourette's syndrome.
9. Anxiety and depressive disorders. The distinction between youths with conduct disorder versus bipolar disorder, or potentially comorbid illnesses is a particular diagnostic challenge.
10. Emerging maladaptive personality traits or personality disorder, including early antisocial personality disorder.
11. Need to assess for possible suicidal ideation and attempts.
12. PTSD.
13. Schizophrenia or early psychotic disorder.

Course and Prognosis

1. Prediction of outcome is difficult. Mild forms show improvement over time; severe forms tend to be chronic. Early age at onset, aggressive behavior predominance, and diverse antisocial acts across multiple settings predict poorer prognosis.
2. Course and prognosis are limited by lack of treatment motivation.
3. Conduct disorder in childhood predicts antisocial behavior, alcohol abuse, and alcohol dependence in adults.

Treatments

1. No single intervention is effective. Multimodal interventions must be individualized to age, ethnicity, and treatment amenability of the youth and family and delivered for an adequate time.
2. Behavioral techniques using problem-solving skills, training to control problematic behavior, and reinforcement of alternative nondestructive behavior may be helpful.
3. Parent management training, including conflict resolution and disciplinary techniques based on positive reinforcement and altering destructive patterns, are needed.
4. Family-focused treatments, therapy, and group therapy may be helpful.
5. Consider more intensive, community-based, and family-centered interventions and structured services such as outreach and tracking, intensive case management, residential and day treatment settings, and school-based interventions.
6. Inpatient psychiatric hospitalization should only be considered for youth with comorbid depression or psychosis who are posing imminent risks of harm to self or others in the community. Hospitalization should be avoided with youth who have pending legal issues (upcoming court appearance), or who present with malingered symptoms or behavior or other secondary-gain issues (e.g., a youth who verbalizes suicidal ideation only in the context of current legal involvement and is otherwise attempting to avoid incarceration or out-of-home placement).
7. Juvenile and family court involvement can result in out-of-home placement into group homes, residential treatment programs, juvenile detention, or other correctional facilities.
8. The role of psychopharmacology is unclear, except for comorbid conditions. Lithium, antidepressants, psychostimulants, anticonvulsants, β-blockers, and clonidine have been used for target symptoms

of aggression and impulsivity with mixed results. Have a high index of suspicion for noncompliance, diversion, and abuse (e.g., psychostimulants) and medicolegal risks. Avoid antipsychotics until the patient is evaluated by a psychiatrist.

OPPOSITIONAL DEFIANT DISORDER

Definition and Identification

1. Oppositional defiant disorder is an enduring pattern of negativistic, hostile, and defiant behavior in the absence of serious violations of social norms or the rights of others.
2. Characteristic symptoms include a pattern of losing temper, arguing with adults, actively defying or refusing to comply with adults' requests or rules, deliberately doing things that annoy other people, and blaming others for one's mistakes or misbehavior.
3. The behavior causes impairment in social, academic, or occupational functioning.

Epidemiology

1. Oppositional and negativistic behavior may be developmentally appropriate.
2. Oppositional defiant disorder is more prevalent in boys than in girls before puberty; the sex ratio is probably equal after puberty.

Diagnosis

1. Oppositional defiant disorder surfaces almost invariably at home, but it might not be present at school or with other adults or peers. It can occur exclusively in interactions with adults or peers whom the child knows well.
2. The child may show little or no sign of the disorder during clinical examination.
3. The disorder might cause more distress to others than to the affected child.
4. Oppositional defiant disorder can result in poor self-esteem, low frustration tolerance, depressed mood, temper outbursts, and impairment in school performance and peer relationships.
5. Adolescents might abuse alcohol and other drugs.
6. Oppositional defiant behavior tends to precede more serious violations.
7. Evaluate parental and family psychopathologic conditions such as antisocial personality disorder, substance abuse, and chaotic or unstable home environments.

Differential Diagnosis

1. Normal, adaptive, developmentally appropriate oppositional behavior (usually of shorter duration, and it is not more intense than that seen in other children of the same mental age).
2. Adjustment disorder when defiant behavior occurs temporarily in reaction to a significant stressor.
3. Conduct disorder.
4. Substance abuse.
5. ADHD.
6. Cognitive disorders, such as learning disorders or mental retardation.

7. Depressive or anxiety disorders.
8. Schizophrenia.

Course and Prognosis

1. Depends on numerous variables, including severity of the disorder, stability over time, comorbid disorders, and family functioning and psychopathologic conditions.
2. Approximately 25% of children no longer qualify for the diagnosis after several years.
3. The child can remain stable or go on to violate societal norms, leading to a diagnosis of conduct disorder. Prognosis is guarded.

Treatments

1. Individual psychotherapy for the child.
2. Family therapy with counseling and direct training of parents in child management skills and parental compliance training.
3. Behavior therapy (i.e., selectively reinforcing and praising appropriate behavior and ignoring or not reinforcing negative behavior) to encourage appropriate behavior and discourage oppositional defiant disorder behavior.

21.5 Depressive Disorders

Depression in youths is a serious illness, sometimes episodic and often chronic. Symptoms can interfere with academic learning, peer relationships, and family interactions. Prompt evaluation of risk of suicide, homicide, tobacco use, and substance abuse are needed.

TYPES OF DEPRESSIVE DISORDER
Major Depressive Disorder

1. Every youth can be sad occasionally and appropriately. However a DSM-IV-TR diagnosis of major depressive disorder (MDD) requires at least 2 weeks of pervasive change in mood manifested by either depressed or irritable mood and/or loss of interest and pleasure. This also represents a change from previous functioning and produces social or academic impairment.
2. Other symptoms include changes in pattern of appetite, weight, sleep (daily insomnia or hypersomnia), activity (psychomotor agitation or retardation), diminished ability to think or concentrate, decreased energy level (daily fatigue or loss of energy), decreased self-esteem (feelings of worthlessness or inappropriate guilt), decreased interest and motivation, and recurrent thoughts of suicide and/or death.
3. Insidious onset may be more difficult to diagnose than acute onset of symptoms. The patient might have previous history of difficulties with hyperactivity, separation anxiety, or intermittent depressive symptoms.
4. Developmental expression of MDD in childhood or adolescence.
   a. Children with MDD might only exhibit irritable mood or feelings of being unloved, anger, self-deprecation, somatic complaints, anxiety, and disobedience.

b. Prepubertal children might have mood-congruent experiences suggestive of hallucinations, inability to sit still, or frequent temper tantrums. These require more detailed assessment.

c. Symptoms such as separation anxiety, phobias, somatic complaints, and behavioral problems seem to occur more often in children.

d. Instead of significant weight loss or weight gain, children with MDD might exhibit failure to make expected weight gains.

e. Seasonal affective disorder, atypical depression (refer to DSM-IV-TR), and premenstrual dysphoric disorder emerge during adolescence. Anhedonia, hopelessness, psychomotor retardation, and delusions (fixed false beliefs) are more common in adolescents and adults with MDD than in young children.

f. Adolescents might exhibit negativistic or antisocial behavior or abuse alcohol or other drugs. Look for increased emotionality or irritability, particular sensitivity to rejection in relationships, poor attention to personal appearance, complaints of restlessness, grouchiness, aggression, reluctance to participate in family activities, withdrawal from usual peer and social activities, desire to leave home, or preoccupation with dark themes.

5. Depressive symptoms must not be attributable only to substance abuse, use of medications, other psychiatric illness, bereavement, or medical illness.

Dysthymic Disorder

1. Dysthymic disorder (DD) is the occurrence of a depressed or irritable mood for most of the day, for more days than not, over a period of 1 year (this is in contrast to adults, who require a 2-year duration of symptoms).

2. Other symptoms include poor self-esteem, pessimism or hopelessness, loss of interest, social withdrawal, chronic fatigue, feelings of guilt or brooding about past events, irritability or excessive anger, decreased activity or productivity, and poor concentration or memory.

Bipolar Disorder

1. Bipolar disorder (formerly manic depression) was once thought to occur only rarely in youth. Whether bipolar disorder has the same clinical presentation, treatment response, and course of illness in children, adolescents, and adults remains a subject of clinical and research debate. There is ongoing controversy in the child mental health community regarding accurate and appropriate recognition, diagnosis, and treatment of bipolar disorder in youths.

a. Approximately 20% of all bipolar patients have their first episode during adolescence, with a peak age of onset between 15 and 19 years of age.

b. Although the same diagnostic criteria are used as for adults (see Chapter 8), youth can differ with regard to the developmental presentation of symptoms and comorbid psychiatric disorders.

c. It can be very difficult to distinguish childhood and adolescent mania, hypomania, and bipolar depression from other substance-related and other emotional and behavior disorders.

2. A multimodal treatment plan, combining medications with psychotherapeutic interventions, is needed to address the symptomatology and confounding psychosocial factors in children and adolescents with bipolar disorder.

   a. Antimanic agents (primarily lithium or valproic acid) are the mainstays of pharmacotherapy (Table 21-4), but the literature regarding medication treatment for children and adolescents with bipolar disorder is limited. Many of the current recommendations are, therefore, based on studies of adults.

   b. Avoid antimanic medications until the patient is evaluated by a psychiatric consultant.

EPIDEMIOLOGY OF MAJOR DEPRESSIVE DISORDER

1. Depression in adults often begins in adolescence.
2. Prevalence of MDD in children ranges from 0.4% to 2.5% and 0.4% to 8.3% in adolescents. Lifetime prevalence of MDD in adolescents has been estimated to range from 15% to 20%, comparable to adults.
3. MDD has a reported point prevalence from 0.6% to 1.7% in children and 1.6% to 8.0% in adolescents.
4. MDD occurs at approximately the same rate in girls and boys in childhood, but in adolescents, there is a female-to-male ratio of approximately 2:1, similar to adults.
5. The median length of an episode of MDD is approximately 7 to 9 months.
6. The existing research examining bipolar disorder in children and adolescents is limited.

DIFFERENTIAL DIAGNOSIS

1. Rule out effects of alcohol, cannabis, or other substances or a medical condition (e.g., thyroid dysfunction).
2. Psychiatric comorbidity is present in 40% to 90% of depressed children and adolescents; at least 20% to 50% have two or more comorbid diagnoses.
3. Psychiatric comorbidity.
   a. Comorbid depression and anxiety disorders can increase severity and duration of depressive symptoms, risk for substance abuse, and suicidality; decrease response to psychotherapy; and worsen psychosocial problems.
   b. Comorbid depression and disruptive disorder (e.g., oppositional defiant disorder, conduct disorder) are associated with poor short-term outcome, fewer melancholic symptoms, fewer recurrences of depression, lower family aggregation of mood disorders, a higher incidence of adult criminality, more suicide attempts, and higher levels of family criticism.
4. "Double depression" (MDD and dysthymia together) can have more severe and longer depressive episodes, higher rates of comorbid disorders, more suicidality, and worse social impairments than youths with MDD or dysthymia alone.
5. Distinguish from bereavement after loss of a loved one.
6. Consider bipolar disorder or psychotic disorders such as schizophrenia.

Table 21-4	Mood Stabilizers				
Drug (Brand)	Preparations	Main Uses	Dosing	Adverse Effects	Comments
Carbamazepine (Tegretol)	Tabs: 100 mg chewable; 100, 200 mg; 100, 200, 400 mg ER Caps: 100, 200, 300 mg Suspension: 100 mg/5 mL	Complex partial seizures Bipolar disorder Adjunct in MDD	100-200 mg/day; then adjust to plasma level. Plasma half-life 13-17 h. Plasma level can vary. This can change from autoinduction of its metabolism Max dose: 1000 mg for children 6-15 y	Bone marrow suppression (requires baseline and close monitoring of blood counts), dizziness, drowsiness, nausea, rashes, liver toxicity (uncommon, but monitor LFTs), skin disorders (Stevens–Johnson), sedation, aplastic anemia, agranulocytosis	Therapeutic plasma level 4-12 µg/mL; monitor blood levels, CBC, LFTs, TFTs, UA, Na$^+$, BUN, creatinine, serum iron, epoxide level
Divalproex sodium (Depakote)	Tabs: 125, 250, 500 mg; 250, 500 mg ER Caps: 125 mg (sprinkle)	Absence seizures; bipolar disorder; adjunct in MDD	125-250 mg/day then adjusted to plasma level Plasma half-life 8-16 h	Sedation, nausea, liver, bone marrow suppression (requires baseline and close monitoring)	Therapeutic plasma level for seizures 50-100 µg/mL; for adult mania 50-125 µg/mL

Table continued on following page

Table 21-4 **Mood Stabilizers** (Continued)

Drug (Brand)	Preparations	Main Uses	Dosing	Adverse Effects	Comments
Valproic acid (Depakene)	Caps: 250 mg Syrup: 250 mg/ 5 mL				Risk of hepatic involvement increases with age < 2 y and use of other drugs Monitor CBC, LFTs, plasma level FDA black box warnings: hepatotoxicity, teratogenicity, pancreatitis No level required for seizure disorders
Gabapentin (Neurontin)	Caps: 100, 300, 400, 600, 800 mg Soln: 250 mg/ 5 mL	Seizure disorders Off label for ped psychiatric use	3-12 y initial dosing: 10-15 mg/kg/day in 3 divided doses. Effective dose: Ages 3-4 y: 40 mg/kg/day in divided doses Ages 5-12 y: 25-35 mg/kg/day in divided doses	Sedation	
Lamotrigine (Lamictal)	Tabs: 25, 100, 150, 200 mg; 2, 5, 25 mg chewable	Seizure disorders Off label for ped psychiatric use	> 12 y: 300-600 mg tid 12.5-25 mg/day; then titrate to 100-400 mg/day Dose differently if pt is on VPA,	Sedation	Potential for serious rashes and Stevens–Johnson syndrome, especially in ped population

| Lithium (Eskalith, Lithobid) | ER Tabs: 300, 450 mg, Caps: 150, 300, 600 mg, Soln: 300 mg/5 mL | Bipolar disorder, manic; prophylaxis of bipolar disorder; adjunct in MDD; hyperaggressive behavior | carbamazepine, phenytoin, phenobarbital Dose adjusted to plasma level | Polyuria, polydipsia, tremors, nausea, diarrhea, weight gain, drowsiness, skin abnormalities, possible hypothyroidism and impaired renal function with long-term use; acne; cognitive dulling Withdrawal effects and rebound; tics, headaches, dizziness, irritability; abdominal discomfort, lethargy, fatigue Cognitive dulling or irritability 1-2 h after dose can indicate excessive dose Can lower seizure threshold | Blood samples for serum lithium levels should be drawn 12 h after last dose Therapy requires monitoring lithium levels, renal functions, TSH at baseline and periodically thereafter Target level for active episode = 0.8-1.2 mEq/L Target level for prophylaxis = 0.6-0.8 mEq/L Drug interactions are common Lithium toxicity is life-threatening |

Table continued on following page

Table 21-4 **Mood Stabilizers** (Continued)

Drug (Brand)	Preparations	Main Uses	Dosing	Adverse Effects	Comments
Oxcarbazepine (Trileptal)	Tabs: 150, 300, 600 mg Susp: 300 mg/ 5 mL	Seizure disorders Off label for ped psychiatric use	Dosing for adjunctive therapy: 150-300 mg/day initially; then ↑ slowly in divided doses to 900 mg/ day for 20-29 kg; 1200 mg/day for 29.1-39 kg; 1800 mg/day for >39 kg		No blood levels required; no epoxide metabolite

| Topiramate (Topamax) | Tabs: 25, 50, 100, 200 mg Caps: 15, 25 mg (sprinkle) | Seizure disorders Off label for ped psychiatric use | No specific recommendation | Appetite suppression, weight loss, potential cognitive dulling | Used off label as adjunct for appetite suppression with atypical antipsychotics (no controlled studies) Can cause metabolic acidosis: baseline and periodic HCO_3^- levels are recommended |

Note: Consult the *Physicians' Desk Reference* for complete listing of adverse effects.

In pediatric psychiatry, mood stabilizers are used for impulse control disorders, bipolar disorder, and severe temper or behavioral dyscontrol. None are currently FDA approved for mental disorders in child/adolescent populations. There are limited controlled studies for mental disorders (i.e., bipolar disorder, aggression, violence) in child and adolescent populations.

BUN, blood urea nitrogen; cap, capsule; CBC, complete blood count; ER, extended release; FDA, United States Food and Drug Administration; LFT, liver function test; MDD, major depressive disorder; ped, pediatric; pt, patient; soln, solution; susp, suspension; tab, tablet; TFT, thyroid function test; TSH, thyroid-stimulating hormone; UA, urinalysis; VPA, valproic acid.

7. School performance impairment may be misdiagnosed as a learning disorder.

Course and Prognosis

1. Both MDD and dysthymia are recurrent (e.g., MDD has a cumulative probability of recurrence of 40% by 2 years and 70% by 5 years) that increase the risk for substance abuse, suicidal behavior, and poor psychosocial and functional outcome.
2. Depression persists into adulthood, with recurrence rates estimated to be 60% to 70%.
3. MDD increases the risk for bipolar disorder, and dysthymia increases the risk for future MDD episodes.
4. After recovery, some children and adolescents continue to exhibit subclinical symptoms of depression, negative attributions, impairment in interpersonal relationships, increased smoking, impairment in global functioning, early pregnancy, and increased physical problems.
5. Course and prognosis depend on the age at onset, severity of symptoms of the episode, and presence of comorbid disorders. Young age of onset and multiple disorders predict a worse prognosis.

TREATMENTS

1. Evidence-based data in children are sparse. Caution must be used in extrapolating adult research to children.
2. Early identification and treatment are essential because of potential for suicide and other significant psychosocial impairments. The frequency of sessions should be based on symptom severity, the age and developmental status, current exposure to negative life events, and other clinical factors.
3. Hospitalization.
   a. Treatment should be provided in the least restrictive setting. Selection of setting depends on symptoms as well as parent's support, motivation for treatment, and safety issues.
   b. Determine if emergency hospitalization is warranted to protect against self-destructive impulses, behavior, and potential for suicide.
   c. The patient may need to be observed as an inpatient for comorbid substance abuse or dependence.
4. Psychotherapy.
   a. Educate patient and family about depression and the combined use of individual or family therapy and medication.
   b. Long-term social skills interventions are often necessary. CBT appears to be effective for reducing symptoms.
5. Pharmacotherapy (Table 21-5).
   a. Medication alone is never considered adequate treatment.
   b. Double-blind, randomized clinical trials of tricyclics have not shown superiority to placebo.
   c. SSRIs. Fluoxetine (Prozac) is the only FDA-approved medication for the treatment of depressive disorders in children and adolescents. Although there are no clearly defined standard dosing strategies for juveniles, the general principle is to start low and

Table 21-5 Antidepressants

Drug (Brand)	Preparations	Main Uses[a]	Typical Starting Dose	Adverse Effects	Comments
Selective Serotonin Reuptake Inhibitors[a]					
Citalopram (Celexa)	Tabs: 10, 20, 40 mg Elixir: 10 mg/5 mL	MDD	10 mg qAM	Irritability, insomnia, GI symptoms, headache, agitation	
Escitalopram (Lexapro)	Tabs: 5, 10, 20 mg Elixir: 5 mg/5 mL	MDD	5-10 mg/day	Irritability, insomnia, GI symptoms, headache, agitation	
Fluoxetine (Prozac)	Tabs: 10, 20, 40 mg IR; 90 mg DR Elixir: 20 mg/5 mL	MDD[†] OCD (7-17 y)[†]	10-20 mg qAM	Irritability, insomnia, GI symptoms, headache, agitation	
Fluvoxamine (Luvox)	Tabs: 25, 50, 100 mg	OCD[†] (> 8 y)	25 mg qhs	Irritability, insomnia, GI symptoms, headache, agitation	
Paroxetine (Paxil)	Tabs: 10, 20, 30, 40 mg IR Tabs: 12.5, 25, 37.5 mg CR Elixir: 10 mg/5 mL	MDD, OCD	5-10 mg qAM	Irritability, insomnia, GI symptoms, headache, agitation	FDA discourages use for depression in patients <18 y

Table 21-5 **Antidepressants** (*Continued*)

Drug (Brand)	Preparations	Main Uses	Typical Starting Dose	Adverse Effects	Comments
Sertraline (Zoloft)	Tabs: 25, 50, 100 mg Elixir: 20 mg/ 5 mL	MDD, OCD (6-18 y)[†]	12.5-50 mg q$_{AM}$	Irritability, insomnia, GI symptoms, headache, agitation	
Tricyclics Clomipramine (Anafranil)	Caps: 25, 50, 75 mg	OCD[†]	Daily dose 2-3 mg/ kg/day OCD: 25 mg/day, gradually ↑ to max 3 mg/kg/ day or 200 mg (whichever is less)	Dangerous in overdose	Slightly increased risk of sudden death associated with the use of desipramine Baseline and serial ECGs throughout treatment are recommended (with dose increases)

| Desipramine (Norpramin, Pertofrane) | Tabs: 10, 25, 50, 75, 100, 150 mg | ADHD, enuresis, MDD, tic disorders | 1-3 mg/kg/day
Max: 5 mg/kg/day
Child 6-12 y:
10-30 mg/day in divided doses
Adolescent:
25-50 mg/day gradually ↑ to 100 mg/day in single or divided doses
Max: 150 mg/day | No known long-term side effects
Dangerous in overdose | Important to *not* miss doses
FDA black box warning: possible risk of suicidal ideation
Same as clomipramine |

Table continued on following page

Table 21-5 **Antidepressants** (Continued)

Drug (Brand)	Preparations	Main Uses	Typical Starting Dose	Adverse Effects	Comments
Imipramine (Tofranil)	Tabs: 10, 25, 50 mg Caps: 75, 100, 125, 150 mg	MDD, ADHD Enuresis[†]	~ 10-25 mg/d; ↑ slowly every wk by 20%-30%. Max/day: lesser of 4 mg/kg or 6-12 y: 50 mg >12 y: 75-100 mg	Anticholinergic (dry mouth, constipation, blurred vision), weight loss Cardiovascular (check conduction parameters) Dangerous in overdose Withdrawal effects and rebound; tics, headache, dizziness, irritability; abdominal discomfort, lethargy, fatigue Cognitive dulling or irritability 1-2 h after dose can indicate excessive dose Can lower seizure threshold	Same as clomipramine

| Nortriptyline (Pamelor, Aventil) | Caps: 10, 25, 50, 75 mg
Soln: 10 mg/5 mL | ADHD, anxiety, tic disorders | Dose adjusted according to serum levels (therapeutic window for nortriptyline) and response
6-12 y: 10-20 mg/day in 3-4 divided doses
Adolescent: 10-25 mg/day in divided doses
Max/day: lesser of 2 mg/kg/day or 100 mg | Withdrawal effects can occur (severe GI symptoms, malaise)
Dangerous in overdose | Same as clomipramine |

*Black box warning: All SSRIs might carry increased risk of suicidal ideation.
†FDA approved use.
Note: Consult the *Physicians' Desk Reference* for complete listing of adverse effects.
ADHD, attention-deficit/hyperactivity disorder; cap: capsule; CR, controlled release; DR, delayed release; FDA, United States Food and Drug Administration; GI, gastrointestinal; IR, immediate release; MDD, major depressive disorder; OCD, obsessive–compulsive disorder; soln, solution; tab, tablet.

make small increases based on effect. For example, start with 10 mg/day in the morning with food, and then slowly increase by 10-mg increments on a biweekly or monthly basis as tolerated to clinical effect (a goal is to typically achieve daily doses in the 20- to 40-mg range for at least 4 to 6 weeks). Monitor for compliance, comorbid substance abuse and other mental disorders, other psychosocial stressors, and overactivating side effects.

6. Antidepressant medications and suicidality.
   a. The FDA now requires a black box for each antidepressant's package insert warning about increased suicidal thinking and suicidal behavior that can occur in children and adolescents during the early phases of treatment.
   b. The FDA has not asserted that the use of these medications in youths with depressive disorders is contraindicated, so physicians may continue to prescribe them.
      (1) The use of an antidepressant must balance risk with clinical need.
      (2) Patients started on therapy should be observed closely for clinical worsening, suicidality, or unusual changes in behavior.
      (3) Families and caregivers should be advised of the need for close observation and communication with the prescriber.
      (4) Untreated depression has potentially greater risks than medication, and medication treatment can be effective, especially when started early.

7. Strategies for antidepressant treatment.
   a. Obtain assent from the youth and thorough informed consent from a parent or legal guardian.
   b. Evaluate first-degree relatives' past response to antidepressants.
   c. Reserve tricyclic antidepressants (TCAs) as second-line agent after SSRIs because of the relatively greater medical risks of TCAs. Check baseline ECG and monitor for ECG changes if using TCAs or MAOIs.
   d. Gradual titration of the drug (start low and go slow) can improve tolerability.
   e. Establish a specific monitoring frequency. Observe for clinical worsening (activation, restlessness, potential for induction of manic symptoms), suicidality, or unusual changes in behavior during the initial few months. There is no accepted standard of care on optimal frequency of visits. Implement, to the extent that is practical, the FDA's most recent specific instruction, including once-a-week visits with the patient the first 4 weeks, and biweekly the next 8 weeks.
   f. When using TCAs, monitor for noradrenergic side effects (e.g., orthostatic symptoms, sedation), or anticholinergic side effects (e.g., dry mouth, blurred vision, constipation), and weight gain. When using SSRIs, monitor for akathisia (inner restlessness, inability to sit still), overactivation, insomnia, and other possible serotoninergic side effects as described above.

g. Enlist the patient and family as allies to monitor status and report any side effects.

h. Consider child psychiatric consultation.

i. Abrupt TCA discontinuation can lead to nausea, vertigo, cholinergic, and withdrawal-like symptoms, particularly if the medication is an SSRI other than fluoxetine (Prozac).

21.6 Learning Disorders

DEFINITION AND IDENTIFICATION

1. Varied definitions exist. The critical elements of all definitions are:
   a. Heterogeneity of learning disabilities.
   b. Intrinsic or neurobiological nature.
   c. Significant discrepancy between learning potential and academic performance.
   d. Exclusion of cultural, educational, environmental, and other etiologies or other impairments as a cause of disability.

2. According to the DSM-IV-TR, learning disorders include reading disorder, mathematics disorder, and disorder of written expression. The diagnosis requires a discrepancy, based on age and intelligence, between potential and achievement.
   a. Reading achievement, mathematical ability, and writing skills as measured by standardized tests are substantially below those expected for age, measured intelligence, and education.
   b. Disturbances significantly interfere with academic achievement or activities of daily living that require reading, writing, and mathematics.
   c. If a sensory deficit is present, the reading, writing, and mathematics difficulties are in excess of those usually associated with it.
   d. Learning disorder, not otherwise specified, is a category for disorders that do not meet criteria for any specific learning disorder but that cause impairment below expected for intelligence, education, and age.

3. Many children referred for evaluation because of school behavior or conflicts around homework have unrecognized language or learning difficulties. Untreated learning problems can lead to decreased self-esteem, school failure, aggression, rule violation, truancy, affiliation with delinquent peers, substance abuse, and family or juvenile court involvements.

EPIDEMIOLOGY

In school-age children, language and learning disorders are among the most common disorders. About 50% of children with a language or learning disorder also have a comorbid psychiatric disorder. Prevalence of learning disorders is listed in Table 21-6.

DIAGNOSIS AND CLINICAL FEATURES

1. The patient is usually referred by school or parents after poor school performance during grades 1 to 3 (ages 6 to 8 years). A learning

21—Child and Adolescent Psychiatry

Table 21-6 **Prevalence of Learning Disorders**

Disorder	Prevalence	Sex Ratio (male to female)
Reading disorder	Estimated 4%; 2% to 8%	3:1 or 4:1
Mathematics disorder	Rough estimate of 6%	Unclear
Disorder of written expression	Estimated 3% to 10%	Unclear

disorder may be compensated for in early grades and might not be apparent until age 9 (fourth grade) or later.

2. Evaluate general health and clarify past or current subject areas of weakness. Pediatric examination within 12 months is indicated. Collaborate with family doctor or pediatrician. Vision and hearing testing should be ordered as indicated. Evaluate for other medical and neurologic conditions.

3. Review standardized intelligence and psychoeducational diagnostic tests. Evaluation should include observation of behavior and a child diagnostic interview.

4. Learning disorders can lead to frustration and anger because of feelings of inadequacy and academic failure.

5. There may be refusal or reluctance to go to school and do homework, poor academic performance, general disinterest in school work, or truancy.

DIFFERENTIAL DIAGNOSIS

1. Rule out pervasive developmental disorders and mental retardation. Consider referral for a special education evaluation.

2. Writing, language, and reading disorders can coexist.

3. Rule out sensory deficits (e.g., hearing and visual impairments) with screening tests.

4. Motor skills disorder.

5. Medical or neurologic primary diagnosis (e.g., fetal alcohol syndrome or effects, prenatal substance abuse, fragile X syndrome).

6. Think about ADHD, disruptive behavior disorders such as conduct disorder, and anxiety and depressive disorders, particularly in older children and adolescents.

COURSE AND PROGNOSIS

Course and prognosis depend on the type and severity of the disorders, the age or grade when the intervention is started, the length and continuity of treatment, motivation, the presence or absence of emotional or behavioral problems, and the presence of a supportive family and school environment.

TREATMENTS

Collaborate with parents and school to clarify diagnosis, provide education and consultation when appropriate, implement treatment and remediation, and monitor progress. Identify and treat comorbid conditions, including determining the appropriateness of medication.

1. Remedial educational approaches and teaching strategies are helpful.
2. If poor coordination is found, physical therapy and sensory integration activities through occupational therapy may be helpful.
3. Psychotherapy may be needed to sustain motivation.
4. Consider referral to an appropriate evaluation center if indicated.
5. Function as an advocate. Build on the family's and child's strengths. Work as a team with teachers, education consultants, community agencies, medical consultants, and families.
6. Monitor progress and appropriateness of school interventions.
7. Be aware of protections afforded under federal law. Youth may qualify under Section 504 of the Rehabilitation Act of 1973 or, alternatively, under the Individuals with Disabilities Education Act (IDEA), which was originally enacted in 1975 as the Education for All Handicapped Children Act (EAHCA). These federal laws provide children with learning disabilities the right to a free and appropriate public education.
8. In many states any *interested party* (i.e., teacher, parent, administrator, physician, school nurse, etc.) may refer a student to the Multi-Disciplinary Team (MDT)/Disability Determination Team (DDT) to evaluate a student for a determination of the presence of a disability. Thus, when indicated, it is appropriate to encourage a parent or guardian to request an evaluation for an individualized education plan (IEP) or a reevaluation of an existing IEP or 504 plan.

21.7 Mental Retardation and Developmental Disabilities

Definition and Identification

1. Developmental delay is a lag in the acquisition of developmental milestones, with skills below those expected of the child's chronologic age.
2. Mental retardation is a heterogeneous disorder defined by significantly below-average intellectual functioning and impairment in adaptive skills that is present before age 18 years.
3. With an approach underscored by principles of normalization and the availability of appropriate education and habilitation, persons with mental retardation generally live, are educated, and work in the community.

EPIDEMIOLOGY

1. Prevalence of mental retardation at any one time is estimated to be about 1% of the population.
2. It is difficult to calculate incidence.

3. The highest incidence is in school-age children, with peaks at ages 10 to 14 years.
4. Mental retardation is about one and a half times more common in men than in women.

EVALUATION

1. Thorough physical and neurologic exam for physical stigmata, dysmorphology, and neurologic abnormalities. Look for motor, language, and global delays. Consider consultation from a geneticist before embarking on expensive genetic laboratory analyses. Consider neuroimaging (computed tomography [CT] or magnetic resonance imaging [MRI]) and electroencephalogram (EEG) after consultation from neurology.
2. If a developmental delay or mental retardation is suspected, refer for standardized psychological testing.
3. Evaluate for comorbid psychiatric disorders such as depressive or anxiety disorders.
4. Children or adolescents with mental retardation can have emotional or behavioral difficulties requiring psychiatric consultation or treatment. Presentations can be modified by poor language skills and by life circumstances, so a diagnosis might hinge more heavily on observable behavioral symptoms.
5. The diagnostic assessment considers and synthesizes the biological, psychological, and psychosocial contexts. Careful past medical history of pregnancy, labor and delivery, family history of MR, consanguinity of parents, history of hereditary disorders, and social history. Get a longitudinal picture of child's development, milestones, and functioning.
6. Evaluate hearing and speech.

DIFFERENTIAL DIAGNOSIS

1. Mental disorders due to a general medical condition (e.g., hypothyroidism).
2. Down's syndrome, fragile X, Turner's syndrome, Klinefelter's syndrome, Prader–Willi, cri-du-chat, and other chromosomal abnormalities.
3. Genetic syndromes such as phenylketonuria, Rett's disorder, neurofibromatosis, tuberous sclerosis, Lesch–Nyhan, muscular dystrophy, adrenoleukodystrophy, maple syrup urine disease, and other enzyme deficiency disorders.
4. Prenatal toxic exposures such as rubella, cytomegalovirus, syphilis, toxoplasmosis, herpes simplex, acquired immunodeficiency syndrome (AIDS), fetal alcohol syndrome, prenatal substance exposure.
5. Complications of pregnancy and other perinatal factors such as anoxia or cerebral palsy.
6. Acquired childhood disorders such as central nervous system infections, head trauma, or subclinical lead intoxication.
7. Learning disorders.
8. Uncontrolled seizure disorders.

9. Environmental and sociocultural factors leading to inadequate stimulation and deprivation.
10. Pervasive developmental disorders and mental retardation often coexist.
11. ADHD.
12. Tic disorders and stereotypic movement disorder.
13. Schizophrenia and other psychotic disorders.
14. Depressive and anxiety disorders.
15. Eating disorders.

COURSE AND PROGNOSIS

1. The more comorbid mental disorders occur, the more guarded is the overall prognosis.
2. In most cases of mental retardation, the underlying intellectual impairment does not improve.

TREATMENTS

1. Comprehensive treatment integrating various approaches, including family counseling, pharmacologic, educational, habilitative, and milieu interventions is the rule.
2. Function as an advocate for the child's family. Build on strengths, and work in a team with teachers, educational consultants, community agencies, medical consultants, and families.
3. Once mental retardation is identified, hereditary metabolic or endocrine disorders, such as phenylketonuria (PKU) and hypothyroidism, should be treated by diet control or hormone replacement therapy.
4. The goal of treatment is to provide enriched and supportive environment to improve level of adaptation.
5. Comprehensive educational programs that address adaptive skills training, social skills training, communication skills, and vocational training are needed. Group therapy is often useful.
6. Public Law 94-142 EAHCA/IDEA guarantees children with disabilities the right to a free and appropriate public education.
   a. Use behavioral, cognitive, and supportive psychotherapies.
   b. Family education and therapy are important.
7. Check the Health Care Financing Administration (HCFA) *Guidelines for Psychotropic Medication Use in Persons with Mental Retardation*, before prescribing psychotropic medication.
   a. Medical, environmental, and other causes of the behavioral problem must be ruled out.
   b. A detailed description of symptoms and differential diagnosis is required.
   c. Behavioral data should be collected.
   d. The least intrusive and most positive interventions should be used, including as applicable behavior therapy, psychotherapy, and habilitation and education. Medications might be the least intrusive and most positive intervention in some cases.
8. When medication is prescribed:
   a. It should be an integral part of an overall active treatment program.
   b. It should not diminish functional status.

Table 21-7 Antipsychotics

Drug (Brand)	Preparations	Main Uses	Typical Starting Dose	Adverse Effects	Comments
Typical Antipsychotics					
Low-Potency Phenothiazines					
Chlorpromazine (Thorazine)	Elixir: 10, 25, 50, 100, 200 mg; Injectable: 10, 25, 50, 100 mg	As last resort for aggressive behavior; severe agitation; severe insomnia; Tourette's syndrome; severe self-abuse in children with developmental disorders, including mental retardation and pervasive developmental disorders	Range varies widely depending on agent, age, and disorder Bedtime dosing might prevent daytime sedation and cognitive impairment in school	Anticholinergic (dry mouth, constipation, blurred vision; more common with low-potency agents), hypotension, sedation, weight gain (↓ risk with molindone), EPS (dystonia, rigidity, tremor, akathisia, ↑ risk with high potency), drowsiness, risk of TD with long-term administration, withdrawal dyskinesia, SMS (muscle rigidity, delirium, autonomic instability, increased CPK levels), withdrawal effects and rebound, tics, headache, dizziness, irritability, abdominal discomfort, lethargy, fatigue	Antipsychotics should not be used to treat anxiety or as a primary agent for behavioral problems EPS can be prevented by avoiding rapid neuroleptization Avoid antiparkinson agents unless strictly necessary because of added adverse effects Treat akathisia by lowering the antipsychotic dose or using β-blockers (propranolol) or high-potency benzodiazepines (clonazepam)
Thioridazine (Mellaril)					
High Potency					
Fluphenazine	Tabs: 1, 2.5, 5, 10 mg; Elixir: 4 mg/mL; Injectable				
Perphenazine	Tabs: 2, 4, 8, 16 mg; Injectable				
Butyrophenones					
Haloperidol (Haldol)	Tabs: 0.5, 1, 2, 5, 10, 20 mg; Soln: 2 mg/mL; Injectable				
Thiothixene (Navane)	Tabs: 1, 2, 5, 10, 20 mg			Cognitive dulling or irritability 1-2 h after dose can indicate excessive dose Withdrawal effects and rebound phenomena.	Because of long-term risks, these agents usually require involvement of specialists
Molindone (indole derivative) (Moban)	Tabs: 5, 10, 25, 50 mg			Rarely, tic disorders. Infrequently, headaches, dizziness, irritability, abdominal discomfort, lethargy, and fatigue. Can lower seizure threshold. QTc prolongation esp. with phenothiazines	QTc prolongation with certain antipsychotics, risk for torsades de pointes, arrhythmias, and sudden death
Pimozide (Orap)	Tabs: 1, 2 mg	Tourette's	Prepubertal: 0.5 mg qd Adolescents: 1-2 mg qd	ECG changes Doses >20 mg/day not recommended due to concerns of sudden death Avoid concurrent use with fluoxetine due to risks of QTc prolongation	Long elimination half-life Requires qd or qod dosing ECG monitoring recommended at baseline and 2-3 d after each dose increase

Atypical Antipsychotics

Drug	Forms	Approval	Dosing	Adverse Effects
Aripiprazole (Abilify)	Tabs: 2, 5, 10, 15, 20, 30 mg; Soln: 1 mg/1 mL	No atypical antipsychotics are approved for use in children or adolescents, despite increased use	Initial: 5-10 mg; Target: 5-20 mg	Low incidence of extrapyramidal adverse effects; does not induce dystonia. Low risk of TD
Clozapine (Clozaril)	Tabs: 25, 100 mg	Treat refractory psychosis; psychotic with serotoninergic, adrenergic, histaminergic activity	Initial: 12.5 mg; Target: 25-400 mg	Cardiac arrhythmias (ECG: elongated QTc), seizures, EPS, drowsiness, TD, withdrawal dyskinesia, sedation, sialorrhea. Granulocytopenia/agranulocytosis (mandatory ongoing monitoring of blood count, reporting to National Clozapine Registry). Higher risk of seizures (dose-related). PDR recommends monitoring for cataracts
Quetiapine (Seroquel)	Tabs: 25, 100, 200, 300, 400 mg	No atypical antipsychotics are approved for use in children or adolescents, despite increased use	Initial: 25 mg; Target: 25-450 mg	
Risperidone (Risperdal)	Tabs: 0.25, 0.5, 1, 2, 3, 4 mg; ODT: 0.5, 1, 2, 3, 4 mg; Elixir: 1 mg/1 mL; LA injectable (Consta)	No atypical antipsychotics are approved for use in children or adolescents, despite increased use	0.25-1 mg	↑ appetite, weight gain, other risks. Can lead to glucose dysregulation, increased prolactin, dyslipidemia
Ziprasidone (Geodon)	Caps: 20, 40, 60, 80 mg; Injectable	No atypical antipsychotics are approved for use in children or adolescents, despite increased use	Initial: 20 mg; Target: 20-160 mg	Monitor potential QTc prolongation

Note: Consult the *Physicians' Desk Reference* for complete listing of adverse effects.
cap, capsule; CPK, creatine phosphokinase; ECG, electrocardiogram; EPS, extrapyramidal symptoms; LA, long acting; ODT, orally disintegrating tablet; soln, solution; tab, tablet; TD, tardive dyskinesia;

  c. The lowest effective dose should be used.
  d. A gradual dose reduction should be periodically considered (at least annually) unless clinically contraindicated.
  e. Adverse drug effects should be monitored.
  f. Data should be collected documenting that the drug achieves the desired outcome (including the patient's quality of life).
9. There are many examples of pharmacologic intervention for aggression and self-injurious behavior (lithium, naltrexone, valproic acid, and carbamazepine; see Table 21-4), stereotyped motor movements (antipsychotics, Table 21-7), explosive rage behavior (mood stabilizers [see Table 21-4], β-blockers, buspirone [see Table 21-1]; limited systematic studies), and ADHD symptoms (stimulants and α_2 agents, see Table 21-3). Avoid antipsychotics in this population without a child psychiatric consultation because of side effects and serious risks.

Acknowledgement

Thanks to Carolyn K. Welch, PharmD, for her invaluable assistance in preparing the tables.

SUGGESTED READINGS

Achenbach TM: Empirically Based Taxonomy: How to Use Syndromes and Profile Types Derived from the CBCL (Child Behavior Checklist) from 4 to 18, TRF (Teacher Rating Form), and WSR. Burlington, University of Vermont, 1993.

American Academy of Child and Adolescent Psychiatry: Policy statement: Prescribing psychoactive medications for children and adolescents. September 20, 2001. Available at http://www.aacap.org/page.ww?section = Policy + Statements&name = Prescribing + Psychoactive + Medication + for + Children + and + Adolescents (accessed October 17, 2006).

American Academy of Child and Adolescent Psychiatry: Practice parameters for the assessment and treatment of children, adolescents, and adults with autism and other pervasive developmental disorders. J Am Acad Child Adolesc Psychiatry 38:32S-54S, 1999.

American Academy of Child and Adolescent Psychiatry: Practice parameters for the assessment and treatment of anxiety disorders. J Am Acad Child Adolesc Psychiatry 36:69S-84S, 1997.

American Academy of Child and Adolescent Psychiatry: Practice parameters for the assessment and treatment of children, adolescents, and adults with attention-deficit/hyperactivity disorder. J Am Acad Child Adolesc Psychiatry 36:85S-121S, 1997.

American Academy of Child and Adolescent Psychiatry: Practice parameters for the assessment and treatment of children and adolescents with bipolar disorder. J Am Acad Child Adolesc Psychiatry 36:157S-176S, 1997.

American Academy of Child and Adolescent Psychiatry: Practice parameters for the assessment and treatment of children and adolescents with conduct disorder. J Am Acad Child Adolesc Psychiatry 36:122S-139S, 1997.

American Academy of Child and Adolescent Psychiatry: Practice parameters for the assessment and treatment of depressive disorders. J Am Acad Child Adolesc Psychiatry 37:63S-83S, 1998.

American Academy of Child and Adolescent Psychiatry: Practice parameters for the assessment and treatment of language and learning disorders. J Am Acad Child Adolesc Psychiatry 37:46S-62S, 1998.

American Academy of Child and Adolescent Psychiatry: Practice parameters for the assessment and treatment of children, adolescents, and adults with mental retardation and comorbid mental disorders. *J Am Acad Child Adolesc Psychiatry* 38:5S-31S, 1999.

American Academy of Child and Adolescent Psychiatry: Practice parameters for the assessment and treatment of obsessive-compulsive disorder. *J Am Acad Child Adolesc Psychiatry* 37:27S-45S, 1998.

American Academy of Child and Adolescent Psychiatry: Practice parameters for the assessment and treatment of posttraumatic stress disorder. *J Am Acad Child Adolesc Psychiatry* 37:4S-26S, 1998.

American Academy of Child and Adolescent Psychiatry: Supplementary talking points for child and adolescent psychiatrists regarding the FDA black box warning on the use of antidepressants for pediatric patients. October 31, 2004. PDF available at http://www.aacap.org/galleries/PsychiatricMedication/Black Box TalkingPoints.pdf (accessed October 17, 2006).

American Psychiatric Association: *Diagnostic and Statistical Manual of Mental Disorders*, 4th ed, text revision. Washington, DC, American Psychiatric Press, 2004.

Bernstein GA, Borchardt CM, Perwien AR: Anxiety disorders in children and adolescents: A review of the past 10 years. *J Am Acad Child Adolesc Psychiatry* 35:1110-1119, 1996.

Birmaher B, Ryan ND, Williamson DE, et al: Childhood and adolescent depression: A review of the past 10 years. Part I. *J Am Acad Child Adolesc Psychiatry* 35(11):1427-1439, 1996.

Birmaher B, Ryan ND, Williamson DE, et al: Childhood and adolescent depression: A review of the past 10 years. Part II. *J Am Acad Child Adolesc Psychiatry* 35(12):1575-1583, 1996.

Cantwell DP: Attention deficit disorder: A review of the past 10 years. *J Am Acad Child Adolesc Psychiatry* 35(8):978-987, 1996.

Capute AJ, Accardo PJ (eds): *Developmental Disabilities in Infancy and Childhood*, ed 2. Baltimore, Brooks, 1996.

Conner K: *Conner's Abbreviated Symptom Questionnaire*. North Tonawanda, NY, Multi Health Systems, 1994.

Golova N, Hojman H: Behavioral and psychiatric disorders of childhood. In Alario AJ (ed): *Practical Guide to the Care of the Pediatric Patient*. St Louis, Mosby, 1997, pp 507-542.

Golova N, Hojman H: Major drug classes used in pediatric psychiatry. In Alario AJ (ed): Practical guide to the care of the pediatric patient. St Louis, Mosby, 1997, pp 542-555.

Health Care Financing Administration (HCFA): *Psychopharmacological Medications: Safety Precautions for Persons with Developmental Disabilities*. Washington, DC, Health Care Financing Administration, 1997.

Penn JV, Leonard HL: Diagnosis and treatment of obsessive–compulsive disorder in children and adolescents. In Pato MT, Zohar J (eds): *Current Treatments of Obsessive–Compulsive Disorder*, 2nd ed. Washington, DC, American Psychiatric Press, 2001, pp 109-132.

Zonfrillo MR, Penn JV, Leonard HL: Pediatric psychotropic polypharmacy. *Psychiatry* 8:14-19, 2005.

Formulary

This chapter provides essential and concise information on more than 170 commonly prescribed medications. For the reader's convenience, the common brand names are cross-indexed to the generic names. Each drug is listed by its principal generic name and is presented in the following format:

1. Generic name (common brand names follow in parentheses)
2. Available form(s) (oral unless otherwise specified)
3. Dosage (adult unless otherwise specified)
4. Indication(s)
5. Action
6. Contraindications and precautions
7. Side effects

Hypersensitivity or an allergic reaction to a medication or any of its components is a definite contraindication to its use. When prescribing multiple medications for the same patient, all the possible drug interactions must be carefully considered.

Every attempt has been made to cover the most important aspects of each drug and to keep medication dosages in conformity with the latest practices of the general medical community. *However, it is strongly recommended that the reader become completely familiar with the manufacturer's product information before prescribing any of these medications.* This is particularly important when prescribing for patients with renal or hepatic impairment and for elderly or debilitated patients.

The use of any drug in women who are pregnant or of childbearing age requires that the anticipated benefit be weighed against the possible hazard. Please note that this section does not list pregnancy as a contraindication to the use of any of these medications. *Refer to the manufacturer's product information for possible warnings, contraindications, or adverse reactions before prescribing any of these medications for pregnant women.*

ABILIFY; *SEE* ARIPIPRAZOLE
ACAMPROSATE CALCIUM (CAMPRAL)
Available Form
Tablet, enteric coated: 333 mg.

Dosage
Two 333-mg tablets (666 mg/dose) tid.

Indication

Maintenance of abstinence from alcohol in patients with alcohol dependence who are abstinent at treatment initiation.

Action

Synthetic compound with a chemical structure similar to that of the endogenous amino acid homotaurine, which is a structural analogue of the amino acid neurotransmitter γ-aminobutyric acid and the amino acid neuromodulator taurine.

Contraindications and Precautions

In patients with severe renal impairment (creatinine clearance < 30 mL/min), does not eliminate or diminish withdrawal symptoms.

Side Effects

Pruritus, abdominal pain, vomiting, nausea, rash, fluctuation in sex drive, diarrhea.

ADDERALL; *SEE* AMPHETAMINE

ALPRAZOLAM (XANAX)

Available Forms

Solution: 0.5 mg/5 mL, 500 mL, 1 mg/mL w/dropper, 30 mL.
Tablet, plain coated: 0.25, 0.5, 1, 2 mg.
Tablet, extended release: 0.5, 1, 2, 3 mg.

Dosage

Anxiety

Initially 0.25 to 0.5 mg tid or extended-release 0.5 to 1 mg qd.
Use lower doses in elderly or debilitated patients.
Maximum daily dose is 4 mg except in panic disorder.

Panic Disorder

Initially 0.5 mg tid or extended-release 0.5 to 1 mg qd.
Increase the dose no more than 1 mg every 3 or 4 days.
Doses >4 mg/day may be necessary.

Indications

Management of anxiety disorders and anxiety associated with depression.
Treatment of panic disorder, with or without agoraphobia.

Action

Benzodiazepine; depresses subcortical levels of central nervous system (CNS), including limbic system, reticular formation.

Contraindications and Precautions

Contraindicated in patients with hypersensitivity to benzodiazepines or untreated narrow-angle glaucoma.
Do not use during activities requiring complete mental alertness.
Contraindicated with concomitant use of ethanol and other CNS depressants or witih itraconazole, ketoconazole, and other azole antifungals.
Alprazolam is metabolized via the cytochrome P450 3A pathway and can interact with other drugs and foods that use this pathway.

Coadministration of cimetidine, sertraline, paroxetine, fluoxetine, nefazodone, propoxyphene, fluvoxamine, diltiazem, macrolide antibiotics, nicardipine, nifedipine, or oral contraceptives can significantly increase the plasma concentration of alprazolam.

Side Effects

Drowsiness, headache, lightheadedness, confusion, dizziness, dry mouth, insomnia, increased anxiety.

AMANTADINE HYDROCHLORIDE (SYMMETREL)

Available Forms

Capsule: 100 mg.
Syrup: 100 mg.
Tablet: 100 mg.

Dosage

Initial: 100 mg bid.
Occasionally, patients whose responses are not optimal at 200 mg/day benefit from an increase up to 300 mg/day in divided doses.

Indication

Drug-induced extrapyramidal symptoms (EPS).

Action

The mechanism of action of amantadine in the treatment of Parkinson's disease and drug-induced EPS is not known.

Contraindications and Precautions

Deaths have been reported from overdose. Suicide attempts, some of which have been fatal, have been reported.
Sporadic cases of possible neuroleptic malignant syndrome (NMS) have been reported in association with dose reduction or withdrawal of amantadine. Therefore, patients should be observed carefully when the dosage of amantadine is reduced abruptly or discontinued, especially if the patient is receiving neuroleptics.

Side Effects

Nausea, dizziness (lightheadedness), and insomnia.

AMBIEN; SEE ZOLPIDEM TARTRATE
AMITRIPTYLINE HYDROCHLORIDE (ELAVIL)

Available Forms

Powder, compounding: 100%.
Solution, injectable (IM): 10 mg/mL.
Tablet: 10, 25, 50, 75, 100, 150 mg.

Dosage

Initial Dosage for Adults

For outpatients, 75 mg/day in divided doses is usually satisfactory. If necessary, this may be increased to a total of 150 mg/day. Increases are made preferably in the late afternoon and/or bedtime doses.

An alternate method of initiating therapy in outpatients is to begin with 50 to 100 mg amitriptyline hs. This may be increased by 25 or 50 mg as necessary in the bedtime dose to a total of 150 mg/day.

A sedative effect may be apparent before the antidepressant effect is noted, but an adequate therapeutic effect can take as long as 30 days to develop.

Hospitalized patients can require 100 mg/day initially. This may be increased gradually to 200 mg/day if necessary. A few hospitalized patients need as much as 300 mg/day.

IM dose is initially 20 to 30 mg (2-3 mL) qid.

Adolescent and Elderly Patients

In general, lower dosages are recommended for these patients.

Amitriptyline 10 mg tid with 20 mg hs may be satisfactory in adolescent and elderly patients who do not tolerate higher doses.

Maintenance

The usual maintenance dosage of amitriptyline is 50 to 100 mg/day. In some patients 40 mg/day is sufficient.

The total maintenance dose may be given in a single dose, preferably at bedtime. When satisfactory improvement has been reached, the dose should be reduced to the lowest amount that will maintain relief of symptoms. It is appropriate to continue maintenance therapy 3 months or longer to lessen the possibility of relapse.

Indication

Depression.

Action

An antidepressant with sedative effects.

Its mechanism of action in humans is not known. It is not a monoamine oxidase inhibitor (MAOI) and it does not act primarily by stimulation of the CNS.

Contraindications and Precautions

Should not be given concomitantly with MAOIs.

Should not be given with cisapride due to the potential for increased QT interval and increased risk of arrhythmia.

Not recommended for use during the acute recovery phase following myocardial infarction.

Amitriptyline can block the antihypertensive action of guanethidine or similarly acting compounds.

Use with caution in patients with a history of seizures, urinary retention, angle-closure glaucoma, or increased intraocular pressure.

Side Effects

Common: Dizziness, drowsiness, dry mouth, headache, increased appetite (can include craving for sweets), nausea, tiredness or weakness (mild), unpleasant taste, and weight gain.

Less common: Diarrhea, heartburn, increased sweating, insomnia, and vomiting.

AMPHETAMINE; DEXTROAMPHETAMINE (ADDERALL, ADDERAL XR)

Available Forms

Capsule, extended release (Adderall XR): 5, 10, 15, 20, 25, 30 mg.
Tablet: 5, 10, 20, 30 mg.

Dosage

For attention-deficit/hyperactivity disorder (ADHD), initial dose in children 3 to 5 years old is 2.5 mg/day.
Daily dose may be increased in 2.5-mg increments at weekly intervals.
For children 6 years and older, the initial dose is 5 mg qd or bid.

Indications

ADHD, narcolepsy, obesity.
Exogenous Adderall XR is indicated for use in children 6 years of age and older.

Action

A single-entity amphetamine product combining the neutral sulfate salts of dextroamphetamine and amphetamine, with the dextro isomer of amphetamine saccharate and D,L-amphetamine aspartate.

Contraindications and Precautions

Do not use in children younger than 3 years.
Contraindicated in patients with advanced arteriosclerosis, symptomatic cardiovascular disease, moderate to severe hypertension, hyperthyroidism, known hypersensitivity or idiosyncrasy to the sympathomimetic amines, glaucoma, agitated states, or a history of drug abuse.
Do not use during or within 14 days following administration of MAOIs (hypertensive crisis can result).
Use caution in prescribing amphetamines for patients with even mild hypertension.
Amphetamines have a high potential for abuse. Administration of amphetamines for prolonged periods can lead to drug dependence and must be avoided. Particular attention should be paid to the possibility of subjects obtaining amphetamines for nontherapeutic use or distribution to others, and the drugs should be prescribed or dispensed sparingly.

Side Effects

Anorexia, insomnia, weight loss, emotional lability, depression.

ANAFRANIL; SEE CLOMIPRAMINE HYDROCHLORIDE

ANTABUSE; SEE DISULFIRAM

ARICEPT; SEE DONEPEZIL

ARIPIPRAZOLE (ABILIFY)

Available Form

Tablet: 5, 10, 15, 20, 30 mg.

Dosage

Recommended starting and target dose is 10 or 15 mg/day administered once a day without regard to meals.

Dosage increases should not be made before 2 weeks, the time needed to achieve steady-state.

Indications

Schizophrenia, bipolar disorder, mania.

Action

Psychotropic.

Contraindications and Precautions

Neuroleptic malignant syndrome (NMS) has been reported in association with administration of antipsychotic drugs.

Side Effects

Common side effects include headache, nausea, constipation, anxiety, restlessness, weakness, nervousness, rash, sleepiness or unusual drowsiness, insomnia, vomiting, and weight gain.

Less common side effects include blurred vision, coughing, fever, runny or stuffy nose, sneezing, and tremor.

ATIVAN; *SEE* LORAZEPAM

ATOMOXETINE HYDROCHLORIDE (STRATTERA)

Available Form

Capsule: 10, 18, 25, 40, 60 mg.

Dosage

For children and adolescents up to 70 kg body weight, initially 0.5 mg/kg, increased after a minimum of 3 days to a maximum of 1.2 mg/kg.

For children and adolescents weighing more than 70 kg and for adults, initially 40 mg/day, increased after at least 3 days to a maximum of 80 mg. In the absence of an optimal response, the daily dose may be increased to 100 mg after 2 to 4 weeks.

The total daily dose in children and adolescents should not exceed 1.4 mg/kg or 100 mg, whichever is less.

Indication

Attention-deficit/hyperactivity disorder.

Action

A selective norepinephrine reuptake inhibitor.

Contraindications and Precautions

Should not be taken with or 2 weeks after discontinuing an MAOI.

Not recommended in patients with narrow-angle glaucoma.

Allergic reactions, including angioneurotic edema, urticaria, and rash, have been reported.

Use with caution in patients with hypertension, tachycardia, or cardiovascular or cerebrovascular disease.

Side Effects

Dyspepsia, nausea, vomiting, fatigue, decreased appetite, dizziness, and mood swings.

BEVITAMEL; *SEE* MELATONIN–B-VITAMIN SUPPLEMENT

BUPRENORPHINE HYDROCHLORIDE (SUBOXONE, SUBUTEX)

Available Forms

Tablet, sublingual disintegrating (Suboxone): 2/0.5, 8/2 mg (buprenorphine HCl/naloxone).

Tablet, sublingual disintegrating (Subutex): 2, 8 mg.

Dosage

Administered sublingually as a single daily dose in the range of 12 to 16 mg/day.

Indication

Treatment of opioid dependence.

Action

Suboxone sublingual tablets contain buprenorphine HCl and naloxone HCl dihydrate in a ratio of 4:1 buprenorphine to naloxone (ratio of free bases). Subutex sublingual tablets contain buprenorphine HCl.

Buprenorphine is a partial agonist at the μ opioid receptor and an antagonist at the κ opioid receptor. Naloxone is an antagonist at the μ opioid receptor

Contraindications and Precautions

Suboxone should not be administered to patients who have been shown to be hypersensitive to naloxone.

Use with caution in patients with compromised respiratory function.

Naloxone might not be effective in reversing the respiratory depression produced by buprenorphine HCl. Therefore, as with other potent opioids, the primary management of overdose should be the reestablishment of adequate ventilation, with mechanical assistance of respiration, if required.

Naloxone should be used with caution in patients with compromised respiratory function (e.g., chronic obstructive pulmonary disease [COPD], cor pulmonale, decreased respiratory reserve, hypoxia, hypercapnia, or preexisting respiratory depression).

Side Effects

Sedation, nausea, dizziness or vertigo, sweating, hypotension, vomiting, miosis, headache, and hypoventilation.

BUPROPION HYDROCHLORIDE (WELLBUTRIN, WELLBUTRIN SR, WELLBUTRIN XL, ZYBAN)

Available Forms

Tablet (Wellbutrin): 75, 100 mg.

Tablet, extended release (Wellbutrin SR): 100, 150, 200 mg.

Tablet, extended release (Wellbutrin XL): 150, 300 mg/24 h.
Tablet, sustained release (Zyban): 150 mg.

Dosage

Wellbutrin: Initially 100–150 mg/day, adjusted to 300 mg/day as needed. Maximum recommended dose is 450 mg/day.

Wellbutrin SR: Initially 150 mg/day with increase to target of 300 mg/day as early as day 4 of dosing. Maximum recommended dose is 450 mg/day.

Wellbutrin XL: Initially 150 mg/day with increase to target 300 mg/day as early as day 4 of dosing. Maximum recommended dose is 450 mg/day.

Indications

Depression, smoking cessation.

Action

An antidepressant of the aminoketone class.

Contraindications and Precautions

Contraindicated in patients with a seizure disorder, patients currently treated with Zyban sustained-release tablets or any other medications that contain bupropion, and patients taking an MAOI.

Contraindicated in those with a current or prior diagnosis of bulimia or anorexia nervosa or patients undergoing abrupt discontinuation of alcohol or sedatives (including benzodiazepines).

The FDA has issued black box warnings for suicidality on all antidepressants (Box 22-1).

Side Effects

Agitation, dry mouth, insomnia, headache or migraine, nausea or vomiting, constipation, and tremor.

BUSPAR; *SEE* BUSPIRONE HYDROCHLORIDE

BUSPIRONE HYDROCHLORIDE (BUSPAR, BUSPAR DIVIDOSE)

Available Form

Tablet: 5, 7.5, 10, 15, 30 mg.

Dosage

Initial dose is 15 mg/day (7.5 mg bid).

At intervals of 2 or 3 days the dose may be increased by 5 mg/day, as needed.

The maximum daily dose should not exceed 60 mg.

Indications

Anxiety disorders.

Action

Antianxiety agent that is not chemically or pharmacologically related to the benzodiazepines, barbiturates, or other sedative or anxiolytic drugs.

Contraindications and Precautions

Administration to a patient taking an MAOI can pose a hazard.

BOX 22-1   FDA Black Box Warning on Antidepressants

Suicidality in Children and Adolescents

Antidepressants increase the risk of suicidal thinking and behavior (suicidality) in children and adolescents with major depressive disorder (MDD) and other psychiatric disorders. Anyone considering the use of [Drug Name] or any other antidepressant in a child or adolescent must balance this risk with the clinical need. Patients who are started on therapy should be observed closely for clinical worsening, suicidality, or unusual changes in behavior. Families and caregivers should be advised of the need for close observation and communication with the prescriber. [Drug Name] is not approved for use in pediatric patients except for patients with [Any approved pediatric claims here]. (See Warnings and Precautions: Pediatric Use)

Pooled analyses of short-term (4 to 16 weeks) placebo-controlled trials of nine antidepressant drugs (SSRIs and others) in children and adolescents with MDD, obsessive–compulsive disorder (OCD), or other psychiatric disorders (a total of 24 trials involving over 4400 patients) have revealed a greater risk of adverse events representing suicidal thinking or behavior (suicidality) during the first few months of treatment in those receiving antidepressants. The average risk of such events on drug was 4%, twice the placebo risk of 2%. No suicides occurred in these trials.

Side Effects

Dizziness, nausea, headache, nervousness, lightheadedness, excitement, and insomnia.

CAFCIT; *SEE* CAFFEINE CITRATE

CAFFEINE CITRATE (CAFCIT)

Available Forms

Liquid, citrate 20 mg/mL: 3 mL × 10.
Powder, compounding, anhydrous, 100%: 125, 500, 2500 g.
Solution, IV, citrate 20 mg/mL: 3 mL.

Dosage

Table 22-1 shows dosing for caffeine citrate.

Indication

Apnea of prematurity in infants 28 to 33 weeks' gestational age.

Action

CNS stimulant.

Contraindications and Precautions

Patients should be carefully monitored for the development of necrotizing enterocolitis.

Table 22-1 **Dosing for Caffeine Citrate**		
Attribute	**Loading Dose**	**Maintenance Dose**
Dose of caffeine citrate (volume)	1 mL/kg	0.25 mL/kg
Dose expressed as caffeine citrate	20 mg/kg	5 mg/kg
Dose expressed as caffeine base	10 mg/kg	2.5 mg/kg
Route	Intravenous* (Over 30 min)	Intravenous* (Over 10 min) or orally
Frequency	Once	Every 24 hours†

*Using a syringe infusion pump.
†Beginning 24 hours after the loading dose.

Rule out all other possible causes of apnea before treatment with caffeine citrate.

Side Effects

General: Diarrhea, dizziness, tachycardia, irritability, nervousness, or severe jitters (in newborn babies), nausea (severe), tremors, trouble sleeping, vomiting.

Hyperglycemia: Symptoms include blurred vision, drowsiness, dry mouth, flushed dry skin, fruit-like breath odor, increased urination, ketones in urine, anorexia, nausea, stomachache, tiredness, troubled breathing, unusual thirst, or vomiting (in neonates).

Hypoglycemia: Symptoms include anxiety, blurred vision, cold sweats, confusion, cool pale skin, drowsiness, excessive hunger, tachycardia, nausea, nervousness, restless sleep, shakiness, or unusual tiredness or weakness (in neonates).

CAMPRAL; *SEE* ACAMPROSATE CALCIUM

CARBAMAZEPINE (CARBATOL, EQUETRO, TEGRETOL, TEGRETOL-XR)

Available Forms

Capsule, extended release: 100, 200, 300, 400 mg.
Powder, compounding: 100%.
Suspension: 100 mg/5 mL.
Tablet: 200 mg.
Tablet, chewable: 100 mg.

Dosage

For treatment of mania and bipolar disorder, the initial dose is 400 mg/day divided bid.

Adjust the dose in 200-mg/day increments to achieve optimal clinical response.

Doses greater than 1600 mg/day have not been studied.

Indications

Glossopharyngeal and trigeminal neuralgia.

Complex partial, generalized tonic–clonic, and mixed-pattern seizures. Bipolar disorder, mania.

Action

Anticonvulsant and specific analgesic for trigeminal neuralgia.

The mechanism of action of carbamazepine in the treatment of bipolar disorder has not been elucidated.

Contraindications and Precautions

Aplastic anemia and agranulocytosis have been reported in association with use.

Carbamazepine should not be used in patients with a history of previous bone marrow depression, hypersensitivity to the drug, or known sensitivity to any of the tricyclic compounds such as amitriptyline, desipramine, imipramine, protriptyline, or nortriptyline. Likewise, on theoretical grounds its use with MAOIs is not recommended.

Patients with a history of adverse hematologic reaction to any drug may be particularly at risk.

Severe dermatologic reactions, including toxic epidermal necrolysis (Lyell's syndrome) and Stevens–Johnson syndrome, have been reported.

Side Effects

Dizziness, drowsiness, unsteadiness, nausea, and vomiting.

CARBATOL; *SEE* CARBAMAZEPINE

CELEXA; *SEE* CITALOPRAM HYDROBROMIDE

CHLORDIAZEPOXIDE HYDROCHLORIDE (LIBRIUM)

Available Form

Capsule, hard gelatin: 5, 10, 25 mg.

Dosage

Adults

Mild and moderate anxiety disorders and symptoms of anxiety: 5 to 10 mg tid or qid.

Severe anxiety and symptoms of anxiety: 20 to 25 mg tid or qid.

Children

Usual dose is 5 mg bid to qid.

Dose may be increased in some pediatric patients to 10 mg bid or tid.

Indications

For management of anxiety disorders or for short-term relief of symptoms of anxiety, withdrawal symptoms of acute alcoholism, and preoperative apprehension and anxiety.

Action

Antianxiety, sedative, appetite-stimulating, and weak analgesic actions.

Contraindications and Precautions

Avoid during pregnancy, because increased risk of congenital malformations has been associated with the use of minor tranquilizers.

Concomitant use of alcohol or other CNS depressants may have an additive effect.

Concomitant administration with other psychotropic medications is not recommended.

Withdrawal symptoms of the barbiturate type have occurred after the discontinuation of benzodiazepines.

Side Effects

Drowsiness, ataxia, confusion.

CITALOPRAM HYDROBROMIDE (CELEXA)

Available Forms

Solution: 10 mg/5 mL.
Tablet: 10, 40 mg.

Dosage

Initially, 20 mg/day in a single dose, with an increase to 40 mg/day.

Indication

Depression.

Action

Selective serotonin reuptake inhibitor.

Contraindications and Precautions

Do not use concurrently with an MAOI.

Side Effects

Asthenia, nausea, dry mouth, vomiting, dizziness, insomnia, somnolence, and agitation.

CLOMIPRAMINE HYDROCHLORIDE (ANAFRANIL)

Available Form

Capsule: 25, 50, 75 mg.

Dosage

Adults

Initial: 25 mg/day; gradually increased, as tolerated, to approximately 100 mg/day during the first 2 weeks.

During initial titration, clomipramine should be given in divided doses with meals to reduce gastrointestinal side effects. Thereafter, the dose may be increased gradually over the next several weeks to a maximum of 250 mg/day.

After titration, the total daily dose may be given once daily at bedtime to minimize daytime sedation.

Children and Adolescents

As with adults, the starting dose is 25 mg/day and should be gradually increased (also given in divided doses with meals to reduce gastrointestinal side effects) during the first 2 weeks, as tolerated, up to a daily maximum of 3 mg/kg or 100 mg, whichever is less.

Thereafter, the dose may be increased gradually over the next several weeks up to a daily maximum of 3 mg/kg or 200 mg, whichever is less.

Indication

Obsessions and compulsions in patients with obsessive—compulsive disorder (OCD).

Action

Clomipramine is an antiobsessional drug that belongs to the class (dibenzazepines) of tricyclic antidepressants.

Contraindications and Precautions

The FDA has issued black box warnings for suicidality on all antidepressants (see Box 22-1).

Clomipramine should not be given in combination, or within 14 days before or after treatment, with an MAOI.

It should not be given during the acute recovery period after a myocardial infarction.

Side Effects

Gastrointestinal: dry mouth, constipation, nausea, dyspepsia, and anorexia.

Genitourinary: changed libido, ejaculatory failure, impotence, and micturition disorder.

Miscellaneous: fatigue, sweating, increased appetite, weight gain, and visual changes.

Nervous system: somnolence, tremor, dizziness, nervousness, and myoclonus.

CLONAZEPAM (KLONOPIN)

Available Forms

Tablet: 0.5, 1, 2 mg.

Tablet, orally disintegrating (Klonopin Wafers): 0.125, 0.25, 0.5, 1, 2 mg.

Dosage

For anxiety, starting dose is usually 0.25 mg bid, increasing if needed to 1 mg/day after 3 days.

Indications

Panic disorder, with or without agoraphobia.

Seizure disorders, alone or as an adjunct in the treatment of the Lennox—Gastaut syndrome (petit mal variant) or akinetic and myoclonic seizures.

Action

A benzodiazepine.

Contraindications and Precautions

Avoid in patients with clinical or biochemical evidence of significant liver disease.

Avoid in patients with acute narrow-angle glaucoma.

Side Effects

Seizure Disorders

The most often seen side effects of clonazepam are referable to CNS depression. Experience in treatment of seizures has shown that

drowsiness has occurred in approximately 50% of patients and ataxia in approximately 30%. In some cases, these effects diminish with time.
Behavior problems have been noted in approximately 25% of patients.

Neurologic Effects

Abnormal eye movements, aphonia, choreiform movements, coma, diplopia, dysarthria, dysdiadochokinesis, glassy-eyed appearance, headache, hemiparesis, hypotonia, nystagmus, respiratory depression, slurred speech, tremor, and vertigo.

Psychiatric Effects

Confusion, depression, amnesia, hallucinations, hysteria, increased libido, insomnia, psychosis, suicide attempt.

The behavior effects are more likely to occur in patients with a history of psychiatric disturbances.

The following paradoxical reactions have been observed: excitability, irritability, aggressive behavior, agitation, nervousness, hostility, anxiety, sleep disturbances, nightmares, and vivid dreams.

CLORAZEPATE DIPOTASSIUM (TRANXENE)

Available Forms

Tablet (Tranxene T-Tab): 3.75, 7.5, 15 mg.
Tablet (Tranxene-SD): 11.25, 22.5 mg.

Dosage

Usual daily dose is 30 mg/day, divided.
Adjust gradually within the range of 15 to 60 mg/day.
The dose for elderly or debilitated patients is 7.5 to 15 mg/day.

Indications

Generalized anxiety disorder, alcohol withdrawal, partial seizures.

Action

A benzodiazepine.

Contraindications and Precautions

Avoid in patients with narrow-angle glaucoma.
Not recommended for patients with depressive neuroses or psychotic reactions.
Should not be used with other CNS-depressant drugs, in children younger than 9 years, or during pregnancy.

Side Effects

Common: Drowsiness is the most common effect.
Less common: Dizziness, various gastrointestinal complaints, nervousness, blurred vision, dry mouth, headache, and mental confusion.

CLOZAPINE (CLOZARIL, FAZACLO)

Available Forms

Tablet (Clozaril): 25, 100 mg.
Tablet, orally disintegrating: 25, 100 mg.

Dosage

Initial dose is one half of a 25-mg tablet (12.5 mg) bid or tid.

Titrate dosage up in increments of 25 to 50 mg/day, if well tolerated, to achieve a target dose of 300 to 450 mg/day by the end of 2 weeks.

Subsequent dosage increments should be made no more than once or twice weekly in increments not to exceed 100 mg.

Cautious titration and a divided dosing schedule are necessary to minimize the risks of hypotension, seizure, and sedation.

Indication

Severely ill schizophrenic patients who fail to respond adequately to standard drug treatment for schizophrenia.

Action

An atypical antipsychotic drug, a tricyclic dibenzodiazepine derivative.

Contraindications and Precautions

Contraindicated in patients with myeloproliferative disorders, uncontrolled epilepsy, or a history of clozapine-induced agranulocytosis or severe granulocytopenia.

Contraindicated in patients with severe CNS depression or comatose states from any cause.

This drug presents a significant risk of agranulocytosis. Avoid concomitant use with agents known to cause agranulocytosis or otherwise suppress bone marrow function.

Can increase risk of seizures, myocarditis, and other adverse cardiovascular and respiratory effects.

Side Effects

Cardiovascular: Primarily tachycardia, hypotension, and electrocardiographic (ECG) changes.

CNS: Primarily drowsiness or sedation, seizures, and dizziness or syncope.

Gastrointestinal: Primarily nausea and vomiting.

Hematologic: Primarily leukopenia, granulocytopenia, agranulocytosis, and fever.

CLOZARIL; *SEE* CLOZAPINE

CONCERTA; *SEE* METHYLPHENIDATE HYDROCHLORIDE

CYMBALTA; *SEE* DULOXETINE HYDROCHLORIDE

DALMANE; *SEE* FLURAZEPAM HYDROCHLORIDE

DEPAKENE; *SEE* VALPROIC ACID

DEPAKOTE; *SEE* DIVALPROEX SODIUM

DESIPRAMINE HYDROCHLORIDE (NORPRAMIN)

Available Form

Tablet: 10, 25, 50, 75, 100, 150 mg.

Dosage

Start with 100 to 200 mg/day.

Dose may be increased to 300 mg/day if necessary.

Indication

Depression.

Action

Antidepressant drug of the tricyclic type.

Contraindications and Precautions

Desipramine is contraindicated in patients taking an MAOI and in patients in the acute recovery period following myocardial infarction.

Extreme caution should be used in patients with cardiovascular disease, in patients with a history of urinary retention or glaucoma, in patients with thyroid disease or those taking thyroid medication, and in patients with a history of seizure disorder.

Not recommended for use in children because its safety and effectiveness in this age group has not been determined.

Side Effects

See imipramine.

DESOXYN; *SEE* METHAMPHETAMINE HYDROCHLORIDE
DEXEDRINE; *SEE* DEXTROAMPHETAMINE SULFATE
DEXMETHYLPHENIDATE HYDROCHLORIDE (FOCALIN)

Available Forms

Tablet: 2, 5, 10 mg.

Dosage

Initial dose is 5 mg/day.

Dose may be adjusted in 2.5- to 5-mg increments to a maximum of 20 mg/day.

Indication

Attention-deficit/hyperactivity disorder.

Action

A CNS stimulant.

Contraindications and Precautions

Contraindicated in patients with marked anxiety, tension, and agitation; glaucoma; motor tics or with a family history or diagnosis of Tourette's syndrome; and during treatment with MAOIs, and also within a minimum of 14 days following discontinuation of an MAOI (hypertensive crisis can result).

Should not be used to treat severe depression, or to prevent or treat normal fatigue states.

It should not be used in children younger than 6 years, because safety and efficacy in this age group have not been established.

Side Effects

Twitching, anorexia, insomnia, and tachycardia.

DEXTROAMPHETAMINE SACCHARATE; SEE AMPHETAMINE

DEXTROAMPHETAMINE SULFATE (DEXEDRINE SPANSULE, DEXTROSTAT)

Available Forms

Capsule, extended release (Dexedrine Spansule): 5, 10, 15 mg.
Tablet (Dexedrine, DextroStat): 5, 10 mg.

Dosage

Narcolepsy

The usual dose is 5 to 60 mg/day in divided doses, depending on the individual patient response.

Attention-Deficit/Hyperactivity Disorder

This drug is not recommended for pediatric patients younger than 3 years.

Pediatric patients 3 to 5 years of age: Start with 2.5 mg/day, by tablet. The daily dosage may be raised in increments of 2.5 mg at weekly intervals until the optimal response is obtained.

Pediatric patients 6 years of age and older: Start with 5 mg once or twice daily. The daily dosage may be raised in increments of 5 mg at weekly intervals until the optimal response is obtained.

Indications

Attention-deficit/hyperactivity disorder, narcolepsy.

Action

A sympathomimetic amine of the amphetamine group.

Contraindications and Precautions

Dextroamphetamine is contraindicated in advanced arteriosclerosis, symptomatic cardiovascular disease, moderate to severe hypertension, hyperthyroidism, known hypersensitivity or idiosyncrasy to the sympathomimetic amines, glaucoma, agitated states, patients with a history of drug abuse, and during or within 14 days following the administration of MAOIs (hypertensive crisis can result).

Exercise caution in prescribing amphetamines for patients with even mild hypertension. The least amount feasible should be prescribed or dispensed at one time to minimize the possibility of overdose.

Side Effects

Allergic: Urticaria.

Cardiovascular: Palpitations, tachycardia, and elevation of blood pressure. There have been isolated reports of cardiomyopathy associated with chronic amphetamine use.

CNS: Psychotic episodes at recommended doses (rare), overstimulation, restlessness, dizziness, insomnia, euphoria, dyskinesia, dysphoria, tremor, headache, and exacerbation of motor and phonic tics and Tourette's syndrome.

Endocrine: Impotence, changes in libido.

Gastrointestinal: Dry mouth, unpleasant taste, diarrhea, constipation, other gastrointestinal disturbances. Anorexia and weight loss can occur as undesirable effects.

DEXTROSTAT; *SEE* DEXTROAMPHETAMINE SULFATE

DIASTAT; *SEE* DIAZEPAM

DIAZEPAM (DIASTAT, DIASTAT PEDIATRIC, VALIUM)

Available Forms

Concentrate: 5 mg/mL.
Gel (rectal): 5 mg/mL.
Solution (injectable): 5 mg/mL, 5 mg/5 mL.
Tablet: 2, 5, 10 mg.

Dosage

Adults: 2 to 10 mg bid to qid.
Geriatric patients: Initially, 2 to 2.5 mg qd or bid. Increase gradually as needed and tolerated.
Pediatric patients: Initially, 1 to 2.5 mg tid or qid. Increase gradually as needed and tolerated.

Indications

Generalized anxiety disorder, preanesthesia, generalized tonic–clonic seizures, alcohol withdrawal, muscle spasm, athetosis, delirium tremens, status epilepticus, stiff-man syndrome, tetanus.

Action

A benzodiazepine derivative.

Contraindications and Precautions

Diazepam is contraindicated in acute narrow-angle glaucoma and in open-angle glaucoma unless patients are receiving appropriate therapy.
Because the diazepam emulsion vehicle contains soybean oil, diazepam injectable emulsion should not be used in patients with known hypersensitivity to soy protein.

Warnings

When diazepam is used intravenously, the following procedures should be undertaken to reduce the possibility of venous thrombosis, phlebitis, local irritation, swelling, and, rarely, vascular impairment.

- Diazepam should be injected slowly, taking at least 1 minute for each 5 mg (1 mL) given.
- Do not use small veins, such as those on the dorsum of the hand or wrist.
- Extreme care should be taken to avoid intra-arterial administration or extravasation.

Do not mix or dilute diazepam with other solutions or drugs in the syringe or infusion container. If it is not feasible to administer diazepam directly IV, it may be injected slowly through the infusion tubing as close as possible to the vein insertion.

Extreme care must be used in administering injectable diazepam by the IV route to the elderly, to very ill patients, and to those with limited pulmonary reserve because apnea and/or cardiac arrest can occur.

Concomitant use of barbiturates, alcohol, or other CNS depressants increases depression with increased risk of apnea. Resuscitative equipment including that necessary to support respiration should be readily available.

When diazepam is used with a narcotic analgesic, the dosage of the narcotic should be reduced by at least one third and administered in small increments. In some cases a narcotic is not necessary with diazepam.

Diazepam should not be administered to patients in shock, coma, or acute alcoholic intoxication with depression of vital signs.

Diazepam should not be used during pregnancy or in neonates aged 30 days or younger.

Side Effects

Drowsiness, fatigue, and ataxia.

Venous thrombosis and phlebitis at the site of injection (injectable solution).

DIPRIVAN; *SEE* PROPOFOL

DISULFIRAM (ANTABUSE)

Available Form

Tablet: 250 mg.

Dosage

Initially, maximum of 500 mg/day in a single dose for 1 to 2 weeks.

The average maintenance dose is 250 mg/day (range, 125-500 mg/day). The maximum dose is 500 mg/day.

Indication

Treatment of chronic alcoholism in patients who want a state of enforced sobriety.

Action

Blocks the oxidation of alcohol at the acetaldehyde stage.

During alcohol metabolism after intake, the concentration of acetaldehyde occurring in the blood may be 5 to 10 times higher than that found during metabolism of the same amount of alcohol alone.

Accumulation of acetaldehyde in the blood produces a complex of highly unpleasant symptoms.

Contraindications and Precautions

Contraindicated in patients who have recently received metronidazole, paraldehyde, alcohol, or alcohol-containing preparations.

Contraindicated in patients with severe myocardial disease or coronary occlusion.

Contraindicated in patients with psychoses.

Contraindicated in patients with hypersensitivity to thiuram derivatives used in pesticides and rubber vulcanization.

Never administer disulfiram to an intoxicated patient or without the patient's full knowledge.

Use with caution in concomitant treatment with phenytoin and its congeners and in patients with diabetes mellitus, hypothyroidism, epilepsy, cerebral damage, chronic and acute nephritis, and hepatic cirrhosis or insufficiency.

Side Effects

Optic neuritis, peripheral neuritis, polyneuritis, peripheral neuropathy, and hepatitis.

DIVALPROEX SODIUM (DEPAKOTE, DEPAKOTE ER, DEPAKOTE SPRINKLES)

Available Forms

Capsule, enteric coated: 125 mg.
Tablet, enteric coated: 125, 250, 500 mg.
Tablet, extended release: 250, 500 mg.

Dosage

For seizures, therapy is initiated at 10 to 15 mg/kg/day and increased by 5 to 10 mg/kg/day every week to achieve the desired response. Response is usually seen when the blood concentration of valproic acid is 50 to 100 μg/mL.

For mania, give 750 mg/day in divided doses and increase until the desired effect or plasma concentration at trough of 50 to 125 μg/mL is achieved. The maximum dose is 60 mg/kg/day.

For migraine, give 250 mg bid. The maximum recommended dose is 1000 mg/day.

Indications

Absence or complex partial seizures.
Migraine headache prophylaxis.
Bipolar disorder, mania.

Action

Divalproex sodium is a stable coordination compound composed of sodium valproate and valproic acid in a 1:1 molar relationship and formed during the partial neutralization of valproic acid with 0.5 equivalent of sodium hydroxide.

Contraindications and Precautions

Contraindicated in patients with hepatic disease and known urea cycle disorders.

Use with caution in patients with renal disease, Addison's disease, or blood dyscrasias.

Side Effects

Nausea, somnolence, dizziness, vomiting, weakness, diarrhea, anorexia, thrombocytopenia, weight gain, tremor, alopecia, diplopia.

DONEPEZIL (ARICEPT)

Available Forms

Tablet: 5, 10 mg.

Dosage

Initially 5 mg hs.

May increase to 10 mg hs after 4 to 6 weeks.

Indication

Mild to moderate dementia of the Alzheimer type.

Action

Reversible acetylcholinesterase inhibitor.

Contraindications and Precautions

Contraindicated in patients with sick sinus syndrome or other supraventricular cardiac conduction abnormalities.

Concomitant treatment with nonsteroidal antiinflammatory drugs (NSAIDs) can increase risk of gastrointestinal bleed.

Side Effects

Nausea, insomnia, diarrhea, vomiting, anorexia, and muscle cramps.

DOXEPIN HYDROCHLORIDE (SINEQUAN)

Available Forms

Capsule: 10, 25, 50, 75, 100, 150 mg.

Concentrate: 10 mg/mL.

Dosage

A starting dose of 75 mg/day is recommended.

Dosage may subsequently be increased or decreased at appropriate intervals and according to individual response.

The usual optimum dose range is 75 to 150 mg/day.

Indication

Depression, anxiety.

Action

One of a class of psychotherapeutic agents known as dibenzoxepin tricyclic compounds.

Contraindications and Precautions

Contraindicated in patients with glaucoma or a tendency to urinary retention.

The once-a-day dosage regimen of doxepin in patients with intercurrent illness or patients taking other medications should be carefully adjusted. This is especially important in patients receiving other medications with anticholinergic effects.

Side Effects

Seizures, fast or irregular heartbeat, heart attack, high blood pressure, tinnitus, nausea, agitation, sweating, difficulty urinating, fever with increased sweating, muscle stiffness or severe muscle weakness, weakness, headache, dizziness or drowsiness, constipation, dry mouth and eyes, blurred vision, tremors or muscle twitches, anorexia, abdominal pain.

DULOXETINE HYDROCHLORIDE (CYMBALTA)
Available Form
Capsule: 20, 30, 60 mg.

Dosage
Standard dose is 40 mg/day (given as 20 mg bid) to 60 mg/day (given either in one dose or as 30 mg bid) without regard to meals.

Indication
Major depressive disorder.

Action
Selective serotonin and norepinephrine reuptake inhibitor.

Contraindications and Precautions
Concurrent use with an MAOI is contraindicated.
Avoid in patients with uncontrolled narrow-angle glaucoma.

Side Effects
Nausea, dry mouth, constipation, diarrhea, vomiting, anorexia, weight decrease, fatigue, dizziness, somnolence, tremor, increased sweating, hot flushes, blurred vision, insomnia, anxiety, decreased libido, abnormal orgasm, erectile dysfunction, delayed ejaculation, ejaculatory dysfunction.

EFFEXOR; SEE VENLAFAXINE HYDROCHLORIDE
ELAVIL; SEE AMITRIPTYLINE HYDROCHLORIDE
ELDEPRYL; SEE SELEGILINE HYDROCHLORIDE
EQUETRO; SEE CARBAMAZEPINE
ESCITALOPRAM (LEXAPRO)
Available Forms
Solution: 1 mg/mL.
Tablet: 5, 10, 20 mg.

Dosage
Initial dose is 10 mg qd.

Indication
Depression.

Action
Selective serotonin reuptake inhibitor.

Contraindications and Precautions
Contraindicated in patients taking MAOIs.
Use with caution in patients with hepatic or renal disease or epilepsy.

Side Effects
Insomnia, somnolence, dizziness, headache, tremor, fatigue, male sexual dysfunction, dry mouth, diarrhea, nausea.

ESKALITH; *SEE* LITHIUM CARBONATE

ESTAZOLAM (PROSOM)

Available Forms

Tablet: 1, 2 mg.

Dosage

Initial dose is 1 mg hs. The dose may be increased to 2 mg if indicated.
In small or debilitated patients, an initial dose of 0.5 mg may be warranted.

Indication

Insomnia.

Action

Triazolobenzodiazepine derivative, oral hypnotic agent.

Contraindications and Precautions

Contraindicated in pregnant women.
Contraindicated in patients using alcohol and other CNS depressants.
Safe and effective use in children younger than 18 years has not been
    established.

Side Effects

Somnolence, hypokinesia, dizziness, and abnormal coordination.

ESZOPICLONE (LUNESTA)

Available Form

Tablet: 1, 2, 3 mg.

Dosage

Dosage should be individualized. The recommended starting dose is
    2 mg hs. Dosing can be initiated at or raised to 3 mg if clinically
    indicated.
For elderly and/or debilitated patients, the suggested starting dose is 1 mg.

Indication

Insomnia.

Action

Nonbenzodiazepine hypnotic agent that is a pyrrolopyrazine derivative of
    the cyclopyrrolone class.

Contraindications and Precautions

There are no known contraindications.
Because sleep disturbances may be the presenting manifestation of a phys-
    ical and/or psychiatric disorder, symptomatic treatment of insomnia
    should be initiated only after a careful evaluation of the patient.
    Sedative—hypnotic drugs should be administered with caution to
    patients exhibiting signs and symptoms of depression.

Side Effects

Unpleasant taste, headache, drowsiness, dizziness.

EXELON; *SEE* RIVASTIGMINE
FAZACLO; *SEE* CLOZAPINE
FLUOXETINE HYDROCHLORIDE (PROZAC, SARAFEM, SYMBYAX)

Available Forms

Capsule (Sarafem): 10, 20 mg.
Capsule, enteric-coated delayed-release (Prozac Weekly): 90 mg.
Capsule, gel: 10, 20, 40 mg.
Solution: 20 mg/5 mL.
Tablet: 10 mg.

Dosage

For depression or OCD, the initial dose is 10 to 20 mg qAM. Increase the
    dose if needed after several weeks. The maximum dose is 80 mg/day.
For bulimia, the initial dose is 60 mg qAM.
For premenstrual dysphoric disorder, the dose is 10 to 20 mg/day.

Indications

Depression, OCD, bulimia, and premenstrual dysphoric disorder.

Action

Selective serotonin reuptake inhibitor.

Contraindications and Precautions

Do not use concurrently with or within 14 days of taking an MAOI.
Fluoxetine inhibits the metabolism of tricyclic antidepressants and possi-
    bly antipsychotic drugs and can increase their toxicity.
Use with caution in patients with renal, hepatic, or cardiac disease
    and in patients with a history of seizures or who are using other CNS
    drugs.
Discontinue if rash occurs.
Fluoxetine increases the international normalized ratio (INR) in patients
    using warfarin; it also increases the digoxin level. Therefore, close
    monitoring is indicated in patients taking these medications.

Side Effects

Anorexia, tremor, nausea, drowsiness, and insomnia.

FLUPHENAZINE HYDROCHLORIDE (PERMITIL, PROLIXIN, PROLIXIN DECANOATE)

Available Forms

Concentrate: 5 mg/mL.
Elixir: 2.5 mg/5 mL.
Solution, injectable: 2.5 mg/mL.
Solution, injectable, decanoate: 25 mg/mL.
Tablet: 1, 2.5, 5, 10 mg.

Dosage

Tablets and Elixir

The initial adult dose is 2.5 to 10 mg divided and given at 6- to 8-hour
    intervals. Treatment is best instituted with a low initial dose, which

may be increased, if necessary, until the desired clinical effects are achieved.

The therapeutic effect is often achieved with doses less than 20 mg/day. Maximum dose is 40 mg/day. Maintenance dose is 1 to 5 mg/day.

For psychotic patients who have been stabilized on a fixed daily dose of oral fluphenazine, conversion to the long-acting injectable fluphenazine decanoate may be indicated.

For geriatric patients, the suggested starting dose is 1.0 to 2.5 mg/day, adjusted according to the response of the patient.

Injection

Initially, 1.25 mg (0.5 mL) IM. Depending on the severity and duration of symptoms, initial total daily dose may range from 2.5 to 10 mg divided and given at 6- to 8-hour intervals.

Doses exceeding 10 mg/day should be used with caution.

Indication

Management of manifestations of psychotic disorders and of behavioral complications in patients with mental retardation.

Action

A trifluoroethyl phenothiazine derivative.

Contraindications and Precautions

Fluphenazine is contraindicated in patients with suspected or established subcortical brain damage, receiving large doses of hypnotics, in comatose or severely depressed states, and with blood dyscrasias or liver damage.

Because of the possibility of cross-sensitivity, fluphenazine should be used cautiously in patients who have developed cholestatic jaundice, dermatoses, or other allergic reactions to phenothiazine derivatives.

Fluphenazine HCl tablets 2.5, 5, and 10 mg contain FD&C yellow no. 5 (tartrazine), which can cause allergic-type reactions (including bronchial asthma) in certain susceptible persons. Although the overall incidence of tartrazine sensitivity in the general population is low, it is often seen in patients who also have aspirin hypersensitivity.

Psychotic patients taking large doses of a phenothiazine drug who are undergoing surgery should be watched carefully for possible hypotensive phenomena. Reduced amounts of anesthetics or CNS depressants may be necessary.

The effects of atropine may be potentiated in some patients receiving fluphenazine because of added anticholinergic effects.

Fluphenazine should be used cautiously in patients exposed to extreme heat or phosphorus insecticides; in patients with a history of convulsive disorders, because grand mal convulsions have been known to occur; and in patients with certain medical disorders, such as mitral valve insufficiency or other cardiovascular diseases and pheochromocytoma.

Liver damage, pigmentary retinopathy, lenticular and corneal deposits, and development of irreversible dyskinesia are possible in patients on prolonged therapy.

Neuroleptic drugs elevate prolactin.

Side Effects

Most common are EPS, including tardive dyskinesia. The frequency and severity of EPS are directly proportional to the dose given and the duration of treatment.

Other side effects (sedation, hypotension, anticholinergic effects such as dry mouth and blurred vision) also vary with the dose given.

As a member of the phenothiazine class of drugs, fluphenazine shares in general all side effects of chlorpromazine. Sedative, allergic–toxic, and anticholinergic or sympatholytic side effects are less likely to occur compared with chlorpromazine.

FLURAZEPAM HYDROCHLORIDE (DALMANE)

Available Form

Capsule: 15, 30 mg.

Dosage

Dosage should be individualized for maximum beneficial effects. Initial dosage is 30 mg hs. In some patients, 15 mg might suffice.

In elderly and/or debilitated patients, 15 mg is usually sufficient for a therapeutic response.

Indication

Insomnia.

Action

A benzodiazepine derivative, oral hypnotic agent.

Contraindications and Precautions

Contraindicated in pregnant women.

Should not be used with alcohol and other CNS depressants.

Should not be given to children younger than 15 years.

Side Effects

Dizziness, drowsiness, lightheadedness, staggering, ataxia, and falling have occurred, particularly in elderly or debilitated persons.

Also reported were headache, heartburn, upset stomach, nausea, vomiting, diarrhea, constipation, gastrointestinal pain, nervousness, talkativeness, apprehension, irritability, weakness, palpitations, chest pains, body and joint pains, and genitourinary complaints.

FOCALIN; SEE DEXMETHYLPHENIDATE HYDROCHLORIDE

GALANTAMINE HYDROBROMIDE (RAZADYNE)

Available Forms

Capsule, extended release: 8, 16, 24 mg.

Solution: 4 mg/mL.

Tablet: 4, 8, 12 mg.

Dosage

Initial dose is 4 mg bid. The usual range is 16 to 32 mg/day.

Indication

Mild to moderate dementia of the Alzheimer type.

Action

Reversible, competitive acetylcholinesterase inhibitor.

Contraindications and Precautions

Galantamine may be expected to increase gastric acid secretion due to increased cholinergic activity.

Monitor for gastrointestinal bleeding with concurrent NSAIDs.

Side Effects

Nausea, vomiting, diarrhea, anorexia, weight loss.

GEODON; *SEE* ZIPRASIDONE HYDROCHLORIDE, ZIPRASIDONE MESYLATE

HALCION; *SEE* TRIAZOLAM

HALOPERIDOL (HALDOL DECANOATE 50, HALDOL DECANOATE 100)

Available Form

Solution (IM): 50 mg haloperidol as 70.5 mg/mL haloperidol decanoate, 10 × 1 mL ampules, 3 × 1 mL ampules, and 5 mL multiple-dose-vials; 100 mg haloperidol as 141.04 mg/mL haloperidol decanoate, 5 × 1 mL ampules and 5 mL multiple-dose vials.

Dosage

Administer by deep IM injection. A 21-gauge needle is recommended. The maximum volume per injection site should not exceed 3 mL.

Do not administer intravenously.

Indication

Schizophrenic patients who require prolonged parenteral antipsychotic therapy.

Action

First of the butyrophenone series of major tranquilizers.

The precise mechanism of action has not been determined.

Contraindications and Precautions

Haloperidol is contraindicated in severe toxic CNS depression or comatose states from any cause and in patients who are hypersensitive to this drug or who have Parkinson's disease.

Side Effects

CNS Effects

EPS have been reported frequently, often during the first few days of treatment. EPS are Parkinson-like symptoms, akathisia, or dystonia (including opisthotonos and oculogyric crisis). EPS can occur at relatively low doses, but they occur more often and with greater severity at higher doses. The symptoms may be controlled with dose reductions or administration of antiparkinsonian drugs such as benztropine mesylate or trihexyphenidyl. Persistent EPS have been reported; the drug might have to be discontinued in such cases.

As with all antipsychotic agents, haloperidol has been associated with persistent dyskinesias. Tardive dyskinesia, which is potentially irreversible, can appear in some patients on long-term therapy with haloperidol decanoate or can occur after drug therapy has been discontinued.

Tardive dystonia, not associated with tardive dyskinesia, has also been reported. Tardive dystonia is characterized by delayed onset of choreic or dystonic movements, is often persistent, and can become irreversible.

Other CNS effects include insomnia, restlessness, anxiety, euphoria, agitation, drowsiness, depression, lethargy, headache, confusion, vertigo, grand mal seizures, exacerbation of psychotic symptoms including hallucinations, and catatonic-like behavioral states, which may be responsive to drug withdrawal and/or treatment with anticholinergic drugs.

Other Effects

Side effects that might go away during treatment include mild drowsiness, dizziness, changes in menstrual cycle, or swelling or pain in the breasts.

Other adverse effects include drowsiness or sleepiness, drooling, difficulty speaking or swallowing, muscle stiffness, fever, restless body movements, mild hand or leg tremors, or other unusual body movements or muscle twitching.

IMIPRAMINE (TOFRANIL, TOFRANIL PM)

Available Forms

Capsule, pamoate (Tofranil PM): 75, 100, 125, 150 mg.
Tablet, HCl: 10, 25, 50 mg.

Dosage

Adults: 25 to 50 mg tid or qid (not to exceed 300 mg/day). Total daily dose may be given at bedtime.

Geriatric patients: 25 mg at bedtime initially, up to 100 mg/day in divided doses.

Children older than 12 years: 25 to 50 mg/day in divided doses (not to exceed 100 mg/day). Children 6 to 12 years: 10 to 30 mg/day in two divided doses.

IM (Adults): Up to 100 mg/day in divided doses (not to exceed 300 mg/day).

Indication

Depression.

Action

Tricyclic antidepressant.

Contraindications and Precautions

Imipramine can cause hypotension, tachycardia, and potentially fatal reactions when used with MAOIs. Do not prescribe imipramine and MAOIs concurrently and discontinue the MAOI 2 weeks before starting imipramine.

Concurrent use with SSRI antidepressants can result in increased toxicity and should be avoided. Fluoxetine should be stopped 5 weeks before starting imipramine.

Concurrent use with clonidine can result in hypertensive crisis and should be avoided.

Side Effects

Sedation, urinary retention, constipation, dry mouth, dizziness, drowsiness, and arrhythmia.

KLONOPIN; *SEE* CLONAZEPAM
LAMICTAL; *SEE* LAMOTRIGINE
LAMOTRIGINE (LAMICTAL)

Available Forms

Tablet: 25, 100, 150, 200 mg.
Tablet, chewable: 2, 5, 25 mg.

Dosage

See manufacturer's product information for proper dosing.

Indications

Bipolar disorder.
Lennox—Gastaut syndrome, partial seizures.

Action

An antiepileptic drug of the phenyltriazine class.

Contraindications and Precautions

Safety and effectiveness of lamotrigine have not been established as initial monotherapy, for conversion to monotherapy from non—enzyme-inducing antiepileptic drugs except valproate, or for simultaneous conversion to monotherapy from two or more concomitant antiepileptic drugs.

Safety and effectiveness in pediatric patients younger than 16 years, other than those with partial seizures and the generalized seizures of Lennox—Gastaut syndrome, have not been established.

Side Effects

Rash

Serious rashes requiring hospitalization and discontinuation of treatment have been reported. Because the rate of serious rash is greater in pediatric patients than in adults, lamotrigine is approved only for use in pediatric patients younger than 16 years who have seizures associated with the Lennox—Gastaut syndrome or in patients with partial seizures.

Other than age, no known factors predict the risk of occurrence or the severity of rash associated with lamotrigine. There are suggestions, yet to be proved, that the risk of rash may also be increased by coadministration of lamotrigine with valproate, exceeding the recommended initial dose of lamotrigine, or exceeding the recommended dose escalation for lamotrigine. However, cases have been reported in the absence of these factors.

Nearly all cases of life-threatening rash associated with lamotrigine have occurred within 2 to 8 weeks of initiating treatment. However, isolated cases have been reported after prolonged treatment (e.g., 6 months).

Accordingly, duration of therapy cannot be relied upon as a means to predict the potential risk heralded by the first appearance of a rash.

Although benign rashes also occur with lamotrigine, it is not possible to predict reliably which rashes will prove to be serious or life-threatening. Accordingly, lamotrigine should ordinarily be discontinued at the first sign of rash, unless the rash is clearly not drug related. Discontinuation of treatment might not prevent a rash from becoming life-threatening or permanently disabling or disfiguring.

Other Adverse Effects

More common: blurred vision, dizziness, double vision, headache, nausea, rash, sleepiness, uncoordinated movements, and vomiting.

Less common: abdominal pain, accidental injury, anxiety, constipation, depression, diarrhea, fever, flulike symptoms, increased cough, inflammation of vagina, irritability, painful menstruation, sore throat, and tremor.

Rare: absence of menstrual periods, chills, confusion, dry mouth, ear pain, emotional changes, heart palpitations, hot flushes, joint disorders, memory decrease, mind racing, muscle weakness, muscle spasm, poor concentration, ringing in ears, sleep disorder, and speech disorder.

Additional side effects in children: bronchitis, convulsions, ear problems, eczema, facial swelling, hemorrhage, infection, indigestion, light sensitivity, lymph node problems, nervousness, penis disorder, sinus infection, swelling, tooth problems, urinary tract infection, vertigo, and vision problems.

LEXAPRO; *SEE* ESCITALOPRAM

LIBRIUM; *SEE* CHLORDIAZEPOXIDE HYDROCHLORIDE

LITHIUM CARBONATE (ESKALITH, ESKALITH CR, LITHOBID)

Available Forms

Capsules (Eskalith): 300 mg.
Tablets, controlled release (Eskalith CR): 450 mg.

Dosage

Adults and Children 12 Years and Older

Tablets or capsules: 300 to 600 mg tid initially. The usual maintenance dose is 300 mg tid or qid.

Slow-release capsules: 200 to 300 mg tid initially. Dose may be increased up to 1800 mg/day in divided doses. Usual maintenance dose is 300 to 400 mg tid.

Extended-release tablets: 450 to 900 mg bid or 300 to 600 mg tid initially. The usual maintenance dose is 450 mg bid or 300 mg tid.

Children Younger than 12 Years

Initial dose is 15 to 20 mg (0.4-0.5 mEq)/kg/day divided bid or tid.
Dosage may be adjusted weekly.

Indication

Manic episodes of manic–depressive illness.

Action

Alters sodium transport in nerve and muscle cells and effects a shift toward intraneuronal metabolism of catecholamines.

Contraindications and Precautions

Lithium toxicity is closely related to serum lithium levels and can occur at doses close to therapeutic levels. Facilities for prompt and accurate serum lithium determinations should be available before initiating therapy.

Lithium should generally not be given to patients with significant renal or cardiovascular disease, severe debilitation or dehydration, or sodium depletion, because such patients have higher risk of lithium toxicity.

Lithium is not recommended for patients younger than 12 years.

Side Effects

Abdominal pain, arthralgia, blackout spells, cavities, changes in taste perception, coma, confusion, dehydration, dizziness, dry hair, dry mouth, fatigue, frequent urination, gas, hair thinning or loss, hallucinations, hand tremor, increased salivation, indigestion, involuntary tongue movements, urinary or fecal incontinence, irregular heartbeat, pruritus, anorexia, hypotension, mild thirst, muscle rigidity, muscle twitching, nausea, poor memory, restlessness, tinnitus, seizures, sexual dysfunction, skin problems, sleepiness, slowed thinking, slurred speech, startle response, swelling, tightness in chest, vision problems, vomiting, weakness, weight gain, weight loss.

LITHOBID; *SEE* LITHIUM CARBONATE

LORAZEPAM (ATIVAN)

Available Forms

Solution, injectable: 2, 4 mg/mL.
Tablet: 0.5, 1, 2 mg.

Dosage

Oral

For optimal results, dose, frequency of administration, and duration of therapy should be individualized according to patient response.

The usual range is 2 to 6 mg/day given in divided doses, the largest dose being taken before bedtime, but the daily dosage may vary from 1 to 10 mg/day.

Intravenous

Recommended initial dose is 2 mg total, or 0.02 mg/lb (0.044 mg/kg), whichever is less. This dose suffices for sedating most adult patients and should not ordinarily be exceeded in patients older than 50 years.

Indication

Anxiety disorder.

Action

Benzodiazepine with antianxiety and sedative effects.

Contraindications and Precautions

Lorazepam is contraindicated in patients with acute narrow-angle glaucoma.

Before injection, lorazepam must be diluted with an equal amount of compatible diluent. IV injection should be made slowly and with repeated aspiration. Care should be taken to determine that any injection will not be intraarterial and that perivascular extravasation will not take place.

Partial airway obstruction can occur in heavily sedated patients. Intravenous lorazepam, when given alone in greater than the recommended dose, or at the recommended dose and accompanied by other drugs used during administration of anesthesia, can produce heavy sedation. Therefore, equipment necessary to maintain a patent airway and to support respiration and ventilation should be available.

Lorazepam can cause fetal damage when administered to pregnant women.

Side Effects

Dizziness, sedation (excessive calm), unsteadiness, weakness.

LUNESTA; SEE ESZOPICLONE
MELATONIN–B-VITAMIN SUPPLEMENT (BEVITAMEL)

Available Form

Tablet: 3 mg melatonin, 1 mg vitamin B_{12}, 400 mg folic acid.

Dosage

One tablet sublingually approximately 30 minutes before bedtime.
Fractional tablets may be taken when indicated.

Indications

Can be used to enhance the natural sleep process.
Vitamin B_{12} and folic acid can be used to assist the metabolism of blood homocysteine.

Action

Not known.

Contraindications and Precautions

This product is not intended to treat pernicious anemia.
The dose size and timing might need to be adjusted to provide maximum effect for individual patients.
Use with caution in patients taking other medications; in patients with autoimmune, seizure, or endocrine disorders; and in pregnant or lactating women.

Side Effects

None known.

MELLARIL; *SEE* THIORIDAZINE HYDROCHLORIDE
MEMANTINE HYDROCHLORIDE (NAMENDA)
Available Forms

Solution: 2 mg/mL.
Tablet: 5, 10 mg; kit containing 49 tablets. 28 × 5 mg and 21 × 10 mg.

Dosage

Initial dose is 5 mg qd.
The recommended target dose is 20 mg/day. Increase in 5-mg increments
to 10 mg/day (5 mg bid), 15 mg/day (5 mg and 10 mg as separate doses),
and 20 mg/day.

Indication

Alzheimer's disease.

Action

NMDA (*N*-methyl-D-aspartate) receptor antagonist.

Contraindications and Precautions

Memantine is contraindicated in patients with known hypersensitivity to
memantine HCl or to any excipients used in the formulation.

Side Effects

Common: Dizziness, confusion, constipation, headaches, and rash.
Less common: Fatigue, back pain, hypertension, insomnia, hallucinations,
vomiting, and shortness of breath.

METADATE; *SEE* METHYLPHENIDATE
HYDROCHLORIDE
METHADONE HYDROCHLORIDE (METHADOSE)
Available Forms

Concentrate: 10 mg/mL.
Powder, compounding: 100%.
Solution: 5, 10 mg/5 mL.
Solution, injectable: 10 mg/mL (20 mL).
Tablet: 5, 10, 40 mg.

Dosage

Concentrate: Initially, a single dose of 20 to 30 mg. The initial dose
should not exceed 30 mg and the daily dose should not exceed 40 mg.
Tablet: 2.5 to 10 mg q3-4h as necessary.

Indications

Moderate to severe pain.
Opiate dependence or withdrawal.

Action

Methadone is a μ opioid agonist. It is a synthetic opioid analgesic with
multiple actions qualitatively similar to those of morphine, the most
prominent of which involve the CNS and organs composed of smooth
muscle.

The principal actions of therapeutic value are analgesia and sedation and detoxification or maintenance in opioid addiction.

Contraindications and Precautions

Can cause respiratory depression, sedation, increased intracranial pressure, hypotension, and bradycardia.

Side Effects

Lightheadedness, dizziness, sedation, nausea, vomiting, sweating, respiratory depression, and circulatory depression.

METHADOSE; *SEE* METHADONE HYDROCHLORIDE
METHAMPHETAMINE HYDROCHLORIDE (DESOXYN)

Available Form

Tablet: 5, 10 mg.

Dosage

For treatment of children 6 years or older with ADHD: initial dose is 5 mg qd or bid. Daily dosage may be raised in increments of 5 mg at weekly intervals until an optimal clinical response is achieved. The usual effective dose is 20 to 25 mg/day.

For obesity: 10 or 15 mg qAM. Treatment should not exceed a few weeks.

Indications

Attention-deficit/hyperactivity disorder.
Exogenous obesity.

Action

A member of the amphetamine group of sympathomimetic amines.

Contraindications and Precautions

Contraindicated during or within 14 days following the administration of MAOIs; hypertensive crisis can result.

Contraindicated in patients with glaucoma, advanced arteriosclerosis, symptomatic cardiovascular disease, moderate to severe hypertension, hyperthyroidism, or known hypersensitivity or idiosyncrasy to sympathomimetic amines.

Methamphetamine should not be given to patients who are in an agitated state or who have a history of drug abuse.

Methamphetamine should be used with caution in patients with even mild hypertension.

Prescribing and dispensing of methamphetamine should be limited to the smallest amount that is feasible at one time in order to minimize the possibility of overdose.

Methamphetamine is not recommended for use as an anorectic agent in children younger than 12 years.

Side Effects

Hypertension, tachycardia, palpitation, dizziness, dysphoria, overstimulation, euphoria, insomnia, tremor, restlessness, headache; exacerbation of motor and phonic tics and Tourette's syndrome; diarrhea, constipation, dry mouth, unpleasant taste, and other gastrointestinal disturbances; urticaria; impotence and changes in libido.

Suppression of growth has been reported with the long-term use of stimulants in children.

METHYLIN; *SEE* METHYLPHENIDATE HYDROCHLORIDE

METHYLPHENIDATE HYDROCHLORIDE (CONCERTA, METADATE, METHYLIN, RITALIN)

Available Forms

Capsule, extended release (Metadate CD): 10, 20, 30 mg.
Capsule, extended release (Ritalin LA): 20, 30, 40 mg.
Tablet (Methylin, Ritalin): 5, 10, 20 mg.
Tablet, extended release (Concerta): 18, 27, 36, 54 mg.
Tablet, extended release (Methylin ER, Metadate ER): 10, 20 mg.
Tablet, extended release (Ritalin SR): 20 mg.

Dosage

Concerta: Initially 18 mg qd. Adjust in 18-mg increments to a maximum of 54 mg/day.

Methylin: Adult average 20 to 30 mg/day in divided doses bid or tid. Children initially 5 mg bid for chewable tablets; adjust gradually in 5- to 10-mg increments weekly. Take with at least 8 oz (250 mL) of water.

Ritalin and Ritalin SR: Adult dose averages 20 to 30 mg/day. Pediatric dose initially is 10 mg/day, not to exceed 60 mg/day. Adjust in weekly 5- to 10-mg increments.

Ritalin LA: Initially 20 mg/day. May adjust in weekly 10-mg increments to maximum of 60 mg/day.

Indications

Attention-deficit/hyperactivity disorder, narcolepsy.

Action

Mild CNS stimulant.

Contraindications and Precautions

Do not use in children younger than 6 years.
Do not use in patients with agitation, glaucoma, motor tics, Tourette's syndrome, or family history of Tourette's.
Should not be used to treat severe depression or fatigue.
Tablets (except chewable) must be swallowed whole, never crushed or chewed.

Side Effects

Nervousness, insomnia, anorexia, abdominal pain, weight loss during prolonged therapy, and tachycardia.

MIRTAZAPINE (REMERON)

Available Forms

Tablet: 15, 30, 45 mg.
Tablet, disintegrating: 30, 45 mg.

Dosage

Initially, 15 mg/day administered in a single dose, preferably in the evening at bedtime.

Patients not responding to the initial 15-mg dose might benefit from dose increases up to a maximum of 45 mg/day.

Dose changes should not be made at less than 1- to 2-week intervals to allow for therapeutic observation.

Indication

Major depressive disorder.

Action

Has a tetracyclic chemical structure and belongs to the piperazine-azepine group of compounds.

Contraindications and Precautions

The FDA has issued black box warnings for suicidality on all antidepressants (see Box 22-1).

Risk of agranulocytosis has been reported. If a patient develops a sore throat, fever, stomatitis, or other signs of infection along with a low WBC count, treatment with mirtazapine should be discontinued and the patient should be closely monitored.

Concomitant treatment with MAOIs is not recommended.

In U.S. controlled studies, somnolence was reported in 54% of patients, dizziness in 7% of patients.

Side Effects

Malaise, abdominal pain, acute abdomen, vomiting, anorexia, hypertension, vasodilation, thirst, myasthenia, arthralgia, hypesthesia, apathy, depression, hypokinesia, vertigo, twitching, agitation, anxiety, amnesia, hyperkinesia, paresthesia, cough, sinusitis, pruritus, rash, urinary tract infection.

MOBAN; SEE MOLINDONE HYDROCHLORIDE
MODAFINIL (PROVIGIL)

Available Form

Tablet: 100, 200 mg.

Dosage

Dose is 200 mg qAM for narcolepsy and sleep apnea–hypopnea syndrome.

For shift-work sleep disorder, 200 mg/day approximately 1 hour before work shift.

Indications

Narcolepsy, obstructive sleep apnea, shift-work sleep disorder.

Action

A wakefulness-promoting agent for oral administration.
Modafinil is a racemic compound.

Contraindications and Precautions

Hypersensitivity to the drug, CYP2C19 interactions; caution when used with other CNS active drugs.

Side Effects

Headache, nausea, nervousness, rhinitis, diarrhea, back pain, anxiety, insomnia, dizziness, and dyspepsia.

MOLINDONE HYDROCHLORIDE (MOBAN)

Available Form

Tablet: 5, 10, 25, 50, 100 mg.

Dosage

Initial

Give 50 to 75 mg/day. Increase to 100 mg/day in 3 or 4 days.

Dosage may be titrated up or down according to individual patient response.

An increase to 225 mg/day may be required in patients with severe symptoms.

Elderly and debilitated patients should start at a lower dose.

Maintenance Dosage Schedule

Mild symptoms: 5 to 15 mg tid or qid.
Moderate symptoms: 10 to 25 mg tid or qid.
Severe symptoms: 225 mg/day may be required.

Indication

Schizophrenia.

Action

Molindone is a dihydroindolone compound that is not structurally related to the phenothiazines, the butyrophenones, or the thioxanthenes.

Contraindications and Precautions

Molindone should not be used in patients with severe CNS depression (e.g., alcohol, barbiturates, narcotics) or comatose states.

Tardive dyskinesia can develop in patients treated with antipsychotic drugs.

Side Effects

Drowsiness (especially at the start of therapy), galactorrhea, blood disorders, blurred vision, gynecomastia, changed mental state, changes in sex drive, constipation, depression, difficulty urinating, drooling, dry mouth, euphoria, excessive sweating, high fever, hyperactivity, irregular or rapid heartbeat, irregular or missed menstrual periods, liver problems, loss of muscle movement, low or irregular blood pressure, muscle contractions, muscle rigidity, nausea, painful erection, rash, restlessness, tardive dyskinesia, tremor, vision problems, weight change.

NALOXONE HYDROCHLORIDE (NARCAN)

Available Form

Solution, injection: 100 μg/mL, 1 mL (blue label); 1 mg/mL, 2 mL (green label).

Dosage

For narcotic overdose, give 0.4 to 2 mg IV; may repeat q2min prn. If there is no response after 10 mg, consider other diagnosis.

For IM or SC administration, give 0.8 mg/dose.

For endotracheal administration, give 0.8 mg/dose.

Indication

Reversal of narcotic depression.

Action

Narcotic antagonist; onset of action is 2 minutes by IV and less than 5 minutes by SC or IM route.

Contraindications and Precautions

Hypersensitivity to naloxone.

Side Effects

Nausea, vomiting, sweating, tachycardia, seizures from abrupt reversal of narcotic depression.

NALTREXONE HYDROCHLORIDE (REVIVA, VIVITROL)

Available Forms

Tablet: 50 mg.

Injection kit: Extended-release injectable suspension: one 380-mg vial of Vivitrol microspheres, 1 vial containing 4 mL (to deliver 3.4 mL) diluent for the suspension of Vivitrol, one 5-mL syringe, one ½" 20-gauge needle, and two 1½" 20-gauge needles with safety device.

Dosage

For injection, 380 mg delivered IM every 4 weeks or once a month by IM gluteal injection *only*, alternating buttocks.

Naltrexone for extended-release injectable suspension must not be administered intravenously.

Instructions for oral titration for drug withdrawal are too complex to list here. See Chapter 15.

Indications

Opiate dependence, alcohol dependence.

Action

An opioid antagonist with little, if any, opioid agonist activity.

Contraindications and Precautions

Contraindicated in patients receiving opioid analgesics and in patients currently dependent on opioids, patients in acute opioid withdrawal, and anyone who has failed the naloxone challenge test or who has a positive urine screen for opioids.

Severe opioid withdrawal syndromes precipitated by the accidental ingestion of naltrexone HCl have been reported in opioid-dependent patients.

The risk of suicide is known to be increased in patients with substance abuse with or without concomitant depression.

Naltrexone is also contraindicated in patients with acute hepatitis or liver failure. There is a risk of dose-related hepatocellular injury when given in excessive doses. Use caution in patients with renal and hepatic impairment.

Side Effects

CNS: Difficulty sleeping, anxiety, nervousness, low energy, headache.

Gastrointestinal: Nausea, abdominal pain or cramps, vomiting.

Musculoskeletal: Include muscle and joint pain.

An opioid withdrawal—like symptom complex has been reported, consisting of tearfulness, mild nausea, abdominal cramps, restlessness, bone or joint pain, myalgia, and nasal symptoms.

In patients treated for alcoholism, effects include nausea, headache, dizziness, nervousness, fatigue, insomnia, vomiting, anxiety, and somnolence.

NAMENDA; *SEE* MEMANTINE HYDROCHLORIDE
NARCAN; *SEE* NALOXONE HYDROCHLORIDE
NARDIL; *SEE* PHENELZINE SULFATE
NAVANE; *SEE* THIOTHIXENE
NORPRAMIN; *SEE* DESIPRAMINE HYDROCHLORIDE
NORTRIPTYLINE HYDROCHLORIDE (PAMELOR)

Available Forms

Capsule: 10, 25, 50, 75 mg.

Solution: 10 mg/5 mL.

Dosage

Usual adult dose is 25 mg tid or qid; dosage should begin at a low level and be increased as required. As an alternate regimen, the total daily dose may be given once a day.

When doses greater than 100 mg/day are administered, plasma levels of nortriptyline should be monitored and maintained in the optimum range of 50 to 150 ng/mL.

Doses greater than 150 mg/day are not recommended.

For elderly and adolescent patients, the dose is 30 to 50 mg/day in divided doses, or the total daily dose may be given once a day.

Indication

Depression.

Action

Inhibits the activity of such diverse agents as histamine, 5-hydroxytryptamine, and acetylcholine.

Increases the pressor effect of norepinephrine but blocks the pressor response of phenethylamine.

Contraindications and Precautions

Nortriptyline is contraindicated in patients taking an MAOI and during the acute recovery phase following myocardial infarction.

The FDA has issued black box warnings for suicidality on all antidepressants (see Box 22-1).

Side Effects

Fast heart rate, blurred vision, urinary retention, dry mouth, constipation, weight gain or loss, and orthostatic hypotension.

OLANZAPINE (ZYDIS ZYPREXA, ZYPREXA, INTRA-MUSCULAR)

Available Forms

Solution, IM injection: 10 mg.
Tablet: 2.5, 5.0, 7.5, 10 mg.
Tablet, orally disintegrating: 5, 10, 15, 20 mg.

Dosage

Initial dose is 5 to 10 mg/day to a target dose of 10 mg/day.
For bipolar monotherapy, begin with 10 or 15 mg/day PO.
For agitation associated with schizophrenia and bipolar I mania, the efficacy of IM olanzapine in controlling agitation was demonstrated in a dose range of 2.5 to 10 mg. The recommended dose in these patients is 10 mg.

Indications

Schizophrenia, bipolar disorder, mania.

Action

A psychotropic agent that belongs to the thienobenzodiazepine class.

Contraindications and Precautions

Hyperglycemia, in some cases extreme and associated with ketoacidosis or hyperosmolar coma or death, has been reported in patients treated with atypical antipsychotics including olanzapine.
Olanzapine can induce orthostatic hypotension associated with dizziness, tachycardia, and, in some patients, syncope, especially during the initial dose-titration period.
Given the primary CNS effects of olanzapine, caution should be used when olanzapine is taken in combination with other centrally acting drugs and alcohol.
Because of its potential for inducing hypotension, olanzapine can enhance the effects of certain antihypertensive agents.
Olanzapine can antagonize the effects of levodopa and dopamine agonists.

Side Effects

Akathisia, constipation, dizziness, drowsiness, objectionable behavior, orthostatic hypotension, and weight gain.

ORAP; SEE PIMOZIDE

OXCARBAZEPINE (TRILEPTAL)

Available Forms

Suspension: 300 mg/5 mL.
Tablet: 150, 300, 600 mg.

Dosage

Adults: Initial dose is 600 mg/day in divided doses. The dose may be increased by a maximum of 600 mg/day at approximately weekly intervals. The recommended daily dose is 1200 mg/day.
Children: 8 to 10 mg/kg bid, not to exceed 600 mg/day.

Indication

Monotherapy or adjunctive therapy in the treatment of partial seizures.

Action

Produces blockade of voltage-sensitive sodium channels, resulting in stabilization of hyperexcited neural membranes, inhibition of repetitive neuronal firing, and diminution of propagation of synaptic impulses.

Contraindications and Precautions

Contraindicated in patients with hypersensitivity, risk of clinically significant hyponatremia, CNS adverse effects, hypothyroidism.

Concomitant use with alcohol or hormonal sedatives should be avoided.

Side Effects

Dizziness, somnolence, diplopia, fatigue, nausea, vomiting, ataxia, abnormal vision, abdominal pain, tremor, dyspepsia, and abnormal gait.

PAMELOR; SEE NORTRIPTYLINE HYDROCHLORIDE
PARNATE; SEE TRANYLCYPROMINE SULFATE
PAXIL; SEE PAROXETINE HYDROCHLORIDE
PAROXETINE HYDROCHLORIDE (PAXIL)

Available Forms

Tablet: 10, 20, 30, 40 mg.
Tablet, controlled release (Paxil CR): 12.5, 25, 37.5 mg.

Dosage

Initial: 10 mg (or 12.5 mg Paxil CR), increasing to 20 mg (25 mg of Paxil CR) after 1 week.

Indications

Depression, OCD, panic disorder, social anxiety disorder.

Action

Selective serotonin reuptake inhibitor.

Contraindications and Precautions

Contraindicated in patients with hypersensitivity and in patients taking MAOIs (or within 14 days of discontinuing an MAOI).

Use with caution in patients with history of mania or of renal or hepatic disease.

Side Effects

Anxiety (can be minimized by starting with a 10-mg dose rather than a 20-mg dose), nausea, anorexia, decreased appetite, delayed ejaculation, weight gain.

PERMITIL; SEE FLUPHENAZINE HYDROCHLORIDE
PERPHENAZINE (TRILAFON)

Available Forms

Concentrate: 16 mg/5 mL.
Solution, injectable: 5 mg/mL.
Tablet: 2, 4, 8 mg.

Dosage

Tablets

Moderately disturbed nonhospitalized patients with schizophrenia: 4 to 8 mg tid initially; reduce as soon as possible to minimum effective dosage.

Hospitalized patients with schizophrenia: Tablets 8 to 16 mg bid to qid; avoid dosages in excess of 64 mg/day.

Intramuscular Injection

For rapid effect and prompt control of acute or intractable conditions or when oral administration is not feasible. Therapeutic effect is usually evidenced in 10 minutes and is maximal in 1 to 2 hours. The average duration of effective action is 6 hours, occasionally 12 to 24 hours.

Pediatric dosage has not yet been established. Pediatric patients older than 12 years may receive the lowest limit of adult dosage.

Give 5 mg (1 mL) initially. This may be repeated every 6 hours. Maximum daily dose is 15 mg in ambulatory patients or 30 mg in hospitalized patients.

When required for satisfactory control of symptoms in severe conditions, an initial 10-mg IM dose may be given.

Treatment should be changed to oral therapy as soon as practicable, generally within 24 hours. In some instances, however, patients have been maintained on injectable therapy for several months.

It has been established that perphenazine injection is more potent than perphenazine tablets. Therefore, equal or higher dosage should be used when the patient is transferred to oral therapy after receiving the injection.

Indication

Schizophrenia.

Action

Dopamine receptor antagonist, with higher affinity for D_2- over D_1-receptors, and variable selectivity among the cortical dopamine tracts.

Contraindications and Precautions

Severe toxic CNS depression, coma, subcortical brain damage, bone marrow depression, blood dyscrasias, liver damage, sulfite sensitivity (injection contains sodium bisulfite).

Use with caution in patients younger than 12 years and in elderly patients.

Use with caution in treatment over prolonged periods and in patients with severe cardiovascular disorders, epilepsy, hepatic or renal disease, glaucoma, prostatic hypertrophy, severe asthma, emphysema, hypocalcemia, and COPD.

Side Effects

Aching or numbness of the limbs, brain swelling, galactorrhea, diarrhea, drowsiness, dry mouth, orthostatic hypotension, nausea, rapid or irregular heartbeat, restlessness, salivation, seizures, vomiting.

Risk of tardive dyskinesia.

PHENELZINE SULFATE (NARDIL)
Available Form
Tablet: 15 mg.
Dosage
Initial dose: The usual starting dose of phenelzine sulfate is 15 mg (one tablet) tid.

Early-phase treatment: Dosage should be increased to at least 60 mg/day at a fairly rapid pace consistent with patient tolerance. It may be necessary to increase the dosage up to 90 mg/day to obtain sufficient MAO inhibition. Many patients do not show a clinical response until treatment at 60 mg has been continued for at least 4 weeks.

Maintenance dose: After maximum benefit from phenelzine sulfate is achieved, dosage should be reduced slowly over several weeks. Maintenance dose may be as low as 15 mg (one tablet) qd or qod and should be continued for as long as required.

Indications
Phenelzine sulfate has been found to be effective in depressed patients clinically characterized as "atypical," "nonendogenous," or "neurotic." These patients often have mixed anxiety and depression and phobic or hypochondriacal features. There is less conclusive evidence of its usefulness with severely depressed patients with endogenous features.

Phenelzine sulfate should rarely be the first antidepressant drug used. Rather, it is more suitable for use with patients who have failed to respond to the drugs more commonly used for these conditions.

Action
A potent inhibitor of monoamine oxidase (MAO).

Chemically, it is a hydrazine derivative.

Contraindications and Precautions
Contraindicated in patients with pheochromocytoma, congestive heart failure, a history of liver disease, or abnormal liver function tests.

Potentiation of sympathomimetic substances and related compounds by MAOIs can result in hypertensive crisis. Therefore, patients being treated with phenelzine sulfate should not take sympathomimetic drugs (including amphetamines, cocaine, methylphenidate, dopamine, epinephrine, and norepinephrine) or related compounds (including methyldopa, L-dopa, L-tryptophan, L-tyrosine, and phenylalanine).

Hypertensive crisis during phenelzine sulfate therapy can also be caused by the ingestion of foods with a high concentration of tyramine or dopamine. Therefore, patients being treated with phenelzine sulfate should avoid high-protein food that has undergone protein breakdown by aging, fermentation, pickling, smoking, or bacterial contamination. Patients should also avoid cheeses (especially aged varieties), pickled herring, beer, wine, liver, yeast extract (including brewer's yeast in large quantities), dry sausage (including Genoa salami, hard salami, pepperoni, and Lebanon bologna), pods of broad beans (fava beans), and yogurt. Excessive amounts of caffeine and chocolate may also cause hypertensive reactions.

Hypertensive crises associated with phenelzine sulfate have sometimes been fatal. These crises are characterized by some or all of the following symptoms:

- Occipital headache, which can radiate frontally.
- Palpitation.
- Neck stiffness or soreness.
- Nausea, vomiting.
- Sweating (sometimes with fever and sometimes with cold, clammy skin).
- Dilated pupils, photophobia.

Either tachycardia or bradycardia may be present and can be associated with constricting chest pain.

Intracranial bleeding has been reported in association with the increase in blood pressure.

Side Effects

Cardiovascular: Postural hypotension, edema.

Gastrointestinal: Constipation, dry mouth, gastrointestinal disturbances, elevated serum transaminases (without accompanying signs and symptoms).

Genitourinary: Anorgasmia and ejaculatory disturbances.

Metabolic: Weight gain.

Nervous system: Dizziness, headache, drowsiness, sleep disturbances (including insomnia and hypersomnia), fatigue, weakness, tremors, twitching, myoclonic movements, hyperreflexia.

PHENERGAN; *SEE* PROMETHAZINE HYDROCHLORIDE

PIMOZIDE (ORAP)

Available Form

Tablet: 1, 2 mg.

Dosage

The suppression of tics by pimozide requires a slow and gradual introduction of the drug. The patient's dose should be carefully adjusted to a point where the suppression of tics and the relief afforded is balanced against the untoward side effects of the drug.

An ECG should be done at baseline and periodically thereafter.

Children

Reliable dose-response data for the effects of pimozide on tic manifestations in Tourette's patients younger than 12 years are not available.

Treatment should be initiated at a dose of 0.05 mg/kg, preferably taken once at bedtime. The dose may be increased every third day to a maximum of 0.2 mg/kg, not to exceed 10 mg/day.

Adults

Initial: 1 to 2 mg a day in divided doses. The dose may be increased thereafter every other day.

Most patients are maintained on less than 0.2 mg/kg/day or 10 mg/day, whichever is less.

Doses greater than 0.2 mg/kg/day or 10 mg/day are not recommended.

Indications

Suppression of motor and phonic tics in patients with Tourette's syndrome who have failed to respond satisfactorily to standard treatment.

Pimozide is not intended as a treatment of first choice, nor is it intended for the treatment of tics that are merely annoying or cosmetically troublesome.

Pimozide should be reserved for use in Tourette's patients whose development and/or daily life function is severely compromised by the presence of motor and phonic tics.

Action

An orally active antipsychotic agent of the diphenylbutylpiperidine series.

Contraindications and Precautions

Contraindicated in the treatment of simple tics or tics other than those associated with Tourette's syndrome.

Should not be used in patients taking drugs that can, themselves, cause motor and phonic tics (e.g., pemoline, methylphenidate, amphetamines) until such patients have been withdrawn from these drugs to determine whether the drugs, rather than Tourette's syndrome, are responsible for the tics.

Because pimozide prolongs the QT interval, it is contraindicated in patients with congenital long QT syndrome, patients with a history of cardiac arrhythmias, and patients taking other drugs that prolong the QT interval.

Contraindicated in patients with severe toxic CNS depression or comatose states from any cause.

Side Effects

Dry mouth, drowsiness, headache, stomach upset, change in appetite, or sleeplessness can occur the first several days as the patient's body adjusts to the medication.

Blurred vision, change in sex drive, nervousness, muscle cramps, behavior changes, or menstrual changes can also occur.

Other effects include mental confusion, difficulty speaking, sweating, tremors, drooling, stiff muscles, difficulty walking, unusual eye movements, chest pain, increased body heat, seizures, and abnormal tongue, face, or jaw movements (puffing cheeks, chewing, puckering mouth).

PROLIXIN; SEE FLUPHENAZINE HYDROCHLORIDE
PROMETHAZINE HYDROCHLORIDE (PHENERGAN)
Available Forms

Solution, injectable: 25, 50 mg/mL.
Suppository, rectal: 25 mg.
Syrup: 6.25 mg/5 mL, 25 mg/5 mL.
Tablet: 12.5, 25, 50 mg.

Dosage

Injectable solution: In concentration no greater than 25 mg/mL at a rate not to exceed 25 mg/min. It is preferable to inject through the tubing of an IV infusion set. Nighttime sedation may be achieved by a dose of 25 to 50 mg.

Oral or rectal suppository: Administration of 12.5 to 25 mg by the oral route or by rectal suppository at bedtime provides sedation in children. Adults usually require 25 to 50 mg for nighttime, presurgical, or obstetric sedation.

Indications

For sedation and relief of apprehension and to produce light sleep from which the patient can be easily aroused.

Action

A phenothiazine derivative that possesses antihistaminic, sedative, anti—motion-sickness, antiemetic, and anticholinergic effects.

Contraindications and Precautions

Never administer by intraarterial injection due to the likelihood of severe arteriospasm and the possibility of resultant gangrene.

Should not be given by the SC route; evidence of chemical irritation has been noted, and necrotic lesions have resulted on rare occasions following SC injection. The preferred parenteral route of administration is by deep IM injection.

Not recommended for use in pediatric patients younger than 2 years.

Drugs having anticholinergic properties should be used with caution in patients with narrow-angle glaucoma, prostatic hypertrophy, stenosing peptic ulcer, pyloroduodenal obstruction, and bladder-neck obstruction.

Should be used cautiously in persons with cardiovascular disease or impairment of liver function.

Side Effects

Dizziness, drowsiness, sleepiness, or confusion; blurred vision or a dry mouth; nausea or vomiting; increased sensitivity to sunlight.

PROSOM; SEE ESTAZOLAM

PROTRIPTYLINE HYDROCHLORIDE (VIVACTIL)

Available Forms

Tablet, film-coated: 5, 10 mg.

Dosage

Initial: 15-40 mg/day divided tid or qid.

May be increased to 60 mg/day. Increases should be made in the morning dose.

Indication

Depression.

Action

Antidepressant agent.

Contraindications and Precautions

Contraindicated with MAOIs.

Contraindicated in patients taking cisapride.

Contraindicated during the acute recovery phase following myocardial infarction.

Can block the antihypertensive effect of guanethidine or similarly acting compounds.

Use with caution in patients with a history of seizures and in patients with a tendency to urinary retention or increased intraocular tension.

Side Effects

Relatively common: Cardiac arrhythmias.

Rare: Drowsiness, orthostatic hypotension, dry mouth, blurred vision, urinary retention, and constipation.

PROVIGIL; *SEE* MODAFINIL
PROZAC; *SEE* FLUOXETINE HYDROCHLORIDE
QUETIAPINE FUMARATE (SEROQUEL)

Available Form

Tablet: 25, 100, 200 mg.

Dosage

Bipolar Mania

Initial: 100 mg/day divided bid on day 1, increased to 400 mg/day on day 4 in increments of up to 100 mg/day divided bid.

Further dosage adjustments up to 800 mg/day by day 6 should be in increments of no greater than 200 mg/day.

Schizophrenia

Initial: 25 mg bid, with increases in increments of 25 to 50 mg bid or tid on the second and third day, as tolerated, to a target dose range of 300 to 400 mg/day by the fourth day, divided bid or tid.

Further dosage adjustments, if indicated, should generally occur at intervals of not less than 2 days, because steady-state for quetiapine fumarate is achieved for approximately 1 or 2 days in the typical patient.

When dosage adjustments are necessary, dose increments or decrements of 25 to 50 mg bid are recommended.

Indications

Acute manic episodes associated with bipolar I disorder, as either monotherapy or adjunct therapy to lithium or divalproex.

Schizophrenia.

Action

Psychotropic drug belonging to the dibenzothiazepine derivatives.

Contraindications and Precautions

As with other antipsychotics, long-term use of quetiapine can lead to tardive dyskinesia, which is potentially irreversible.

There is a risk of NMS.

Quetiapine can increase blood concentrations of cholesterol and triglycerides by 11% and 17%, respectively.

Side Effects

Dizziness, dry mouth, stomach upset, and lightheadedness.

RAMELTEON (ROZEREM)

Available Form

Tablet: 8 mg.

Dosage

Give 8 mg within 30 minutes of bedtime.
Avoid taking with or immediately after a high-fat meal.

Indication

Insomnia.

Action

A melatonin receptor agonist with both affinity for melatonin MT_1 and MT_2 receptors and selectivity over the MT_3 receptor.

Contraindications and Precautions

Contraindicated in hypersensitivity, severe hepatic impairment, concomitant use with fluvoxamine.
Not recommended for use in patients with severe sleep apnea or severe COPD.

Side Effects

Headache, somnolence, fatigue, dizziness, nausea, exacerbated insomnia, respiratory infection.

RAZADYNE; SEE GALANTAMINE HYDROBROMIDE

REMERON; SEE MIRTAZAPINE

RESTORIL; SEE TEMAZEPAM

REVIVA; SEE NALTREXONE HYDROCHLORIDE

RISPERDAL; SEE RISPERIDONE

RISPERIDONE (RISPERDAL, RISPERDAL CONSTA, RISPERDAL M-TAB)

Available Forms

Injection kit, IM (Risperdal Consta): 25, 37.5, 50 mg.
Solution: 1 mg/mL.
Tablet: 0.25, 0.5, 1, 2, 3, 4 mg.
Tablet, disintegrating (Risperdal M-Tab): 0.5, 1, 2 mg.

Dosage

Injection

Injection should be administered every 2 weeks by deep IM gluteal injection, alternating between the two buttocks.
Do not administer intravenously.
The recommended dose is 25 mg IM q2wk.

Oral

Schizophrenia: 4 to 6 mg/day on either a bid or a qd schedule.
Bipolar mania: 2 to 3 mg/day once daily.

Indications

Schizophrenia, bipolar disorder, mania, psychosis.

Action

Psychotropic agent belonging to the chemical class of benzisoxazole derivatives.

Contraindications and Precautions

NMS, which is potentially fatal, has been reported in association with antipsychotic drugs.

Potentially irreversible tardive dyskinesia can develop in patients treated with antipsychotic drugs. Although the prevalence of the syndrome appears to be highest among the elderly, especially elderly women, it is impossible to rely upon prevalence estimates to predict, at the inception of antipsychotic treatment, which patients are likely to develop tardive dyskinesia.

Side Effects

Application site: Injection site pain, reaction.

Blood: Anemia, purpura, epistaxis, pulmonary embolism, hematoma, thrombocytopenia.

Cardiovascular: Tachycardia, bradycardia, atrioventricular (AV) block, palpitation, bundle branch block, T-wave inversion, hypotension, postural hypotension, myocardial ischemia, angina pectoris, myocardial infarction, intermittent claudication, flushing, thrombophlebitis.

Endocrine: Hyperprolactinemia, gynecomastia, hypothyroidism.

Gastrointestinal: Nausea, vomiting, abdominal pain, gastritis, gastroesophageal reflux, flatulence, hemorrhoids, melena, dysphagia, rectal hemorrhage, stomatitis, colitis, gastric ulcer, gingivitis, irritable bowel syndrome, ulcerative stomatitis.

General: Back pain, chest pain, asthenia, malaise, choking.

Hearing and vestibular: Earache, deafness, decreased hearing.

Liver and biliary: Increased hepatic enzymes (frequent); hepatomegaly, increased serum glutamic-pyruvic transaminase (SGPT) (infrequent); bilirubinemia, increased gamma glutamyl transpeptidase (GGT), hepatitis, hepatocellular damage, jaundice, fatty liver, increased serum glutamic-oxaloacetic transaminase (SGOT) (rare).

Metabolic and nutritional (infrequent): Hyperuricemia, hyperglycemia, hyperlipemia, hypokalemia, glycosuria, hypercholesterolemia, obesity, dehydration, diabetes mellitus, hyponatremia.

Musculoskeletal: Arthralgia, skeletal pain (frequent), torticollis, arthrosis, muscle weakness, tendinitis, arthritis, arthropathy (infrequent).

Nervous system: Hypertonia, dystonia, dyskinesia, vertigo, leg cramps, tardive dyskinesia,* involuntary muscle contractions, paresthesias, abnormal gait, bradykinesia, convulsions, hypokinesia, ataxia, fecal incontinence, oculogyric crisis, tetany, apraxia, dementia, migraine, NMS (rare).

---

*In the integrated database of multiple-dose studies (1499 patients with schizophrenia or schizoaffective disorder), nine patients (0.6%) treated with risperidone injection (all dosages combined) experienced an adverse event of tardive dyskinesia.

Resistance and white cell (infrequent): Lymphadenopathy, leukopenia, cervical lymphadenopathy, granulocytopenia, leukocytosis, lymphopenia, abscess.

Psychiatric: Anxiety, psychosis, depression, agitation, nervousness, paranoid reaction, delusion, apathy (frequent); anorexia, impaired concentration, impotence, emotional lability, manic reaction, decreased libido, increased appetite, amnesia, confusion, euphoria, depersonalization, nightmares, delirium, psychotic depression (infrequent).

Reproductive disorders: Amenorrhea, nonpuerperal lactation, vaginitis, dysmenorrhea, breast pain, leukorrhea, ejaculation failure.

Respiratory: Dyspnea, pneumonia, stridor, hemoptysis, pulmonary edema.

Skin: Rash, eczema, pruritus, dermatitis, alopecia, seborrhea, photosensitivity reaction, increased sweating.

Urinary: Urinary incontinence, hematuria, micturition frequency, renal pain, urinary retention.

Vision: Conjunctivitis, eye pain, abnormal accommodation.

RITALIN; *SEE* METHYLPHENIDATE HYDROCHLORIDE
RIVASTIGMINE (EXELON)
Available Forms

Solution: 2 mg/mL.
Tablet: 1.5, 3, 4.5, 6 mg.

Dosage

In adults, average dose is 20-30 mg/day given in divided doses, preferably before meals. In children, usual starting dose may be 5 mg bid with gradual increments of 5-10 mg weekly.

Indication

Mild to moderate dementia of the Alzheimer type.

Action

Reversible acetylcholinesterase inhibitor.

Contraindications and Precautions

Antagonizes anticholinergics.
Monitor for gastrointestinal bleeding with nonsteroidal antiinflammatory drugs.

Side Effects

Nausea, vomiting, anorexia, weight loss.

ROZEREM; *SEE* RAMELTEON
SARAFEM; *SEE* FLUOXETINE HYDROCHLORIDE
SELEGILINE HYDROCHLORIDE (ELDEPRYL)
Available Forms

Capsule: 5 mg.
Tablet: 5 mg.

Transdermal system: 6 mg/24 h (20 mg/20 cm^2), 9 mg/24 h (30 mg/30 cm^2), 12 mg/24 h (40 mg/40 cm^2).

Dosage

Transdermal: Initially, 6 mg/24 h. As necessary, increase dose in increments of 3 mg/24 h (up to a maximum dose of 12 mg/24 h) at intervals of no less than 2 weeks.

Tablet: 10 mg/day administered as divided doses of 5 mg each taken at breakfast and lunch.

Indications

Adjunct in the management of Parkinson's patients being treated with levodopa—carbidopa who exhibit deterioration in the quality of their response to this therapy.

Major depressive disorder (transdermal system).

Action

Inhibition of MAO type B, which blocks the catabolism of dopamine.

Contraindications and Precautions

Contraindicated in hypersensitive patients.

Contraindicated in patients taking SSRIs or other MAOIs, carbamazepine and oxcarbazepine, sympathomimetic amines.

Contraindicated in patients with pheochromocytoma.

Patients should avoid tyramine-rich foods and beverages.

Side Effects

Abdominal pain, confusion, dizziness, dry mouth, fainting, hallucinations, nausea.

SEROQUEL; *SEE* QUETIAPINE FUMARATE

SERTRALINE HYDROCHLORIDE (ZOLOFT)

Available Forms

Concentrate: 20 mg/mL.
Tablet: 50, 100 mg.

Dosage

Initial: 50 mg PO qd. Maximum dosage is 200 mg/day.
Do not change dose at intervals of less than 1 week.

Indications

Depression, panic disorder, posttraumatic stress disorder, OCD.

Action

Selective serotonin reuptake inhibitor.

Contraindications and Precautions

Contraindicated in patients taking MAOIs.

Use with caution in patients with hepatic or renal disease and patients with epilepsy.

Side Effects

Insomnia, somnolence, dizziness, headache, tremor, fatigue, male sexual
dysfunction, dry mouth, diarrhea, nausea.

SINEQUAN; *SEE* DOXEPIN HYDROCHLORIDE

SONATA; *SEE* ZALEPLON

SPANSULE; *SEE* DEXTROAMPHETAMINE SULFATE

**STRATTERA; *SEE* ATOMOXETINE
HYDROCHLORIDE**

**SUBOXONE; *SEE* BUPRENORPHINE
HYDROCHLORIDE**

SUBUTEX; *SEE* BUPRENORPHINE HYDROCHLORIDE

SURMONTIL; *SEE* TRIMIPRAMINE MALEATE

SYMBYAX; *SEE* FLUOXETINE HYDROCHLORIDE

SYMMETREL; *SEE* AMANTADINE HYDROCHLORIDE

TEGRETOL; *SEE* CARBAMAZEPINE

TEMAZEPAM (RESTORIL)

Available Form

Capsule: 7.5, 15 mg.

Dosage

Usual dose is 15 to 30 mg PO hs.
Half dose of 7.5 mg may be sufficient in some patients and is recommended in elderly and debilitated patients.

Indication

Short-term treatment of insomnia.

Action

Benzodiazepine hypnotic agent.

Contraindications and Precautions

Contraindicated in patients with anemia, hepatic disease, renal disease,
acute narrow-angle glaucoma, seizure disorders, or lung disease.
Contraindicated in suicidal patients, drug-abusing patients, those with
depression, and those with psychosis.
Contraindicated in elderly patients and children younger than 18 years.

Side Effects

Drowsiness, headache, fatigue, nervousness, lethargy, dizziness, nausea,
hangover, anxiety.

THIORIDAZINE HYDROCHLORIDE (MELLARIL)

Available Form

Tablet: 10, 25, 50, 100 mg.

Dosage

50-100 mg tid, with maximum of 800 mg/day.

Indication

Schizophrenic patients who fail to respond adequately to treatment with other antipsychotic drugs.

Action

A 2-methylmercapto-10-[2-(N-methyl-2-piperidyl)ethyl] phenothiazine.

Contraindications and Precautions

General

Can prolong the QTc interval in a dose-dependent fashion, which can increase the risk of serious, potentially fatal, ventricular arrhythmias.

Contraindicated in schizophrenic patients who fail to respond adequately to treatment with other antipsychotic drugs.

Contraindicated in severe CNS depression or comatose states from any cause including drug-induced CNS depression and in patients with hypertensive and hypotensive heart disease of extreme degree.

Reduced Cytochrome P450 2D6 Isozyme Activity

Drugs that inhibit P450 2D6 (e.g., fluoxetine and paroxetine) and certain other drugs (e.g., fluvoxamine, propranolol, and pindolol) appear to appreciably inhibit the metabolism of thioridazine. The resulting elevated levels of thioridazine would be expected to augment the prolongation of the QTc interval associated with thioridazine and can increase the risk of serious, potentially fatal, cardiac arrhythmias, such as torsades de pointes–type arrhythmias. Such an increased risk can result also from the additive effect of coadministering thioridazine with other agents that prolong the QTc interval.

Thioridazine is contraindicated with these drugs as well as in patients (about 7% of the normal population) who are known to have a genetic defect leading to reduced levels of activity of P450 2D6.

Side Effects

Drowsiness, dizziness, blurred vision, dry mouth, upset stomach, vomiting, diarrhea, constipation, restlessness, headache, weight gain.

THIOTHIXENE (NAVANE)

Available Forms

Capsule: 1, 2, 5, 10, 20 mg.
Concentrate: 5 mg/mL.

Dosage

Dosage of thiothixene should be individually adjusted depending on the chronicity and severity of the schizophrenia.

In general, small doses should be used initially and gradually increased to the optimal effective level based on patient response.

Indication

Schizophrenia.

Action

Psychotropic agent of the thioxanthene series.

Contraindications and Precautions

Contraindicated in patients with circulatory collapse, comatose states, CNS depression due to any cause, and blood dyscrasias.

As with other antipsychotics, long-term use can lead to potentially irreversible tardive dyskinesia.

NMS, which is potentially fatal, has been reported with antipsychotic drugs.

The use of thiothixene in children younger than 12 years is not recommended because safe conditions for its use have not been established.

Side Effects

Drowsiness, dizziness, blurred vision, stomach upset, increased appetite, headache, dry mouth, sweating, sleep disturbances, restlessness.

TOFRANIL; *SEE* IMIPRAMINE
TOPAMAX; *SEE* TOPIRAMATE
TOPIRAMATE (TOPAMAX, TOPAMAX SPRINKLE)

Available Forms

Capsule: 15, 25 mg.
Tablet: 25, 100, 200 mg.

Dosage

Epilepsy

Initial dose: 400 mg/day.

Monotherapy in adults and children older than 9 years: 400 mg/day in two divided doses. The dose should be achieved by titrating according to the schedule in Table 22-2.

Adjunctive therapy use in patients 17 years and older with partial seizures, primary generalized tonic–clonic seizures, or Lennox–Gastaut syndrome:

- Give 200 to 400 mg/day in two divided doses, and 400 mg/day in two divided doses as adjunctive treatment in adults with primary generalized tonic–clonic seizures.
- Initiate therapy at 25 to 50 mg/day followed by titration to an effective dose in increments of 25 to 50 mg/week.
- Titrating in increments of 25 mg/week can delay the time to reach an effective dose.
- Maximum recommended dose is 1600 mg/day.

Pediatric patients (ages 2-16 years) with partial seizures, primary generalized tonic–clonic seizures, or Lennox–Gastaut syndrome:

- Give 5 to 9 mg/kg/day divided bid.
- Titration should begin at 25 mg (or less, based on a range of 1-3 mg/kg/day) nightly for the first week.
- The dosage should then be increased at 1- or 2-week intervals by increments of 1 to 3 mg/kg/day (divided bid).
- Dose titration should be guided by clinical outcome.

Table 22-2	**Topiramate Titration Schedule for Epilepsy Monotherapy**	
Week	**Morning Dose**	**Evening Dose**
Week 1	25 mg	25 mg
Week 2	50 mg	50 mg
Week 3	75 mg	75 mg
Week 4	100 mg	100 mg
Week 5	150 mg	150 mg
Week 6	200 mg	200 mg

Table 22-3	**Topiramate Titration Schedule for Migraine Prophylaxis**	
Week	**Morning Dose**	**Evening Dose**
Week 1	None	25 mg
Week 2	25 mg	25 mg
Week 3	25 mg	50 mg
Week 4	50 mg	50 mg

Migraine Prophylaxis

The recommended total daily dose is 100 mg/day divided bid.
The recommended titration rate to 100 mg/day is shown in Table 22-3.
Dose and titration rate should be guided by clinical outcome. If required, longer intervals between dose adjustments may be used.

Indications

Migraine headache prophylaxis.
Generalized tonic–clonic or partial seizures; Lennox–Gastaut syndrome.

Action

Blocks voltage-dependent sodium channels, augments the activity of the neurotransmitter γ-aminobutyric acid (GABA) at some subtypes of the GABA-A receptor, antagonizes the AMPA/kainate subtype of the glutamate receptor, and inhibits the carbonic anhydrase enzyme, particularly isozymes II and IV

Contraindications and Precautions

Contraindicated in hypersensitive patients.
Avoid concomitant use with valproic acid.
Hyperchloremic, non–anion-gap metabolic acidosis (i.e., decreased serum bicarbonate below the normal reference range in the absence of chronic respiratory alkalosis) is associated with topiramate treatment.

Use with caution in patients with renal and hepatic dysfunction (decreased clearance) and sulfa hypersensitivity. Reduce dose by 50% when creatinine clearance is less than 70 mL/min.

Side Effects

Ataxia, cognitive dysfunction, dizziness, nystagmus, paresthesia, sedation, visual disturbances, nausea, dyspepsia, kidney stones.

TRANYLCYPROMINE SULFATE (PARNATE)

Available Form

Tablet: 10 mg.

Dosage

Initial: 30 mg/day, usually in divided doses.
May be increased in increments of 10 mg/day at intervals of 1 to 3 weeks, to a maximum of 60 mg/day.

Indication

Major depressive episode without melancholia.

Action

A nonhydrazine MAOI with a rapid onset of activity.

Contraindications and Precautions

Tranylcypromine sulfate should be used in adults who can be closely supervised. It should rarely be the first antidepressant drug given. Rather, the drug is suited for patients who have failed to respond to the drugs more commonly administered for depression.

Tranylcypromine sulfate should not be administered in combination with any of the following:
- MAOIs or dibenzazepine derivatives.
- Sympathomimetics (including amphetamines).
- Some CNS depressants (including narcotics and alcohol).
- Antihypertensive, diuretic, antihistaminic, sedative, or anesthetic drugs.
- Bupropion.
- Buspirone.
- Dextromethorphan.
- Cheese or other foods with a high tyramine content.
- Excessive quantities of caffeine.

Tranylcypromine sulfate should not be administered to any patient with a confirmed or suspected cerebrovascular defect or to any patient with cardiovascular disease, hypertension, or history of headache.

Side Effects

Overstimulation, which can include increased anxiety, agitation, and manic symptoms, is usually evidence of excessive therapeutic action. Dosage should be reduced, or a phenothiazine tranquilizer should be administered concomitantly.

Other effects include restlessness or insomnia; weakness, drowsiness, episodes of dizziness, or dry mouth; and nausea, diarrhea, abdominal pain,
or constipation. Most of these effects can be relieved by lowering the
dosage or by giving suitable concomitant medication.

TRANXENE; *SEE* CLORAZEPATE DIPOTASSIUM
TRIAZOLAM (HALCION)
Available Form
Tablet: 0.125, 0.25 mg.

Dosage
Give 0.25 mg hs; maximum dose 0.5 mg. Some patients (e.g., low body
weight) might respond to 0.125 mg.
Geriatric or debilitated patients: 0.125 to 0.25 mg (0.125 initially); maximum 0.25 mg.

Indication
Short-term treatment of insomnia.

Action
A triazolobenzodiazepine hypnotic agent.

Contraindications and Precautions
Contraindicated in patients with narrow-angle glaucoma or psychosis, in
children younger than 18 years, and in pregnant women.
Concomitant use with ketoconazole, itraconazole, and nefazodone is
contraindicated.
Use with caution in elderly and debilitated patients and in patients with
hepatic disease, renal disease, history of drug abuse, or respiratory
depression.
Avoid abrupt withdrawal and prolonged use.

Side Effects
Drowsiness, headache, dizziness, nervousness, lightheadedness, coordination disorders or ataxia, nausea and vomiting.

TRILAFON; *SEE* PERPHENAZINE
TRILEPTAL; *SEE* OXCARBAZEPINE
TRIMIPRAMINE MALEATE (SURMONTIL)
Available Form
Capsule: 25, 50, 100 mg.

Dosage
Initial: 75 mg/day in divided doses, increased to 150 mg/day.
Dosages greater than 200 mg are not recommended.

Indication
Depression.

Action
Antidepressant with an anxiety-reducing sedative component to its
action.

Contraindications and Precautions

Not for concurrent use with an MAOI.

Contraindicated in the acute recovery period following myocardial infarction.

Use with extreme caution in patients with any evidence of cardiovascular disease.

Use with caution in patients with increased intraocular pressure, history of urinary retention, or history of narrow-angle glaucoma; hyperthyroid patients or those on thyroid medication; patients with a history of seizure disorder; patients receiving guanethidine or similar agents.

Not recommended for use in children.

Side Effects

Dry mouth, blurred vision, urinary retention, constipation, drowsiness, weight gain, cardiac arrhythmias, and orthostatic hypotension are relatively common side effects.

VALIUM; SEE DIAZEPAM
VALPROIC ACID (DEPAKENE)

Available Forms

Capsule: 250 mg.
Solution, injectable: 100 mg/mL.
Syrup: 250 mg/5 mL.

Dosage

Complex Partial Seizures

For monotherapy or adjunctive therapy in adults and children 10 years of age or older.

Initial: 10-15 mg/kg/day.

Increase by 5-10 mg/kg/week until the desired effect or plasma concentration trough of 50 to 100 μg/mL is achieved.

The maximum dose is 60 mg/kg/day.

Give in divided doses if the daily dose exceeds 250 mg.

Simple and Complex Absence Seizures

Initial: 15 mg/kg/day.

Increase by 5-10 mg/kg/day at 1-week intervals until desired effects are achieved.

The maximum dose is 60 mg/kg/day.

Give in divided doses if the daily dose exceeds 250 mg.

Indication

Treatment of seizures.

Action

Anticonvulsant.

Contraindications and Precautions

Valproic acid is contraindicated in patients with hepatic disease and known urea cycle disorders.

Pediatric patients younger than 2 years are at a considerably increased risk for developing fatal hepatotoxicity.

Side Effects

Gastrointestinal, liver, blood, and CNS toxicity; weight gain; transient alopecia; acute pancreatitis; nausea; sedation; vomiting; headache; thrombocytopenia; platelet dysfunction; rash; and hyperammonemia.

VENLAFAXINE HYDROCHLORIDE (EFFEXOR)

Available Forms

Capsule, sustained release (Effexor XR): 37.5, 75, 150 mg.
Tablet: 25, 37.5, 50, 75, 100 mg.

Dosage

Initial: 75 mg bid or tid (qd for sustained-release capsule). The dose may be increased at intervals of no less than 4 days.
The maximum dose is 375 mg/day for severe depression.
Reduce the total daily dose 25% in patients with mild to moderate renal impairment, 50% in patients with severe renal impairment, and 50% in patients with moderate hepatic impairment.
Dialysis patients should receive their dose after dialysis.

Indications

Major depression, generalized anxiety disorder.

Action

Strong inhibition of serotonin and norepinephrine reuptake and weak inhibition of dopamine reuptake.

Contraindications and Precautions

Do not use concurrently with MAOIs. At least 14 days should elapse between discontinuing an MAOI and initiating venlafaxine. At least 7 days should be allowed after stopping venlafaxine before starting an MAOI.
Do not use in children younger than 18 years.
Use caution with other CNS drugs and avoid alcohol.
When discontinuing the drug, taper over 2 weeks.

Side Effects

Hypertension, anxiety, seizures, anorexia, asthenia, dizziness, blurred vision, dry mouth, sweating.

VIVACTIL; *SEE* PROTRIPTYLINE HYDROCHLORIDE

VIVITROL; *SEE* NALTREXONE HYDROCHLORIDE

WELLBUTRIN; *SEE* BUPROPION HYDROCHLORIDE

XANAX; *SEE* ALPRAZOLAM

ZALEPLON (SONATA)

Available Form

Capsule: 5, 10 mg.

Dosage

For most nonelderly adults: 10 mg.
For certain low-weight, elderly, or debilitated patients: 5 mg.

Although the risk of certain adverse events associated with the use of zaleplon appears to be dose dependent, the 20-mg dose has been shown to be adequately tolerated and may be considered for the occasional patient who does not benefit from a trial of a lower dose.

Doses greater than 20 mg have not been adequately evaluated and are not recommended.

Indication

Insomnia.

Action

Nonbenzodiazepine hypnotic from the pyrazolopyrimidine class.

Contraindications and Precautions

None.

Side Effects

Drowsiness, dizziness.

ZIPRASIDONE HYDROCHLORIDE (GEODON), ZIPRASIDONE MESYLATE (GEODON FOR INJECTION)

Available Forms

Capsule: 20, 40, 60, 80 mg.
Solution, IM injection: 20 mg/mL.

Dosage

Capsule: Initially, 20 mg bid, up to 80 mg/day.
Injection: 10 to 20 mg, up to a maximum dose of 40 mg/day; 10-mg doses q2h or 20-mg doses q4h.

Indication

Schizophrenia.

Action

Antipsychotic agent.

Contraindications and Precautions

Avoid in combination with other drugs that are known to prolong the QTc interval. Additionally, clinicians should be alert to the identification of other drugs that have been consistently observed to prolong the QTc interval. Such drugs should not be prescribed with ziprasidone.

Avoid in patients with congenital long QT syndrome and in patients with a history of cardiac arrhythmias.

Contraindicated in patients with a known history of QT prolongation (including congenital long QT syndrome), with recent acute myocardial infarction, or with uncompensated heart failure.

Side Effects

Common

Accidental injury, cold symptoms, constipation, cough, diarrhea, dizziness, drowsiness, dry mouth, indigestion, muscle tightness, nausea, rash, stuffy and runny nose, upper respiratory infection, vision problems, weakness.

Other

Abdominal pain, abnormal body movements, abnormal ejaculation, galactorrhea, abnormal walk, abnormally low cholesterol, agitation, amnesia, anemia, bleeding gums, bleeding in the eye, blood clots, blood disorders, hematuria, body spasms, gynecomastia, bruising or purple spots, cataracts, angina, chills, clogged bowels, confusion, conjunctivitis, coordination problems, decreased blood flow to the heart, delirium, dyspnea, dysphagia, difficulty with orgasm, diplopia, dry eyes, cardiomegaly, eyelid inflammation, female sexual problems, fever, flank pain, flulike symptoms, fungal infections, gout, alopecia, menorrhagia, metrorrhagia, hypertension, hyperglycemia, hives, hostility, impotence, increased reflexes, increased sensitivity to touch or sound, inflammation of the cornea, inflammation of the heart, involuntary or jerky movements, cardiac arrhythmia, liver problems, lockjaw, anorexia, amenorrhea, hypoglycemia, hypotension, hypothermia, lymph disorders, male sexual problems, muscle disorders, muscle pain, muscle weakness, nighttime urination, nosebleed, pneumonia, paresthesias, tachycardia, rectal bleeding, rigid muscle movement, tinnitus, rolling of the eyeballs, sensitivity to sunlight, skin problems, bradycardia, bradykinesia, speech problems, stroke, orthostatic hypotension, swelling in the arms and legs, swelling in the face, swollen lymph nodes, swollen tongue, melena, tendon inflammation, thirst, throat spasms, thyroid disorders, tremor, twitching, uncontrolled eye movement, urination decrease or increase, vaginal bleeding, vein inflammation, vertigo, vision disorders, vomiting, hematemesis, jaundice, weight gain, white spots in the mouth.

ZOLOFT; *SEE* SERTRALINE HYDROCHLORIDE
ZOLPIDEM TARTRATE (AMBIEN)
Available Form
Tablet: 5, 10 mg.

Dosage
The dose of zolpidem tartrate should be individualized.

Initial adult dose is 10 mg immediately before bedtime.

Elderly or debilitated patients: 5 mg initially.

Downward dosage adjustment may be necessary when zolpidem is administered with agents having known CNS-depressant effects because of the potentially additive effects.

The total zolpidem tartrate dose should not exceed 10 mg.

Indication
Insomnia.

Action
Nonbenzodiazepine hypnotic of the imidazopyridine class.

Contraindications and Precautions
None.

Side Effects
Drowsiness, dizziness, diarrhea.

ZYBAN; *SEE* **BUPROPION HYDROCHLORIDE**

ZYPREXA; *SEE* **OLANZAPINE**

Index

Note: Page numbers followed by the letter f refer to figures; those followed by t refer to tables; and those followed by b refer to boxed material.

Abdominal assessment, in narcotics withdrawal, 309b
ABGs (arterial blood gases), 46
Abnormal Involuntary Movement Scale (AIMS), 70, 238, 240b
Absorption, of medications. *See specific drug classification or agent.*
Abstinence, from alcohol
  major syndrome of, 295–300
  withdrawal signs of, 293–294, 294b
Abstraction, in cognitive examination, 63
Abuse
  of alcohol. *See* Alcohol use/abuse.
  of drugs. *See* Drug abuse.
  of substances. *See* Substance abuse.
  sexual, 255
Abuse history, in psychiatric database, 23
Academic achievement
  in ADHD, 410, 411
  in learning disorders, 433–434
Acamprosate calcium (Campral), 289, 442–443
Accessibility, to integrated care, 9
Acetylcholinesterase inhibitors
  ECT interaction with, 321
  for Alzheimer's disease, 76, 77–78
Achenbach's Child Behavior Checklist and Teacher Report Form, 411
Acquired immunodeficiency syndrome (AIDS)
  dementia associated with, 57
  psychiatric symptoms caused by, 35b, 40b, 41, 41b

Acquired immunodeficiency syndrome (AIDS)—cont'd
  sexual dysfunction associated with, 373
  temperature with, lumbar puncture for, 44
Activation medications, 116, 117
Activities of daily living, in psychiatric database, 25–26
Acute anxiety
  benzodiazepines for, 178
  in stress disorder, 173–175
Acute dystonic reaction, to antipsychotics, 235–236, 276
Acute pain paradigm, for chronic pain management, 313
Acute psychotic phase, of schizophrenia, 217
  antipsychotic choices for, 230, 232t, 234
Acute somatized symptoms, 257–258
  definition of, 257
  differential diagnosis of, 257
  prevalence of, 257
  prognosis of, 257
  treatment of, 258
Acute stress disorder (ASD), 173–175
  definition of, 173
  differential diagnosis of, 173–174
  medical causes of, 174
  prognosis of, 174
  treatment of, 174–175
AD. *See* Alzheimer's disease (AD).
ADDA (Attention Deficit Disorder Association), 414

Addiction
    chronic pain and, 313
    in narcotic use, 307, 311
    to nicotine, 356
ADEAR (Alzheimer's Disease
    Education and Referral
    Center), 65b
ADHD. See Attention-deficit/
    hyperactivity disorder
    (ADHD).
Adjustment disorder
    definition of, 172
    depression associated with,
        89, 100, 101–102
    differential diagnosis of, 173
    identification of, 172
    oppositional defiant disorder
        versus, 417
    posttraumatic stress disorder
        and, 176
    prevalence of, 173
    treatment of, 173
    with anxiety, 172–173
Admiration, need for, in
    narcissistic personality
    disorder, 336–337
Adolescents, psychiatry for,
    389–440
    ADHD, 409–414
    antisocial personality disorder,
        333
    anxiety disorders, 390–409
        generalized, 169
    depressive disorders, 418–433
    developmental disabilities,
        435–440
    diagnostic assessment of,
        389–390
    disruptive behavior, 414–418
    learning disorders, 433–435
    mental retardation, 435–440
    overview of, 389
    suicidality, 449, 450b
Advocacy, for children,
    435, 437
Affect
    in borderline personality
        disorder, 334–335
    in hypochondriasis, 264
    in personality disorder, 328

Affect—cont'd
    in psychiatric examination, 18, 31
    in schizophrenia, 216
Affective disorders
    acute stress disorder related
        to, 174
    bulimia nervosa versus, 350
    depression associated with, 88
    prevalence of, 2t
    sleep problems associated
        with, 203
Against medical advice (AMA)
    as patient's choice, 267, 268
    commitment and, 285
Aggression
    azapirones for, 185
    by intoxicated patients, 290, 291
    delirium and, 50, 51
    in Alzheimer's patients, 65, 67t
    in mental retardation,
        421t–425t, 440
    in violent patient, 282, 283b
Aggressive play, in children, 400
Agitation
    acute, in schizophrenia, 234
    delirium and, 50, 52
        medical management of,
            249–250
    in alcohol withdrawal delirium,
        297b
    in Alzheimer's patients, 65, 67
        drugs that produce, 68, 69b
    in children, 400
    in dementia, 60
    psychomotor, as major depression
        criteria, 91b, 92
Agoraphobia, 160, 162, 163, 170
    identification of, 170–171
    in children, 397–398
    treatment of, 165, 171, 193
Agranulocytosis, clozapine
    associated with, 247–248
AIDS. See Acquired
    immunodeficiency syndrome
    (AIDS).
AIMS (Abnormal Involuntary
    Movement Scale), 70,
    238, 240b
Airway management, for ECT,
    323, 325

Akathisia
  antipsychotics causing, 236, 276
  SSRIs causing, 129, 432
  with Alzheimer's treatment,
    70, 84
ALA (aminolevulinic acid), 47
Alcohol amnestic syndrome, 291,
  291b
Alcohol dependence, 288–289
Alcohol intoxication, 272, 290
  anxiety associated with, 158,
    161b
  pathologic, 291
Alcohol levels, blood, 45,
  300–301, 301t
Alcohol use/abuse, 287–301
  abuse parameters, 287–288
  bipolar disorder *versus*, 140
  blood levels with, 300–301, 301t
  comorbidities of, 292–293
  dependence parameters,
    288–289
  economic costs of, 3t, 9
  generalized anxiety disorder
    and, 169
  in primary medical care, 6t, 7
  cost-benefit issues of, 9
  intoxication with. See Alcohol
    intoxication.
  medical costs of, 5, 8
  nicotine dependence associated
    with, 357
  patient history of, 28
  prevalence of, 2t
  schizophrenia associated with,
    217
  sexual dysfunction related to,
    364, 367t
  sleep problems associated
    with, 203
Alcohol Use Disorders
  Identification Test, 288, 289b
Alcohol withdrawal, 293–300
  delirium associated with, 53
  ECT for, 325
  major abstinence syndrome of,
    295–300
  overview of, 293
  seizures associated with, 300
  symptoms of, 293–294, 294b

Alcohol withdrawal delirium
    (AWD), 295–300
  risk factors for, 295
  symptoms of, 294b, 295,
    296b–298b
  timing of, 295
  treatment of, 295, 298–300
Alcohol withdrawal seizures, 300
Alcoholic dementia, 292
Alcoholic hallucinosis, 291–292
Alcoholic paranoia, 290–291
Alcoholics Anonymous, 288
Alcoholism, 287–288
  definition of, 287
  morbidity of, 287–288
  mortality of, 287–288, 293
  prevalence of, 287
  treatment of, 288
Allergies, drug
  hepatic responses with, 45–46
  patient history of, 28
α-Adrenergic agonists
  for ADHD, 402t–407t, 414
    posttraumatic stress disorder
      and, 401
  for narcotics addiction,
    310–312
α_1-Antagonists, neuroreceptor
    effects of, 114t
α_2-Antagonists, neuroreceptor
    effects of, 114t
Alprazolam (Xanax)
  for Alzheimer's disease,
    69t, 75
  for anxiety, 184
    in children, 392t
  for panic disorder, 163–164
  for posttraumatic stress disorder,
    177
  for premenstrual dysphoric
    disorder, 106
  formulary, 443–444
  pharmacokinetics of, 179t, 180,
    181b
Alzheimer's Association, 65b
Alzheimer's disease (AD),
    64–84
  anxiety with, 78–79
  behavioral symptoms of, 65, 66t,
    67–68

Alzheimer's disease (AD)—cont'd
  rating scale for disruptive,
    65, 67, 67b
  treatment of, 68–70, 69t, 71t,
    72–76, 74t
  cognitive impairment with, 76
    treatment of, 77–78
  communicating with patients,
    64
  depression with, 79–80, 81t
  description of, 5, 55–56
  diagnostic evaluation of,
    64–65
  differential diagnosis of, 64
  EEG evaluation of, 42
  functional impairment with, 65,
    66b
  lumbar puncture for, 44
  medical causes of, 68, 69b
  medical issues associated with,
    80, 82–83, 83b
  neuroimaging of, 44
  OBRA guidelines for, 79, 83–84
  prevalence of, 64
  professional resources for, 65,
    65b
  psychiatric symptoms caused by,
    40b, 41, 41b
  recognition of, 64–65
  treatment of
    cognitive focus of, 77–78
    medications for, 68–70, 69t,
      71t, 72–76, 74t, 250
    resources for, 65, 65b
Alzheimer's Disease Education and
  Referral Center (ADEAR),
  65b
AMA (against medical advice)
  as patient's choice, 267, 268
  commitment and, 285
Amantadine hydrochloride
  (Symmetrel)
  for medication-induced
    parkinsonism, 236, 237t
  for neuroleptic malignant
    syndrome, 241
  for substance abuse, 304
  formulary, 444
Ambiguous genitalia, in gender
  identity disorder, 376

Ambulatory EEG, 42
American Medical Association
  (AMA), on alcoholism, 287
American Psychiatric Association
  (APA)
  on antipsychotic therapy
    monitoring, 244, 245t, 246
  on bipolar disorder treatment,
    140, 143, 144–145, 150
  on schizophrenia treatment, 230
Amino acids
  branched-chain, for tardive
    dyskinesia, 239
  in P450 system, 378
γ-Aminobutyric acid (GABA)-A
  receptors, sleep problems and,
  206–207, 208
Aminolevulinic acid (ALA), 47
Amiodarone
  antipsychotics interactions with,
    229t
  P450 system inhibition by,
    379b, 383
Amitriptyline hydrochloride
  (Elavil)
  analgesic properties of, 314
  as antidepressant, 111t, 113, 121
  for sleep problems, 206
  formulary, 444–445
Ammonia level, valproic acid
  effect on, 149
Amnesia, ECT causing, 319
Amnestic disorders, 54, 60–61.
  See also Memory impairment.
Amobarbital interview
  contraindications to, 260–261
  for conversion disorder, 260–262
  procedure for, 261–262
  risks of, 261
Amphetamine (Adderall)
  abuse of, symptoms of, 302t, 304
  for ADHD, 403t, 412–413
  formulary, 446
Amplification, in somatization
  process, 253
Analgesics
  as P450 system substrate,
    380b–381b, 384–385
  common problems with use of,
    305–306

Analgesics—cont'd
  for chronic malignant pain, 312, 313t
  for narcotics addicts, 312
  patient-controlled, 306
  psychiatric symptoms caused by, 35b
  psychotropics augmentation of, 314
Anatomic patterns
  in conversion disorder, 258, 259
  in pain disorder, 263
  in somatization disorder, 254
Androgen insensitivity syndrome, 376
Anemia, aplastic, carbamazepine and, 152
Anesthesia
  benzodiazepines use with, 178
  for ECT, 322
    monitoring during, 323
    risks with, 318, 320, 326
    seizure threshold and, 324
    short-acting agents for, 322
  MAOIs interactions with, 134, 135b
Anger
  in borderline personality disorder, 334
  in factitious disorder, 266–267
  in malingering, 268
  in obsessive–compulsive personality disorder, 339
Anhedonia
  in children, 419
  in depression, 91b, 106
  in schizophrenia, 216
Anorexia, drug-induced, in Alzheimer's patients, 80, 82
Anorexia nervosa, 343–348
  body dysmorphic disorder versus, 266
  definition of, 343
  differential diagnosis of, 344, 346
  epidemiology of, 343
  etiology of, 343
  laboratory evaluation of, 344, 344b, 345b
  medical disorders in, 344, 345b

Anorexia nervosa—cont'd
  prognosis of, 348
  recognition of, 343–344
  subtypes of, 343
  treatment of, 346–348, 347b
Anterograde amnesia, ECT causing, 319
Anti-AIDS agents, 35b, 57
Antiandrogens
  for paraphilias, 375–376
  long-term side effects of, 376
  sexual dysfunction related to, 374
Antianxiety agents, 178–189. See also specific classification or drug.
  antidepressants, 187–188, 189t
  azapirones, 185–187, 187t
  behavioral therapies versus, 189–194
  benzodiazepines, 178–185, 179t
    azapirones versus, 186–187, 187t
  for Alzheimer's disease, 78–79
  for borderline personality disorder, 335
  for children, 391, 392t–393t, 394t–395t
  sedative-hypnotics, 188
Antiarrhythmics
  as P450 system substrate, 381b, 384–385
  psychiatric symptoms caused by, 35b
Antibiotics
  as P450 system inducer, 386, 387b
  P450 system inhibition by, 379b, 383
  psychiatric symptoms caused by, 35b
Anticholinergic side effects, of antidepressants, in children, 432
Anticholinergics
  agitation related to, in Alzheimer's patients, 68, 69b, 76, 91t
  antipsychotics and, 229t, 242
  anxiety caused by, 161b

Anticholinergics—cont'd
  for akathisia, 236
  for ECT, 322, 326
  for medication-induced
      parkinsonism, 236, 237t
  for tardive dyskinesia, 239
  neuroreceptor effects of, 114t
  psychiatric symptoms caused by,
      35b–36b
  sexual dysfunction related to,
      365t
  side effects of, 113, 114t, 116
Anticipatory anxiety, 166
Anticoagulants, as P450 system
    substrate, 380b, 385
Anticonvulsants
  analgesic properties of, 314
  ECT and, 322, 324
  for alcohol seizures, 300
  for Alzheimer's disease,
      74–75, 74b
  for borderline personality
      disorder, 335
  for bulimia nervosa, 351
  for generalized anxiety disorder,
      165t
  psychiatric symptoms caused by,
      34, 36b
  sexual dysfunction related to,
      365t
Antidepressants, 108–135
  analgesic properties of, 314
  anxiety caused by, 161b
  as P450 system substrate,
      380b–381b, 384–386
  breast-feeding and, 120
  choosing which to use, 113
  continued treatment guidelines
      for, 110
  ECT and, 321, 324
  effects on EEG, 42
  FDA black box warning on, 432,
      449, 450b
  for ADHD, 413
  for adjustment disorder, 102
  for Alzheimer's disease, 80, 81t
  for anorexia nervosa, 347
  for anxiety disorders, 187–188,
      189t
    generalized, 169, 170

Antidepressants—cont'd
  for avoidant personality
      disorder, 338
  for bipolar depression, 143, 144
  for body dysmorphic disorder,
      266
  for borderline personality
      disorder, 335
  for bulimia nervosa, 350–351
  for dementia, 59–60
    HIV-associated, 57
  for depression
    major, 100–101
    with mixed anxiety, 104
  for dysthymia, 103
  for hypochondriasis, 265
  for major depression, 100–101
    in children, 426, 427t–431t,
        432
    strategies for, 432–433
    suicidality and, 432
  for nicotine dependence, 360
  for obsessive–compulsive
      disorder, 167
  for panic disorder, 163,
      164, 166
  for posttraumatic stress disorder,
      176
    in children, 401, 427t–431t
  for premenstrual dysphoric
      disorder, 106
  for psychosis of schizophrenia,
      251
  for sleep problems, 206
  for social phobia, 171
  guidelines for using, 108–109
  mania and, 143
  monamine oxidase inhibitors as,
      132–135, 133t, 135b
  neuroreceptor effects of,
      113, 114t
  norepinephrine reuptake
      inhibitors, 123–125
  P450 system inhibition by, 378,
      379b, 383
  pharmacokinetics of, 119–120
  pregnancy and, 120
  principles for using, 109–110
  profiles of specific, 110,
      111t–112t, 113

Antidepressants—cont'd
  psychotherapy indications
      with, 110
  second-generation,
      121–127.
    See also Second-generation
      antidepressants.
  selective serotonin reuptake
      inhibitors, 121–123.
    See also Selective
      serotonin reuptake
      inhibitors (SSRIs).
  medical complications of,
      127–131, 130b, 131b
  serotonin reuptake
      inhibitors, 123–125.
    See also Serotonin
      reuptake inhibitors (SRIs).
  sexual dysfunction related to,
      365t–366t
  side effects of, 113–119, 115t
    activation as, 116
    anticholinergic, 113, 116
    cardiac, 117, 118t, 119b
    gastrointestinal, 117
    orthostatic hypotension as,
        116–117, 118t
    sedation as, 116
    seizures as, 117
    sexual, 119
    suicide as, 117, 119
  stimulants as, 131–132
  switching guidelines for, 109
  therapeutic levels of, 108,
      111t, 120
  tricyclic. See Tricyclic
      antidepressants (TCAs).
  when to use, 108
Antiemetic agents, antipsychotics
    as, 250
Antifungal agents
  P450 system inhibition by,
      379b, 383
  psychiatric symptoms caused by,
      36b
Antihistamines
  analgesic properties of, 314
  for anxiety disorders, 188
  sexual dysfunction related to,
      365t

Antihypertensives
  antipsychotics interactions with,
      229t
  MAOIs interactions with, 134,
      135b
  psychiatric symptoms caused by,
      36b
Antiinflammatory agents
  nonsteroidal, 77, 78, 129, 314
  psychiatric symptoms caused by,
      36b
Antimanic agents, for bipolar
    disorder, 420, 421t–425t
Antipanic agents, for
    hypochondriasis, 265
Antipsychotic agents, 219–229
  adverse effects of, 235–248
    cardiovascular, 242–243
    endocrine, 243–244
    metabolic, 243–246
    miscellaneous other, 247–348
    neurologic, 235–242
    sexual, 246–247
  analgesic properties of, 314
  as P450 system substrate,
      380b–381b, 384
  atypical. See Atypical
      antipsychotics.
  chlorpromazine versus, 219, 220t
  depot, 219–220, 235
  drug interactions with, 228, 229t
  first versus second generation,
      219, 220t, 232t
  for Alzheimer's disease, 250
    agent-specific effects of, 70,
        71t, 72–73
    atypical, 68–73, 69t, 79
    conventional neuroleptics,
        68, 70
    parkinsonian symptoms and,
        70, 74, 74t
  for anorexia nervosa, 347
  for anxiety disorders, 188
  for behavioral emergencies, 274,
      275t, 276
  for bipolar disorder, 250
  for body dysmorphic disorder,
      266
  for borderline personality
      disorder, 335

Antipsychotic agents—cont'd
    for delirium, 249–250
    for dementia, 59, 60, 250
    for histrionic personality
        disorder, 336
    for hypochondriasis, 265
    for mental retardation,
        438t–439t, 440
    for paranoid personality
        disorder, 332
    for psychotic depression, 250
    for psychotic symptoms, 219–229
        alternatives to, 251
    for schizoid personality disorder,
        333
    for schizophrenia, 219–229
        alternatives to, 251
        atypical, 217, 218
        clinical guidelines for,
            230–248
    for sleep problems, 206
    intramuscular, 219, 223t, 234
    maintenance guidelines for,
        234–235
    monitoring protocol for, 244,
        245t, 246
    other indications for, 249–251
    overdose of, 248
    overview of, 219, 220t
    pharmacodynamics of, 221t,
        222t, 228
    pharmacokinetics of, 220, 223,
        224t–226t
    pregnancy and, 249
    resistance to, 234, 250
    response rating of, 234, 250
    side effects of, 230, 233t, 234, 276
    switching, 248–249
    typical, 219, 220t
Antiretroviral agents, 35b, 57
Antisocial personality disorder, 24,
    331t, 333
Antitubercular agents, psychiatric
    symptoms caused by, 36b
Antiviral agents
    for amnestic disorders, 61
    P450 system inhibition by, 379b,
        383
    psychiatric symptoms caused by,
        35b

Anxiety
    acute
        benzodiazepines for, 178
        in stress disorder, 173–175
    adjustment disorder with,
        172–173
    alcohol use associated
        with, 293
    alprazolam for, 443
    anticipatory, 166
    azapirones for, 185
    excessive
        in children, 390, 399
        in generalized
            anxiety disorder,
            167, 168, 169
        obsessive–compulsive
            disorder versus, 167
    hypochondriasis associated with,
        264, 265
    in alcohol withdrawal delirium,
        297b
    in Alzheimer's patients, 78
        treatment of, 78–79
    in dementia, 60
    in schizoid personality disorder,
        332
    mixed, depression and,
        103–104
    normative, 171, 173, 192
    performance, 171–172
    physical symptoms of, 158–159,
        159b
    reactive, 174
    situational, 174
    social, exposure therapy for,
        193–194
    substance-induced, 158, 161b
Anxiety disorders, 158–177
    acute stress disorder, 173–175
    adjustment disorder, 172–173
    antidepressants for, 108
    depressive disorders associated
        with, 420
    diagnostic approach to,
        158–159, 159b
    generalized anxiety disorder,
        168–170.
        See also Generalized
        anxiety disorder (GAD).

Anxiety disorders—cont'd
  in children, 390–409
    attention-deficit/hyperactivity
        with, 401,
        402t–407t, 411
    depression with, 401,
        427t–431t
    generalized, 169, 399, 427t
    mutism, 396–397
    obsessive–compulsive, 401,
        408–409
    panic, 397–398
    phobias, 391, 396
    posttraumatic stress, 399–401
    separation-related, 390–391,
        392t–395t
    social phobia, 398
  lack of recognition, 4, 4t
  obsessive–compulsive disorder,
        166–168
  overview of, 158
  panic disorder, 159–166
  personality disorders associated
        with, 328
  phobias, 170–172
  posttraumatic stress disorder,
        175–177
  prevalence of, 2t
    as medical care comorbidity,
        5, 6, 6t
  separation, 390–391, 392t–395t
  treatment of
    nonpharmacologic, 159, 163,
        189–194
    pharmacologic, 178–189.
        See also Antianxiety
        agents.
Anxiety-reduction strategies, 175
Anxiolytics
  for acute stress disorder, 175
  for adjustment disorder, 102
  for anorexia nervosa, 347
  for anxiety disorders, 185–186,
        187t
    generalized, 165t, 166
  for avoidant personality
        disorder, 338
APA. See American Psychiatric
        Association (APA).
Apathy, dementia and, 57

Aphasia, 62
Aplastic anemia, carbamazepine
        and, 152
Apnea
  ECT causing, 321, 322
  obstructive sleep, 195, 197,
        198–199
Apomorphine, for male erectile
        disorder, 371
Appetite change, as major
        depression criteria, 91b, 92, 98
Appetite suppressants, 244
Apprehensive expectation, 399
Aripiprazole (Abilify)
  dose recommendations for, 220t,
        224t
  for acute schizophrenia, 230,
        232t
  for Alzheimer's disease,
        69, 71t, 72
  for destructive behavior,
    in mental retardation,
        422t, 439t
  for mania, 141t, 143, 144
  for schizophrenia, 217
  formulary, 446–447
  pharmacokinetics of, 223, 224t
  pregnancy and, 249
  receptor affinities of, 221t
  side effects of, 233t, 244
Arousal, sexual, antipsychotics
        and, 246
Arrhythmias. See Cardiac
        arrhythmias.
Arterial blood gases (ABGs), 46
Arterial disorders, psychiatric
        symptoms caused by,
        39b, 40, 41b
Arthritis
  obesity associated with, 353
  rheumatoid, schizophrenia and,
        218
ASD. See Acute stress disorder
        (ASD).
Assault, anxiety disorders
        associated with, 173, 175
Asystole, ECT causing, 320, 322,
        324
Atenolol, for anxiety disorders,
        188

Atomoxetine hydrochloride
    (Strattera)
  for ADHD, 406t–407t, 413
  formulary, 447–448
Atropine, for ECT, 322
Attachment
  in dependent personality
    disorder, 338
  in separation anxiety disorder,
    390
Attention
  in cognitive examination,
    61–62
  in passive–aggressive
    personality disorder, 341
Attention Deficit
    Disorder Association
    (ADDA), 414
Attention-deficit/hyperactivity
    disorder (ADHD), 409–414
  anxiety disorders with, 401, 411
  bipolar disorder versus, 140
  comorbidities of, 411–412
  core symptoms of, 409–410
  course and prognosis of, 412
  definition of, 409
  developmental disabilities and,
    402t–407t, 440
  dextroamphetamine for, 458
  diagnostic evaluation of,
    410–411
  differential diagnosis of,
    411–412
  epidemiology of, 410
  learning disorder versus, 434
  subtypes of, 409
  treatment of, 412–414
    family interventions, 412,
      414
    individual interventions, 414
    pharmacotherapy, 402t–407,
      412–414
    school interventions, 414
    support groups, 414
Atypical antipsychotics
  adverse effects of, 219, 222t,
    235, 238
  as P450 system substrate,
    380b–381b, 384
  common, 219, 220t

Atypical antipsychotics—cont'd
  for Alzheimer's disease, 68–73,
    69t
    agent-specific effects of, 70,
      71t, 72–73
    anxiety and, 79
    parkinsonian symptoms and,
      70, 74, 74t
  for antidepressant
    augmentation, 110
  for bipolar depression, 143, 144,
    155, 250
  for destructive behavior, in
    mental retardation, 422t,
    439t, 440
  for mania, 141t, 143, 155, 250
  for posttraumatic stress disorder,
    176
  for schizophrenia, 217, 218
  receptor affinities of, 219, 221t
  therapeutic effects of, 219, 222t
Audiology testing
  for ADHD, 411
  for developmental disabilities,
    436
  for learning disorders, 434
Auditory hallucinations, 211
  alcoholic, 291
  in alcohol withdrawal delirium,
    297b–298b
  in major depression, 96
Authority figures, conduct disorder
    and, 415
Autism, psychotic symptoms
    versus, 213–214
Autoimmune disorders,
    depression associated
    with, 88b
Automatic behavior, in
    narcolepsy, 199
Autonomic nervous system
  anxiety symptoms in, 159b
  delirium and, 51
  ECT impact on, 320
Avoidant personality disorder,
    171, 331t, 337–338
AWD. See Alcohol withdrawal
    delirium (AWD).
Axis I, of DSM-IV, 21b, 22b
Axis II, of DSM-IV, 21b, 22b

Axis III, of DSM-IV, 21b, 22b
Axis IV, of DSM-IV,
    21b, 24, 24b
Axis V, of DSM-IV, 21b, 22b, 26,
    26b–27b
Azapirones
    benzodiazepines *versus*,
        186–187, 187t
    drug interactions with, 186
    for anxiety disorders, 185–187
        generalized, 165t, 169, 170
    indications for, 185–186
    side effects of, 186

BALs (blood alcohol levels)
    factors influencing, 300–301
    interpretation of, 45, 301, 301t
Barbiturates
    effects on EEG, 42
    for anxiety disorders, 188
Bariatric surgery, for obesity, 355
Barriers, in psychiatric interview,
    12, 13
BDD. *See* Body dysmorphic
    disorder (BDD).
Beck Depression Inventory (BDI),
    93, 94f–95f
Behavior disorders/problems
    chronic pain as, 313
    developmental determinants
        of, 23
    disruptive, 414–418.
        See also Disruptive
        behavior disorders.
    in dementia, 54
        treatment of, 59–60
    learning disorders associated
        with, 433, 434
    mental retardation associated
        with, 436
Behavior exaggeration, in
    personality disorders, 328,
    329, 332
Behavior rating scales, for
    ADHD, 411
Behavioral component
    of mental status examination,
        31–32
    of obesity, 351

Behavioral emergencies, 271–286
    acute mania as, 140, 272, 273,
        277
    commitment statutes for,
        284–285
    competence evaluations in,
        285–286
    data summary sheet for,
        collateral, 272t
    definition of, 271
    delirium as, 272, 273, 276
    differential diagnosis of, 272–273
    escalation management in,
        271, 274
    history taking in, 273
        brief initial, 271, 272t
    medication strategies for,
        274–277
        benzodiazepines *versus*
            antipsychotics, 274, 275t
        β-blockers, 277
        buspirone, 277
        divalproex, 277
        dosing of, 274, 276
        narcotics, 277
        preventive, 274
        rapid use, 274
        side effects of, 276–277
    mental status examination in, 273
    neurologic examination in, 274
    physical examination in, 272t,
        273–274
    physical restraint use, 283–284
    safe environment for, 271
    situational handling of,
        271–274
    suicide evaluation in, 277–281
    violent or homicidal patient as,
        281–283
Behavioral symptoms, of
    Alzheimer's disease, 65, 66t,
    67–68
    rating scale for disruptive, 65,
        67, 67b
    treatment of, 68–70, 69t, 71t,
        72–76, 74t
Behavioral therapy(ies)
    cognitive. *See* Cognitive
        behavioral therapy (CBT).
    cost-benefit issues involving, 9

Index

Behavioral therapy(ies)—cont'd
  for ADHD, 414
  for anxiety, 159, 189–194
    anticipatory, 166
  for anxiety disorders, 192–194
  for borderline personality
    disorder, 335
  for bulimia nervosa, 350
  for circadian rhythm sleep
    disorders, 201–202
  for conduct disorder, 416
  for obesity, 353
  for obsessive–compulsive
    disorder, 168
  for oppositional defiant disorder,
    418
  for pain disorders, 263
  for primary insomnia, 200, 201b
  for selective mutism, 396
  for separation anxiety disorder,
    391
  for simple phobias, 172
  for specific phobia, in children,
    391
  for substance abuse, 304
Beliefs, fixed false.
    See also Delusions.
  in children, 419
Benign prostatic hyperplasia,
    antipsychotic selection and,
    234
Benzodiazepines (BZs)
  abuse issues with, 182
    azapirones versus, 186
  as hypnotics, 178, 185, 206–208
  as P450 system substrate,
    380b–382b, 384–385
    azapirones versus, 186–187, 187t
  dependence on, pain disorder
    associated with, 262, 263
  differences among, 184–185
  discontinuing guidelines, 182
  drug interactions with, 183
  ECT interaction with, 322
  for acute stress disorder, 175
  for Alzheimer's disease, 69t, 75
    anxiety and, 79
    cognitive impairment related
      to, 76
    OBRA guidelines for, 83–84

Benzodiazepines (BZs)—cont'd
  for anxiety
    in children, 391, 392t–393t
    with alcoholism, 293
  for anxiety disorders, 178–185,
    179t, 187t
    generalized, 169
  for behavioral emergencies, 274,
    275t, 276
  for borderline personality
    disorder, 335
  for delirium tremens, 299
  for dementia, 60
  for histrionic personality
    disorder, 336
  for mania, 143, 155
  for obsessive–compulsive
    personality disorder, 340
  for panic disorder, 163–164,
    165t
    in children, 398
  for posttraumatic stress disorder,
    177
  for psychosis of schizophrenia,
    251
  for sleep problems, 206–208
  for social phobia, 171
  for tardive dyskinesia, 239
  for withdrawal-associated
    delirium, 53
  indications for, 178
  overdose of, 184
  pharmacokinetics of, 179t, 180,
    181b
  pregnancy and, 184
  psychiatric symptoms caused by,
    33
  side effects of, 181–182,
    276–277
  withdrawal issues, 182–183,
    183b
Benztropine (Cogentin), 235–236,
    276
Bereavement
  adjustment disorder versus, 173
  major depression associated
    with, 100, 420
β-Blockers
  ECT indications for, 325
  for akathisia, 236

β-Blockers—cont'd
  for Alzheimer's disease, 69t
  for anxiety disorders, 188
    performance, 171–172
  for behavioral emergencies, 277
  for mental retardation, 440
  for sedative withdrawal, 295
  for serotonin syndrome, 131
  for substance abuse, 304, 305
  SSRIs interaction with, 130
Bethanechol (Urecholine), 113
Binge-eating and purging
  in anorexia nervosa, 343
  in bulimia nervosa, 348–349
Biological context, in mental
    retardation evaluation, 436
Biperiden (Akineton), 237t
Bipolar disorder(s), 137–156
  ADHD versus, 411
  antipsychotics for, 250
  cyclothymic disorder in,
    138, 139
  definition of, 137–138
  depressive episodes in, 137–138
    major, 99–100, 108
    treatment of, 108, 143–144
    maintenance, 144
  hypomanic episode in, 137,
    138–139
  in children, 419
    treatment of, 420, 421t–425t
  manic episode in, 137, 138
    differential diagnosis of,
      139–140
    treatment of, 140, 141t, 142t,
      143
    maintenance, 144
  mixed episode in, 139
  obesity associated with, 352
  quetiapine for, 489
  rapid cycling in, 138, 139
  treatment of
    atypical antipsychotics for,
      155
    benzodiazepines for, 155
    carbamazepine for, 150–153,
      151b
    ECT for, 143, 156, 256, 317
    general issues for, 140–144
    lamotrigine, 154–155

Bipolar disorder(s)—cont'd
    lithium for, 144–147,
      145b
    maintenance, 144
    nonmedication dimensions of,
      156
    oxcarbazepine for, 153–154
    valproic acid for, 147–150
Bipolar I disorder, 137
Bipolar II disorder, 137–138
Birth defects, teratogens
    causing, 48, 147, 150,
      153, 154, 249
Bite block, for ECT, 323
Black box warning, on
    antidepressants, 432, 449,
      450b
Bleeding
  as SSRIs complication, 129
  intracranial versus subarachnoid,
    277
Blood alcohol levels (BALs)
  factors influencing, 300–301
  interpretation of, 45, 301, 301t
Blood glucose, screening tests
    for, 45
Blood pressure
  decrease. See Hypotension.
  in behavioral emergencies, 273
  in narcotics assessment, 309b
  increase. See Hypertensive crisis.
Blood urea nitrogen (BUN), 46
Blunts, abuse of, 315
BMI. See Body mass index (BMI).
Body dysmorphic disorder (BDD),
    265–266
  definition of, 265
  differential diagnosis of,
    265–266
  obsessive–compulsive disorder
    versus, 167
  premenstrual, 105–106
  treatment of, 266
Body mass index (BMI)
  antipsychotics effect on, 244,
    245t, 246
  in anorexia nervosa, 346
  in obesity, 351, 352, 353
    surgery indications based on,
      355

Body weight
    in anorexia nervosa, 343
    major depressive disorder and,
        418–419
Borderline personality disorder,
        334–335
    alcohol use associated with, 293
    as chronic suicidal, 280
    definition of, 334
    interventions for, 334–335
    major depression associated
        with, 92, 100
    medical management of, 331t
Boundaries, drawing, for
        personality disorders, 335, 339
BPRS (Brief Psychiatric Rating
        Scale), 234
Bradycardia
    ECT causing, 320, 322, 324, 325
    SSRIs causing, 130
Brain, ECT impact on, 317, 318,
        320, 324–325
Brain impairment/injury
    hemorrhagic. See Hematomas.
    ischemic. See Stroke.
    neuroimaging of, 42–44
    symptoms associated with, 38
    traumatic. See Head trauma.
Breast cancer, antipsychotic
        selection and, 230
Breast-feeding, medications and,
        120, 153, 249
Breathing problems, sleep
        problems associated with,
        195–196
Breathing training, diaphragmatic,
        for anxiety disorders, 189
Brief Psychiatric Rating Scale
        (BPRS), 234
Brief psychotic disorder, psychotic
        symptoms versus, 212
Bright light stimulation, for
        seasonal depression, 99
Brompton's mixture, 314
Bronchodilators, ECT indications
        for, 325
Bulimia nervosa, 348–351
    comorbidities of, 349
    definition of, 348–349
    differential diagnosis of, 350

Bulimia nervosa—cont'd
    epidemiology of, 349
    laboratory evaluation of, 344b,
        350
    medical disorders in, 344, 345b,
        349
    prognosis of, 351
    recognition of, 349
    treatment of, 350–351
BUN (blood urea nitrogen), 46
Buprenorphine hydrochloride
        (Suboxone, Subutex),
        311–312, 448
Bupropion hydrochloride
        (Wellbutrin, Zyban), 112t,
        125
    adverse effects of, 115t, 117,
        118t
    for Alzheimer's disease, 81t
    for anxiety disorders, 189t
    for bipolar depression, 143
    for nicotine dependence,
        359–360
    for obesity, 355
    formulary, 448–449
    neuroceptor effects of, 114t
    P450 system inhibition by, 379b,
        383
Buspirone hydrochloride (BuSpar)
    for Alzheimer's disease, 69t
    anxiety and, 79
    for anxiety, in children, 392t
    for anxiety disorders, 166,
        185–186
    for behavioral emergencies, 277
    for generalized anxiety disorder,
        165t, 166, 170
    in children, 392t, 427t–431t
    with alcoholism, 293
    for mental retardation, 440
    for mixed anxiety with
        depression, 104
    for obsessive–compulsive
        disorder, 167–168
    formulary, 449–450
Butorphanol nasal spray, for
        chronic malignant pain, 312
Butyrophenones, as antipsychotics,
        220t, 421t
BZs. See Benzodiazepines (BZs).

Caffeine citrate (Cafcit),
    450–451, 451t
Caffeine use, 28, 223
CAGE questionnaire, 28, 288, 288b
Calcium channel blockers, as P450
    system substrate, 381b, 385
Calorie restriction, 244
Cancer(s)
    breast, antipsychotic selection
        and, 230
    depression associated with, 88b,
        89
    mood disorder associated with,
        89–90
    obesity associated with, 353
    psychiatric symptoms caused by,
        33, 34t, 39b
    sexual dysfunction associated
        with, 373
Cannabis abuse, 315–316
    schizophrenia associated with, 217
Carbamazepine (Carbatol,
        Equetro, Tegretol)
    analgesic properties of, 314
    drug interactions with,
        150–151, 151b, 183
    for Alzheimer's disease, 69t,
        74–75, 74b, 74t
    for bipolar disorder, 150
        in children, 421t
    for borderline personality
        disorder, 335
    for mania, 142t, 143, 144, 150
    for sedative withdrawal, 295
    formulary, 151–152, 451–452
    formulations of, 151
    laboratory monitoring of, 152
    lamotrigine combined with, 155
    P450 system implications of, 387
    pharmacology of, 150
    side effects of, 152–153
Carbidopa-levodopa (Sinemet),
    134, 135b
Carbon dioxide (CO$_2$) retention, 46
    benzodiazepines and, 181
        azapirones versus, 186
Cardiac arrhythmias
    antidepressants causing, 117,
        118t, 119b
    antipsychotic selection and, 234

Cardiac arrhythmias—cont'd
    as SSRIs complication, 129–130
    carbamazepine causing, 153
    ECT and, 318, 322, 325
    in behavioral emergencies, 274
    lithium causing, 147
Cardiac/cardiovascular disorders
    alcohol use associated with, 287
    anorexia nervosa associated
        with, 345b, 346
        refeeding impact on, 347
    anxiety caused by, 160b
    ECT and, 318, 325
    marijuana abuse associated with,
        315
    obesity associated with, 352
    sexual dysfunction associated
        with, 372
    stimulant use cautions with, 413
Cardiac pacemakers, ECT and, 325
Cardiovascular medications
    as P450 system substrate,
        380b–381b, 385
    sexual dysfunction related to,
        366t–367t
Cardiovascular system
    antipsychotics effect on, 242–243
    anxiety symptoms in, 159b, 162
    ECT impact on, 318, 319, 320,
        324–325
"Care not cure" approach,
    256, 263
Case management, for conduct
    disorder, 416
Cataplexy, 199, 200
Catecholamines
    ECT impact on, 320
    MAOIs effect on, 134, 135b
CBC (complete blood count), 46
CBT. See Cognitive behavioral
        therapy (CBT).
CD4 count, in HIV-associated
        dementia, 56, 57
Central nervous system (CNS)
        disorders
    eating disorders and, 345b, 346
    fetal alcohol syndrome and, 292,
        434, 436
    infections, behavioral
        emergencies related to, 273

Central nervous system (CNS)
    disorders—cont'd
  lumbar puncture indications for,
    44
  mania associated with, 140
  neuroimaging of, 42–44
  psychiatric symptoms caused by,
    33, 34, 34t, 38, 40–41
  sexual dysfunction associated
    with, 373, 374
  space-occupying lesions, ECT
    and, 318, 326
Cerebral blood flow, ECT impact
    on, 320, 325
Cerebral infarction, neuroimaging
    of, 44
Cerebrovascular accident.
    See Stroke.
Cerebrovascular disease
  amnestic disorders and, 61
  antipsychotics associated with,
    243
  depression associated with, 88b
  ECT and, 318, 320, 325
  mania associated with, 140
  neuroimaging of, 43, 44
Ceruloplasmin levels, 47
CHADD (Children with
    Attention Deficit Disorder),
    414
Chemotherapy
  psychiatric symptoms caused by,
    33, 36b
  sexual dysfunction related to,
    366t
Chest pain
  panic disorder manifesting as,
    7, 8
  somatoform disorders
    manifesting as, 258, 259
Chief complaint, 14f, 19–22
Child Attention Profile, 411
Children, psychiatry for, 389–440
  ADHD, 409–414
  antisocial personality disorder,
    333
  anxiety disorders, 390–409
  depressive disorders, 418–433
  developmental disabilities,
    435–440

Children, psychiatry for—cont'd
  diagnostic assessment of,
    389–390
  disruptive behavior, 414–418
  learning disorders, 433–435
  mental retardation, 435–440
  overanxious disorder, 168
  overview of, 389
  suicidality, 449, 450b
Children with Attention Deficit
    Disorder (CHADD), 414
Chloral hydrate, for sedative
    withdrawal, 295
Chlordiazepoxide hydrochloride
    (Librium)
  for anxiety, 184
  for delirium tremens, 299
  for sleep problems, 206
  for withdrawal-associated
    delirium, 53
  formulary, 452–453
  pharmacokinetics of,
    179t, 180, 181b
Chlorpromazine (Thorazine)
  antipsychotic equivalents of, 220t
  dose recommendations for, 220t
  ECT interaction with, 321
  for destructive behavior, in
    mental retardation,
    421t, 438t
  neonatal jaundice from, 249
  P450 system inhibition by, 379b
Cholinergic antagonists.
    See Anticholinergics.
Cholinesterase inhibitors, 59, 61,
    239
Chronic fatigue syndrome,
    hypochondriasis versus, 264
Chronic medical conditions
  in primary medical care, 5, 6t
  suicidality related to, 277
Chronic obstructive pulmonary
    disease (COPD), ECT and,
    318, 325
Chronic pain
  malignant, management of, 312,
    313t
  medical history of, 28
  nonmalignant, management of,
    312–313

Cigarettes. See Nicotine dependence; Nicotine use.
Cimetidine (Tagamet), 379b, 383, 387
CINA (Clinical Institute Narcotic Assessment), 308b–309b, 310
Ciprofloxacin, P450 system inhibition by, 379b, 383
Circadian rhythm sleep disorders, 201–202
Citalopram hydrobromide (Celexa), 109, 111t, 122
  adverse effects of, 115t
  for anxiety disorders, 188
  for generalized anxiety disorder, 165t
  for major depression, in children, 427t
  formulary, 453
  P450 system inhibition by, 379b, 383
CIWA-A (Clinical Institute Withdrawal Assessment for Alcohol), 295, 296b–298b
CK (creatine kinase), 47
CK isoenzymes, in myocardial infarction, 47
Classroom interventions. See School interventions.
Claustrophobia, 172
Clinical disorders, in psychiatric database, 13, 21b, 22b
Clinical Institute Narcotic Assessment (CINA), 308b–309b, 310
Clinical Institute Withdrawal Assessment for Alcohol (CIWA-A), 295, 296b–298b
Clinically Useful Depression Outcome Scale (CUDOS), 94
Clomipramine hydrochloride (Anafranil), 111t, 121
  for anxiety disorders, 187
  for body dysmorphic disorder, 266
  for hypochondriasis, 265
  for major depression, in children, 428t–429t
  for obsessive–compulsive disorder, 167

Clomipramine hydrochloride (Anafranil)—cont'd
  for premenstrual dysphoric disorder, 106
  formulary, 453–454
Clonazepam (Klonopin)
  for anxiety, 184–185
    in children, 392t–393t
  for generalized anxiety disorder, 165t
  for mania, 143, 155
  for panic disorder, 163, 164, 165t
  for posttraumatic stress disorder, 177
  for serotonin syndrome, 131
  formulary, 454–455
  pharmacokinetics of, 179t, 180, 181b
  side effects of, 454–455
Clonidine (Catapres)
  for ADHD, 414
  for anxiety, in children, 394t
  for narcotics withdrawal, 310
  for nicotine dependence, 360
Clorazepate dipotassium (Tranxene), 179t, 180, 181b, 455
Clozapine (Clozaril, Fazaclo)
  contraindications to, 247
  dose recommendations for, 220t, 224t
  for acute schizophrenia, 230, 232t
  for Alzheimer's disease, 69, 71t, 72–73, 74, 74t
  for bipolar disorder, 144
  for destructive behavior, in mental retardation, 422t, 439t
  for schizophrenia, 217, 218, 234
  for seizure risk, with antipsychotics, 242
  for tardive dyskinesia, 239
  formulary, 455–456
  P450 system and, 223, 227t, 387
  pharmacokinetics of, 224t
  pregnancy and, 249
  receptor affinities of, 221t
  side effects of, 233t, 235, 244
    unusual, 247–248
  therapeutic level of, 228

CNS. *See* Central nervous system (CNS) disorders.
CNS depressants. *See also* Alcohol use/abuse; Barbiturates; Benzodiazepines (BZs).
  antipsychotics interactions with, 229t
  as P450 system inducer, 386, 387b
CNS stimulants. *See* Stimulants.
Cocaine level, 45, 304
Cocaine use/abuse, 301–305
  analgesic properties of, 314
  medical treatment of, 304–305
  prevalence of, 301
  recognition of, 304
  schizophrenia associated with, 217
  symptoms of, 301, 302t, 304
Codeine, half-life of, 310t
Cognitive assessment.
  See also Thought *entries.*
  for ADHD, 410, 411
  of sober alcoholics, 292
Cognitive behavioral therapy (CBT)
  for anorexia nervosa, 348
  for anxiety disorders, 159, 163, 189–194
    behavior interventions, 192–194
    cognitive interventions, 192
    contraindications for, 192
    physical interventions, 189–190, 190b, 191b, 192
  for avoidant personality disorder, 338
  for bipolar depression, 144
  for body dysmorphic disorder, 266
  for generalized anxiety disorder, 166, 170
  for hypochondriasis, 265
  for major depression, 101
    in children, 426
  for nicotine dependence, 360
  for obsessive–compulsive disorder, 408–409
  for panic disorder, 163, 164–165
    in children, 397

Cognitive behavioral therapy (CBT)—cont'd
  for psychosis of schizophrenia, 251
  for separation anxiety disorder, 391
  for social phobia, in children, 398
  for somatization disorder, 257
  for specific phobia, in children, 391
Cognitive impairment
  antipsychotics causing, 242
  benzodiazepines causing, 181
    azapirones *versus*, 186
  delirium and, 50, 51
  dementia and, 54, 55, 56, 57
  ECT causing, 319–320
  in Alzheimer's patients, 76
    treatment of, 77–78
  in hypochondriasis, 264
  in personality disorder, 328
  in posttraumatic stress disorder, 176
  in psychosis, 210, 211b
  in schizophrenia, 215, 251
  suicide risk related to, 278
Cognitive mental status examination, 61–63
  components of, 61–63
    higher functions, 63
  for dementia, 58
  overview of, 61
Cognitive restructuring, for anxiety disorders, 192
Collateral information
  for ADHD evaluation, 410
  for conduct disorder diagnosis, 415
COMA, 291, 291b
Command hallucinations, 211
Commitment
  of suicidal patient, 280
  under mental health statutes, 284–285
Commitment hearing, 284
Communication
  in psychiatric interview, 12–13
  with Alzheimer's patients, 64

Community-based interventions, for psychosis of schizophrenia, 251

Comorbidities
  in medical care
    evaluation of, 33–48.
      See also Medical evaluation.
    prevalence of, 5, 6–7 6t.
      See also Primary care.
  national survey on, 1, 2t
  of ADHD, 411–412
  of alcohol use/abuse, 292–293
  of bulimia nervosa, 349
  of child and adolescent conditions, 389, 411
  of ECT, 318–319
  of major depression, 95–96
    in children, 420
  of obesity, 352
  of personality disorders, 328
  of schizophrenia, 217–218
    antipsychotic choices based on, 230, 233t

Compensatory behaviors, in bulimia nervosa, 348–349

Competence
  evaluation of, 285–286
  implied consent and, 285

Complaints/complaining, in passive–aggressive personality disorder, 341

Complete blood count (CBC), 46

Complex absence seizures, 499

Complex partial seizures, 499

Comprehension, in cognitive examination, 62

Compulsions, definition of, 166, 401

Computed tomography (CT) scan
  contrast versus noncontrast, 43, 44
  for developmental disabilities, 436
  MRI versus, 43
  single positron emission, 44

Concentration, poor
  as major depression criteria, 91b, 92
  posttraumatic stress disorder and, 175, 176

Conduct disorder, 333, 414–417
  ADHD versus, 411
  course and prognosis of, 416
  definition of, 414
  diagnosis of, 415
  differential diagnosis of, 415–416
  epidemiology of, 415
  identification of, 414–415
  treatment of, 416–417

Conduction delay, cardiac.
  See Heart block.

Confabulation, alcohol intoxication and, 291

Confidentiality, 13, 22, 30

Confrontation
  of antisocial personality disorder, 333
  of factitious disorder, 267

Confusion, ECT causing, 320

Congenital adrenal hypoplasia, 376

Connor's Parent and Teacher Questionnaires, 411

Consent
  for obtaining medical records, 13
  for third party confirmation, 280
  implied, 285
  informed
    for antipsychotics, 238
    for ECT, 321
    in child and adolescent psychiatry, 389

Constipation, with narcotics use, 306

Consultations
  for generalized anxiety disorder, in children, 399
  for homicidal patient, 282
  for learning disorder treatment, 435
  for suicidal patient, 280
  legal, for commitment, 284–285
  specialist, for ECT, 322

Contract for safety, with suicidal patient, 281

Control issues, in personality disorders, 337, 339–340

Conversion disorder, 258–262
  definition of, 258
  diagnostic criteria for, 258
  differential diagnosis of, 259
  factitious disorder *versus*, 267
  identification of, 258
  malingering *versus*, 268
  multiple sclerosis manifesting
    as, 33
  pain disorder *versus*, 263
  prevalence of, 259
  prognosis of, 259
  treatment of, 259–262
COPD (chronic
    obstructive pulmonary
    disease), ECT and,
    318, 325
Copper, serum level of, 47
Coproporphyrins, 47
Correctional facilities, conduct
    disorder and, 416
Cortical dementia, 55
Cosmetic surgery, body
    dysmorphic disorder and,
    265, 266
Costs
  economic, of psychiatric
    disorders, 2, 3t
  medical. *See* Medical costs.
Counseling
  for nicotine dependence, 360
  for obesity, 353
  psychosocial, for depression, 87
Courtesy, in psychiatric
    interview, 12
Creatine kinase (CK), 47
Creatinine, 46
Criticism, fear of, 337–338
Cross-gender identification, 376
Cross-titration, of antipsychotics,
    249
CT scan. *See* Computed
    tomography (CT) scan.
CUDOS (Clinically Useful
    Depression Outcome
    Scale), 94
Cushing's syndrome, obesity
    and, 352
Cyclothymia, 138
Cyclothymic disorder, 139

CYP 1A2
  genetics of, 382
  inducers of, 386, 387b
  inhibitors of, 379b, 383
  substrate competition with,
    380b, 385
CYP 2D6
  age effects on, 383
  genetics of, 382
  inhibitors of, 379b, 383
  substrate competition with,
    381b, 384–385
CYP 2C9
  genetics of, 382
  inducers of, 386, 387b
  inhibitors of, 379b, 383
  substrate competition with,
    380b, 385
CYP 2C19
  age effects on, 383
  genetics of, 382
  inducers of, 386, 387b
  inhibitors of, 379b, 383–384
  substrate competition with,
    380b, 386
CYP 3A4
  age effects on, 383
  genetics of, 382
  inducers of, 386, 387b
  inhibitors of, 379b, 383
  QT prolongation associated
    with, 243
  substrate competition with,
    381b–382b, 385
Cyproheptadine, for anorexia
    nervosa, 347
Cytochrome P450 enzymes.
    See CYP *entries;* P450 system.

Daily activity history, in
    psychiatric database, 25
Data summary sheet, for behavioral
    emergencies, 271, 272t
Database
  for ADHD evaluation, 410
  for conduct disorder diagnosis,
    415
  psychiatric, 13–32. *See also*
    Psychiatric database.

DBRS (Disruptive Behavior
    Rating Scale), for Alzheimer's
    patients, 65, 67, 67b
DD. See Dysthymic disorder (DD).
DDT (Disability Determination
    Team), 435
Deafness, in Alzheimer's patients, 76
Decision making, impaired, in
    personality disorders, 338, 340
Defensive behavior
  in conversion disorder, 259
  in passive–aggressive
    personality disorder, 341
Defibrillators, ECT and, 325
Deficit state, in schizophrenia, 216
Degenerative disorders
  EEG evaluation of, 42
  psychiatric symptoms caused by,
    40b, 41b
Delinquency, 333, 414
Delirium, 50–54
  alcohol withdrawal, 295–300.
    See also Alcohol with-
    drawal delirium (AWD).
  antipsychotics for, 249
  anxiety secondary to, 158
  as behavioral emergencies, 272,
    273, 276
  definition of, 50
  dementia and, 51, 54
  DSM categories of, 50
  ECT for, 317, 322, 325–326
  EEG evaluation of, 41
  in Alzheimer's patients, 67, 68
  incidence of, 52
  medical etiologies of, 34t, 38,
    46, 50, 51b
  miscellaneous conditions
    versus, 52
  prevalence of, 52
  prognosis of, 52
  recognition of, 51
  risk factors for, 52
  sleep problems associated
    with, 203
  symptoms of, 50–51
  treatment of, 52–54
    for alcohol or sedative
      withdrawal, 53, 298–300
    for all other etiologies, 53–54

Delirium tremens (DTs),
    292, 293, 295
  treatment of, 298–300
Delusional disorder
  body dysmorphic disorder
    versus, 266
  diagnosis of, 213, 213b
  hypochondriasis versus, 264
  somatization disorder versus, 255
Delusions
  delirium and, 50
  in Alzheimer's patients, 66t,
    67–68
  in major depression, 96
  in psychosis, 210–211
  medical etiologies of, 34t
  prevalence in dementias, 5
  social phobia and, 171
Dementia
  alcoholic, 292
  antipsychotics for, 59, 60, 250
  personality disorders associated
    with, 328, 329
  sexual disinhibition and, 60, 374
Dementia(s), 5, 54–60. See also
    specific disorder.
  antipsychotics for, 250
  as medical care comorbidity, 5
  behavioral problems in, 54
    treatment of, 59–60
  cause by age of onset,
    54–55, 55t
  cortical versus subcortical, 55, 56
  definition of, 54
  delirium and, 51, 54
  differential diagnosis of,
    54–55, 166, 176
  EEG evaluation of, 41
  evaluation of, 57–59, 58b
  identification of, 54
  neuroimaging of, 42, 44
  psychiatric problems in, 54
    treatment of, 59–60
  selected disorders of, 55–57
  sleep problems associated with,
    203
Demographics, in psychiatric
    database, 13–19, 17f, 19f
Dependence, in narcotic use, 306,
    308b–309b

Dependent personality disorder, 331t, 338–339
Depot antipsychotics, for schizophrenia, 219–220, 235
Depression, 86–106
   ADHD versus, 411
   adjustment disorder associated with, 89, 101–102
   alcohol use associated with, 292–293
   benzodiazepines causing, 181
   body dysmorphic disorder and, 265, 266
   chronic, somatization disorder versus, 256
   "double," 420
   dysthymia associated with, 100, 102–103
   EEG evaluation of, 41
   endogenous versus exogenous, 90–91
   evaluation strategy for, 86–89
   functional impact of, 1–2
   hypochondriasis associated with, 264, 265
   identification of
      general issues in, 86
      lack of in medical practice, 4, 4t
   in Alzheimer's patients, 78, 79, 80
   in bipolar disorder, 137–138
      major, 99–100
      treatment of, 108, 143–144
      maintenance, 144
   in children, 418–433
      anxiety disorders with, 401, 427t–431t
      course and prognosis of, 426
      differential diagnosis of, 420, 426
      epidemiology of, 420
      treatment of
         antidepressants for, 426, 427t–431t, 432–433
         mood stabilizers for, 420, 421t–425t
      types of, 418–420
   in dementia, 54, 59

Depression—cont'd
   in generalized anxiety disorder, 169
   in schizophrenia, 218
   major, 90–101. See also Major depressive disorder.
   medical costs of, 8
   medical problems triggering, 33, 38, 47
      examples of, 34t, 86, 88b
   minor (subthreshold), 106
   mixed anxiety and, 103–104
   mood disorders and, 86, 89–90
   myocardial infarction and, 5, 6, 6t
   nicotine dependence associated with, 356–357
   obesity associated with, 352
   panic disorders in, 162, 166
   premenstrual dysphoric disorder and, 105–106
   prevalence of, 2t
      as medical care comorbidity, 5, 6–7 6t
   psychotic, 212, 250
   symptom database for, 86, 87f
Depressive personality disorder, 331t, 340
DES (diethylstilbestrol), for Alzheimer's disease, 76
Descriptive component, of mental status examination, 30–31
Desensitization, for anxiety disorders, 193
Desipramine hydrochloride (Norpramin)
   as antidepressant, 111t, 121, 429t
   formulary, 456–457
Detention period, in commitment, 285
Detoxification
   for alcoholism, 288, 290
   for narcotics addiction, 311
Developmental delay, 435
   of speech, 396
Developmental disabilities, 435–440
   course and prognosis of, 437
   definition of, 432
   differential diagnosis of, 436–437

Developmental disabilities—
    cont'd
  epidemiology of, 435—436
  evaluation of, 436
  identification of, 396, 435
  treatment of
    nonpharmacologic, 437
    psychotropics for, 437,
      438t—439t, 440
Developmental history, 16f, 23
Dexmethylphenidate
    hydrochloride (Focalin), 457
Dextroamphetamine mixed salts.
    See Amphetamine (Adderall).
Dextroamphetamine sulfate
    (Dexedrine Spansule,
    Dextrostat)
  analgesic properties of, 314
  as antidepressant, 131—132
  for ADHD, 403t, 413
  for antidepressant
    augmentation, 110
  for narcolepsy, 199
  formulary, 446, 458—459
Dextromethorphan, 33, 384
Diabetes insipidus, nephrogenic,
    lithium causing, 147
Diabetes mellitus
  antipsychotics associated with,
    244
    monitoring guidelines for,
      244, 245t, 246
  ECT and, 322
  obesity associated with, 353
  sexual dysfunction associated
    with, 373
Diagnostic and Statistical Manual of
    Mental Disorders, 4th edition
    (DSM-IV)
  axes of, 13, 21b, 22b, 24, 24b
  learning disorder criteria, 433
  multiaxial report form, 13, 21b
  personality disorder criteria,
    328—329
  psychosocial function
    assessment in, 26,
      26b—27b
  somatoform disorder criteria,
    253—255, 268
  V codes of, 173

Diagnostic Interview for
    Personality Disorders
    (DIPD-IV), 330
Diagnostic testing, for
    psychiatric symptoms,
    41—48
Dialectical behavior therapy, for
    borderline personality
    disorder, 335
DIAPERS, for incontinence
    diagnosis, in Alzheimer's
    patients, 82, 83b
Diaphragmatic breathing
    training, for anxiety
    disorders, 189
Diazepam (Diastat, Valium)
  for acute stress disorder, 175
  for akathisia, 236
  for anxiety, 185
  for delirium tremens, 299
  for generalized anxiety
    disorder, 169
  for prolonged seizures, with
    ECT, 324
  for sleep problems, 206
  formulary, 459—460
  pharmacokinetics of, 179t,
    180, 181b
  pregnancy cautions with, 184
Diet modifications
  for obesity, 353
  for premenstrual dysphoric
    disorder, 106
Diethylstilbestrol (DES), for
    Alzheimer's disease, 76
Digoxin, Alzheimer's disease and,
    69t, 76
Diltiazem, P450 system inhibition
    by, 379b, 383
Dimethyltryptamine (DMT),
    302t, 305
DIPD-IV (Diagnostic
    Interview for Personality
    Disorders), 330
Diphenhydramine (Benadryl)
  for acute dystonic reaction, 236
  for anxiety disorders, 188
  for medication-induced
    parkinsonism, 237t
  for sleep problems, 205—206

Disability(ies)
    developmental.
        See Developmental
        disabilities.
    learning. See Learning
        disorders/disabilities.
    mental. See Mental disability.
    psychosocial, 24–25
    self-care, 25, 338
Disability Determination Team
        (DDT), 435
Disapproval, fear of, 337–338
Discharge, AMA
    as patient's choice, 267, 268
    commitment and, 285
Discipline techniques, for
        conduct disorder, 416
Disease, fear of, 263.
        See also Hypochondriasis.
Disinhibition
    in borderline personality
        disorder, 335
    in dementia, 60, 374
    personality disorders associated
        with, 328
Disinterest, as major depression
        criteria, 91
Dislocations, musculoskeletal,
        ECT causing, 321
Dismissal, of somatization
        disorder, 256
Disorganization
    in psychosis, 210, 211b
    in schizophrenia, 215–216
Disruptive behavior disorders
    depressive disorders associated
        with, 420
    in children, 414–418
        conduct, 414–417
        oppositional defiant, 417–418
Disruptive Behavior Rating Scale
        (DBRS), for Alzheimer's
        patients, 65, 67, 67b
Distractibility, in ADHD, 409
Distress. See Stress/stressors.
Distribution, of medications.
        See specific drug classification or
        agent.
Disulfiram (Antabuse), 289,
        460–461

Diuretic abuse
    in anorexia nervosa, 345b, 347
    in bulimia nervosa, 348–349
Diuretics, psychiatric symptoms
        caused by, 37b
Divalproex sodium (Depakote)
    for Alzheimer's disease, 75
    for behavioral emergencies, 277
    for bipolar depression, 143, 144
    for bipolar disorder, in
        children, 421t
    for mania, 142t, 143
    for posttraumatic stress
        disorder, 176
    formulary, 461
DMT (dimethyltryptamine),
        302t, 305
Doctor-patient relationship,
        personality disorders
        complication of, 329, 337
Donepezil (Aricept), 77, 461–462
Dopamine agonists.
        See Dopaminergics.
Dopamine receptors, atypical
        antipsychotics affinity for,
        219, 221t
    therapeutic versus adverse
        effects, 222t
Dopamine uptake
    inhibitors, 114t
Dopaminergics
    agitation related to, in
        Alzheimer's patients, 68,
        69b, 76
    anxiety caused by, 161b
    for medication-induced
        parkinsonism, 236
    for periodic limb movement
        disorders, 202
    psychiatric symptoms caused
        by, 37b
    sexual dysfunction related
        to, 367t
    sleep problems associated
        with, 203
Dose conversions
    for narcotics, 306, 307b
        to fentanyl patch,
            312, 313t
    for sedative-hypnotics, 299t

Dose–response relationship
  in smoking cessation therapies,
    357
  of antidepressants, 109
  of tetrahydrocannabinol, 315
"Double depression," in children,
    420
Doxepin hydrochloride
    (Sinequan), 111t, 462
Drooling, clozapine associated
    with, 247
Droperidol, MAOIs interactions
    with, 134, 135b
Drowsiness, benzodiazepines
    causing, 181, 186
Drug abuse
  bipolar disorder *versus*, 140
  economic costs of, 3t
  illicit street drugs, patient
    history of, 28
  in primary medical care, 6t, 7
  medical costs of, 5, 8, 355
  of diuretics, 345b, 347, 348–349
  of laxatives, 345b, 347, 348–349
  of narcotics, 305–314
  of nitrous oxide, 301, 303t, 304
  of psychotropics, 314–316
  of stimulants. *See* Stimulant
    abuse.
  psychiatric symptoms caused by,
    34t, 35, 38
Drug allergies
  hepatic responses with, 45–46
  patient history of, 28
Drug challenge tests, for "poor"
    metabolism, 382
Drug interactions
  in nicotine dependence, 356,
    356b
  in psychiatric database, 20
  with antipsychotics, 228, 229t
  with azapirones, 186
  with benzodiazepines, 183
  with carbamazepine, 150–151,
    151b, 183
  with ECT, 321, 322
  with lithium, 145, 145b
  with MAOIs, 134, 135b
  with P450 system, 74, 74t, 123,
    130

Drug interactions—cont'd
  with SSRIs, 130
  with TCAs, 118t, 121, 122b
  with valproate/valproic acid, 148
Drug levels
  in substance use screening, 28, 29
  therapeutic. *See* Therapeutic
    levels.
Drug reactions, patient history of, 28
Drug resistance, 234, 250, 317
Drug withdrawal
  anxiety caused by, 158, 161b
  management of. *See* Withdrawal.
  patient history of, 28
  sleep problems associated
    with, 203
DSM-IV. *See Diagnostic and
    Statistical Manual of Mental
    Disorders, 4th edition*
    (DSM-IV).
DTs (delirium tremens),
    292, 293, 295
  treatment of, 298–300
Duloxetine hydrochloride
    (Cymbalta), 112t, 124–125
  adverse effects of, 115t
  analgesic properties of, 314
  formulary, 463
  neuroceptor effects of, 114t
  P450 system inhibition by,
    379b, 383
Durable powers of attorney, 286
Dyslipidemia, antipsychotics
    associated with, 70, 72, 244
  monitoring guidelines for, 244,
    245t, 246
Dyspareunia, 371–372
Dysphoric disorder
  body. *See* Body dysmorphic
    disorder.
  premenstrual, 105–106, 419
Dysphoric response, to
    antidepressants, 164
Dyspnea, panic-related, 162
Dysthymic disorder (DD)
  depression associated with, 100,
    102–103
  in children, 419
  sleep problems associated with,
    203

Dystonia, tardive, 240
Dystonic reaction, acute, to
    antipsychotics, 235–236, 276

EAHCA (Education for
    All Handicapped Children
    Act) of 1975, 435, 437
Eating disorder not otherwise
    specified, 343
Eating disorders, 343–355
    anorexia nervosa, 343–348
    bulimia nervosa, 348–351
    in Alzheimer's patients, 80, 82
    laboratory evaluation of, 344,
        344b
    medical disorders in, 344, 345b
    obesity related to, 351–355
Eccentricities, in schizoid
    personality disorder, 332
ECG (electrocardiogram), for
    children, on antidepressants,
    432–433
Economic costs, of psychiatric
    disorders, 2, 3t
"Ecstasy," 302t, 305, 385
ECT. See Electroconvulsive
    therapy (ECT).
ED (emergency department),
    psychiatric comorbidity
    screening in, 7, 8.
    See also Emergencies.
Education, of patients and
    families. See Patient teaching.
Education for All Handicapped
    Children Act (EAHCA) of
    1975, 435, 437
Educational level, in psychiatric
    database, 14, 23–24
Educational therapies. See School
    interventions.
EEG. See Electroencephalogram
    (EEG).
Ego functions, in schizophrenia, 216
Ejaculation, 363
    premature, 371
Elderly patients. See Geriatric
    patients.
Electrical stimulus parameters, in
    ECT, 323

Electrocardiogram (ECG), for
    children, on antidepressants,
    432–433
Electroconvulsive therapy (ECT),
    317–326
    adverse effects of, 318–321
        cardiovascular, 320
        cerebrovascular, 320
        cognitive, 319–320
        intragastric, 320
        intraocular, 320
        miscellaneous other, 321
        overall mortality, 318–319
        pulmonary, 320
    common complaints following,
        319
    contraindications to, 318
    drug interactions with, 321, 322
    for bipolar disorder, 143, 156
        antipsychotics versus, 250
    for major depression, 97, 100,
        101, 317
        as drug augmentation, 110
        in pregnancy, 120
    for neuroleptic malignant
        syndrome, 242, 325
    for psychosis of schizophrenia, 251
    indications for, 317
    maintenance, 324
    medical disease considerations
        for, 318, 324–326
        cardiovascular, 318, 325
        CNS space-occupying lesions,
            318, 326
        COPD, 318, 325
        CVA, 318, 325
        delirium, 317, 325–326
        epilepsy, 326
        neuroleptic malignant
            syndrome, 325
        Parkinson's disease, 325
    overview of, 317
    physiologic effects of, 324–325
    pregnancy and, 120, 318, 326
    procedure for, 321–324
        consent, 321
        pre-therapy assessment,
            321–322
        pre-therapy orders, 322
        technique, 322–324

Electrode placement, for ECT, 319, 323
Electroencephalogram (EEG), 41–42
    effect of drugs on, 42, 117
    for mental retardation, 436
    in polysomnography, 48, 197
Electrolyte disturbances
    in eating disorders, 345b, 346, 347, 349
    psychiatric symptoms caused by, 39b, 40, 41b, 46–47
Electrolytes, 46–47
Electromyography (EMG), in polysomnography, 197
EMDR (eye movement desensitization and reprocessing), 401
Emergencies
    alcohol amnestic syndrome as, 291, 291b
    alcoholic hallucinosis as, 292
    behavioral, 271–286
        commitment statutes for, 284–285
        competence evaluations in, 285–286
        management of, 271–277. *See also* Behavioral emergencies.
        physical restraint use, 283–284
        suicide evaluation in, 277–281
        violent or homicidal patient as, 281–283
Emergency department (ED), psychiatric comorbidity screening in, 7, 8
Emesis, antipsychotics for, 250
EMG (electromyography), in polysomnography, 197
Emotional detachment, in personality disorders, 332
Emotional safety, acute stress disorder and, 174–175
Emotional situations, somatized symptoms associated with, 257
Emotions, anxiety caused by, 192

Emptiness, chronic
    in major depression, 91b, 92, 100
    in personality disorders, 334
Encephalopathy, hepatic, 292
Endocrine disorders
    anxiety caused by, 160b
    depression associated with, 88b, 89
    eating disorders associated with, 344, 345b
    hypochondriasis *versus*, 264
    mood disorder associated with, 89–90
    mood stabilizers causing, 147, 152, 153
    psychiatric symptoms caused by, 39b, 40, 41b
    sexual dysfunction associated with, 374
Endocrine effects, of antipsychotics, 243–244
Endocrinology consultation, 30
Endogenous depression, 90–91
Entitlement programs, patient participation in, 25
Enuresis, 400
Environmental interventions
    for delirium, 52
    for dementia, 59
Environmental problems
    developmental disabilities associated with, 434, 436–437
    DSM-IV axis IV for, 21b, 24, 24b
    in psychiatric database, 24–26
    obesity related to, 351
Eosinophilia, clozapine associated with, 248
Epilepsy
    ECT for, 326
        refractory, 317
    temporal lobe epilepsy, bipolar disorder *versus*, 139–140
    topiramate for, 495–496
        titration schedule, 495, 496t
    violence associated with, 281
EPS. *See* Extrapyramidal symptoms/effects (EPS).
Epworth sleepiness scale, 196, 196b

Erectile disorder, male,
    370–371
  neurogenic, 373
Escalation management, in
    behavioral emergencies,
    271, 274
Escitalopram (Lexapro),
    109, 111t, 122–123
  adverse effects of, 115t
  for anxiety disorders, 188, 189t
  for generalized anxiety
    disorder, 165t
  for major depression, in
    children, 427t
  formulary, 463
  P450 system inhibition by,
    379b, 383
Esmolol, ECT indications for, 325
Estazolam (Prosom), 464
Estrogen therapy
  for Alzheimer's disease,
    75–76, 78
  for paraphilias, 376
Eszopiclone (Lunesta), 208, 464
Exaggeration, of behavior,
    in personality disorders,
    328, 329
Excretion, of medications. See
    specific drug classification
    or agent.
Exercise
  excessive, in eating disorders,
    344, 349
  for acute stress disorder, 175
  for adjustment disorder, 173
  for generalized anxiety
    disorder, 170
  for obesity, 353
  lack of, obesity related to, 351
Exhibitionism, 375
Exogenous depression, 90–91
Explosive behavior, in
    mental retardation,
    421t–425t, 440
Exposure therapy
  for anxiety disorders, 193–194
  for obsessive–compulsive
    disorder, 168
  for phobias, 165, 171, 193
Expression disorders, 411, 433

Extrapyramidal symptoms/effects
    (EPS)
  of antipsychotics, 219, 233t,
    235, 249
    acute dystonic reactions,
      235–236
    in Alzheimer's disease, 69t,
      70, 74
  of schizophrenia, 216
  of SSRIs, 129, 131
Eye contact, with Alzheimer's
    patients, 64
Eye movement desensitization and
    reprocessing (EMDR), 401
Eyes
  disorders of. See Ocular disorders.
  ECT impact on, 320

Factitious disorder, 266–267
  clinical presentation of, 266–267
  definition of, 266
  differential diagnosis of, 267, 268
  pain disorder versus, 263
  severe form of, 266
  somatization disorder versus, 256
  treatment of, 267
Family assessment, 13, 22, 30
  in child and adolescent
    psychiatry, 389–390
Family history
  in conduct disorder, 415
  in psychiatric database, 16f,
    26–27
Family therapy
  for ADHD, 412, 414
  for anorexia nervosa, 348
  for bipolar depression, 144
  for bulimia nervosa, 350
  for conduct disorder, 416
  for major depression, in
    children, 426
  for obsessive–compulsive
    disorder, 168, 409
  for oppositional defiant
    disorder, 418
  for panic disorder, in
    children, 397
  for psychosis of
    schizophrenia, 251

Fantasies, sexual, 375
Fasting, in bulimia nervosa, 349
Fasting blood glucose (FBG),
    45, 246
Fatigue
    as major depression criteria,
        91b, 92
    in primary medical care, 5, 6t
FBG (fasting blood glucose),
    45, 246
FDA (Food and Drug
    Administration)
    approval status. See specific drug.
    warning on antidepressants,
        432, 449, 450b
Fear(s)
    cognitive behavioral therapy
        for, 165
    in children, 390, 399, 401
    of criticism, disapproval, and
        rejection, 337–338
    of disease, 263. See also
        Hypochondriasis.
    of inability to care for self, 338
    phobic. See specific phobias.
Feigning, of symptomatology,
    266–267
Female orgasmic disorder, 371
Female sexual arousal disorder,
    370
Fentanyl patch, for chronic
    malignant pain, 312, 313t
Fertility disorders, antipsychotic
    selection and, 230
Fetal alcohol syndrome, 292,
    434, 436
Fetal heart rate, ECT and, 326
Fetishism, 375
Fetus
    ECT impact on, 326
    TCAs effect on, 120
    teratogenic drug effects on, 48,
        147, 150, 153, 154, 249
Fever
    CBC and, 46
    clozapine associated with, 248
    in behavioral emergencies, 274
    lumbar puncture for, 44
Fibromyalgia, hypochondriasis
    versus, 264

Fight-or-flight reflex, 192
5-HT$_2$ antagonists, 112t, 114t, 116
Floppy baby syndrome, 184
Fluconazole (Diflucan), 379b, 383
Fluoroquinolone antibiotics, P450
    system inhibition by, 379b,
    383
Fluoxetine hydrochloride (Prozac,
    Sarafem, Symbyax)
    adverse effects of, 115t, 117, 130
        cardiac, 117, 118t, 119b, 130
    as antidepressant, 109, 112t, 121
    as P450 system substrate, 381b,
        384
    for anxiety disorders, 187, 189t
    for hypochondriasis, 265
    for major depression, in
        children, 426, 427t, 432,
        433
    for obsessive–compulsive
        disorder, 167
    for panic disorder, 164
    formulary, 465
    obstetrical patients and, 120
    olanzapine with, for bipolar
        depression, 155
    P450 system inhibition by, 379b,
        383, 387
    pharmacokinetics of, 119–120,
        123
Fluoxetine once a week (Serafim),
    120
Fluphenazine hydrochloride
    (Permitil, Prolixin)
    dose recommendations for, 220t,
        224t
    for destructive behavior, in
        mental retardation,
        421t, 438t
    for schizophrenia, 219
    formulary, 465–467
    pharmacokinetics of, 224t
    side effects of, 233t
Flurazepam hydrochloride
    (Dalmane), 206, 467
Fluvastatin (Lescol), 379b
Fluvoxamine (Luvox)
    for anxiety disorders, 189t
    for major depression, in
        children, 427t

Fluvoxamine (Luvox)—cont'd
    for obsessive–compulsive
        disorder, 167
    P450 system inhibition by, 379b,
        383, 387
Folate
    deficiency of, 48
    for alcohol intoxication, 291
Food
    as P450 system inducer, 386
    as P450 system inhibitor, 379b,
        383
Food and Drug Administration
        (FDA)
    approval status.
        See specific drug.
    warning on antidepressants, 432,
        449, 450b
Food buying, in bulimia nervosa,
        349
Food interactions, with MAOIs,
        134, 135b
Forced feeding, for anorexia
        nervosa, 347
Forensic issues
    in behavioral emergencies,
        271–277
    in commitment statutes,
        284–285
    in competence evaluations,
        285–286
    in physical restraint use,
        283–284
    in suicide evaluation, 277–281
    in violent or homicidal patients,
        281–283
Formal thought disorder, 211b, 215
Formulary, 442–503
Fractures
    ECT causing, 321
    hip, in geriatric patients, 9
Fragile X syndrome, 434
Frontal lobe disease, 329
Frontotemporal dementia, 54
Frotteurism, 375
Frustration level, in children, 417,
        434
Functional impairment
    in ADHD, 411
    in Alzheimer's disease, 65, 66b

Functional impairment—cont'd
    in dementia, 54, 57
    in depressive disorders, of
        children, 418–419, 426
    in gender identity disorder, 376
    in generalized anxiety disorder,
        168
    in personality disorders,
        328–329
    in schizophrenia, 214b, 215
        residual, 217
    psychiatric disorders associated
        with, 1–2
Functional optimization, for
        somatization disorder, 256–257
Fungal infection, CNS, lumbar
        puncture for, 44
Future orientation, signs of, in
        suicide evaluation, 280

GABA (γ-aminobutyric acid)-A
        receptors, sleep problems and,
        206–207, 208
Gabapentin
    for bipolar disorder, in children,
        422t
    for dementia, 60
GAD. See Generalized anxiety
        disorder (GAD).
Galantamine hydrobromide
        (Razadyne, Reminyl), 77, 78,
        467–468
Gallstones, obesity associated with,
        353
γ-Aminobutyric acid (GABA)-A
        receptors, sleep problems and,
        206–207, 208
Gastric banding, for obesity,
        adjustable versus vertical, 355
Gastric bypass, for obesity, 355
Gastroesophageal reflux disease
        (GERD)
    antidepressants causing, 117
    sleep problems associated with,
        195–196, 202
Gastrointestinal bleeding
    alcohol use associated with, 287
    antidepressants associated with,
        117, 129

Gastrointestinal system
    anxiety symptoms in, 159b, 162
    eating disorders and, 344, 345b,
        346
    ECT impact on, 320
    in somatization disorder, 254
    lithium effects on, 147
    valproic acid effects on, 149
Gatekeepers, for mental health
    problems, 10
Gatifloxacin, antipsychotics
    interactions with, 229t
Gender, suicide risk related to, 278
Gender identity disorder, 376–377
    diagnostic criteria for, 376
    sexual ambiguity and, 376
    treatment of, 376–377
Generalized anxiety disorder
    (GAD), 168–170
    alcohol use associated
        with, 293
    antidepressants for, 108
    azapirones for, 185
    benzodiazepines for, 178, 182
    course of, 168–169
    definition of, 168, 399
    differential diagnosis of, 169,
        256, 399
    identification of, 168
    in children, 392t, 399
    in primary medical care, 6, 6t
    prevalence of, 169
    prognosis of, 169
    sleep problems associated with,
        203
    treatment of
        exposure therapy, 194
        pharmacologic, 165t, 166,
            169–170, 399
        psychotherapies, 170, 399
Genetics
    in eating disorders, 343, 346,
        349
    in mental retardation, 436–437
    in obesity, 351, 352
    in panic disorders, 162
    polymorphism, in P450 system,
        382–383
    psychiatric symptoms related
        to, 47

Genitalia
    ambiguous, in gender identity
        disorder, 376
    dysfunction of. See Sexual
        disorders/dysfunction.
    self-mutilation of, 376
Genitourinary system
    anxiety symptoms in, 159b
    sexual dysfunction related to, 374
Genogram, for family history, 27
GERD (gastroesophageal reflux
    disease)
    antidepressants causing, 117
    sleep problems associated with,
        195–196, 202
Geriatric Depression Scale, 93, 97b
Geriatric patients
    antipsychotics metabolism in,
        228, 230
    cognitive decline in. See
        Alzheimer's disease (AD);
        Dementia.
    personality disorders in, 328,
        329
    psychiatric disorders in
        as overlooked, 6t
        hip fracture and, 9
    suicide risk in, 278
Gilles de la Tourette's syndrome,
    167
Gingko, for Alzheimer's disease, 78
Glaucoma
    anticholinergics contradicted
        with, 113, 114t
    antipsychotic selection and, 234
    stimulant use cautions with, 413
Global Assessment of
    Functioning scale, 21b, 22b,
    26, 26b–27b
Glucose dysregulation
    antipsychotics associated with,
        244
        monitoring guidelines for,
            244, 245t, 246
    antipsychotics causing, 70, 72
Glucose screening, 45
Glucose tolerance test (GTT), 45
Glycopyrrolate, for ECT, 322
Goose flesh, in narcotics
    assessment, 308b

Grandiosity, in narcissistic
    personality disorder,
    336–337
Grapefruit juice, P450 system
    inhibition by, 379b, 383
Grief/grieving
    adjustment disorder versus, 173
    major depression associated
        with, 100, 420
Group therapy
    for anorexia nervosa, 348
    for antisocial personality
        disorder, 333
    for anxiety disorders, 194
    for avoidant personality
        disorder, 338
    for bipolar depression, 144
    for borderline personality
        disorder, 335
    for bulimia nervosa, 350
    for conduct disorder, 416
    for panic disorder, in children,
        397
    for social phobia, in children, 398
    for somatization disorder, 257
GTT (glucose tolerance test), 45
Guanfacine (Tenex), 394t–395t,
    414
Guilt, excessive, as major
    depression criteria, 91b, 92
Gynecology consultation, 30

Habilitation, for mental
    retardation, 435, 437
HAD (HIV-associated dementia),
    56–57
Hallucinations
    alcoholic, 291–292
    auditory, 96, 211
    command, 211
    hypnagogic, 199, 200
    in alcohol withdrawal delirium,
        297b–298b
    in Alzheimer's patients, 66t, 68
    in major depression, 96
    in psychosis, 211–212
    olfactory, 212
    prevalence in dementias, 5
    social phobia and, 171

Hallucinations—cont'd
    tactile, 212
    visual, 34, 67, 76, 212
Hallucinogen use/abuse
    symptoms of, 301, 302t, 304
    treatment of, 305
Haloperidol, depot (Haldol
    decanoate), 219, 468–469
Haloperidol (Haldol)
    dose recommendations for, 220t,
        225t
    for Alzheimer's disease, 70, 71t,
        84
    for anxiety disorders, 188
    for behavioral emergencies, 274,
        275t, 276
    for delirium, 53, 249
    for destructive behavior,
        in mental retardation,
        421t, 438t
    intramuscular, 219, 223t, 234
    intravenous, 219
    P450 system and, 223, 227t
    pharmacokinetics of, 225t
    receptor affinities of, 221t
    side effects of, 233t, 276
    therapeutic level of, 228
Hamilton Depression Rating Scale
    (HDRS), 93
Harmful behavior
    commitment for, 284–285
    delirium and, 51
    to self versus others, 282, 283b,
        285
Hashish, 315
HCFA (Health Care Financing
    Administration), on
    psychotropics for mental
    retardation, 437, 438t–439t,
    440
HDRS (Hamilton Depression
    Rating Scale), 93
Head trauma
    amnestic disorders and, 61
    behavioral emergencies related
        to, 273, 274
    psychotropic contraindications
        with, 277
    delirium and, 51
    dementia associated with, 55t

Head trauma—cont'd
  medical history of, 28
  neuroimaging of, 44
  obesity and, 352
  psychiatric symptoms caused by,
      33, 40b
Headache. *See also* Migraines.
  ECT causing, 319, 321
  in alcohol withdrawal delirium,
      298b
  medical history of, 28
  psychiatric symptoms caused by,
      34
  sleep problems associated with,
      196, 202
Health Care Financing
      Administration (HCFA), on
      psychotropics for mental
      retardation, 437, 438t–439t,
      440
Hearing loss, in Alzheimer's
      patients, 76
Hearing testing
  for ADHD, 411
  for developmental disabilities, 436
  for learning disorders, 434
Heart block
  antidepressants causing, 117,
      118t, 119b, 130
  antipsychotics associated with,
      234, 243
  carbamazepine causing, 153
  lithium causing, 147
Heart rate, in narcotics
      assessment, 309b
Hematologic system
  alcohol use impact on, 287
  eating disorders and, 345b
Hematomas
  brain, neuroimaging of, 43
  subdural, psychiatric symptoms
      caused by, 33
Hemoglobin A1c, 246
Hemorrhage
  as SSRIs complication, 129
  intracranial *versus*
      subarachnoid, 277
Hepatic encephalopathy, 292
Hepatic impairment. *See* Liver
      function tests (LFTs).

Hepatitis, carbamazepine
      associated with, 152–153
Heroin
  half-life of, 310t
  overdose of, 310–311
Herpes, CNS, lumbar puncture
      for, 44
Hiccups, antipsychotics for, 250
High-risk behavior, in children,
      390, 400
Hip fracture, psychiatric
      interventions for, 9
Histamine 2 (H$_2$) antagonists
  Alzheimer's disease and, 69t, 76
  mood disorders caused by, 90
  neuroreceptor effects of, 114t
  sexual dysfunction related to,
      367t
Histamine receptors, atypical
      antipsychotics affinity for,
      219, 221t
  therapeutic *versus* adverse
      effects, 222t
History of present illness (HPI)
  in ADHD, 410
  in behavioral emergencies, 273
    brief initial, 271, 272t
  in dementia evaluation, 57, 58b
  in depression evaluation,
      86, 87f
  in evaluation of symptoms,
      33–35, 38
  in mental retardation
      evaluation, 436
  in psychiatric interview, 14f, 22
  in sexual disorders, 363–364
  in sleep disorders, 195–196, 196b
  in violent patient, 281–282
  suicide risk related to, 278
Histrionic personality disorder,
      331t, 335–336
HIV. *See* Human
      immunodeficiency virus
      (HIV) infection.
HIV-associated dementia (HAD),
      56–57
Homicidal patient
  alcohol use in, 288
  evaluation of, 279t, 281–282
  management of, 282

Hormone therapy
  for Alzheimer's disease, 75–76, 78
  for gender identity disorder, 376–377
  for paraphilias, 375–376
  for premenstrual dysphoric disorder, 106
  sexual dysfunction related to, 368t, 374
Hospital risk manager, 286
Hospitalizations
  for alcohol withdrawal, 292, 293, 294
    delirium tremens management, 298–300
  for anorexia nervosa, 346–348
    indications for, 346–347
    interventions during, 347–348
    refeeding protocol, 347, 347b
    complications of, 347
  for conduct disorder, 416
  for major depression, in children, 426
  for suicidal patient, 280
    chronic, 280
  past history of, 23
HPI. See History of present illness (HPI).
Human immunodeficiency virus (HIV) infection
  dementia associated with, 55, 55t, 56
  psychiatric symptoms caused by, 40b, 41, 41b
  sexual dysfunction associated with, 373
Hydrocarbons, volatile, symptoms of use, 301, 303t, 304
Hydrocodone (Vicodin), 202
Hydromorphone, half-life of, 310t
Hydroxyzine (Vistaril), 188, 205–206, 314
Hyperactivity
  developmental determinants of, 23
  eating disorders and, 344
  in ADHD, 409

Hyperglycemia, glucose testing for, 45
Hyperlipidemia, antipsychotics associated with, 70, 72, 244
  monitoring guidelines for, 244, 245t, 246
Hyperphagia, compulsive, 350
Hypersomnia, 197–200
  causes of, 197–199
    insufficient sleep, 197
    narcolepsy, 199–200
    obstructive sleep apnea, 198–199
    shift-work sleep disorder, 197–198
  idiopathic, 200
Hypertension
  ECT impact on, 320, 324
  in behavioral emergencies, 273
Hypertensive crisis, MAOIs causing, 133
Hyperthyroidism, 39b, 40, 41b, 45
Hypervigilance, 175, 400
Hypnagogic hallucinations, 199, 200
Hypnosis, for conversion disorder, 259, 260–261
Hypnotics. See also Sedatives.
  benzodiazepines as, 178, 185, 206–208
  cross-tolerant, for sedative withdrawal, 295, 299t
  dose conversions for, 299t
  for anxiety disorders, 188
  for sleep problems, 205–208
  OBRA regulations on, Alzheimer's disease and, 79, 84
  sleep problems associated with, 203
Hypoactive sexual desire, 364
Hypochondriasis, 263–265
  definition of, 263
  differential diagnosis of, 264
  obsessive–compulsive disorder versus, 166, 167
  pain disorder versus, 263
  prevalence of, 263
  prognosis of, 264
  treatment of, 264–265

Hypogeusia, drug-induced, in Alzheimer's patients, 82
Hypoglycemia, glucose testing for, 45
Hypoglycemic agents, as P450 system substrate, 380b, 385
Hypogonadism, 376
Hypokalemia, 47
Hypomanic episode, in bipolar disorder, 137, 138–139
in children, 419
Hyponatremia, 47
Hypotension
ECT causing, 324
orthostatic
anorexia nervosa associated with, 345b, 346
antipsychotics associated with, 234, 242–243
from antidepressants, 116–117, 118t, 133
Hypothalamic tumor, obesity and, 352
Hypothyroidism
mood stabilizers causing, 147, 153
obesity and, 352
symptoms associated with, 39b, 40, 41b, 45
Hypoxia, 46
Hypoxic drive, benzodiazepines depression of, 181
azapirones versus, 186

Iatrogenic dependence, pain disorder associated with, 262, 263
ICP (intracerebral pressure), ECT impact on, 326
ICU (intensive care unit), substance abuse patients in, 7, 8
IDEA (Individuals with Disabilities Education Act) of 1975, 435, 437
IDS (Inventory for Depressive Symptomatology), 93
IEP (individualized education plan), 435

Illicit street drugs, in patient history, 28
Illness behavior, abnormal, 253
IM. See Intramuscular (IM) agents.
Imipramine (Tofranil), 111t, 121
analgesic properties of, 314
for anxiety disorders, 187
for generalized anxiety disorder, 165t, 170
for major depression, in children, 430t
for panic disorder, 164, 165t
formulary, 469–470
Immunologic approach, to nicotine abstinence, 361
Impairment. See also Disability(ies).
cerebral. See Brain impairment/injury.
cognitive. See Cognitive impairment.
functional. See Functional impairment.
hepatic. See Liver function tests (LFTs).
of memory. See Memory impairment.
of mobility, in Alzheimer's patients, 82–83
psychomotor, benzodiazepines causing, 181, 186
psychosocial, 24–26, 24b
self-care
in dependent personality disorder, 338
in psychiatric database, 25–26
Implied consent, 285
Impotence, antipsychotics causing, 246
Impulse control/impulsivity
in ADHD, 409, 412
in personality disorders, 329, 334–335
Inattention, in ADHD, 409
Income source, in psychiatric database, 25
Incontinence, in Alzheimer's patients, 82, 83b
Indecisiveness, as major depression criteria, 91b, 92

Indinavir, P450 system inhibition
by, 379b, 383
Individual psychotherapy
for ADHD, 414
for anorexia nervosa, 348
for borderline personality
disorder, 335
for bulimia nervosa, 350
for conduct disorder, 416
for narcissistic personality
disorder, 337
for obsessive–compulsive
disorder, 409
for oppositional defiant disorder,
418
for panic disorder, in children,
397
for selective mutism, 396
for separation anxiety disorder,
391
for social phobia, in children,
398
for specific phobia, in children,
391
Individualized education plan
(IEP), 435
Individuals with Disabilities
Education Act (IDEA) of
1975, 435, 437
Infancy history, in psychiatric
database, 23
Infections
chronic, hypochondriasis versus,
264
CNS, behavioral emergencies
related to, 273
dementia associated with, 55, 55t
opportunistic, 56–57
depression associated with, 88b
lumbar puncture indications
for, 44
neuroimaging indications for,
42–44
prenatal, developmental
disabilities associated with,
436–437
psychiatric symptoms caused by,
40b, 41, 41b
Inflexibility, in personality
disorders, 328, 329

Informed consent
for antipsychotics, 238
for ECT, 321
in child and adolescent
psychiatry, 389
Inhalant abuse, symptoms of,
301, 303t, 304
Inhaler, nicotine, for smoking
cessation, 359
Inpatient treatment
medical, psychiatric
consultation for, 5
past history of psychiatric, 23
Insight, in cognitive
examination, 63
Insomnia, 200–202
affective disorders associated
with, 203
circadian rhythm and,
201–202
delirium and, 51
in primary medical care, 5, 6t
MAOIs causing, 133
periodic limb movements and,
202
primary, 200, 201b
sleep state misperception and,
200–201
Insulin therapy, ECT and, 322
Insurance reimbursement, for
smoking cessation therapies,
357
Insurance status, in psychiatric
database, 15–16
Integrated services, medical and
psychiatric, 9–10
Intelligence, in schizophrenia, 216,
217, 218
Intelligence testing, in children,
410, 434
Intensive care unit (ICU),
substance abuse patients
in, 7, 8
Interactions
drug. See Drug interactions.
food, with MAOIs, 134, 135b
Interpersonal behavior
in personality disorders, 328,
329–330
in schizophrenia, 216–217

Interpersonal psychotherapy
  for bipolar disorders, 144,
    155, 156
  for major depression, 101
Interpersonal relationships
  ADHD and, 410
  in borderline personality
    disorder, 334–335
  in psychiatric database, 23
  schizoid personality disorder
    and, 332–333
  somatization disorder and, 256
Intersex conditions, 376
Interviews/interviewing
  amobarbital, for conversion
    disorder, 260–262
  for ADHD, 410
  for personality disorders, 329–330
  psychiatric, 12–13
    for suicidal ideation
      evaluation, 92, 93b
    in primary medical care, 4,
      4t, 10
Intolerance, in
    obsessive–compulsive
    personality disorder, 339
Intoxication
  as behavioral emergency, 272,
    290
  substance, anxiety associated
    with, 158, 161b
Intracerebral/intracranial pressure
    (ICP), ECT impact on, 320,
    325, 326
Intracranial bleeding, 277
Intramuscular (IM) agents
  antipsychotics as, 219, 223t, 234
  for behavioral emergencies, 274,
    275t, 276
  perphenazine as, 482–483
Intraocular pressure, ECT impact
    on, 318, 320, 325
Intravenous (IV) agents, for
    behavioral emergencies, 276
Inventory for Depressive
    Symptomatology (IDS), 93
Irritability, in posttraumatic stress
    disorder, 175, 176
Irritable bowel syndrome,
    hypochondriasis versus, 264

Isoenzymes, in oxidative metabolism,
    378, 382. See also CYP entries;
    P450 system.

Jaundice, antipsychotics associated
    with, 247
Jet lag, 202
Joint Commission for
    Accreditation of Hospitals
    (JCAH), physical restraint
    rules of, 284
Judgment
  in cognitive examination, 63
  in schizophrenia, 216
Juvenile detention, conduct
    disorder and, 416

Ketamine, 303t
  for ECT, 322
Kinetics, in mental status
    examination, 31
Kleine–Levin syndrome,
    203, 350
Klüver–Bucy syndrome, 350

Labetalol, ECT indications for,
    325
Laboratory evaluation
  for ECT, 322
  of Alzheimer's disease, 64–65
  of dementia, 58b, 59
  of eating disorders, 344, 344b,
    345b, 350
  of intoxicated patient, 290
  of psychiatric symptoms,
    41–48
  of schizophrenia, 230, 231b
  of somatization disorder, 257
Lacrimation, in narcotics
    assessment, 308b
Lactation, medications and, 120,
    153, 249
Lamotrigine (Lamictal)
  administration guidelines for,
    154–155
  for bipolar depression, 143, 144,
    154

Lamotrigine (Lamictal)—cont'd
  for bipolar disorder, in children,
    422t
  formulary, 470–471
  side effects of, 155, 470–471
Language
  Alzheimer's disease and, 64, 67
  in ADHD evaluation, 410, 411
  in cognitive examination, 62
  in mental status examination,
    30, 31
  in selective mutism, 396
Lansoprazole (Prevacid), 379b
Laryngeal dystonia, as
    antipsychotics reaction, 235
Laryngospasm, ECT causing, 321
Laxative abuse
  in anorexia nervosa, 345b,
    347
  in bulimia nervosa, 348–349
Learning disorder not otherwise
    specified, 433
Learning disorders/disabilities,
    433–435
  ADHD and, 411, 412, 414
  course and prognosis of, 434
  definition of, 433
  developmental determinants
    of, 23
  diagnostic features of, 433–434
  differential diagnosis of, 434
  epidemiology of, 433, 434t
  identification of, 433
  treatment of, 435
Legal aspects
  of commitment, 284–285
  of competence determination,
    285–286
  of conduct disorder
    interventions, 416
  of learning disorder treatment,
    435
  of mental retardation programs,
    437
Length of stay (LOS), medical,
    psychiatric comorbidity
    impact on, 5, 8, 9
Lesions, spinal cord, sexual
    dysfunction associated with,
    374

Leukotomy, stereotactic limbic,
    for obsessive–compulsive dis-
    order, 168
Leuprolide, for paraphilias, 376
Level of consciousness
  in cognitive examination, 61
  in delirium, 50
  in head trauma, 277
  in mental status examination,
    30–31
Levomethadyl acetate, half-life of,
    310t
Lewy bodies, dementia with, 55t, 56
LFTs. See Liver function tests
    (LFTs).
Libido, decrease in, with
    antipsychotics, 246
Lidocaine, Alzheimer's disease
    and, 69t
Life-threatening events, exposure
    in childhood, 400
Lifestyle
  management, for premenstrual
    dysphoric disorder, 105–106
  obesity related to, 351
Light therapy, for circadian
    rhythm sleep disorder, 201
Limb movement disorders,
    periodic, 202
Limbic leukotomy, stereotactic,
    for obsessive–compulsive
    disorder, 168
Limit setting, for personality
    disorders, 335, 339
Lingual dystonia, as antipsychotics
    reaction, 235
Lipid dysregulation
  antipsychotics associated with,
    monitoring guidelines for,
    244, 245t, 246
  antipsychotics causing, 70, 72,
    244
Lipophilic property, of
    antipsychotics, 223, 234
Listening, to Alzheimer's patients,
    64
Lithium carbonate (Eskalith,
    Lithobid)
  dosing of, 146
  drug interactions with, 145, 145b

Lithium carbonate (Eskalith,
    Lithobid)—cont'd
  ECT interaction with, 321, 322
  effects on EEG, 42
  for antidepressant
    augmentation, 110
  for bipolar depression, 143, 144
  for bipolar disorder, in children,
    420, 423t
  for borderline personality
    disorder, 335
  for mania, 142t, 143, 144
  formulary, 471–472
  formulations of, 146
  laboratory monitoring of, 146
  pharmacology of, 145
  side effects of, 146–147
  toxic effects of, 46, 47, 145b
Liver function tests (LFTs), 45–46
  alcohol use impact on, 287, 288
  antipsychotics metabolism and,
    228
  carbamazepine effects on, 152
  oxcarbazepine effects on, 154
  valproic acid effects on, 148, 149
Living arrangements, in
    psychiatric database, 25
Living will, 286
Logical reasoning, in borderline
    personality disorder, 335
Long-term memory
  ECT and, 319
  in cognitive examination, 62–63
Lorazepam (Ativan)
  for alcohol intoxication, 290
  for Alzheimer's disease, 69t, 75,
    79
  for anxiety, 185, 393t
  for behavioral emergencies, 274,
    275t
  for delirium tremens, 299
  for generalized anxiety disorder,
    165t
  for mania, 155
  for sleep problems, 206
  for withdrawal-associated
    delirium, 53
  formulary, 472–473
  pharmacokinetics of, 179t, 180,
    181b

LOS (length of stay), medical,
    psychiatric comorbidity
    impact on, 5, 8, 9
Loss(es)
  adjustment disorder and, 173
  major depression associated
    with, 100, 420
  personality disorders associated
    with, 328
Loxapine (Loxitane), 220t
Lozenges, nicotine, for smoking
    cessation, 359
Lumbar puncture, 44
Lysergic acid diethylamide
    (LSD), 301, 302t, 304, 305

Macrolide antibiotics, P450
    system inhibition by, 379b,
    383
MADRS (Montgomery–Asberg
    Depression Rating Scale), 93
Magnesium, for delirium tremens,
    300
Magnesium-depleting drugs,
    antipsychotics interactions
    with, 229t
Magnesium pemoline (Cylert),
    406t, 413
Magnetic resonance imaging
    (MRI)
  advantages versus disadvantages
    of, 43
  diagnostic indications for, 43,
    436
Maintenance ECT, 324
Maintenance therapies
  antipsychotic guidelines in,
    234–235
  for bipolar depressive episodes,
    144
  for sobriety, 288
  methadone as, 311
Major abstinence syndrome,
    295–300
  risk factors for, 295
  symptoms of, 294b, 295,
    296b–298b
  timing of, 295
  treatment of, 295, 298–300

Major depressive disorder (MDD),
    90–101
  atypical features with, 98
  comorbidities of, 95–96, 420
  definition of, 90–91
  depressed mood associated with,
      86, 88–89, 91, 100
    antidepressants for, 108
  diagnostic criteria for, 91–92,
      91b
  diagnostic modifiers for, 96–99
  differential diagnosis of, 99–100
  ECT for, 317
  generalized anxiety disorder and,
      169
  in children, 418–419
    antidepressants for, 426,
        427t–431t, 432
    strategies for, 432–433
    suicidality and, 432
    course and prognosis of, 426
    differential diagnosis of, 420,
        426
    epidemiology of, 420
    symptoms of, 418–419
    treatment of, 426, 427t–431t,
        432–433
  melancholic features with,
      97–98
  obsessive–compulsive disorder
      versus, 166
  panic attacks in, 162, 166
  personality disorders associated
      with, 328
  postpartum onset of, 98
  prevalence of, 94–95, 97t
  prognosis for, 100
  psychotic features with, 96–97
  rating scales for
    clinician-administered, 93
    self-administered, 93–94,
        94f–96f, 97b
  recognition of, 95
  recurrent, 96, 100
  screening for, 92–94
    interview protocol, 92, 93b
  seasonal pattern of, 98–99
  sleep problems associated with,
      203
  treatment of, 100–101

Maladaptation, in personality
    disorders, 328
Male erectile disorder, 370–371
  neurogenic, 373
Male orgasmic disorder, 371
Malignancies, hypochondriasis
    versus, 264
Malignant pain, chronic, in
    narcotics addicts, 312
Malingering, 268
  clinical characteristics of, 268
  definition of, 268
  differential diagnosis of, 268
  factitious disorder versus, 266,
      267, 268
  pain disorder versus, 263
  secondary gain in, 258, 263,
      264, 266
  somatization disorder versus, 255
  treatment of, 268
  with psychotic symptoms, 214
Mania
  as behavioral emergency, 140,
      272, 273
    management of, 274–277, 275t
  bipolar, 138
    differential diagnosis of,
        139–140
    in children, 419–420,
        421t–425t
    medical causes of, 139, 139b
    quetiapine for, 489
    treatment of, 140, 141t,
        142t, 143
  in dementia
    HIV-associated, 57
    treatment of, 59–60
  in major depression, 99
  psychotic symptoms versus, 212
Manipulation, in personality
    disorders, 329, 333, 335
MAOIs. See Monoamine oxidase
    inhibitors (MAOIs).
Marijuana
  abuse of, 315–316
    schizophrenia associated with,
        217
  withdrawal from, 315
Marital status, in psychiatric
    database, 14

Masochism, 350
  sexual, 375
Mathematic disorder, 411, 433,
    434, 434t
MDD. See Major depressive
    disorder (MDD).
MDMA (methylenedioxy-
    methamphetamine), 302t,
    305, 385
Mechanical injuries, psychiatric
    symptoms caused by, 40b, 41,
    41b
Medical condition/illness
  acute somatized symptoms
    versus, 257
  acute stress disorder caused by,
    174
  ADHD versus, 411
  alcohol use associated with,
    287–288
  anxiety disorders caused by, 158,
    160b, 169
  chronic
    in primary medical care, 5, 6t
    suicidality related to, 277
  conversion disorder versus, 259
  depression associated with, 33,
    38, 47
    examples of, 34t, 86, 88b
    prevalence of, 94–95, 97t
  developmental disabilities
    associated with, 436–437
  eating disorders associated with,
    344, 345b, 349
  hypochondriasis versus, 264
  in psychiatric database, 13, 21b,
    22b, 27–29
  mania caused by, 139, 139b, 140
  mental retardation associated
    with, 436–437
  obesity and, 352–353
  pain disorder associated with,
    262–263
  psychiatric disorders with
    as comorbidities, 5, 6–7, 6t
    symptoms produced by, 33,
      34t, 38, 39b–41b, 40–41
  psychiatric problems versus, 4
  psychotic symptoms associated
    with, 212

Medical condition/illness—cont'd
  schizophrenia associated with,
    218
    antipsychotic choices based
      on, 230, 233t
  sexual dysfunction associated
    with, 370, 372–374
  sleep problems associated with,
    195–196, 202
  somatization disorder versus,
    254–255
  violence associated with, 281
Medical costs
  of nicotine dependence, 355
  of psychiatric disorders, in
    primary care, 5, 7, 8–9
Medical evaluation
  in ADHD, 410–411
  of psychiatric symptoms, 33–48
    anxiety disorders and, 158,
      160b
    diagnostic testing, 41–48
    etiologic factors, 5–8, 6t, 33,
      34t
    physical examination, 41
    principles of, 33–41
Medical history, 15f–16f, 27–29
  misreporting by patient, 266
Medical outcomes, with
    psychiatric disorder
    comorbidities, 5, 10
Medical practice. See Primary care.
Medical records, privacy
    protection for, 13
Medications. See also specific agent
    or classification.
  acute stress disorder caused
    by, 174
  ADHD associated with, 411
  Alzheimer's disease and
    approved therapies, 68–70,
      69t, 71t, 72–76, 74t
    symptoms related to, 68, 69b
  anxiety disorders caused by,
    158, 161b
  depression associated
    with, 88b
  disease indications for. See
    specific disorder.
  effects on EEG, 42

Medications—cont'd
  electrolyte imbalances caused
      by, 46–47
  formulary for, 442–503
  mania caused by, 139, 139b, 140
  metabolism of
      drug challenge tests for, 382
      nicotine impact on, 228, 356,
          356b
      oxidative. See CYP entries;
          P450 system.
  patient history of, 28, 29
  psychiatric symptoms caused by,
      34, 34t, 35b–38b, 41b
  sexual dysfunction related to,
      364, 365t–369t, 370
  sleep problems associated with,
      203–204
  teratogenic, 48, 147, 150, 153,
      154, 249
Meditation, mindfulness, for
      anxiety disorders, 189, 191b
Medroxyprogesterone acetate, for
      hypersexual dementia, 374
Melancholy, in major depression,
      97–98
Melatonin, for sleep disorders, 201,
      205
Melatonin–B-vitamin supplement
      (Bevitamel), 473
Memantine hydrochloride
      (Namenda)
  for Alzheimer's disease, 76, 77,
      78
  for dementia, 57, 59
  formulary, 474
Memory
  in cognitive examination,
      62–63
  in posttraumatic stress disorder,
      175, 176
Memory impairment
  age-associated, 54
  alcohol intoxication and, 291
  definition of, 60
  dementia and, 54, 56, 57
  ECT causing, 319
  etiology of, 61
  identification of, 61
  isolated, 60

Memory impairment—cont'd
  substance-induced, 61
  treatment of, 61
MEND A MIND, 40, 41b
Menopause, patient history of, 30
Menses/menstrual cycle
  disorders of, antipsychotic
      selection and, 230
  in anorexia nervosa, 343
  patient history of, 29–30
Mental disability, functional
      impact of, 1–2
Mental health disorders.
      See Psychiatric disorders.
Mental health services.
      See also Psychiatry.
  cost-benefit issues involving, 9
  strategic integration of, 9–10
Mental Health Services
      Administration (MHSA),
      integration assessment of,
      9–10
Mental health statutes,
      commitment under, 284–285
Mental retardation, 435–440
  ADHD versus, 412
  course and prognosis of, 437
  definition of, 435
  differential diagnosis of,
      436–437
  epidemiology of, 435–436
  evaluation of, 436
  identification of, 432
  psychotic symptoms versus, 214
  treatment of
      nonpharmacologic, 437
      psychotropics for, 437,
          438t–439t, 440
Mental status examination, 30–32
  affective component. See Affect.
  anxiety component. See Anxiety.
  basic components of, 22, 30
  behavioral component, 31–32
  cognitive component.
      See Cognitive mental status
      examination.
  descriptive component, 30–31
  for ECT, 321
  for psychosis/psychotic
      symptoms, 210, 211b

Mental status examination—
    cont'd
  for violent patient, 279t, 281, 282
  in behavioral emergencies, 273
  in child and adolescent
      psychiatry, 389
  in suicide evaluation, 278, 279t,
      280
  personality component.
      See Personality entries.
  psychosis component.
      See Psychiatric assessment/
      consultation; Psychosis
      entries.
Meperidine, half-life of, 310t
Meprobamate (Miltown, Equanil),
    188
Mescaline, 302t, 305
Mesoridazine (Serentil), 220t
Metabolic disorders
  antipsychotics causing, 70, 72,
      243–246, 245t
  anxiety caused by, 160b
  depression associated with, 88b
  psychiatric symptoms caused by,
      39b, 40, 41b
Metabolic syndrome,
    antipsychotics associated
    with, 244
  monitoring guidelines for, 244,
      245t, 246
Metabolism, of medications.
    See also specific drug
    classification or agent.
  drug challenge tests for, 382
  nicotine impact on, 228, 356,
      356b
  oxidative, isoenzymes in, 378,
      382. See also CYP entries;
      P450 system.
Methadone hydrochloride
    (Methadose)
  for narcotics addiction, 310, 311
  formulary, 474–475
  half-life of, 310t
Methamphetamine hydrochloride
    (Desoxyn), 475–476
Methohexital, for ECT, 322
Methylenedioxymethamphetamine
    (MDMA), 302t, 305, 385

Methylmalonic acid assay, 48
Methylphenidate hydrochloride
    (Concerta, Focalin, Metadate,
    Methylin, Ritalin)
  as antidepressant, 131–132
  for ADHD, 404t–406t,
      412–414
  for antidepressant
      augmentation, 110
  for narcolepsy, 199
  formulary, 476
Metoclopramide (Reglan), 236,
    379b
Mexiletine, P450 system
    inhibition by, 379b, 383
MHSA (Mental Health Services
    Administration), integration
    assessment of, 9–10
MI. See Myocardial infarction
    (MI).
Michigan Alcohol Screening Test,
    28, 288, 289b
Midazolam (Versed), 179t, 180,
    181b, 324
Migraines, 34
  topiramate prophylaxis for, 496
  titration schedule, 496, 496t
"Mind–body" approach
  to conversion disorder, 260
  to somatization disorder, 256,
      257
Mindfulness meditation, for
    anxiety disorders, 189, 191b
Mineral deficiencies,
    drug-induced, in Alzheimer's
    patients, 82
Mini Mental State Examination
    (MMSE), 58, 62–63
Minnesota Multiphasic
    Personality Inventory
    (MMPI), 330
Minor depression, 106
Mirtazapine (Remeron)
  adverse effects of, 115t
  as antidepressant, 112t,
      126–127
  for Alzheimer's disease, 81t
  for anxiety disorders, 189t
  for sleep problems, 206
  formulary, 476–477

Mirtazapine (Remeron)—cont'd
  neuroceptor effects of, 114t
  P450 system inhibition by,
    379b, 383
Mixed anxiety, depression and,
  103–104
Mixed episode, in bipolar disorder,
  137, 139
MMPI (Minnesota Multiphasic
  Personality Inventory), 330
MMSE (Mini Mental State
  Examination), 58, 62–63
Mobility impairment, in
  Alzheimer's patients, 82–83
Modafinil (Provigil)
  for ADHD, 414
  for narcolepsy, 199–200
  formulary, 477–478
  P450 system inhibition by, 379b,
    383, 387
Molindone hydrochloride
  (Moban), 220t, 421t, 478
Monitoring guidelines, for
  children, on antidepressants,
  432–433
Monoamine oxidase inhibitors
  (MAOIs)
  as antidepressants, 132–135
    dosing of, 133, 133t
    drug interactions with, 134,
      135b
    food interactions with, 134,
      135b
    indications for, 98, 113,
      132–133
    principles of using, 109
    side effects of, 133–134
  ECT interaction with, 321, 322
  for Alzheimer's disease, 78
  for bipolar depression, 143
  for borderline personality
    disorder, 335
  for bulimia nervosa, 350
  for panic disorder, 163, 164
  for social phobia, 171
  stimulant use cautions with, 413
Montgomery–Asberg Depression
  Rating Scale (MADRS), 93
Mood
  in psychiatric examination, 18, 31

Mood-congruent experiences, in
  children, 419
Mood disorders
  alcohol use associated with, 293
  as medical care comorbidity, 5
  depression associated with, 86,
    89–90
  in children, 418, 419
  in major depression, 100, 418
  obesity associated with, 352
Mood hygiene, for bipolar
  disorder, 156
Mood stabilizers
  for bipolar disorder,
    in children, 420,
      421t–425t
  for major depression, 100
  for mania, 140, 142t, 143
  for mental retardation,
    421t–425t, 440
  for psychosis of schizophrenia,
    251
Mood swings
  in bipolar disorder, 137–139
  major depression and, in
    children, 418–419
Morbidity. See also Comorbidities.
  of alcoholism, 287–288
  of ECT, 318–319
  of marijuana abuse, 315
  of obesity, 352–353
Morphine
  dose conversion to fentanyl
    patch, 312, 313t
  for behavioral emergencies, 277
  for chronic malignant pain, 312
  half-life of, 310t
Mortality
  of alcoholism, 287–288, 293
  of ECT, 318–319
  of marijuana abuse, 315
  of obesity, 352
Motor behavior/disturbances.
    See also Mobility impairment.
  as major depression criteria,
    91b, 92
  delirium and, 51
  dementia and, 57
  in children, 411, 434
  in conversion disorder, 258

Motor behavior/disturbances—
    cont'd
  in mental retardation,
      pharmacologic interven-
      tion for, 438t–439t, 440
  in schizophrenia, 216
  in somatization disorder, 254
Motor tics, 408
Motor vehicle accidents
  anxiety disorders associated
      with, 173, 175
  substance use associated with,
      288, 315
Mouth injuries, ECT causing, 321,
    323
MRI. See Magnetic resonance
    imaging (MRI).
MSLT (multiple sleep latency
    testing), 197, 199, 200
Multiaxial Evaluation Report
    Form, 13, 21b
Multidisciplinary approach, to
    treatments, 263, 389, 435
Multiple sclerosis, 44, 374
Multiple sleep latency testing
    (MSLT), 197, 199, 200
Munchausen syndrome, 266
Muscarinic receptors, atypical
    antipsychotics affinity for,
    219, 221t
  therapeutic versus adverse
      effects, 222t
Muscle aches, in narcotics
    assessment, 309b
Muscle relaxants, for ECT, 322
Muscle relaxation
  benzodiazepines for, 206–207
  progressive, for anxiety
      disorders, 189, 190b
Musculoskeletal disorders
  benzodiazepines for, 178
  ECT causing, 319, 321, 322
Musculoskeletal system, anxiety
    symptoms in, 159b
Mutilation, of self, 334
Mutism, selective, in children,
    396–397
Myocardial depression,
    antidepressants causing, 117,
    118t

Myocardial infarction (MI)
  CK isoenzymes in, 47
  ECT and, 318, 325
  in primary medical care, 5, 6, 6t
Myocarditis, clozapine associated
    with, 248

Nadolol, for anxiety disorders, 188
Naloxone hydrochloride (Narcan)
  for heroin overdose, 310–311
  for narcotics addiction, 311–312
  formulary, 478–479
Naltrexone hydrochloride (Reviva,
    Vivitrol)
  for alcoholism, 288–289
  for anorexia nervosa, 347
  for bulimia nervosa, 351
  formulary, 479–480
Naming, in cognitive examination,
    62
Narcissistic personality disorder,
    331t, 336–337
Narcolepsy, 199–200, 458
Narcotics
  Alzheimer's disease and, 69t
  for behavioral emergencies, 277
  issues with use of, 305–314
    addiction, 307
    analgesia for addicts, 312
    buprenorphine for addicts,
        311–312
    constipation, 306
    dependence, 306,
        308b–309b
    dose conversion, 306, 307b
    half-life of, 306, 310t
    methadone maintenance
        programs, 311
    pain management problems,
        305–306
    patient-controlled, 306
    psychiatric effects, 306
    respiratory depression, 305
    tolerance, 306
    withdrawal, 307, 309–311
  psychiatric symptoms caused by,
      37b
  sexual dysfunction related to,
      368t

Narcotics withdrawal, 309–311
    multiple drug abuse in, 309–310
    onset and duration of, 307
    recognition of, 310
    severity issues, 309–310
    treatment of, 310–311
Nasal congestion, in narcotics
        assessment, 309b
Nasal spray, butorphanol, for
        malignant pain, 312
National Comorbidity Survey, 1, 2t
National Institutes of Health
        (NIH), obesity trials review,
        353, 355
National Mental Health Survey, 2
Nausea
    antidepressants causing, 117
    antipsychotics for, 250
    in withdrawal syndromes, 296b,
        308b
Need expression, in personality
        disorders, 329
Needle phobia, 172
Nefazodone (Serzone), 112t,
        125–126
    analgesic properties of, 314
    as P450 system substrate, 381b,
        384
    cardiac effects of, 118t
    dose-response relationship of, 109
    for Alzheimer's disease, 81t
    for anxiety disorders, 188, 189t
    P450 system inhibition by, 379b,
        383
Negative symptoms, of
        schizophrenia, primary versus
        secondary, 216
Negativistic behavior, in children,
        417–418
Negativistic personality disorder,
        331t, 340–341
Neoplasms
    malignant. See Cancer(s).
    psychiatric symptoms caused by,
        33, 34t, 39b, 40, 41b
Neurochemical imbalance,
        symptoms associated with, 38
Neurodevelopment, in
        child and adolescent
        psychiatry, 389, 401

Neuroimaging
    contraindications for, 43
    for developmental disabilities,
        436
    in Alzheimer's disease, 65
    in depression evaluation, 89
    indications for, 42–44
Neuroleptic agents
    as P450 system substrate, 380b,
        384
    effects on EEG, 42
    for acute stress disorder, 175
    for Alzheimer's disease
        agent-specific effects of, 70,
            71t, 72–73
        conventional, 68, 70
        OBRA guidelines for, 84
    for cocaine abuse, 304
    for delirium tremens, 300
    pregnancy and, 184
    sexual dysfunction related to,
        368t–369t
Neuroleptic malignant syndrome
        (NMS)
    antipsychotics causing,
        241–242, 276
    differential diagnosis of, 241, 241b
    ECT and, 317, 325
    identification of, 241
    incidence of, 47, 241
    natural course of, 241
    serotonin syndrome versus, 131
    treatment of, 241–242
Neurologic disorders
    anxiety associated with, 159b,
        160b, 162
    depression associated with, 88b
    hypochondriasis versus, 264
    in somatization disorder, 254
    psychiatric symptoms caused
        by, 40b
        CNS-related, 33, 34, 34t, 38,
            40–41
Neurologic effects
    of antipsychotics, 241–242
        extrapyramidal symptoms,
            235–240
        neuroleptic malignant
            syndrome, 241–424
    of clonazepam, 455

Neurologic examination, 17f, 29
  for ADHD, 411
  for dementia, 57
  for ECT, 321
  for mental retardation, 436
  in behavioral emergencies, 274
Neuromuscular blockade, for ECT,
    321, 322–323
  pregnancy and, 326
Neurontin, analgesic properties
    of, 314
Neuropathic pain syndromes, 314
Neuropsychological testing
  for dementia, 58
  in ADHD, 411
Neuroreceptors, antidepressants
    effects on, 113, 114t
Neurosarcoidosis, lumbar
    puncture for, 44
Neurotensin neuropeptide, in
    psychosis of schizophrenia, 251
Newborns, diazepam effects on, 184
Nicotine abstinence. See Smoking
    cessation.
Nicotine dependence, 355–361
  drug interactions in, 356, 356b
  health expenditures related to,
    355
  pharmacology of, 355–356
  prevalence of, 355
  psychiatric disorders associated
    with, 356–357
  treatment of, 357–360
    buproprion SR for, 359–360
    cognitive behavior therapies,
      360
    miscellaneous medications, 360
    nicotine replacement trials,
      358–359
    overview of, 357
    vaccine trials, 361
Nicotine gum (Nicorette), 358
Nicotine inhaler, 359
Nicotine lozenges, 359
Nicotine replacement therapies,
    358–359
Nicotine resin complex, 358
Nicotine transdermal patches
    (Habitrol, Nicoderm,
    Nicotrol), 358–359
Nicotine use
  drug metabolism and, 228, 356,
    356b
  generalized anxiety disorder and,
    169
  in primary medical care, 6t, 7
  P450 system and, 386, 387
  patient history of, 28
  schizophrenia associated with,
    217
Nicotine withdrawal syndrome,
    356
Night terrors, 204
Nightmares, 196, 205, 400
NIH (National Institutes of
    Health), obesity trials review,
    353, 355
Nitrates, ECT indications for, 325
Nitroglycerin, ECT indications for,
    325
Nitrous oxide abuse, 301, 303t, 304
NMDA receptor antagonist.
    See Memantine hydrochloride
    (Namenda).
NMS. See Neuroleptic malignant
    syndrome (NMS).
Noncompliance, in
    obsessive–compulsive
    personality disorder, 339–340
Nonsteroidal antiinflammatory
    drugs (NSAIDs), 314
  for Alzheimer's disease, 77, 78
  GI bleeding associated with,
    129
Noradrenergic agents, for anxiety,
    in children, 391, 394t–395t
Noradrenergic side effects, of
    antidepressants, in children,
    432
Norepinephrine receptors, atypical
    antipsychotics affinity for,
    219, 221t
  therapeutic versus adverse
    effects, 222t
Norepinephrine reuptake
    inhibitors, 123–125
  medical complications of,
    127–131
  neuroceptor effects of, 114t
  profiles of specific, 112t

Norfluoxetine, P450 system
    inhibition by, 379b, 383
Normative anxiety, 171, 173, 192
Nortriptyline hydrochloride
    (Pamelor), 111t, 121
    for generalized anxiety disorder,
        165t
    for major depression, in
        children, 431t
    for nicotine dependence, 360
    formulary, 480
    P450 system implications of, 387
Nothing by mouth (NPO), for
    ECT, 322
NSAIDs. See Nonsteroidal
    antiinflammatory drugs
    (NSAIDs).
Nursing home care
    hypnotic drug use in, 206
    OBRA regulations for
        Alzheimer's patients, 79,
        83–84
Nutrition counseling
    for bulimia nervosa, 350
    for obesity, 246, 353
Nutritional deficiencies
    in Alzheimer's patients, 80, 82
    psychiatric symptoms caused by,
        40b, 41, 41b

Obesity, 351–355
    antipsychotics causing, 244
        in Alzheimer's disease, 72
        monitoring guidelines for,
            244, 245t, 246
    course of, 352–353
    definition of, 351
    differential diagnosis of, 352
    ECT and, 318
    epidemiology of, 351
    etiology of, 351–352
    major depression associated
        with, 98
    mood stabilizers causing, 147,
        153
    prognosis of, 352–353
    psychiatric comorbidities of, 352
    secondary causes of, 352
    treatment of, 353–355

Obesity—cont'd
    nonpharmacologic, 353
    pharmacologic, 353–355
OBRA. See Omnibus Budget
    Reconciliation Act (OBRA)
    of 1987.
Observation, of ADHD
    direct, 410
    parent-child interaction, 410
Obsessions, definition of,
    166, 401
Obsessive–compulsive behavior,
    166
    in eating disorders, 344, 345b,
        346, 350
Obsessive–compulsive disorder
    (OCD), 166–168
    body dysmorphic disorder versus,
        265
    course of, 167
    definition of, 166, 401
    differential diagnosis of,
        166–167, 408
    hypochondriasis versus, 264,
        265
    identification of, 166, 401, 408
    in children, 401, 408–409
    in schizophrenia, 218
    panic attacks with, 160
    prevalence of, 166
    prognosis of, 167
    psychotic symptoms
        versus, 213
    sleep problems associated
        with, 203
    treatment of, 167–168, 193
        in children, 408–409,
            427t–431t
Obsessive–compulsive (OC)
    personality disorder, 331t,
    339–340
Obstructive sleep apnea (OSA)
    consequences of, 195, 198
    diagnosis of, 197, 198
    identification of, 198
    treatment of, 198–199
Occupational dysfunction, in
    schizophrenia, 214b, 215
OCD. See Obsessive–compulsive
    disorder (OCD).

Ocular disorders
    ECT and, 320
    in Alzheimer's patients, 67, 76
    psychiatric symptoms caused
        by, 33
Oculogyric crisis, 235
Olanzapine (Zyprexa)
    dose recommendations for, 220t,
        226t
    for acute schizophrenia, 230, 232t
    for Alzheimer's disease, 69, 71t,
        73, 74t
    for behavioral emergencies,
        275t, 276
    for bipolar mania, 250
    for mania, 141t, 143, 144, 155
    for schizophrenia, 217
    for tardive dyskinesia, 239
    formulary, 481
    intramuscular, 219, 223t, 234
    P450 system and, 227t
    pharmacokinetics of, 226t
    pregnancy and, 249
    receptor affinities of, 221t
    side effects of, 233t, 244
Olanzapine-fluoxetine, for bipolar
        depression, 155
Olfactory hallucinations, 212
Omeprazole (Prilosec), 379b, 384,
        387
Omnibus Budget Reconciliation
        Act (OBRA) of 1987,
        Alzheimer's treatment
        guidelines, 83–84
    for anxiety, 79
Ondansetron, 289, 351
1A2 enzyme, antipsychotics
        metabolism role, 223, 227t,
        228
Opioids
    dependence on, pain disorder
        associated with, 262, 263
    for periodic limb movement
        disorders, 202
    issues with use of. See Narcotics.
    withdrawal from. See Narcotics
        withdrawal.
Opisthotonus, 235
Opportunistic diseases, dementia
        associated with, 56–57

Oppositional defiant disorder,
        417–418
    ADHD versus, 411
    course and prognosis of, 418
    definition of, 417
    diagnosis of, 417
    differential diagnosis of, 417–418
    epidemiology of, 417
    identification of, 417
    treatment of, 418
Optimization therapy, for
        somatization disorder,
        256–257
Oral injuries, ECT causing, 321, 323
Organic affective disorder, 89
Orgasm, 363
    disorders of, 246, 371
Orientation, loss of, in alcohol
        withdrawal delirium, 298b
Orlistat, for obesity, 354
Orthostatic hypotension
    anorexia nervosa associated
        with, 345b, 346
    antipsychotics associated with,
        234, 242–243, 276
    from antidepressants, 116–117,
        118t, 133
OSA. See Obstructive sleep
        apnea (OSA).
Osteoarthritis, obesity associated
        with, 353
Osteopenia, antipsychotic
        selection and, 230
Osteoporosis, antipsychotic
        selection and, 230
Out-of-home placement, conduct
        disorder and, 416
Outpatient treatment
    for alcohol withdrawal, 294
    for posttraumatic stress disorder,
        in children, 401
    for suicidal patient, 280
    in primary care, 2, 4
    past history of, 23
Outreach services, for conduct
        disorder, 416
Over-the-counter (OTC) drugs,
        patient history of, 28
Overanxious disorder of
        childhood, 168, 399

Overdose
    of antipsychotics, 248
    of benzodiazepines, 184
    of heroin, 310–311
Overt Aggression Scale, 282, 283b
Oxazepam (Serax)
    for Alzheimer's disease, 69t, 75
    pharmacokinetics of, 179t, 180,
        181b
Oxcarbazepine (Trileptal)
    administration guidelines for,
        153–154
    for bipolar disorder, in children,
        424t
    for mania, 142t, 143, 144, 153
    formulary, 481–482
    side effects of, 154
Oxidative metabolism, isoenzymes
    in, 378, 382. See also CYP
    entries; P450 system.
Oxycodone, half-life of, 310t
Oxygen consumption, ECT impact
    on, 320
Oxygen saturation, 46, 48
Oxygen therapy, for ECT, 323, 325

P450 system, 378–387
    age effects on, 383
    antidepressants interactions
        with, 123, 130
    antipsychotics metabolism role,
        223, 227t, 228
    atypical antipsychotics
        interactions with, 74, 74t
    definition of, 378
    genetic polymorphism of,
        382–383
    inducers of, 386, 387b
    inhibition of
        drug interactions causing,
            379b, 383–384
        onset and termination, 378
    isoenzymes of, 378, 382.
        See also CYP entries.
    substrates, 380b–382b, 384–386
        competition of, 378
    terminology for, 378, 382
    therapeutic implications of,
        386–387

Pacemakers, cardiac, ECT and, 325
PACT (Program for Assertive
    Community Treatment), 230
Pain
    acute paradigm of, for chronic
        management, 313
    chronic
        malignant versus nonmalignant,
            312–313, 313t
        medical history of, 28
    in conversion disorder, 258
    in somatization disorder, 254
Pain clinics, multidisciplinary
    approach in, 263
Pain disorder, 262–263
Pain management, common
    narcotic problems in,
    305–306, 312
Pain syndromes
    neuropathic, 314
    sleep problems associated with,
        196, 202
Panic attacks
    criteria for, 160, 161b
    definition of, 160
    in acute stress disorder, 174
    in posttraumatic stress disorder,
        176
    medical problems
        manifesting as, 33, 34,
        162, 163b
    recurring, 166
    sleep problems associated with,
        196
Panic disorder, 159–166
    agoraphobia and, 170–171
    alprazolam for, 443
    benzodiazepines for, 178
    course of, 163
    definition of, 159–160
    differential diagnosis of,
        162–163, 163b
    generalized anxiety disorder and,
        169
    hypochondriasis associated with,
        264, 265
    identification of, 160, 161b
    in children, 397–398
    in primary medical care, 6t, 7
    medical costs of, 7, 8

Panic disorder—cont'd
  prevalence of, 162
  prognosis of, 163
  sleep problems associated with,
    203
  somatization disorder *versus*, 255
  treatment of, 163–166
    for comorbidities, 165–166
    nonpharmacologic, 163, 193
    psychopharmacology,
      163–165, 165t
PANSS (Positive and Negative
    Syndrome Scale), 234
PAP (positive airway pressure), for
    obstructive sleep apnea, 199,
    205
Paradoxical effects, of
    benzodiazepines, 182
Paranoia, alcoholic, 290–291
Paranoid delusions, 210
Paranoid personality disorder, 330,
    331t, 332
Paranoid schizophrenia, 217
Paraphilias, 375–376
Paraplegia, sexual dysfunction
    associated with, 373
Parasomnias, 204–205
  night terrors, 204
  nightmares, 205
  REM sleep behavior disorder,
    205
  sleepwalking, 204
Parasympathetic nervous system,
    ECT stimulation of, 320, 324
Parent-child interaction
  in ADHD, 410
  in conduct disorder, 415, 416
Parent management training, for
    conduct disorder, 416
Parkinsonism
  antipsychotics causing, 236
  dementia with, 56, 57, 60
  in Alzheimer's disease, 84
    antipsychotics and, 70,
      74, 74t
Parkinson's disease
  ECT and, 317, 325
  sleep problems associated with,
    203
Parotids, swelling of, 349

Paroxetine hydrochloride (Paxil),
    109, 112t, 121–122
  adverse effects of, 115t, 123
  as P450 system substrate, 381b,
    384
  for anxiety disorders, 187–188,
    189t
  for generalized anxiety disorder,
    165t
  for hypochondriasis, 265
  for major depression, in
    children, 427t
  for obsessive–compulsive
    disorder, 167
  for panic disorder, 164, 165t
  for posttraumatic stress disorder,
    176
  formulary, 482
  P450 system inhibition by, 379b,
    383, 386
Paroxysmal sweats, in alcohol
    withdrawal delirium, 296b
Participants/participation, in
    mental status examination, 30
Passive–aggressive personality
    disorder, 331t, 340–341
Pathologic intoxication, with
    alcohol, 291
Patience, for hypochondriacal
    patients, 264
Patient appearance. *See* Personal
    appearance.
Patient-controlled analgesia
    (PCA), 306
Patient teaching
  database for, 13
  for acute somatized symptoms,
    257–258
  for ADHD, 412, 414
  for anxiety disorders, 192
  for conversion disorder, 260
  for factitious disorder, 267
  for generalized anxiety
    disorder, in children, 399
  for major depression, in
    children, 426
  for panic disorder, in children,
    397
  for posttraumatic stress disorder,
    401

Patient teaching—cont'd
  for separation anxiety disorder, 390
  for somatization disorder, 257
Payment responsibility, in psychiatric database, 16–17
PBG (porphobilinogen), 47
PCA (patient-controlled analgesia), 306
PCP (phencyclidine) use, 301, 303t, 304
PDSQ (Psychiatric Diagnostic Screening Questionnaire), 93
Pedophilia, 375
Peer relations, in conduct disorder, 415
Penile implants, for erectile disorder, 371
Penile injection (Alprostadil Caverject), 371
Penile suppository (Alprostadil), 371
Penile tumescence studies, nocturnal, 370
Pentazocine, half-life of, 310t
Pentobarbital, for delirium tremens, 299
Peptide chains, in P450 system, 378
Perceptual disturbances
  delirium and, 50
  in psychosis, 210, 211b
  in schizophrenia, 216
Performance anxiety, 171–172
Perinatal history, in psychiatric database, 23
Periodic limb movement disorders, 202
Perphenazine (Trilafon)
  dose recommendations for, 220t
  for Alzheimer's disease, 84
  for anxiety disorders, 188
  for destructive behavior, in mental retardation, 421t, 438t
  formulary, 482–483
  side effects of, 233t
Personal appearance
  in histrionic personality disorder, 336
  in hypochondriasis, 264

Personal appearance—cont'd
  in mental status examination, 30
  preoccupation with. See also Body dysmorphic disorder (BDD).
  in eating disorders, 343, 348
Personality changes, obsessive–compulsive disorder versus, 167
Personality disorders, 328–341
  antisocial, 333
  as behavioral emergency, 273
  avoidant, 171, 337–338
  borderline, 334–335
  comorbidity of, 328
  definition of, 328–329
  dementia and, 54
  dependent, 338–339
  depressive, 340
  developmental determinants of, 24
  doctor-patient relationship and, 329, 337
  histrionic, 335–336
  in medical management, 330, 331t
  in psychiatric database, 13, 21b, 22b
  narcissistic, 336–337
  obsessive–compulsive, 339–340
  paranoid, 330, 332
  passive–aggressive (negativistic), 340–341
  prevalence of, 328
  recognition of, 329–330
  schizoid, 332–333
  schizotypal, 171, 213
Personality traits, 328
PET (positron emission tomography), 44
PFAMC (psychological factors affecting medical condition), 173
Pharmacokinetics. See specific drug classification or agent.
Pharmacology. See Medications.
Phencyclidine (PCP), use of, 301, 303t, 304, 305

Phenelzine sulfate (Nardil), 133, 133t, 134
  formulary, 484–485
Phenothiazines
  as antipsychotics, 220t
    adverse effects of, 247
  for destructive behavior, in mental retardation, 421t, 438t, 440
Phentermine
  as P450 system substrate, 385
  indications for, 130, 354
Phentolamine, for male erectile disorder, 371
Phenylalanine, for tardive dyskinesia, 239
Phenytoin
  Alzheimer's disease and, 69t, 76
  as P450 system substrate, 380b, 385
  for alcohol seizures, 300
Phobia(s)
  social, 171–172. See also Social phobia.
    in children, 398
  specific, 170–172. See also Specific phobias.
    in children, 391, 396
Phonic tics, 408
Physical activity counseling, for obesity, 246
Physical aggression
  against objects, 283b
  against others, 283b
  against self, 283b
Physical complaints, in somatization disorder, 254
  undifferentiated, 254–255
Physical defects, in body dysmorphic disorder, 265, 266
Physical disorders. See Medical condition/illness.
Physical examination
  for acute somatized symptoms, 258
  for anorexia nervosa, 344
  for dementia, 57–58, 58b
  for developmental disabilities, 436
  for ECT, 321

Physical examination—cont'd
  for psychiatric symptoms evaluation, 41
  for schizophrenia, 230, 231b
  for sleep disorders, 197
  in behavioral emergencies, 272t, 273–274
  in psychiatric database, 17f, 29
  of violent patient, 282
Physical interventions, for anxiety disorders, 189–190, 190b, 191b, 192
Physical restraints, 283–284
  guidelines for use, 284
  indications for, 283–284
  JCAH rules for, 284
Physical setting, in mental status examination, 30
Physician gatekeepers, 10
Physiologic mechanisms
  in conversion disorder, 258, 259
  in somatization disorder, 254
  of nicotine addition, 355–356
  pain disorder versus, 263
Pick's disease, 54, 55t
Pimozide (Orap)
  for destructive behavior, in mental retardation, 421t, 438t
  for Tourette's syndrome, 250
  formulary, 485–486
  P450 system and, 223, 227t
  QT prolongation associated with, 243
PMDD (premenstrual dysphoric disorder), 105–106, 419
PMR (progressive muscle relaxation), for anxiety disorders, 189, 190b
PMS (premenstrual syndrome), 30
Polypharmacy, in child and adolescent psychiatry, 389
Polysomnography (PSG), 48, 197, 198
Porphobilinogen (PBG), 47
Porphyria, 47
Porphyrins, 47
Positive airway pressure (PAP), for obstructive sleep apnea, 199, 205

Positive and Negative Syndrome Scale (PANSS), 234
Positive reinforcement techniques
   for ADHD management, 414
   for behavior disorders, 416, 418
Positive symptoms, of schizophrenia, 216, 230
Positive thinking, for anxiety disorders, 192
Positron emission tomography (PET), 44
Postpartum period, depression associated with, 98, 137
Posttraumatic stress disorder (PTSD), 175–177
   course and prognosis of, 400–401
   definition of, 175, 399
   diagnostic criteria for, 175, 400
   differential diagnosis of, 173, 176, 400
   identification of, 175, 400
   in children, 399–401
   in schizophrenia, 218
   panic attacks with, 160
   prevalence of, 175
   prognosis of, 176
   sleep problems associated with, 203
   treatment of, 176–177, 193
      in children, 401, 402t, 427t
Potassium-depleting drugs, antipsychotics interaction with, 229t
Power struggles, in narcissistic personality disorder, 337
Prader–Willi syndrome, 352
Pramipexole (Mirapex), 202
Pregnancy
   antidepressants and, 120
   antipsychotics and, 249
   as MRI contraindication, 43
   benzodiazepines and, 184
   bipolar depression during, 137, 143, 156
   ECT and, 120, 318, 326
   teratogenic drugs and, 48, 147, 150, 153, 154, 249

Pregnancy history, in psychiatric database, 23, 29
Pregnancy test, 48
Premature ejaculation, 371
Premenstrual dysphoric disorder (PMDD), 105–106, 419
Premenstrual syndrome (PMS), 30, 105
Premorbid phase, of schizophrenia, 216
Prenatal conditions, developmental disabilities associated with, 434, 436–437
Preoccupation
   in hypochondriasis, 264
   in narcissistic personality disorder, 336–337
   pathologic. See Obsessive–compulsive disorder (OCD).
   with personal appearance. See also Body dysmorphic disorder (BDD).
   in eating disorders, 343, 348
Prescription medications, patient history of, 28
Prevention–intervention model, for posttraumatic stress disorder, 401
Primary care
   anxiety disorders in, 158, 159b, 160b, 162
   major depressive disorder in
      prevalence of, 94–95, 97t
      recognition of, 95–96
   personality disorders in, 330, 331t
   psychiatric comorbidity in
      as first treatment source, 2, 3t, 4
      cost-benefit issues of, 9
      examples of, 5–8, 6t
      impact of, 5
      lack of recognition, 4, 4t, 95
      screening prevalence, 4, 4t, 10
      strategic integration of services, 9–10
Primary Care Evaluation of Mental Disorders (PRIME-MD), 93

Primary gain, in conversion
    disorder, 258
Primary insomnia, 200, 201b
Privacy, in psychiatric interview,
    12, 13
Prodromal phase, of schizophrenia,
    216–217
Program for Assertive
    Community Treatment
    (PACT), 230
Progressive muscle relaxation
    (PMR), for anxiety disorders,
    189, 190b
Prolactin, antipsychotics effect on,
    243–244
Promethazine hydrochloride
    (Phenergan), 486–487
Propafenone, P450 system
    inhibition by, 379b, 383
Propofol (Diprivan), 299, 487–488
Propoxyphene, half-life of, 310t
Propranolol (Inderal), 60, 188,
    395t
Protriptyline hydrochloride
    (Vivactil), 487–488
Pseudoneurologic symptoms
    in conversion disorder, 258, 259
    in somatization disorder, 254
    pain disorder versus, 263
Pseudoseizures, in conversion
    disorder, 259
PSG (polysomnography), 48, 197,
    198
Psilocybin, 302t, 305
Psychiatric assessment/
    consultation
    for ECT, 321
    for medical inpatients, 5
Psychiatric database, 13–32
    chief complaint, 14f, 19–22
    developmental history, 16f, 23
    DSM-IV formulation from, 13,
        21b, 22b, 24b, 26b–27b
    family history, 16f, 26–27
    history of present illness, 14f, 22
    in child and adolescent
        psychiatry, 389–390
    medical history, 15f–16f, 27–29
    neurologic examination, 17f, 29
    overview of, 13, 14f

Psychiatric database—cont'd
    past psychiatric history, 14f, 23
    physical examination, 17f, 29
    psychosocial review, 17f–19f,
        24–26
    sexual history, 29–30
    sociodemographics, 13–19,
        17f, 19f
    vital signs, 29
Psychiatric Diagnostic Screening
    Questionnaire (PDSQ), 93
Psychiatric disorders
    acute somatized symptoms
        versus, 257
    acute stress disorder related to,
        174
    chronic, alcohol use associated
        with, 293
    clonazepam causing, 455
    conversion disorder versus, 259
    eating disorders associated with,
        345b, 346
    economic costs of, 2, 3t
    functional impact of, 1–2
    hypochondriasis versus, 264
    in children, 389–440
        anxiety as, 390–409
        attention-deficit/hyper-
            activity as, 409–414
        depression as, 418–433
        developmental disabilities as,
            435–440
        diagnostic principles of,
            389–390
        disruptive behavior as,
            414–418
        learning problems, 433–435
        mental retardation as,
            435–440
    in dementia, 54
        treatment of, 59–60
    in medical practice. See Primary
        care.
    medical costs of, 5, 7, 8–9, 355
    medical illness versus, 4
    narcotics and, 306
    nicotine dependence associated
        with, 356–357
    panic attacks associated with,
        162–163

Psychiatric disorders—cont'd
    prevalence of, 1, 2t
        in primary care, 5–8, 6t
    primary care gatekeepers for, 10
    sexual disorders associated with,
        364, 370, 371, 372
    sleep problems associated with,
        203
    somatization disorder
        versus, 255
    treatment success rates for, 2, 3t
    violence associated with, 281
Psychiatric history
    family, 16f, 27
    past, 14f, 23
Psychiatric interview, 12–13
    in primary medical care, 4,
        4t, 10
Psychiatry
    cost-benefit issues involving, 9
    for children, 389–440
        diagnostic assessment of,
            389–390
        overview of, 389
        specific disorders in, 390–440
    medical practice utilization
        versus, 2, 3t, 4, 4t
    strategic integration of, 1, 9–10
Psychoactive substance abuse, 314,
    315–316
Psychobiological mechanisms, of
    ECT, 317
Psychodynamic psychotherapy,
    337, 348
Psychodynamic theories, of eating
    disorders, 343, 349, 352
Psychoeducational tests,
    diagnostic, 434
Psychogenic nonepileptic seizures,
    259
Psychological factors, pain
    disorder associated with, 262
Psychological factors affecting
    medical condition (PFAMC),
    173
Psychological testing, for mental
    retardation, 436
Psychomotor impairment,
    benzodiazepines causing, 181
    azapirones *versus*, 186

Psychopaths, 333
Psychosis/psychotic symptoms,
    210–251
    antipsychotics for, 219–229.
        See also Antipsychotic
        agents.
    alternatives to, 251
    bipolar disorder and, 139, 140,
        143, 156
    definition of, 210
    differential diagnosis of, 212–214
    ECT for, 317
    identification of, 210–212, 211b
    in Alzheimer's patients, 66t, 67
    in borderline personality
        disorder, 334–335
    in dementia, 59
    in major depression, 96–97
    in schizophrenia, 214–218.
        See also Schizophrenia.
    exacerbations of, 217
    mental status examination for,
        210, 211b
    suicide risk related to, 278
Psychosocial assessment
    in psychiatric database, 17f–19f,
        24–26
    of anxiety symptoms, 158
Psychosocial interventions
    for bipolar disorder, 144, 156
    for delirium, 53
    for psychosis of schizophrenia, 251
Psychosocial problems
    diagnoses associated with. *See*
        Stress/stressors.
    DSM-IV axis IV for, 21b,
        24–25, 24b
    in primary medical care, 6t, 7–8
    psychiatric symptoms caused by,
        33
Psychostimulants. *See* Stimulants.
Psychosurgery, for obsessive–
    compulsive disorder, 168
Psychotherapy(ies)
    antidepressant indications for, 110
    cost-benefit issues involving, 9
    for adjustment disorder, 173
    for anorexia nervosa, 348
    for anxiety, 159
    for bipolar depression, 144

Psychotherapy(ies)—cont'd
    for body dysmorphic disorder, 266
    for borderline personality
        disorder, 335
    for bulimia nervosa, 350
    for children. See specific disorder.
    for dependent personality
        disorder, 339
    for depression, 87, 102, 103
    for generalized anxiety disorder,
        supportive versus focused,
        170
    for hypochondriasis, 264–265
    for major depression, 100–101
    for marijuana abuse, 316
    for narcissistic personality
        disorder, 337
    for obsessive–compulsive
        disorder, 168
    for paraphilias, 376
    for posttraumatic stress disorder,
        176
    for substance abuse, 304–305
    initial plan for, 20
Psychotic depression, 212, 250
Psychotic disorder, brief, 212
Psychotic phase, of schizophrenia,
    217
Psychotropic agents
    abuse issues with, 314, 315–316
    as analgesic augmenters, 314
    ECT and, 322
    effects on EEG, 42
    effects on fetus, 48
    factitious disorder and, 267
    for chronic suicidal patient, 280
    for premenstrual dysphoric
        disorder, 106
    in child and adolescent
        psychiatry, 389
    mental retardation and, 437,
        438t–439t, 440
    P450 system inhibition by, 378,
        379b, 383–384
PTSD. See Posttraumatic stress
    disorder (PTSD).
Pulmonary system. See Respiratory
    tract/system.
Pulses, in behavioral emergencies,
    274

Punishment, physical restraint as, 284
Punishment structures, for ADHD
    management, 414
Purging, binge-eating and, 343,
    348–349
Pyridoxine deficiency, MAOIs
    causing, 133

QT prolongation, antipsychotics
    associated with, 234, 243, 276
Quadriplegia, sexual dysfunction
    associated with, 373
Quality assurance, database for, 13
Questionnaires, standardized
    for ADHD, 411
    for alcohol use, 28, 288, 288b
    for psychiatric screening, 93
Quetiapine furmarate (Seroquel)
    dose recommendations for, 220t,
        226t
    for acute schizophrenia, 230,
        232t
    for Alzheimer's disease, 70, 71t,
        73, 74
    for bipolar mania, 250
    for delirium, 53–54
    for dementia, 60
    for destructive behavior, in
        mental retardation, 422t,
        439t
    for mania, 141t, 143, 144
    for tardive dyskinesia, 239
    formulary, 488
    P450 system and, 223, 227t
    pharmacokinetics of, 226t
    pregnancy and, 249
    receptor affinities of, 221t
    side effects of, 233t, 244
Quinidine
    antipsychotics interactions with,
        229t
    P450 system inhibition by, 379b,
        383

Rage behavior, in mental
    retardation, 421t–425t, 440
Ramalteon/ramelteon (Rozerem),
    208, 489

Rape, 173, 175, 375
Rapid cycling, in bipolar disorder, 138, 139, 143
Rash
  lamotrigine-related, 470–471
  mood stabilizers causing, 153, 155
Rating scales, for major depression
  clinician-administered, 93
  self-administered, 93–94, 94f–96f, 97b
Rauwolfia alkaloids, ECT and, 322
Re-experiencing, posttraumatic stress disorder and, 175, 176
Reactions
  drug, patient history of, 28
  excessive. See Adjustment disorder.
Reactive anxiety, 174
Reading, in cognitive examination, 62
Reading disorder, 411, 433, 434, 434t
Reason, for psychiatric consultation, 12, 16–17
Reasoning
  emotional, anxiety caused by, 192
  in cognitive examination, 63
  logical, in borderline personality disorder, 335
Reassurance
  for acute stress disorder, 175
  for hypochondriasis, 264
  for somatization disorders, 256, 258
Refeeding protocol, for anorexia nervosa, 347, 347b
Referrer, in psychiatric database, 16, 17
Refusal, of treatment
  commitment and, 285
  competence and, 286
Rehabilitation Act (1973), 435
Rejection sensitivity, 98
  in avoidant personality disorder, 337–338
  in dependent personality disorder, 338–339
Relapse, after ECT, 324

Relapse prevention programs
  for alcoholism, 288–289
  for paraphilias, 376
Relaxation therapy(ies)
  contraindications for, 192
  for adjustment disorder, 173
  for anxiety disorders, 189–190, 190b, 191b, 192
  generalized, 159, 170
  for simple phobias, 172
  guidelines for starting, 189–190
Religion, in psychiatric database, 14
REM sleep, in sleep disorders, 199–200, 203
REM sleep behavior disorder, 205
Remediation programs, for learning disorders, 435
Renal function/failure
  antipsychotics metabolism and, 228
  eating disorders and, 345b
  psychiatric symptoms caused by, 46
  sexual dysfunction associated with, 373
Repetition, in cognitive examination, 62
Reserpine, ECT interaction with, 321, 322
Residential treatment programs, for conduct disorder, 416
Resistance, in passive–aggressive personality disorder, 341
Resocialization, for schizoid personality disorder, 333
Resolution phase, of sexual function, 363
Respect, in psychiatric interview, 12
Respiratory depression
  amobarbital risks for, 261
  benzodiazepines causing, 181, 276
  azapirones versus, 186
  with narcotics use, 305
Respiratory disorders, anxiety caused by, 160b
Respiratory rate, in behavioral emergencies, 274

Respiratory tract/system
  anxiety symptoms in, 159b
  ECT impact on, 318–319, 320
  marijuana abuse impact on, 315
Responsible person, in psychiatric
    database, 15
Restless leg syndrome, 178, 195, 202
Restlessness, in narcotics
    assessment, 308b
Restricting anorexia nervosa, 343
Retinitis pigmentosa, antipsychotics
    associated with, 247
Retrograde amnesia, ECT causing,
    319
Review of systems (ROS)
  in dementia evaluation, 57
  in psychiatric interview, 17f, 33
Reward structures, for ADHD
    management, 414
Rheumatoid arthritis,
    schizophrenia and, 218
Rheumatologic conditions,
    hypochondriasis versus, 264
Rifampin, as P450 system inducer,
    386, 387b
Rimonabant, for obesity, 354
Risperidone, depot
    (Risperdal Consta), 219–220,
    489–491
Risperidone (Risperdal)
  dose recommendations for, 220t,
    225t
  for acute schizophrenia, 230,
    232t
  for Alzheimer's disease, 70, 71t,
    73, 74t, 79, 250
  for anxiety disorders, 188
  for behavioral emergencies, 274,
    275t
  for delirium, 54, 249
  for destructive behavior, in
    mental retardation,
    421t–439t
  for mania, 141t, 143, 144
  for schizophrenia, 217
  formulary, 489–491
  P450 system and, 223, 227t
  pharmacokinetics of, 225t
  receptor affinities of, 221t
  side effects of, 233t, 235, 244

Ritonavir
  as P450 system inducer, 386,
    387b
  P450 system inhibition by, 379b,
    383, 384
Rituals, common developmental,
    401
Rivastigmine (Exelon), 77–78,
    491
Ropinirole (Requip), 202
ROS. See Review of systems (ROS).
Ruminative worry, 169

Sadism, 350
  sexual, 375
Safety
  for intoxicated patients, 290
  in behavioral emergencies, 271,
    283, 285
  in psychiatric interview, 12
Safety contract, for suicidal
    patient, 281
St. John's wort, HIV-associated
    dementia and, 57
Salicylates, Alzheimer's disease
    and, 69t, 76
SAMHSA (Substance Abuse and
    Mental Health Services
    Administration), 9
Schilling's test, 48
Schizoaffective disorder, 99, 212,
    213b, 317
Schizoid personality disorder, 331t,
    332–333
Schizophrenia, 214–218
  antipsychotics for, 219–229.
    See also Antipsychotic
    agents.
  acute phase choices, 230, 232t
  alternatives to, 251
  atypical, 217, 218
  clinical guidelines for,
    230–248
  body dysmorphic disorder versus,
    266
  clinical features of, 215–216
  comorbidity of, 217–218, 244
  antipsychotic choices based
    on, 230, 233t

Schizophrenia—cont'd
  decompensation of, as
      behavioral emergency, 273
  definition of, 214
  diagnostic criteria for, 214–215,
      214b
  eating disorders associated with,
      345b, 346
  epidemiology of, 215
  hypochondriasis versus, 264
  incidence of, 214, 215
  lifetime prevalence of, 215
  medical problems manifesting
      as, 34
  natural history of, 216–217
  nicotine dependence associated
      with, 357
  nonpharmacologic treatment
      of, 251
  obsessive–compulsive disorder
      versus, 166
  outcomes of, good versus poor,
      217
  paranoid, 217
  psychotic symptoms versus, 214
  quetiapine for, 489
  risk factors of, 215
  sleep problems associated with,
      203
  somatization disorder versus, 255
  suicide associated with, 218
  treatment planning for
    goals of, 230
    initial assessment in, 230,
        231b
  treatment setting for, 230
Schizophreniform disorder, 213
Schizotypal personality disorder,
    171, 213
School history, in psychiatric
    database, 23
School interventions
  for ADHD, 414
  for conduct disorder, 416
  for learning disorders, 435
  for mental retardation, 435, 437
School performance.
    See Academic achievement.
School refusal, in children, 343,
    390–391

Screening
  cognitive, 61–63
    for dementia, 58
  for alcoholism, 28, 288, 288b,
      289b
  for major depression, 92–94,
      93b
  for psychiatric disorders, 93
    in emergency department,
        7, 8
    in medical practice, 4, 4t, 10
  neuroimaging as, 42–44
  for substance use, 28, 29,
      44–45
  for Wilson's disease, 47
  of blood glucose level, 45
Search/searching, of patient and
    belongings, 267, 268
Seasonal affective disorder, in
    children, 419
Seasonal pattern, of major
    depression, 98–99
Second-generation anti-
    depressants, 121–127
  norepinephrine reuptake
      inhibitors as, 123–125
  other agents as, 125–127
  profiles of specific, 111t–112t
  selective serotonin reuptake
      inhibitors as, 121–123.
      See also Selective serotonin
      reuptake inhibitors
      (SSRIs).
  serotonin reuptake inhibitors as,
      123–125
Secondary gain, in malingering,
    258, 263, 264, 266
Security guards, for behavioral
    emergencies, 271
Sedative withdrawal syndromes,
    293
  benzodiazepines for, 178
    azapirones versus, 186
  treatment of, 295
Sedatives. See also Hypnotics.
  abuse of, bipolar disorder versus,
      140
  agitation related to, in
      Alzheimer's patients, 68,
      69b, 81t

Sedatives—cont'd
  antidepressants as, 116
  antipsychotics as, 242
  as P450 system substrate, 382b,
      385–386
  benzodiazepines augmentation
      of, 183
    azapirones *versus*, 186
  cross-tolerant, for sedative
      withdrawal, 295, 299t
  dose conversions for, 299t
  for Alzheimer's disease, OBRA
      guidelines for, 83
  for anxiety disorders, 188
  for sleep problems, 202, 205
  psychiatric symptoms caused by,
      37b
  sexual dysfunction related to,
      369t
  sleep problems associated with,
      203
  withdrawal from, delirium
      associated with, 53
Seductive behavior, 336
Seizure disorders
  benzodiazepines for, 178
  bipolar disorder *versus*,
      139–140
  clonazepam causing, 454–455
  EEG evaluation of, 42
  psychiatric symptoms caused by,
      34–35, 39b
Seizure duration, in ECT, 324
Seizure threshold, 242, 324
Seizures
  alcohol withdrawal, 300
  antidepressants causing, 117
  ECT and, 317, 321
    missed, 323–324
    prolonged, 324
  medical history of, 28
  psychogenic nonepileptic, 259
  valproic acid for, 499–500
Selective mutism, in children,
      396–397
Selective norepinephrine reuptake
      inhibitors (SNRIs), 123–125
  for ADHD, 406t–407t, 413
  for borderline personality
      disorder, 335

Selective norepinephrine reuptake
      inhibitors (SNRIs)—cont'd
  for generalized anxiety disorder,
      165t, 170
  medical complications of,
      127–131
  neuroceptor effects of, 114t
  profiles of specific, 112t
  sexual dysfunction and, 119
Selective serotonin reuptake
      inhibitors (SSRIs)
  as P450 system substrate,
      380b–381b, 384–386
  cardiac effects of, 117, 118t,
      129–130
  continued use guidelines for,
      110
  for ADHD, 406t–407t
  for alcoholism, 289
  for Alzheimer's disease, 76, 80,
      81t
  for anxiety disorders, 187–188
  for bipolar depression, 143
  for body dysmorphic disorder,
      266
  for borderline personality
      disorder, 335
  for bulimia nervosa, 350
  for dementia, 59, 60
  for generalized anxiety disorder,
      170
    in children, 399, 427t–431t
  for hypochondriasis, 265
  for major depression, 98
    in children, 426, 427t–428t,
        432–433
  for narcolepsy, 200
  for obsessive–compulsive
      disorder, 167, 408–409,
      427t–431t
  for panic disorder, 163, 164, 165t
    in children, 398, 427t–431t
  for posttraumatic stress disorder,
      176
  for premenstrual dysphoric
      disorder, 106
  for selective mutism, 397, 427t
  for social phobia, 171
    in children, 398, 427t–431t
  loss of effectiveness, 123

Selective serotonin reuptake
    inhibitors (SSRIs)—cont'd
  lower dose effectiveness of, 109
  medical complications of,
      127–131
    bleeding as, 129
    cardiac arrhythmias as,
        129–130
    extrapyramidal side effects,
        129
    serotonin syndrome as,
        130–131, 130b, 131b
    SIADH as, 127–129
  P450 system inhibition by, 378,
      379b, 383
  profiles of specific, 111t–112t
  withdrawal symptoms of, 109
Selegiline hydrochloride
    (Eldepryl), 133, 133t, 492
Selegiline transdermal patch
    (ENSAM), 133, 133t
Self-care impairments, 25, 338
Self-destructive behavior
  commitment for, 284–285
  in borderline personality
      disorder, 334
  in mental retardation,
      421t–425t, 440
  in violent patient, 282, 283b
Self-esteem
  in avoidant personality disorder,
      337–338
  in oppositional defiant disorder,
      417
  loss of, as major depression
      criteria, 91b, 92
Self-identification, in psychiatric
    interview, 12
Self-image
  in borderline personality
      disorder, 334–335
  in histrionic personality
      disorder, 336
Self-importance, in narcissistic
    personality disorder, 336–337
Self-injury. See Self-destructive
    behavior.
Self-mutilation
  genital, 376
  in children, 400

Self-perception, in eating
    disorders, 343, 348
Self-rating scales, for major
    depression, 93–94, 94f–96f,
    97b
Self-referrals, 16
Self-regulation, of anxiety
    symptoms, 159, 170, 172
Self-report instruments, for
    personality disorders, 330
Semantics, in mental status
    examination, 32
Semi-structured interviews, for
    personality disorders, 330
Sensory disturbances
  in alcohol withdrawal, 291,
      297b, 298b
  in conversion disorder, 258
  in somatization disorder, 254
Separation anxiety disorder,
    390–391
  course and prognosis of, 390
  definition of, 390
  differential diagnosis of, 390
  epidemiology of, 390
  in dependent personality
      disorder, 338
  panic attacks with, 160
  treatment of, 390–391,
      392t–395t
Serotonin dysregulation, depression
    linked to, 105–106
Serotonin receptors, atypical
    antipsychotics affinity for,
    219, 221t
  therapeutic versus adverse
      effects, 222t
Serotonin reuptake inhibitors
    (SRIs), 123–125
  for borderline personality
      disorder, 335
  for generalized anxiety disorder,
      170
  for obsessive–compulsive
      disorder, 167
  neuroceptor effects of, 114t
  profiles of specific, 112t
Serotonin syndrome
  differential diagnosis of, 130–131
  MAOIs and, 134, 135b

Serotonin syndrome—cont'd
  medical management of, 131
  medications causing, 130, 131b
  symptoms of, 130, 130b
Serotoninergic agents, 37b, 265
Sertraline hydrochloride (Zoloft),
    109, 112t, 121
  adverse effects of, 115t
  for anxiety disorders, 187, 189t
  for generalized anxiety disorder,
    165t
  for hypochondriasis, 265
  for major depression, in
    children, 428t
  for obsessive–compulsive
    disorder, 167
  for posttraumatic stress disorder,
    176
  formulary, 492–493
  P450 system inhibition by, 379b,
    383, 387
SES (socioeconomic status),
    conduct disorder and, 415
Sexual abuse, 255
Sexual ambiguity, in gender
    identity disorder, 376
Sexual arousal, 363
  disorders of, 364, 370–371
  in paraphilias, 375–376
Sexual aversion disorder,
    364, 370
Sexual desire, 363
  disorders of, 364, 370
Sexual disinhibition, dementia
    and, 60, 374
Sexual disorders/dysfunction, 119,
    134, 363–377
  antidepressants causing, 119, 134
  antipsychotics causing, 246–247
  functional phases in, 363
  in conversion disorder, 258
  in somatization disorder, 254
  medical conditions associated
    with, 370, 372–374
  medications associated with,
    364, 365t–369t, 370
  of gender identity, 376–377
  of sexual arousal, 364, 370–371
  of sexual desire, 364, 370
  orgasmic, 246, 371

Sexual disorders/dysfunction—
    cont'd
  pain-related, 371–372
  paraphilias, 375–376
  patient history of, 29–30
  psychiatric disorders associated
    with, 364, 370, 371, 372
  sexual history in, 363–364
Sexual excitement, 363
Sexual function, phases in, 363
Sexual history, 29–30
  aspects to include in, 363
  how to obtain, 363–364
  medical factors, 364, 365t–369t
Sexual masochism, 375
Sexual play, in children, 400
Sexual sadism, 375
Sexually transmitted diseases
    (STDs), 29
Shift-work sleep disorder, 195,
    197–198, 205
Short-term memory
  impairment of, ECT causing,
    319
  in cognitive examination, 62
SIADH. See Syndrome of
    inappropriate antidiuretic
    hormone (SIADH).
Sialorrhea, clozapine associated
    with, 247
Sibutramine, for obesity, 353–354
Sick role, 266, 337
Side effects, of medications. See
    specific drug classification or
    agent.
Sildenafil (Viagra), 371
Simple phobias, 172, 391
Simple seizures, 499
Single positron emission computed
    tomography (SPECT), 44
SIPD-IV (Structured Interview for
    DSM Personality IV), 330
Situational anxiety, 174
Sleep apnea
  depression associated with, 88b
  obstructive, 195, 197, 198–199
  symptoms associated with, 46, 48
Sleep EEG, for seizure evaluation,
    42
Sleep history, 195–196, 196b

Sleep hygiene, improving, 200, 201b
Sleep log, 196
Sleep paralysis, 199, 200
Sleep phase
   advanced, 201–202
   delayed, 201
Sleep problems, 195–208
   as major depression criteria, 91b, 92, 98–99
   circadian rhythm in, 201–202
   evaluation of, 195–197, 196b
   hypersomnia, 197–200
   in Alzheimer's patients, 80
   in children, 400
   insomnia, 200–202
   medications associated with, 203–204
   mental disorders associated with, 203
   overview of, 195
   parasomnias, 204–205
   shift-work causing, 195, 197–198
   treatment of
      antidepressants in, 206
      benzodiazepines in, 178, 185, 206–208
      hypnotics in, 205–208
      over-the-counter medications, 201, 205–206
      sedatives in, 202, 205
Sleep state, misperception of, 200–201
Sleep studies, 42, 48, 197
Sleepiness scale, Epworth, 196, 196b
Sleepwalking, 204
Smoking. See Nicotine use.
Smoking cessation, 357–360
   buproprion SR for, 359–360
   cognitive behavior therapies for, 360
   immunologic approaches to, 361
   miscellaneous medications for, 360
   nicotine replacement for, 358–359
   overview of, 357
   vaccines for, 361

Snoring, apnea with, 195, 197, 198
SNRIs. See Selective norepinephrine reuptake inhibitors (SNRIs).
Sobriety maintenance, for alcoholism, 288
Social anxiety, exposure therapy for, 193–194
Social context
   in mental retardation evaluation, 436
   of child and adolescent psychiatry, 389, 415, 417
   of intoxicated patients, 290
Social dysfunction
   eating disorders and, 344
   in conduct disorder, 415
   in oppositional defiant disorder, 417
   in schizophrenia, 214b, 215
Social isolation, in schizoid personality disorder, 332
Social phobia, 171–172
   course and prognosis of, 171, 398
   definition of, 398
   differential diagnosis of, 171, 398
   epidemiology of, 171, 398
   identification of, 171, 398
   in children, 398, 427t–431t
   in schizophrenia, 218
   panic attacks with, 160
   treatment of, 171–172, 398, 427t
Social skills training. See Socialization.
Social support. See also Support groups.
   for acute stress disorder, 175
   in psychiatric database, 25
   intra- versus extratreatment, for smoking cessation, 360
Social withdrawal, dementia and, 54, 57
Socialization
   developmental determinants of, 24
   for ADHD, 414
   for major depression, in children, 426

Socialization—cont'd
  for psychosis of schizophrenia,
    251
  in selective mutism, 396
  psychiatric determinants of, 391
Sociodemographics
  conversion disorder associated
    with, 259
  in factitious disorder, 267
  in psychiatric database, 13–19,
    17f, 19f
Socioeconomic status
  (SES), conduct disorder
    and, 415
Sociopaths, 333
Socratic cognitive restructuring,
    192
Sodium imbalance, 46, 47
Sodium oxybate (Xyrem), 200
Soft signs, neurologic, for ADHD,
    411
Somatic delusions, 210
Somatization disorder, 254–257
  definition of, 254
  diagnostic criteria for, 254
  differential diagnosis of,
    255–256
  factitious disorder versus, 256,
    266–267
  generalized anxiety disorder
    versus, 169, 256
  identification of, 254
  in primary medical care, 6, 6t, 7
    cost-benefit issues of, 9
  malingering versus, 255,
    267–268
  pain disorder versus, 263
  prevalence of, 254–255
  prognosis of, 256
  treatment of, 256–257
  undifferentiated, 254–255
Somatization process, 253
Somatized symptoms
  acute, 257–258
  in children. See specific
    psychiatric disorder.
  in hypochondriasis, 264
  in primary medical care, 6, 6t
  in somatization disorder, 254
  of anxiety, 158–159, 159b

Somatoform disorders, 253–268
  acute somatized symptoms,
    257–258
  body dysmorphic disorder, 167,
    265–266
    premenstrual, 105–106
  conversion disorder, 258–262
  definition of, 253
  factitious disorder, 266–267
  hypochondriasis, 166, 167,
    263–265
  malingering, 214, 267–268
  not otherwise specified, 268
  overview of, 253
  pain disorder, 262–263
  somatization disorder, 169,
    254–257
    in primary medical care, 6, 6t,
      7, 9
Specialist consultations, for ECT,
    322
Specific phobias
  agoraphobia, 160, 162, 163, 165,
    170–171
  as medical care comorbidity, 5
  definition of, 170
  developmental determinants of,
    24
  eating disorders associated with,
    345b, 346
  exposure therapy for, 193
  identification of, 170
  in children, 391, 396
  obsessive–compulsive disorder
    versus, 167
  panic attacks in, 160
  simple, 172, 391
  social, 160, 171–172
SPECT (single positron emission
    computed tomography), 44
Speech
  delayed, 396
  in ADHD evaluation, 410, 411
  in mental status examination,
    31, 62
  in schizophrenia, 215–216
Spinal cord injury, sexual
    dysfunction and, 373
Spinal cord lesions, in sexual
    dysfunction, 374

Splitting, in borderline personality disorder, 334, 335
SRIs. *See* Serotonin reuptake inhibitors (SRIs).
SSRIs. *See* Selective serotonin reuptake inhibitors (SSRIs).
Stabilization psychotic phase, of schizophrenia, 217
  antipsychotics continuation in, 234–235
Stable psychotic phase, of schizophrenia, 217
  antipsychotics continuation in, 234–235
Status epilepticus, ECT causing, 321
STDs (sexually transmitted diseases), 29
Steroids
  Alzheimer's disease and, 69t
  analgesic properties of, 314
  depression associated with, 90
  exogenous
    as P450 system inducer, 386, 387b
    as P450 system substrate, 380b, 385
  psychiatric symptoms caused by, 37b
Stevens–Johnson syndrome, 153, 155
Stimulant abuse
  bipolar disorder *versus*, 140
  prevalence of, 301
  symptoms of, 301, 302t–303t, 304–305
Stimulants
  agitation related to, in Alzheimer's patients, 68, 69b
  analgesic properties of, 314
  anxiety caused by, 161b
  as antidepressants, 131–132
  as P450 system substrate, 381b, 384–385
  effects on EEG, 42
  for ADHD, 402t–407t, 414
    posttraumatic stress disorder and, 401

Stimulants—cont'd
  for antidepressant augmentation, 110
  for narcolepsy, 199
  MAOIs interactions with, 134, 135b
  psychiatric symptoms caused by, 37b
  sleep problems associated with, 203
Stimulus dosing, for ECT, 323
Stimulus threshold, in ECT, 323
Street drugs, illicit, in patient history, 28
Stress disorders
  acute, 173–175
  posttraumatic, 175–177
Stress management/reduction
  for dementia, 59
  for posttraumatic stress disorder, 401
  for premenstrual dysphoric disorder, 105–106
Stress/stressors
  excessive reactions to. *See* Adjustment disorder.
  in acute stress disorder, 173, 174
  in posttraumatic stress disorder, 175, 176, 400
  normal reaction to, adjustment disorder *versus*, 173
  personality disorders associated with, 328
  psychological/psychosocial, 174
    conversion disorder associated with, 259
    depression associated with, 87, 90, 101
    somatized symptoms associated with, 257, 258
  with medical problems, 33
  somatized symptoms associated with, 257
  sources of, in psychiatric database, 25, 26
Stroke
  depression associated with, 88b
  ECT and, 318, 320, 325
  mania associated with, 140

Stroke—cont'd
  neuroimaging of, 43, 44
  sexual dysfunction associated
      with, 373–374
Structured Interview for DSM
      Personality IV (SIPD-IV),
      330
Subarachnoid hemorrhage, 277
Subcortical dementia, 55, 56
Subdural hematoma, psychiatric
      symptoms caused by, 33
Substance abuse, 301–316. *See also
      specific substance.*
  acute stress disorder related to,
      174
  ADHD associated with, 411,
      412
  antisocial personality disorder
      associated with, 333
  as behavioral emergency, 272
  conduct disorder associated
      with, 415
  half-life of common drugs, 306,
      310t
  in children, 390, 419, 420
  in personality disorders, 329
  in schizophrenia, 217–218
  nicotine dependence associated
      with, 357
  P450 system substrates and, 385
  posttraumatic stress disorder
      and, 176
  prenatal, 434
  psychoactive, 314, 315–316
  sexual dysfunction related to,
      364, 367t
  somatization disorder *versus*, 256
  violence associated with, 281
Substance Abuse and Mental
      Health Services
      Administration (SAMHSA), 9
Substance abuse disorders
  anxiety symptoms associated
      with, 158–159, 159b
  economic costs of, 2, 3t
  functional impact of, 1–2
  in primary medical care, 6t, 7
      cost-benefit issues of, 9
  medical costs of, 5, 8, 355
  mood disorder associated with, 89

Substance abuse disorders—cont'd
  panic disorder associated with,
      162, 163
  prevalence of, 1, 2t
  psychiatric symptoms
      associated with, 34t, 35, 38
  treatment success rates for, 2, 3t
Substance abuse services,
      cost-benefit issues of, 9
Substance dependence, pain
      disorder associated with, 262,
      263
Substance use, patient history of, 28
Subthreshold depression, 106
Succinylcholine, for ECT, 321,
      322–323, 325
Suicidal ideation
  as major depression criteria, 91b,
      92, 100
  cocaine abuse associated with,
      304
  evaluation and documentation
      of, 277–281
  in children, 400
  interview protocol for, 92, 93b
  mental status examination for,
      278, 279t, 280
Suicidality
  assessment of
    clinical questions for, 278,
        279t, 280
    individual, 277–278
  chronic, 280
  dementia and, 54
  in children, 449, 450b
    antidepressants and, 432
  panic disorders and, 163
  personality disorders
      associated with, 328, 334,
      335
Suicide
  alcohol use associated with, 288,
      293
  antidepressants associated with
    in children, 117, 119
    in pregnancy, 120
  bipolar disorders and, 137, 143,
      156
  completion rates for, 277
  in schizophrenia, 218

Suicide attempts. *See* Suicidality.
Suicide plan, evaluation and
    documentation of, 278, 279t,
    280
Sulfamethoxazole (Bactrim,
    Septra), 379b
Sulfonylurea hypoglycemics, as
    P450 system substrate, 380b,
    385
Sundowning, 50, 52
    treatment of, 60, 249–250
Support groups
    for ADHD, 414
    for alcoholism, 288
    for bipolar disorder, 144, 156
    for posttraumatic stress disorder,
        176
Supportive care/therapy
    for hypochondriasis, 264
    for neuroleptic malignant
        syndrome, 241–242
    for schizoid personality disorder,
        333
Surgery
    for gender identity disorder,
        376–377
    for male erectile disorder, 371
    for obesity, 355
    patient history of, 28
Swallowing mechanism, clozapine
    impact on, 247
Sweating
    in narcotics assessment, 308b
    paroxysmal, in alcohol
        withdrawal delirium, 296b
Sympathetic nervous system, ECT
    impact on, 324–325
Sympathomimetics
    abuse of, symptoms of, 302t, 304
    anxiety caused by, 161b
    MAOIs interactions with, 134,
        135b
    psychiatric symptoms caused by,
        38b
Symptomatology, psychiatric
    feigning of, 266–267
    in database, 22, 23
    medical evaluation of, 33–48.
        See also Medical
        evaluation.

Syndrome of inappropriate
    antidiuretic hormone
    (SIADH)
    as antidepressant complication,
        127–128
    clinical presentations of, 46,
        127–128
    differential diagnosis of, 128
    medical management of,
        128–129
Syntax, in mental status
    examination, 32
Systematic evaluation,
    of psychiatric symptoms,
    40, 41b

T_3 (triiodothyronine), for
    antidepressant augmentation,
    110
Tachyarrhythmias, ECT causing,
    320, 324, 325
Tacrine (Cognex), 77
Tactile hallucinations, 212
    alcohol abuse and, 291, 297b
Tadalafil (Cialis), 371
Tardive dyskinesia (TD)
    antipsychotics causing, 230,
        231b, 233t, 236–241
    definition of, 236, 238
    differential diagnosis of, 238,
        239b
    identification of, 238
    incidence of, 238
    monitoring guidelines for, 238
        AIMS for, 238, 240b
    prevention of, 238
    treatment of, 238–240
    with Alzheimer's treatment, 70,
        74, 84
Tardive dystonia, 240
TCAs. *See* Tricyclic
    antidepressants (TCAs).
TD. *See* Tardive dyskinesia (TD).
Temazepam (Restoril), 206, 493
Temper, in oppositional defiant
    disorder, 417
Temperature
    elevation of. *See* Fever.
    in narcotics assessment, 309b

Temporal lobe epilepsy, bipolar disorder *versus*, 139–140
Temporal onset, of psychiatric symptoms, 34
Temporomandibular joint syndrome, hypochondriasis *versus*, 264
Teratogens, 48, 147, 150, 153, 154, 249
Terbinafine (Lamisil), 379b, 383
Terminal patients, pain management in, 312
Tetrahydrocannabinol (THC), 303t, 315
Theophylline
    Alzheimer's disease and, 76
    ECT and, 322, 325
    psychiatric symptoms caused by, 33
Therapeutic levels
    for antipsychotics, 228
    of antidepressants, 108, 111t, 120
Therapeutic nursery, for selective mutism, 396
Thiamine replacement
    for alcohol intoxication, 290, 291
    for amnestic disorders, 61
    for delirium tremens, 300
Thioridazine hydrochloride (Mellaril)
    dose recommendations for, 220t
    for Alzheimer's disease, 70, 84
    for destructive behavior, in mental retardation, 421t, 438t
    formulary, 493–494
    QT prolongation associated with, 243
    side effects of, 233t
Thiothixene (Navane), 220t, 494–495
Third party confirmation, in suicide evaluation, 280
Thought content
    anxiety caused by, 192
    in psychosis, 210, 211b
    in schizophrenia, 215
Thought monitoring, for anxiety disorders, 192

Thought process. *See also* Cognitive *entries.*
    in psychosis, 210, 211b
    in schizophrenia, 215
3A4 enzyme, antipsychotics metabolism role, 223, 227t, 228
Thumb sucking, 400
Thyroid-stimulating hormone (TSH), 45
Thyroid tests, 45
TIA (transient ischemic attack), antipsychotics associated with, 243
Tiagabine (Gabatril), 165t
Tic disorders
    ADHD *versus*, 411, 413
    complex, compulsive habits *versus*, 408
Ticlopidine (Ticlid), 379b, 383, 384
Time frame, in psychiatric interview, 12
Tobacco dependence. *See* Nicotine dependence.
Tobacco use. *See* Nicotine use.
Tolerance, in narcotics use, 306
Tolerance level, in oppositional defiant disorder, 417
Topiramate (Topamax)
    for bipolar disorder, in children, 425t
    for bulimia nervosa, 351
    for obesity, 354
    formulary, 495–497
    P450 system inhibition by, 379b
    titration schedule
        for epilepsy, 495, 496t
        for migraine prophylaxis, 496, 496t
Torsades de pointes, antipsychotic selection and, 234, 276
Torticollis, as antipsychotics reaction, 235
Touch/touching, with Alzheimer's patients, 64
Tourette's syndrome, 250, 411, 413
Toxic exposures, developmental disabilities associated with, 436–437

Toxicology screens
  for stimulant abuse, 304
  in behavioral emergencies, 273
  indications for, 29, 38, 44–45
Transaminase enzyme,
    antipsychotics effect on, 247
Transdermal patches, nicotine,
    for smoking cessation,
    358–359
Transient global amnesia, 61
Transient ischemic attack (TIA),
    antipsychotics associated
    with, 243
Translator, for mental status
    examination, 30
Transsexualism, 266
Transvestic fetishism, 375
Tranylcypromine sulfate (Parnate),
    133, 133t, 497–498
Trauma
  alcohol use associated with, 288
  psychiatric disorders related
    to, 8
  spinal cord, sexual dysfunction
    associated with, 373
  stress disorder related to. See
    Posttraumatic stress
    disorder (PTSD).
  to head. See Head trauma.
Trazodone (Desyrel)
  as antidepressant, 112t, 125
  as P450 system substrate, 381b,
    384
  for Alzheimer's disease, 69t, 75,
    79, 81t
  for anxiety disorders, 188
  for dementia, 60
  for sleep problems, 206
Treatment
  for medical inpatients, 5
  indications for. See specific
    disorder.
  initial plan for, 20
  integration assessment of, 10
  medical care as.
    See Primary care.
  psychiatric. See Psychiatry.
  success rates for, 2, 3t
Treatment contracts, for pain
    disorders, 263

Treatment refusal
  commitment and, 285
  competence and, 286
Tremor
  fine, lithium causing, 146
  in alcohol withdrawal delirium,
    296b
  in narcotics assessment, 308b
Triazolam (Halcion), 206, 498
Trichotillomania, 167
Tricyclic antidepressants (TCAs),
    120–121
  as P450 system substrate,
    380b–381b, 384–386, 387
  cardiac effects of, 117, 118t
  drug interactions with, 118t,
    121, 122b
  ECT interaction with, 321
  effects on EEG, 42, 117
  fetal effects of, 120
  for Alzheimer's disease, 80, 81t
  for anxiety disorders, 187
  for bipolar depression, 143
  for borderline personality
    disorder, 335
  for bulimia nervosa, 350
  for generalized anxiety disorder,
    170
  for major depression, in children,
    428t–431t, 432–433
  for narcolepsy, 200
  for obsessive–compulsive
    disorder, 167
  for panic disorder, 163, 164, 165t
  for posttraumatic stress disorder,
    176
  neuroceptor effects of, 114t
  pregnancy and, 184
  profiles of specific, 111t
  sexual dysfunction and, 119
Trifluoperazine (Stelazine), 220t
Trihexyphenidyl (Artane), for
    parkinsonism, 237t
Triiodothyronine (T₃), for
    antidepressant augmentation,
    110
Trimipramine maleate
    (Surmontil), 111t, 498–499
Trust/mistrust, in paranoid
    personality disorder, 330, 332

TSH (thyroid-stimulating
    hormone), 45
Tumors, hypothalamic, obesity
    and, 352
2D6 enzyme, antipsychotics
    metabolism role, 223, 227t,
    228

Urine screen, for substance use, 29,
    38, 44–45
Uroporphyrinogen I synthetase, 47
Uroproporphyrins, 47

V codes, of DSM-IV, 173
Vaccine, for nicotine abstinence,
    361
Vaginismus, 372
Valproic acid/valproate
    (Depakene)
    dosing of, 149
    drug interactions with, 148
    for Alzheimer's disease, 69t,
        74b, 75
    for bipolar depression, 143, 144
    for bipolar disorder, in children,
        420, 422t
    for borderline personality
        disorder, 335
    for dementia, 60
    for mania, 143, 147–148
    formulary, 499–500
    formulations of, 148
    laboratory monitoring of, 148
    lamotrigine combined with, 155
    pharmacology of, 148
    side effects of, 149–150
Vascular dementia, 56
Vasomotor collapse, amobarbital
    risks for, 261
Vasopressors, MAOIs
    interactions with, 134, 135b
Vegetative symptoms, in
    psychiatric database, 18
Venlafaxine hydrochloride
    (Effexor), 112t, 123–124
    adverse effects of, 115t
    as P450 system substrate, 381b,
        384

Venlafaxine hydrochloride
    (Effexor)—cont'd
    cardiac effects of, 118t
    dose-response relationship of,
        109
    for Alzheimer's disease, 81t
    for anxiety disorders, 188, 189t
    for bipolar depression, 143
    for generalized anxiety disorder,
        165t
    for panic disorder, 164, 165t
    for posttraumatic stress disorder,
        176
    formulary, 500
    neuroceptor effects of, 114t
    P450 system inhibition by, 379b,
        383
    sexual dysfunction and, 119
Verapamil, P450 system inhibition
    by, 379b
Verbal aggression, 283b
Verbal behavior, in schizophrenia,
    215–216
Verbal fluency, in cognitive
    examination, 62
Verdenafil (Levitra), 371
Vertical banded gastroplasty, for
    obesity, 355
Veterans, posttraumatic stress
    disorder in, 175
Violent patient
    aggression signs in, 282, 283b
    anxiety disorders and, 173, 175
    history taking for, 281–282
    medical disorders associated
        with, 281
    mental status examination for,
        279t, 281, 282
    physical examination of, 282
    psychiatric disorders associated
        with, 281
    risk factors for, 281
    substance abuse in, 288, 305
Vision disorders. See Ocular
    disorders.
Vision testing
    for ADHD, 411
    for developmental disabilities,
        436
    for learning disorders, 434

Visual hallucinations, 34, 212
    in alcohol withdrawal delirium,
        298b
    in Alzheimer's patients, 67, 76
Visuospatial function, in cognitive
        examination, 63
Vital signs, 29
    in behavioral emergencies,
        273–274
Vitamin B_{12} deficiency, 48, 55
Vitamin deficiencies
    drug-induced, in Alzheimer's
        patients, 82
    MAOIs causing, 133
    psychiatric symptoms caused by,
        40b, 41, 41b
Vitamin E
    for Alzheimer's disease, 78
    for tardive dyskinesia, 239
Vitamin supplements
    for alcohol intoxication, 290,
        291
    for delirium tremens, 300
Voice tone, caution with
        Alzheimer's patients, 64
Voices, hearing. See Auditory
        hallucinations.
Volatile hydrocarbons, symptoms
        of use, 301, 303t, 304
Volitional symptoms, of
        schizophrenia, 216
Vomiting
    in alcohol withdrawal delirium,
        296b
    self-induced, 343, 348–349
Voyeurism, 375

Waking, after ECT, 324
Wandering, by Alzheimer's
        patients, 65, 66t
Warfarin (Coumadin), ECT
        interaction with, 321
Wars, posttraumatic stress disorder
        associated with, 175
Weight gain
    antipsychotics causing, 244
    in Alzheimer's disease, 72
    monitoring guidelines for,
        244, 245t, 246

Weight gain—cont'd
    extreme fear of, 343. See also
        Anorexia nervosa.
    major depression associated
        with, 98
    mood stabilizers causing, 147,
        153
Weight goals, in anorexia nervosa
        treatment, 347
Weight loss
    in Alzheimer's patients, 82
    in anorexia nervosa, 346
Weight management counseling,
        244
Wernicke–Korsakoff syndrome,
        291
White blood cell (WBC) count,
        clozapine effects on, 247–248
Wilson's disease, 47
Withdrawal
    from alcohol, 293–300.
        See also Alcohol
        withdrawal.
    from antidepressants, 109
    from benzodiazepines, 182–183,
        183b
        azapirones versus, 186
    from marijuana, 315
    from narcotics, 307, 309–311.
        See also Narcotics
        withdrawal.
    from sedatives, 53, 293
    from SSRIs, 109
    of physical restraints, 284
    social, dementia and, 54, 57
    substance. See Alcohol
        withdrawal; Drug
        withdrawal.
Withdrawal arousal,
        sleep problems
        associated with, 203
Withdrawal syndrome, in
        newborns, 184
Work history, 25, 351
Worry, excessive
    in children, 390, 399
    in generalized anxiety disorder,
        167, 168, 169
    obsessive–compulsive disorder
        versus, 167

Writing, in cognitive
    examination, 62
Written expression
    disorder, 411, 433, 434, 434t

Xanthines, as P450 system
    substrate, 380b, 385

Yawning, in narcotics assessment,
    309b
Yoga, for generalized anxiety
    disorder, 170

Zafirlukast (Accolate), 379b
Zaleplon (Sonata), 207, 500–501
Ziprasidone hydrochloride/mesylate
    (Geodon)
    dose recommendations for, 220t,
        226t
    for acute schizophrenia, 230, 232t

Ziprasidone hydrochloride/mesylate
    (Geodon)—cont'd
    for Alzheimer's disease, 70, 71t,
        73, 74t
    for behavioral emergencies,
        275t, 276
    for destructive behavior, in mental
        retardation, 422t, 439t
    for mania, 141t, 143, 144
    for schizophrenia, 217
    formulary, 501–502
    intramuscular, 219, 223t, 234
    P450 system and, 223, 227t
    pharmacokinetics of, 223, 226t
    pregnancy and, 249
    QT prolongation associated
        with, 243
    receptor affinities of, 221t
    side effects of, 233t, 244
Zolpidem tartrate (Ambien), 207,
    502–503
Zonisamide, for obesity, 355
Zung Depression Scale, 93, 96f

Key Telephone Numbers

This is a listing of the phone numbers of departments and individuals in the hospital who might be needed for immediate consultation.

Department

Admitting _____

Anesthesia _____

CCU _____

ECG _____

EEG _____

ER _____

ICU _____

Information _____

IV Team _____

Laboratory _____

    Chemistry _____

    Hematology _____

    Microbiology _____

    Other _____

Medical Records _____

Nuclear Medicine _____

Paging _____

Pathology _____

Pharmacy _____

Physical Therapy _____

Pulmonary Function _____

Radiology _____

Recovery Room _____

Respiratory Therapy _____

Security _____

Social Service _____

Sonography _____

Other _____

Nursing Stations

_____
_____
_____
_____
_____
_____
_____
_____

House Staff

_____
_____
_____
_____
_____
_____
_____
_____

Attending Staff

_____
_____
_____
_____
_____
_____
_____
_____
_____
_____
_____
_____
_____